ACCP-SEEK®

PULMONARY MEDICINE

Assessment in Critical Care and Pulmonology
Self-Education and Evaluation of Knowledge

Volume
XIX

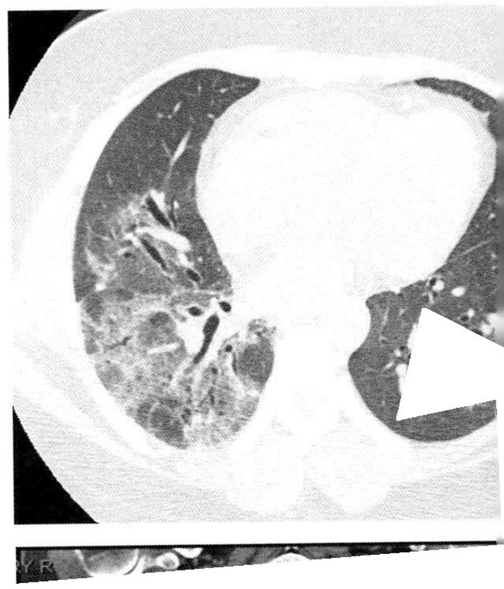

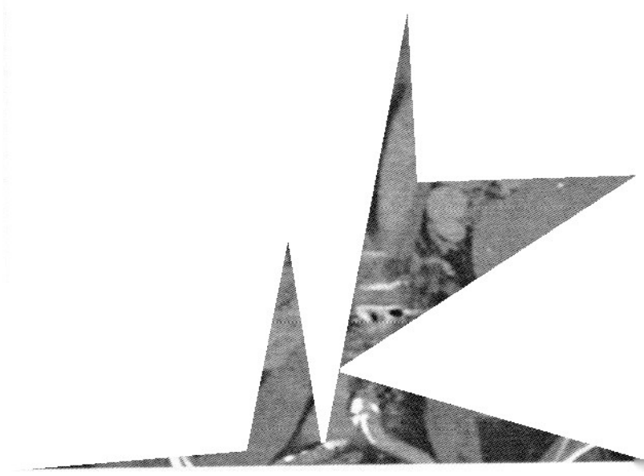

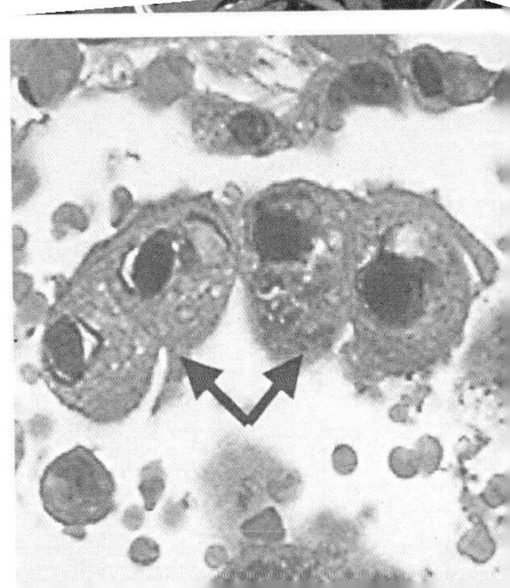

AMERICAN COLLEGE OF CHEST PHYSICIANS®

ISBN - 978-0-916609-78-8

Printed in the USA

Table of Contents

ACCP-SEEK Volume XIX Editorial Board

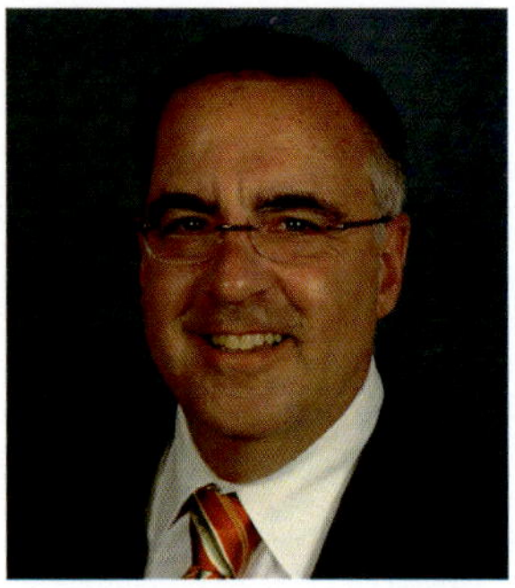

Mark J. Rosen, MD, FCCP

Dr. Rosen is Past-President of the American College of Chest Physicians, Chief of the Division of Pulmonary, Critical Care, and Sleep Medicine at North Shore University Hospital and Long Island Jewish Medical Center in New York, Professor of Medicine at Albert Einstein College of Medicine, and Adjunct Professor of Medicine at New York University School of Medicine. Dr. Rosen authored more than 30 book chapters and monographs and more than 100 peer-review publications and was co-editor of the textbook *HIV and the Lung*. His major research interest is in pulmonary complications and critical care in patients with HIV infection, along with investigating and implementing programs on patient safety, communication, and teamwork among health-care staff in the inpatient and ICU settings. His clinical accomplishments are recognized by repeated citations in Best Doctors in New York and Best Doctors in America.

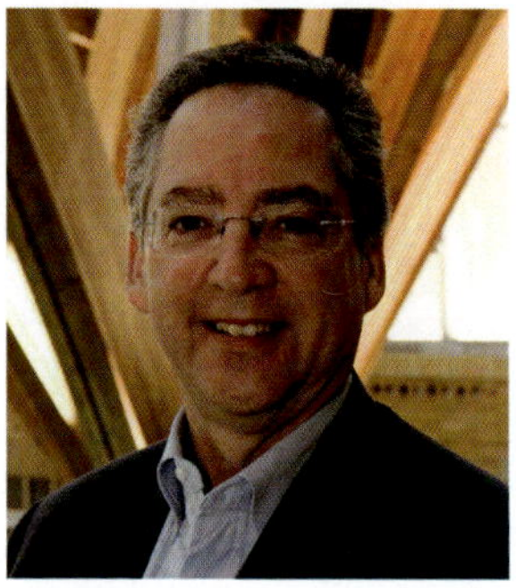

Ronald F. Grossman, MD, FCCP

Dr. Grossman is Professor of Medicine at the University of Toronto, and Respirologist at Credit Valley Hospital, Mississauga, ON, Canada. He has published more than 80 articles in a wide number of medical journals, including *The New England Journal of Medicine*, *Chest*, *American Journal of Respiratory Critical Care Medicine*, and *The American Journal of Medicine*. His major research and teaching interests are in respiratory tract infections. Dr. Grossman has participated in the creation of Canadian and American guidelines for the management of community-acquired pneumonia, Canadian guidelines for the management of hospital-acquired pneumonia, and Canadian and international guidelines for the management of acute exacerbations of chronic obstructive lung disease. He has served as the chairman of the National Information Program on Antibiotics (NIPA), a coalition of many medical and public health societies. This coalition has been established to encourage the appropriate use of antibiotics among physicians and patients.

Continuing Medical Education

The Assessment in Critical Care and Pulmonology Self-Education and Evaluation of Knowledge (ACCP-SEEK) is a self-study opportunity in printed format for pulmonary and critical care physicians and fellows-in-training that fulfills an educational need by providing the latest advances in pulmonary and critical care medicine posed to the learner by case-based questions on a variety of diseases, procedures, and disorders. The American College of Chest Physicians (ACCP) has identified an educational need to update and review existing knowledge and skills, present new information, and provide a preparation tool for board examinations. Each question should take the user approximately 15 to 20 minutes to review thoroughly, research the appropriate response, identify the corresponding correct response, and review the rationale of the correct response. Each ACCP-SEEK volume for pulmonary and critical care medicine has 200 questions.

The ACCP is accredited by the Accreditation Council for Continuing Medical Education to provide continuing medical education for physicians.

The ACCP designates this educational activity for a maximum of fifty (50) *AMA PRA Category 1 Credits*™. Physicians should only claim credit commensurate with the extent of their participation in the activity. This product fulfills ACCP Learning Category IV – Case- and Problem-Based Learning.

To obtain a CME certificate:

1. Go to www.chestnet.org, and click on the "CME Certificates" icon.
2. Log in using your ACCP ID number or e-mail address on file with the ACCP. Enter your ACCP ID number, and click submit, OR, if you do not have an ACCP ID number, click on the link "Create an account here."
3. To locate the product for which you want to claim CME credit, look under the "Available CME" tab on the left navigation bar.
4. Click the "Claim Credit" link next to the product to begin the certificate process.
5. Complete any required posttest and evaluation. Please be sure to check the box that states you are finished with the evaluation.
6. Once you submit the evaluation, your CME certificate will be created and show under the tab, "My CME History." You can print it at any time by clicking the "Certificate" link.

If you need help, please contact the CME Administrator via e-mail at CME@chestnet.org, or leave a voice mail message at (847) 498-8376. For faster assistance, please outline the specific problem you are having and provide your ACCP ID and contact information.

This volume of ACCP-SEEK was made available in August 2009. The CME for this product is valid through December 31, 2011.

Product Description

ACCP-SEEK is designed to stimulate and challenge the learner's clinical thought processes regarding recall, interpretation, and problem-solving skills. The case-based questions contain histories, laboratory results, and images, and they provide education concerning current diagnostic and treatment strategies. Each volume contains 75% new questions, answers, and rationales, in addition to selections from the previous volumes considered by the editors to be among the best designed and written items. The rationales provide thorough explanations and reasoning for the correct and incorrect answers. The ACCP-SEEK series is used most commonly as an invaluable study tool for physicians interested in certifying and recertifying in sleep, pulmonary, and critical care subspecialties.

Goals

The goals of the ACCP-SEEK program are the following:

- Provide a self-assessment program for practicing specialists in pulmonary, critical care, and sleep medicine designed to reinforce training and experience, disseminate important new knowledge in the fields, and identify areas of strengths and weaknesses within specific areas of disease and/or procedural knowledge.

- Assist the practicing specialist and individual in training with preparing for certification and recertification examinations sponsored by the medical specialty board.

Objectives

By completing the questions and reviewing the rationales, participants should be able to:

1. Facilitate self-directed learning efforts, targeting content areas from the pulmonary medicine or the critical care medicine board examination.

2. Compare their responses to the case-based questions in pulmonary and critical care medicine with those of the authors.

3. Appraise management differences in patient cases depicted in the questions through utilization of the provided rationale.

Financial Disclosure

The American College of Chest Physicians (ACCP) remains strongly committed to providing the best available evidence-based clinical information to participants of this educational activity and requires an open disclosure of any potential conflict of interest identified by our committee members. It is not the intent of the ACCP to eliminate all situations of potential conflict of interest, but rather to enable those who are working with the ACCP to recognize situations that may be subject to question by others. All disclosed conflicts of interest are reviewed by the educational activity course director/chair, the Education Committee, or the Conflict of Interest Review Committee to ensure that such situations are properly evaluated and, if necessary, resolved. The ACCP educational standards pertaining to conflict of interest are intended to maintain the professional autonomy of the clinical experts inherent in promoting a balanced presentation of science. Through our review process, all ACCP CME activities are ensured of independent, objective, scientifically balanced information. Disclosure of any or no relationships is made available for all educational activities.

The following committee members of the ACCP-SEEK XIX edition have disclosed to the ACCP that a relationship does exist with the respective company/organization as it relates to their question content material and should be communicated to the participants of this educational activity:

Meyer S. Balter, MD, FCCP
Advisory board: AstraZeneca, Bayer, Boehringer-Ingelheim, GlaxoSmithKline, Pfizer
Speaking honoraria: AstraZeneca, Bayer, Boehringer-Ingelheim, GlaxoSmithKline, Merck, Pfizer

Brian W. Carlin, MD, FCCP
Speaker bureau: GlaxoSmithKline, Sepracor

Ronald F. Grossman, MD, FCCP
Grant monies: Novartis, Replidyne
Consultant fee: Bayer, Schering-Plough, GlaxoSmithKline, Ortho-McNeil, Novartis
Speaker bureau: Bayer, Schering-Plough, Novartis, GlaxoSmithKline, Boehringer-Ingelheim

Teofilo L. Lee-Chiong, Jr., MD, FCCP
University grant monies: University of Colorado
Grant monies (non-industry): National Institutes of Health
Grant monies (industry): Respironics, Restore, Takeda
Consultant fee: Elsevier
Other: Chair, Nosology Committee, American Academy of Sleep Medicine; Program Committee Member, Association of Professional Sleep Societies

Stephanie M. Levine, MD, FCCP
Speaker bureau: Pfizer

Neil R. MacIntyre, MD, FCCP
Consultant fee: Viasys/Cardinal Health Care, Trudell Medical

Darcy D. Marciniuk, MD, FCCP
University grant monies: University of Saskatchewan
Grant monies (non-industry): Canadian Institute of Health Research, Saskatchewan Health Research Foundation, Royal University Hospital Foundation
Grant monies (industry): AstraZeneca, GlaxoSmithKline, Boehringer-Ingelheim, Pfizer, Novartis, Forest, Topigen
Consultant fee: Public Health Agency of Canada, Canadian Pension Approval Board, Saskatchewan Health Quality Council
Speaker bureau: Altana, AstraZeneca, Boehringer-Ingelheim, GlaxoSmithKline, Pfizer, Merck
Advisory committee: GlaxoSmithKline, Boehringer-Ingelheim, AstraZeneca, Pfizer
Fiduciary position: Canadian Thoracic Society

Christian E. Sandrock, MD, MPH FCCP
Grant monies (non-industry): Department of Health and Human Services, Department of Homeland Security, Centers for Disease Control and Prevention, National Institutes of Health
Consultant fee: Pfizer, Astellas, Roche, Merck
Speaker bureau: Pfizer, Astellas, Roche, Merck
Advisory committee: Pfizer
Fiduciary position: American Thoracic Society, Infectious Diseases Society of America

Curtis N. Sessler, MD, FCCP
Advisory committee: Hospira

The following committee members of the ACCP-SEEK XIX program have indicated to the ACCP that no potential conflict of interest exists with any respective company/organization, and this should be communicated to the participants of this educational activity:

Michael H. Baumann, MD, MS, FCCP
Gregory P. Cosgrove, MD, FCCP
Jesse B. Hall, MD, FCCP
Jess Mandell, MD
COL Lisa K. Moores, MC, USA, FCCP
Mark J. Rosen, MD, FCCP

Abbreviations

A-a = alveolar-to-arterial
A1AT = α_1-antitrypsin
ABPA = allergic bronchopulmonary aspergillosis
ACR = acetylcholine receptor
ACS = acute chest syndrome
AFB = acid-fast bacilli
AHI = apnea-hypopnea index
ALI = acute lung injury
ALL = acute lymphoblastic leukemia
ANCA = antineutrophil cytoplasmic antibody
AP = anteroposterior
APAP = autotitrating positive airway pressure
aPTT = activated partial thromboplastin time
ARR = absolute risk reduction
ART = antiretroviral therapy
ASV = adaptive servoventilation
ATC = automatic tube compensation
AUC = area under the curve
AV = atrioventricular
AVM = arteriovenous malformation
BAL = bronchoalveolar lavage
BCG = bacilli Calmette-Guérin
BMI = body mass index
BMT = bone marrow transplantation
BO = bronchiolitis obliterans
BOOP = bronchiolitis obliterans organizing pneumonia
BOS = bronchiolitis obliterans syndrome
BP = blood pressure
BPAP = bilevel positive airway pressure
BUN = blood urea nitrogen
CABG = coronary artery bypass graft
c-ANCA = cytoplasmic antineutrophil cytoplasmic antibody
CBC = complete blood count
CCHS = congenital central hypoventilation syndrome
CCRT = continuous renal replacement therapy
CF = cystic fibrosis
CFTR = cystic fibrosis transmembrane conductance regulator
CI = confidence interval
CKIε = casein kinase I epsilon
CMV = cytomegalovirus
COP = cryptogenic organizing pneumonia
CPAP = continuous positive airway pressure
CSA = central sleep apnea
CT_{min} = minimum core temperature
CVC = central venous catheter
CVID = common variable immune deficiency
DAD = diffuse alveolar damage
DIP = desquamative interstitial pneumonia
DLCO = diffusing capacity of the lung for carbon monoxide
DM = dermatomyositis
DOT = directly observed therapy
DPB = diffuse panbronchiolitis
DSPS = delayed sleep phase syndrome
DTI = direct thrombin inhibitor
EBV = Epstein-Barr virus
EBUS-TBNA = endobronchial ultrasound-guided transbronchial needle aspiration
ED = emergency department
EOG = electrooculography
ET = endotracheal tube
EUS = endoscopic ultrasound
FACTT = Fluid and Catheter Therapy Trial (NIH)
FDA = US Food and Drug Administration
FIN_2 = inspired nitrogen concentration
FIO_2 = inspired oxygen fraction
FRC = functional residual capacity
GM-CSF = granulocyte-monocyte colony-stimulating factor
GVHD = graft-vs-host disease
HELLP = hemolysis, elevated liver enzymes, and low platelets
HHT = hereditary hemorrhagic telangiectasia
HIT = heparin-induced thrombocytopenia
HLA = human leukocyte antigen
HR = heart rate
HRCT = high-resolution CT
HPO = hypertrophic pulmonary osteoarthropathy
HU = Hounsfield units
IBW = ideal body weight
IFN-γ = interferon-γ
IGRA = IFN-γ release assay
ILD = interstitial lung disease
INH = isoniazid
INR = international normalized ratio
IPAH = idiopathic pulmonary arterial hypertension
IPF = idiopathic pulmonary fibrosis
IVIG = IV immunoglobulin
JVP = jugular venous pressure
LAM = lymphangioleiomyomatosis
LDH = lactate dehydrogenase
LIP = lymphocytic interstitial pneumonia
LMWH = low-molecular-weight heparin
LT = lung transplant
LTBI = latent tuberculosis infection
LVRS = lung volume reduction surgery
MAC = *Mycobacterium avium* complex
MALT = mucosa-associated lymphoid tissues
MDR = multidrug resistant
MDR-TB = multidrug-resistant tuberculosis
MG = myasthenia gravis
MGC = myasthenia gravis crisis
MIC_{90} = 90% minimum inhibitory concentration
MRI = magnetic resonance imaging
MRSA = methicillin-resistant *Staphylococcus aureus*
MSLT = multiple sleep latency test
MuSK = muscle-specific kinase
MV = minute ventilation
NBBRA = nonbenzodiazepine benzodiazepine receptor agonist
NETT = National Emphysema Treatment Trial
NIH = National Institutes of Health
NNT = number needed to treat
NSIP = nonspecific interstitial pneumonia
NREM = nonrapid eye movement
OB = obstructive bronchiolitis
OSA = overlap syndrome
OSA = obstructive sleep apnea
PA = posteroanterior
PAC = pulmonary artery catheter

Pa_{CO_2} = arterial carbon dioxide tension
$P_{A}CO_2$ = alveolar carbon dioxide tension
PAH = pulmonary arterial hypertension
p-ANCA = perinuclear antineutrophil cytoplasmic antibody
PAP = pulmonary alveolar proteinosis
PAP = positive airway pressure
PAS = periodic acid-Schiff
PAVM = pulmonary arteriovenous malformation
PCIS = postcardiac injury syndrome
PDH = progressive disseminated histoplasmosis
PE = pulmonary embolism
PEEP = positive end-expiratory pressure
PET = positron emission tomography
PF = pleural fluid
PF4 = platelet factor 4
PFT = pulmonary function test
PICC = peripherally inserted central catheter
PM = polymyositis
PMNs = polymorphonuclear leukocytes
PPD = purified protein derivative
PSI = pectus severity index
PTLD = posttransplant lymphoproliferative disease
PVL = Panton-Valentine leukocidin
PZA = pyrazinamide
QRDR = quinolone resistance-determining region
RA = rheumatoid arthritis
RADS = reactive airways dysfunction syndrome
RB = respiratory bronchiolitis
RCT = randomized controlled trial
REM = rapid eye movement
RM = recruitment maneuver
RV = residual volume
SBT = spontaneous breathing trial
SC = technetium-99m sulfur-colloid
SD = sleep deprivation
Sa_{O_2} = arterial oxygen saturation
Sp_{O_2} = oxygen saturation as measured by pulse oximetry
SFTP = solitary fibrous tumor of the pleura
SLE = systemic lupus erythematosus
SMRP = soluble mesothelin-related peptide
SPN = solitary pulmonary nodule
SPM = spontaneous pneumomediastinum
SWSD = shift work sleep disorder
TB = tuberculosis
TC = total capacity
TEE = transesophageal echocardiography
TES = tumor emboli syndrome
TLC = total lung capacity
TNF-α = tumor necrosis factor-α
TO = tracheobronchopathia osteochondroplastica
TST = total sleep time
TST = tuberculin skin test
TU = tuberculin unit
UFH = unfractionated heparin
UIP = usual interstitial pneumonia
VAP = ventilator-associated pneumonia
VC = vital capacity
V_D/V_T = physiologic dead space ventilation
$\dot{V}/\dot{Q}$ = ventilation-perfusion
VILI = ventilator-induced lung injury
XDR-TB = extensively drug-resistant tuberculosis

Examination Key

Each item on the ACCP-SEEK examination contains four response choices. One of the choices constitutes the correct answer to the question. For most questions, the ACCP-SEEK editorial committee has verified that the answer is factually correct, or it has been determined by consensus that the answer is the best choice among those provided. For a small number of items, the committee acknowledges that valid disagreement about the best answer may exist. These questions have been included because they address significant topics with educational value.

This examination consists of 200 multiple-choice test questions. The questions are numbered, and the possible choices are lettered. For some questions, images are provided for your reference. For each question, decide which choice is the best.

A table of normal laboratory values is provided in the back of this book for your reference.

Part I

Study Questions

1. Which of the following is most effective for improving exercise performance in a pulmonary rehabilitation program for patients with COPD?

A. Strength training.
B. Administer growth hormone.
C. Inspiratory muscle training.
D. High-intensity exercise.

2. A 66-year-old man was assessed for cough and dyspnea. He had a 45 pack-year smoking history and was well until 5 months earlier when he began to have difficulty swallowing and had weight loss. Radiographic and endoscopic studies indicated squamous cell carcinoma of the esophagus with mediastinal nodal involvement precluding surgical resection. He was treated with radiotherapy with shrinkage of the tumor. He was able to swallow after radiotherapy. He now has a 2-week history of cough productive of yellow sputum, further weight loss, and for the past 24 h, has been unable to swallow anything other than saliva. He has had no fever, hemoptysis, or chest pain. Endoscopic examination revealed a food bolus and narrowing of the esophagus with mucosal inflammation. Physical examination indicated that he was afebrile but had left basal crackles. His hemoglobin level was 10.1 g/dL (101 g/L), and his WBC count was 10,500/μL (10.5×10^9/L) with a slight left shift. A chest radiograph (see Figure 2-A) and representative images of the chest CT scan (see Figures 2-B and 2-C) are shown. At this point, what would you suggest?

A. Ceftriaxone plus azithromycin.
B. Placement of an esophageal stent.
C. Initiation of cancer chemotherapy.
D. Further radiotherapy.

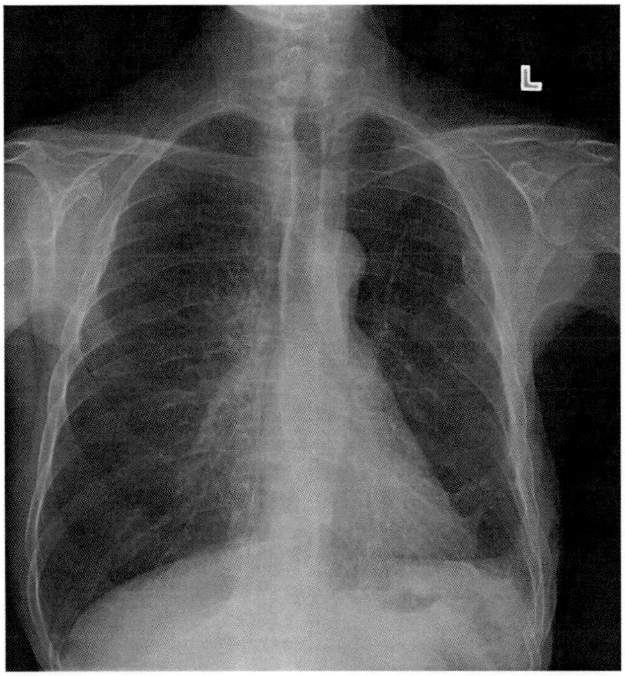

Figure 2-A

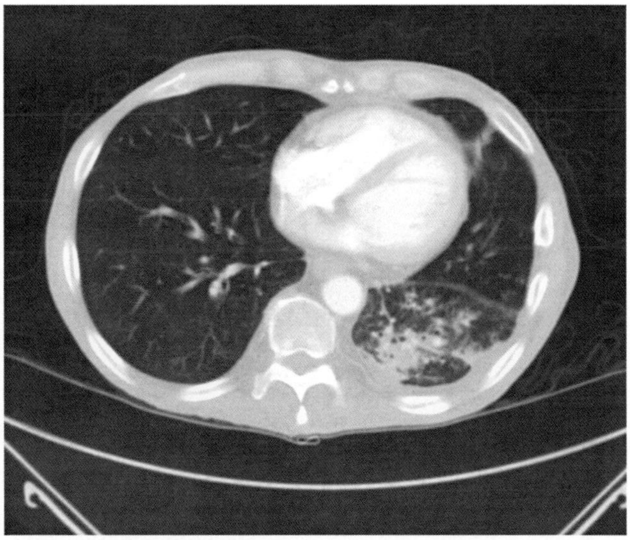

Figure 2-B

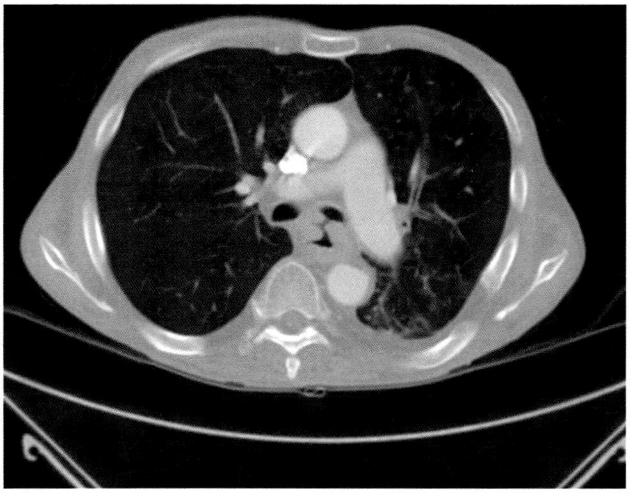

Figure 2-C

3. A 36-year-old woman is referred for evaluation of an abnormal chest CT scan. She had a history of recurrent sinusitis, otitis media, and bronchitis dating back to childhood and had received numerous courses of antibiotics. She improved in her teens, but following the birth of her first child 8 years ago, again began to develop recurrent episodes of bronchitis and pneumonia. She was noted to have an abnormal CT scan (see Figures 3-A and 3-B) that led to the performance of a mediastinoscopy (see Figure 3-C) and a video-assisted thoracoscopic lung biopsy (see Figure 3-D).

She complained of some mild dyspnea on exertion. She was a lifetime nonsmoker. There was a family history of asthma (her father and her brother). She denied arthralgias, visual symptoms, or current skin rashes. Her physical examination revealed a few midinspiratory crackles over the left lower lobe but was otherwise unremarkable.

Which of the following is the most likely explanation for her pulmonary disease?

A. Sarcoidosis.
B. Cryptogenic organizing pneumonia (COP).
C. Common variable immune deficiency (CVID).
D. Wegener granulomatosis.

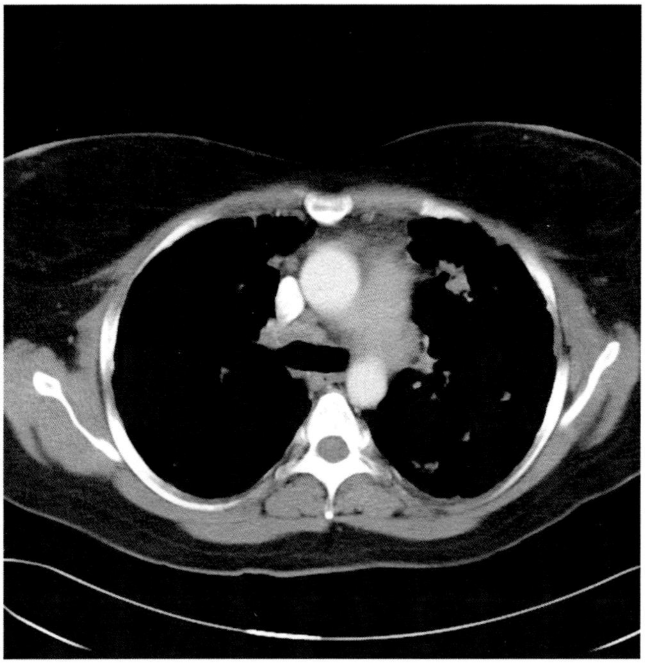

Figure 3-A

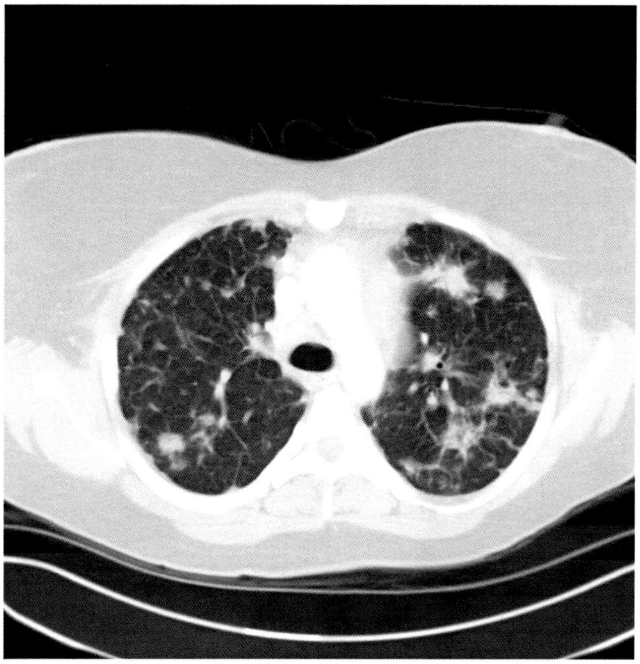

Figure 3-B

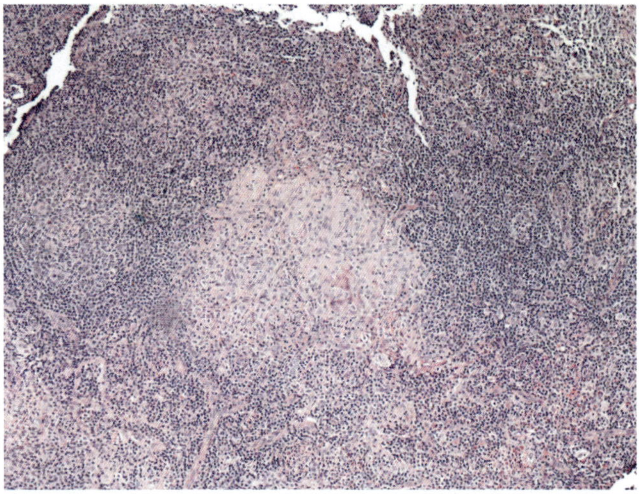

Figure 3-C
Hematoxylin-eosin

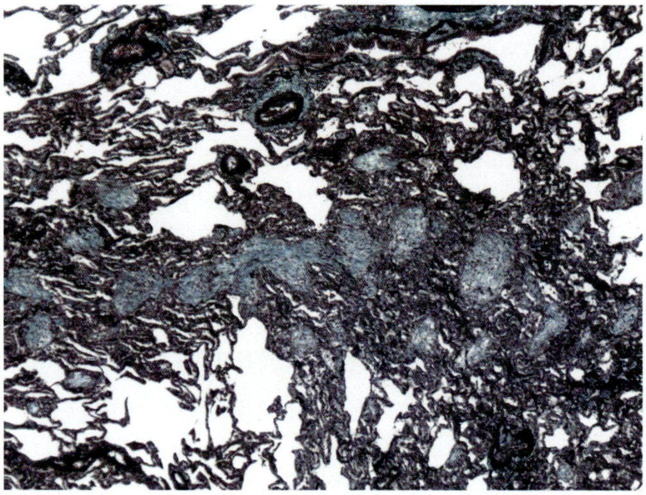

Figure 3-D
Elastic trichrome

4. A 52-year-old man enters the ED complaining of a cough productive of purulent sputum and intermittent fever for 3 days. Posterior-anterior and lateral chest radiographs reveal a right lower lobe infiltrate with an accompanying pleural effusion. An ultrasound of the chest confirms a pleural effusion in the right chest with multiple loculations. A diagnostic thoracentesis is performed using local lidocaine anesthesia. Laboratory analysis of the pleural fluid, including pH, is performed 30 min later.

Which of the following is unlikely to alter the pleural fluid pH result in a clinically significant fashion?

A. Lidocaine in the pH syringe.
B. 30-min delay to analysis.
C. Analysis by a pH meter.
D. Retained air in the pH syringe.

5. A 68-year-old smoker with COPD is referred for pulmonary rehabilitation. His FEV_1 is 55% of predicted, with an FEV_1/FVC of 40%. He was admitted to the hospital 1 month ago with a COPD exacerbation and has lost 15 lbs over the month. He is able to perform his activities of daily living at approximately 50% of his prehospitalization state. His BMI is 19 kg/m^2. He has generalized muscle weakness over all muscle groups. In addition to providing lower and upper extremity training and education regarding his disease process, which of the following has the most proven benefit to add as part of the rehabilitation program at this time?

A. Strength training.
B. Nutritional supplementation.
C. Anabolic steroid administration.
D. Antidepressant therapy.

6. A 28-year-old man is admitted to the ED with crushing, substernal chest discomfort; dyspnea; and lightheadedness after playing soccer earlier in the day. He did not have any recent trauma, history of substance abuse or tobacco use, weight loss, fevers, or hemoptysis. He recalls similar symptoms with activity over the past 6 months, with a progressive increase in intensity.

Upon evaluation in the ED, laboratory results, including a urine drug screen and an ECG, are unremarkable. A chest radiograph (see Figure 6-A) and CT with contrast (see Figure 6-B) were obtained, revealing a mediastinal density. The next course of management would be:

A. Conservative management with serial observation.
B. Esophagram to assess for esophageal perforation.
C. Endobronchial ultrasound-guided needle aspiration.
D. Surgical consultation for resection of the lesion.

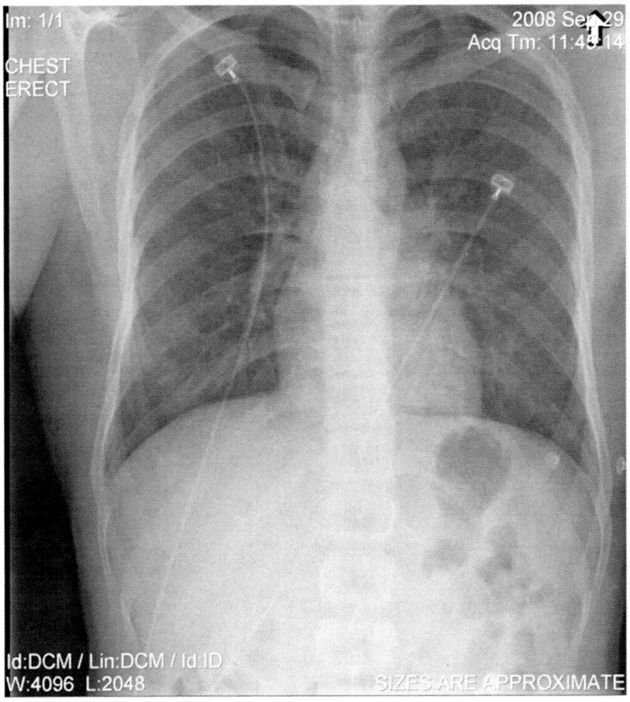

Figure 6-A

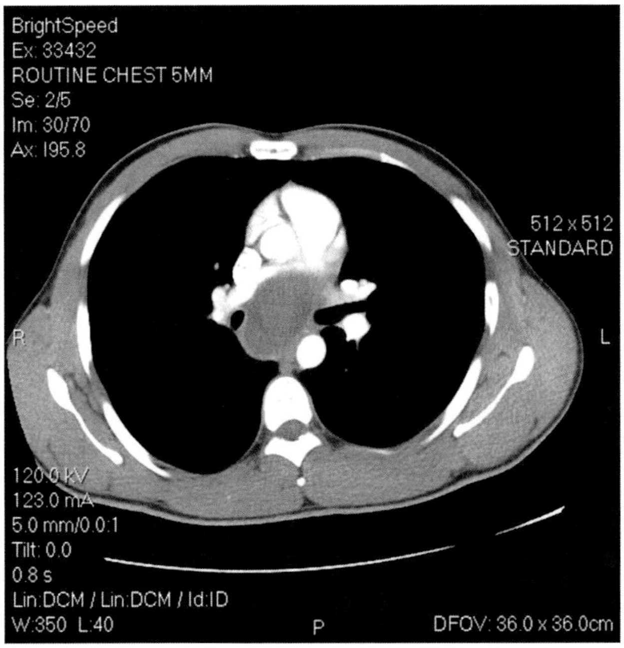

Figure 6-B

7. A 58-year-old man is referred to you because of an abnormal CT scan. He came to the ED 2 weeks earlier with abdominal pain that resolved spontaneously over a day, but as part of his evaluation, an abdominal CT scan was done that revealed absence of the spleen and thoracic abnormalities, which led to a dedicated chest CT scan. This scan showed a complex lobulated left lower lobe mass of uniform consistency (see Figure 7-A, arrow), with posterior pleural-based nodular densities (see Figure 7-B, arrow), and soft tissue masses involving the posterior chest wall (see Figure 7-C, arrow).

The patient states he has never had prior lung disease to his knowledge. He has no known asbestos or other industrial exposures. He smoked one pack of cigarettes a day for 30 years and stopped smoking 5 years ago.

On physical examination, his vital signs are normal, and his heart and lung examinations are unremarkable. He does have a palpable firm subcutaneous mass left of the spine at the level of the eleventh and twelfth ribs. He also has midline and left upper quadrant laparotomy scars. When asked about this, he states that he suffered a gunshot wound to his left upper abdomen as a teenager, which required emergency surgery, and that he was in the ICU for several days. He noticed that the chest wall mass present on examination arose in the months following his injury.

The most appropriate follow-up test to assess the CT scan abnormalities is:

A. CT-guided needle aspiration of the pleural mass.
B. Bronchoscopy with left lower lobe biopsy.
C. Technetium-99m sulfur-colloid (SC) scan.
D. Serum antineutrophil cytoplasmic antibody determination.

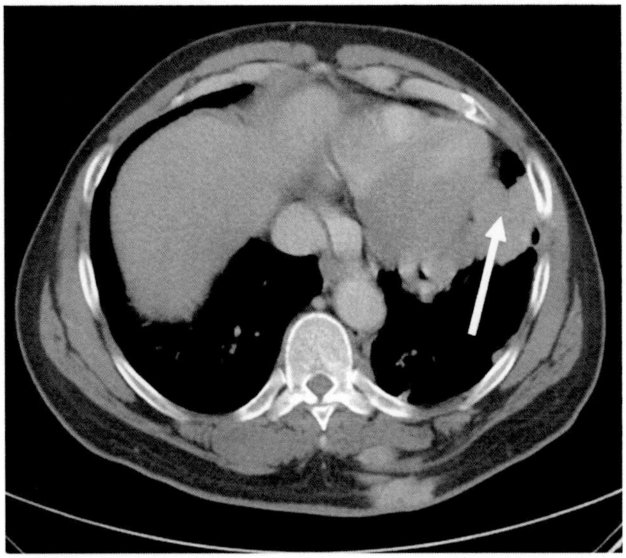

Figure 7-A

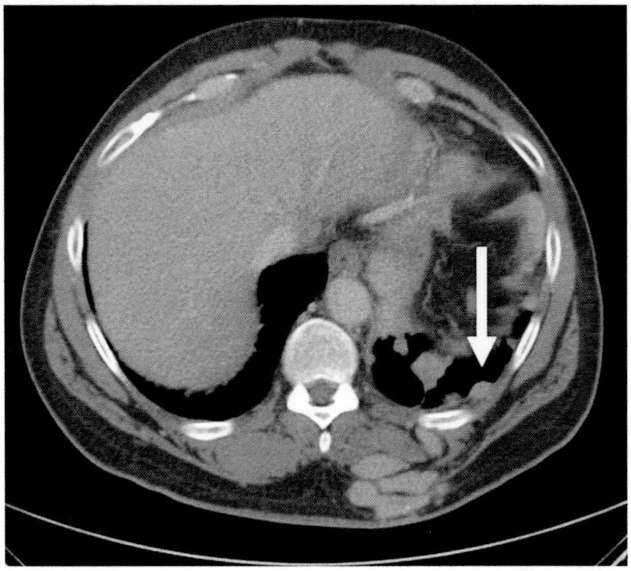

Figure 7-B

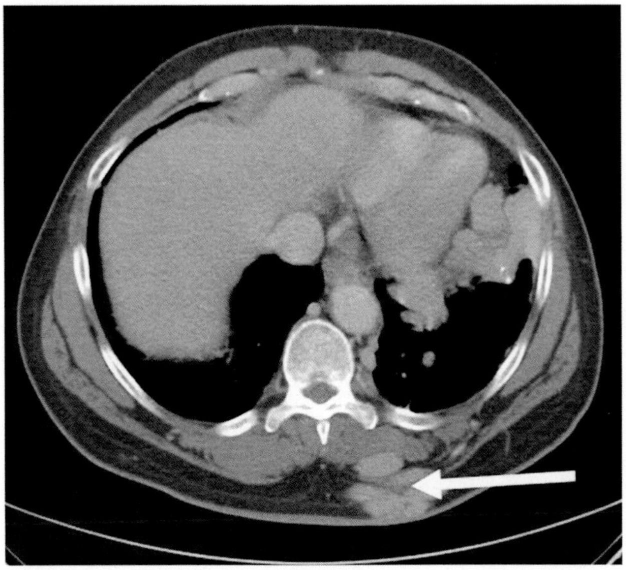

Figure 7-C

8. A 17-year-old high school senior requires evaluation of persistent daytime sleepiness. He is unable to wake up each morning early enough to get to school on time. In school, he is constantly yawning and experiences difficulty staying awake during his classes. He describes being most sleepy in the morning but seems to get a "second wind" at night. He cannot fall asleep when he goes to bed at 10:00 PM on school nights, habitually falling asleep at 2:00 AM to 3:00 AM. If undisturbed, he will sleep until 11:00 AM to 1:00 PM, a pattern he follows on weekends and during vacations.

He denies snoring, witnessed apneas, cataplexy, sleep paralysis, or restless legs. He has a history of depression for which he has been prescribed a selective serotonin reuptake inhibitor. He also has taken several sleep aids, including melatonin, diphenhydramine, and zolpidem, but these medications have no effect on his sleep and make him sleepier the morning after he takes them. He drinks a cup of coffee each morning and has several cans of beer on weekends. He does not

smoke and denies illicit drug use. Physical examination is normal, as are his weight and vital signs. The following 2-week sleep diary completed by the patient is shown in Table 8-1.

Table 8-1. Patient 2-Week Sleep Diary*

	Afternoon						Evening				Midnight			Morning									Noon	
	1	2	3	4	5	6	7	8	9	10	11	12	1	2	3	4	5	6	7	8	9	10	11	12
Day																								
M										↓				X	X	X	X		X	↑				
T											↓			X	X	X	X	X	↑					
W										↓			X	X	X	X	X	X	↑					
Th						N						↓			X	X	X	X	↑					
F								N						↓		X	X	X	X	X	X	X	↑	
S															↓	X	X	X	X	X	X	X	X	X
Sn	↑										↓					X	X	X	↑					
M											↓			X		X	X	X	X	↑				
T												↓		X	X	X	X	X	X	↑				
W						N					↓			X	X	X	X	X	↑					
Th												↓		X	X	X	X	X	↑					
F																↓	X	X	X	X	X	X	X	↑
S														↓		X	X	X	X	X	X	X	↑	
Sn										↓					X		X	X	↑					

*↓ = bedtime; X = sleep; ↑ = time out of bed; N = naps.

Which of the following is the most appropriate management at this time?

A. Stimulant therapy.
B. Hypnotic therapy.
C. Bright light exposure during the morning.
D. Cognitive behavioral therapy for insomnia.

9. A 25-year-old woman with cystic fibrosis who is awaiting lung transplantation is admitted for mildly increased shortness of breath, purulent sputum production, and low-grade fever for 3 days. Her maintenance regimen includes dornase alfa, inhaled tobramycin, and bronchodilators. She has had no recent respiratory infections. She has no known drug allergies. Physical examination reveals a heart rate of 90/min, respiratory rate of 18/min, and a temperature of 38°C. Her oxygen saturation on her home oxygen prescription of 2 L/min is 90%. She is in no acute distress. Lung examination reveals diffuse wheezing and rhonchi. Laboratory examination is notable for a leukocyte count of 13,000/µL (13.0×10^9/L). Her chest radiograph is shown in Figure 9-A and is comparable to her recent chest radiographs. Sputum culture from a clinic visit 48 h before admission is growing a Gram-negative rod identified as *Stenotrophomonas maltophilia.* The best treatment regimen is:

A. Trimethoprim-sulfamethoxazole.
B. Cefepime and IV amikacin.
C. Imipenem-cilastatin.
D. Vancomycin and cefepime.

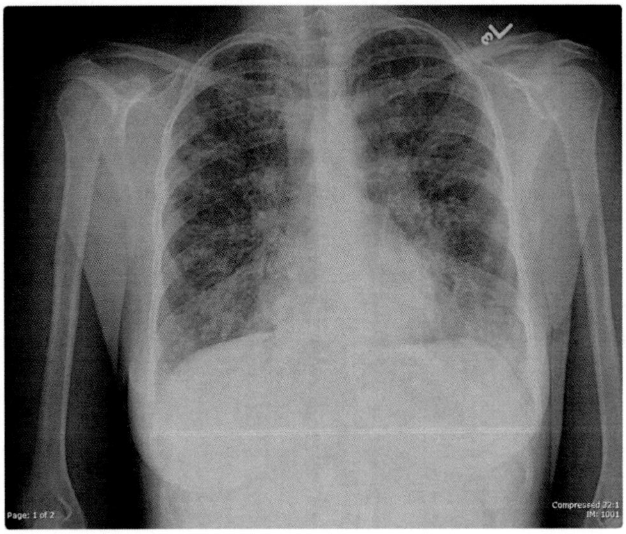

Figure 9-A

10. A 45-year-old alcoholic patient experienced a massive aspiration and develops severe ARDS. He is transferred to the ICU and receives volume-assist control ventilation with a tidal volume of 720 mL (12 mL/kg ideal body weight [IBW]), a respiratory rate of 12/min, a PEEP of 8 cm H_2O, and an FIO_2 of 0.4. His plateau pressure is 36 cm H_2O, pH is 7.38, PCO_2 is 44 mm Hg, and PaO_2 is 68 mm Hg. You elect to follow the National Institutes of Health ARDS Network protocol and reduce his tidal volume to 6 mL/kg IBW in a stepwise fashion while maintaining an acceptable $PaCO_2$ and pH, with an accompanying increase in respiratory rate. According to recent clinical trial results, these changes for 48 to 72 h are likely to lead to which of the following?

A. Improving lung compliance and oxygenation.
B. Worsening lung compliance and oxygenation.
C. Improving lung compliance but no effect on oxygenation.
D. No effect on compliance or oxygenation.

11. A 52-year-old man is rescued from a fire at a factory that used plastic (polyacrylonitrile) resins. He is unconscious and, after rapid transport to a nearby ED, has a pulse of 52/min, BP of 86/48 mm Hg, and respiratory rate of 10/min. Arterial blood gas tests with the patient breathing 100% oxygen by face mask revealed the following:

pH	7.16
$PaCO_2$	36 mm Hg
PaO_2	327 mm Hg
Carboxyhemoglobin	22%

The patient is intubated, and preparations are made to initiate hyperbaric oxygen therapy for carbon monoxide poisoning. Which other agent should be administered immediately?

A. Amyl nitrite.
B. Hydroxocobalamin.
C. Pralidoxime.
D. Sodium nitrate.

12. A 57-year-old man with COPD is referred to you because of worsening shortness of breath. He has a prior 60 pack-year smoking history but has been a nonsmoker for 4 years. He has never been hospitalized or received antibiotics as a result of his COPD. He gets short of breath and has to stop walking after about 200 m. There is no

history of heart failure or ischemic heart disease. His current medications include tiotropium and salmeterol, as well as salbutamol as needed. Physical examination results reveal that his Sao_2 while breathing room air is 93%, breath sounds are decreased to both lung fields, and there are no crackles or wheezes. Heart sounds are normal, there are no murmurs, and there is no peripheral edema. A chest radiograph, revealing hyperinflation and reduced vascular markings but no masses or adenopathy, is unchanged from a radiograph taken 1 year previously. Results of an ECG show sinus rhythm with low voltages. Spirometry reveals an FEV_1 of 1.70 L (55% of predicted) with an FEV_1/FVC ratio of 0.56. What would you recommend?

A. Prescribe supplemental oxygen 2 L/min continuously at rest and 3 L/min with activity.
B. Prescribe participation in a pulmonary rehabilitation program.
C. Discontinue the salmeterol and prescribe a combination inhaled corticosteroid with long-acting inhaled β-agonist.
D. Discontinue the salmeterol and prescribe formoterol.

13. In patients with a first acute pulmonary embolism, the factor that is most predictive of recurrence after completion of a 6-month course of therapy with warfarin is:

A. A homozygous factor V Leiden mutation.
B. Female gender.
C. An unprovoked initial event.
D. A perioperative initial event.

14. An 18-year-old man requests your opinion on surgical treatment for his chest wall abnormality. His posteroanterior and lateral chest radiographs are shown in Figures 14-A and 14-B. His FVC and FEV_1 are 82% and 83% of predicted with a normal FEV_1/FVC. Which of the following best describes the results of a surgical intervention in patients with this deformity?

A. Improved total lung capacity (TLC), FVC, and FEV_1.
B. Improved self-perception of body image and perception of level of physical activity.
C. Improved TLC, FVC, and FEV_1, and a reduced risk of respiratory failure later in life.
D. Reduced risk of acquiring pulmonary nontuberculous mycobacterial disease.

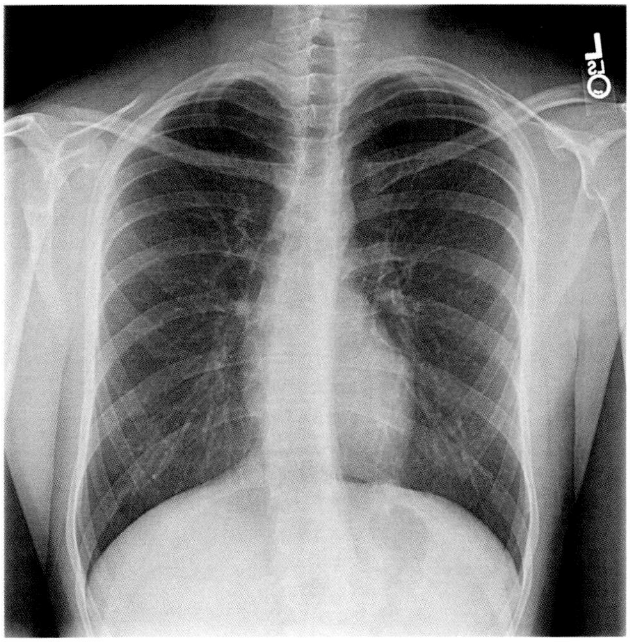

Figure 14-A

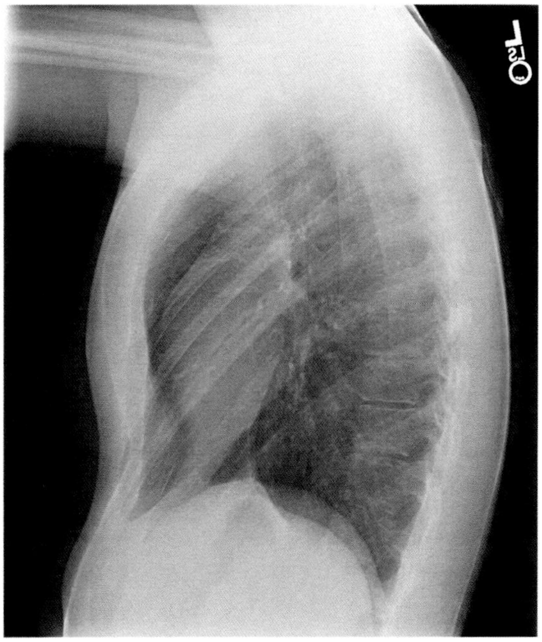

Figure 14-B

15. A 65-year-old man was endotracheally intubated 7 days ago for pneumonia. He self-extubated 3 days ago and was reintubated with a 7.0-mm endotracheal tube (ET) as a result of stridor. Today he passed a 120-min spontaneous breathing trial, is alert, has a strong cough, and is requiring suctioning every 3 to 4 h. He has no discernable audible leak when the cuff is deflated and volume-targeted breaths are administered.

Which of the following approaches performed prior to extubation is the most likely to reduce the likelihood of postextubation stridor?

A. No therapy.
B. Dexamethasone, 10 mg IV once 60 min before extubation.
C. Methylprednisolone, 250 mg IV every 6 h for eight doses.
D. Methylprednisolone, 20 mg IV every 4 h for four doses.

16. A 27-year-old woman comes for evaluation of recurrent episodes of severe and disabling chest pain. Her first episode occurred while traveling at age 15, and a second episode started after an airplane flight at age 17. Subsequently, they occurred approximately every 2 years, often starting after airplane flights. The pain is always very severe, pleuritic in nature, and requires narcotics for relief. The pain usually clears within a few days. She often feels warm when she develops the pain, but a low-grade fever has only been documented on a single occasion.

Her only medication is a low-dose estrogen-containing (20 µg) birth control pill to control severe pelvic pain attributable to endometriosis associated with her menses. Prior attempts at stopping this therapy led to a recurrence of her pelvic pain. She has had two normal ventilation-perfusion scans, normal bilateral leg Doppler arterial ultrasounds, and a normal CT angiogram during episodes of chest pain. Her parents were both born in Egypt, and her grandparents were from Turkey and Greece. There is no family history of thromboembolic disease. A molecular hypercoagulability workup revealed heterozygosity for factor V Leiden. On two occasions, a very small amount of pericardial fluid was seen on echocardiograms done during episodes of chest pain.

Her physical examination at the present time is completely normal. Blood work, including a CBC, serum electrolytes, liver function tests, antineutrophil cytoplasmic antibodies, and antinuclear antibodies, is normal. Her erythrocyte sedimentation rate (ESR) is slightly elevated to 30 mm/h. Complete pulmonary function testing, including measurement of her diffusing capacity, is normal. DNA analysis indicates that she is a heterozygous carrier of the M694V mutation in exon 10 of the *MEFV* gene. Which of the following would you recommend?

A. Initiation of warfarin therapy.
B. Discontinuation of her oral contraceptive tablet.
C. Initiation of colchicine therapy.
D. Initiation of low-dose aspirin therapy.

17. A 55-year-old woman is referred to you due to an abnormal chest radiograph (see Figure 17-A) and CT scan of the chest (see Figure 17-B). A prior chest radiograph from a year ago is no different than Figure 17-A. The patient had a right calf mass ("about the size of my fist") removed 10 months earlier. The lesion was asymptomatic but cosmetically noticeable. The lesion has now recurred but is only about half the size of the prior lesion. The patient has no accompanying local or systemic symptoms. Physical examination is completely normal except for a palpable and easily visible right calf mass beneath a well-healed incision scar. The mass is under the skin and unattached, firm, and nontender. A pathology slide of the lesion that was removed 10 months ago is shown in Figure 17-C. Which of the following best describes this particular manifestation of the disease?

A. Lower extremity involvement is common.
B. Corticosteroid treatment is quite successful.
C. The chest radiographic abnormality is uncommon.
D. Creatinine phosphokinase level is likely elevated.

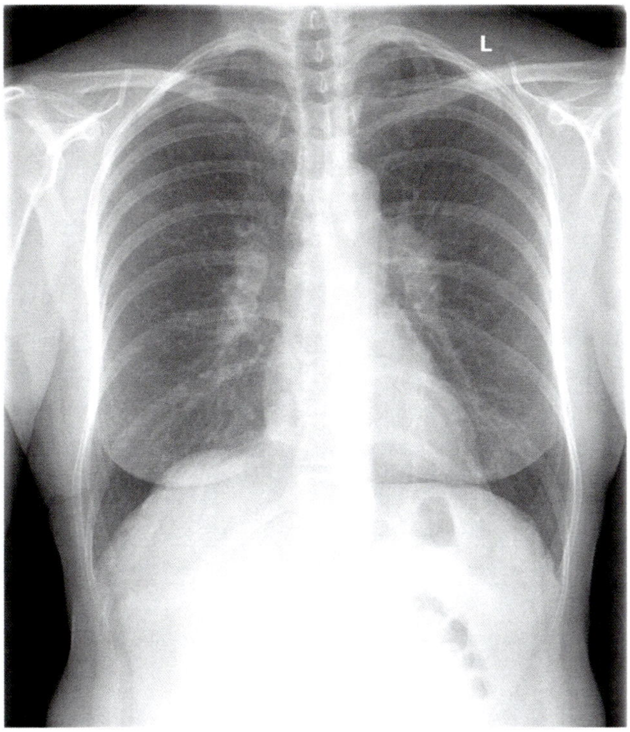

Figure 17-A

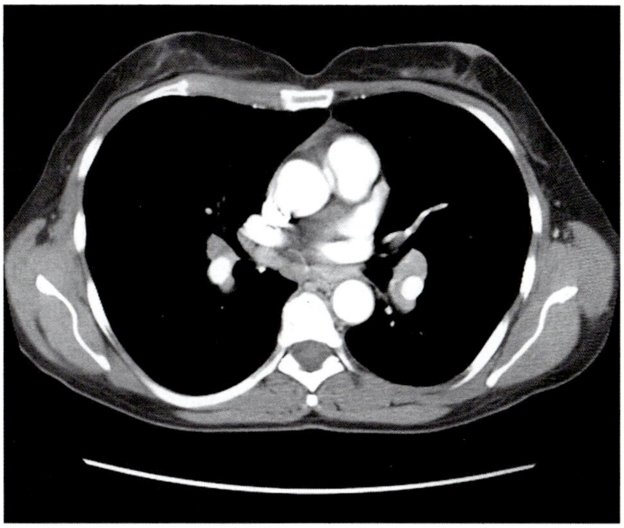

Figure 17-B

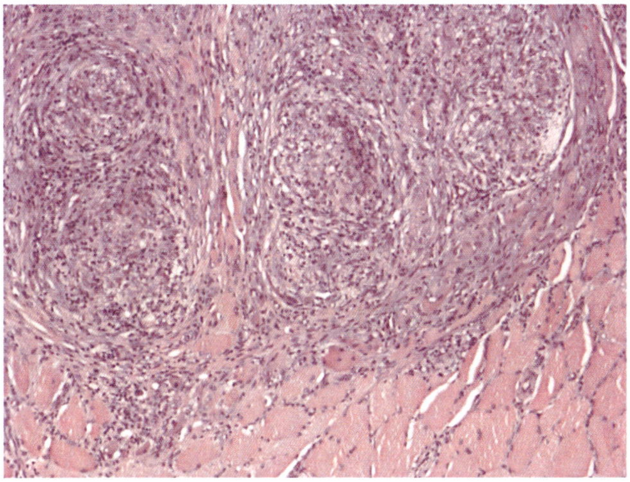

Figure 17-C
Hematoxylin-eosin

18. A 45-year-old previously healthy nonsmoker has a 2-week history of cough productive of light yellow phlegm. It developed acutely 2 days after a sore throat, rhinorrhea, nasal stuffiness, postnasal drip, and throat clearing. After 2 days, the sore throat and rhinorrhea disappeared and nasal stuffiness decreased. Vital signs and examination of the chest are normal. Which of the following medications is most likely to have a favorable effect on the cough?

A. A macrolide antibiotic.
B. Inhaled albuterol.
C. Dexbrompheniramine with pseudoephedrine.
D. Loratadine.

19. A 27-year-old man is referred to you for evaluation of an abnormal chest radiograph. About 5 months ago, he consulted a doctor because of excessive thirst. Evaluation resulted in the diagnosis of diabetes insipidus, which responded favorably to desmopressin administered nasally. Recently, he started to notice shortness of breath when climbing stairs, and a chest radiograph was obtained (see Figure 19-A).

History obtained by you reveals significant tobacco smoking, up to two packs daily, for at least 14 years. The patient noticed the shortness of breath for at least 2 years, and, recently, he noted a point of tenderness over the chest wall, lateral to the posterior axillary line on the left.

Oxygen saturation while breathing room air is 94%, and the rest of the vital signs are normal. Auscultation reveals only rare crackles without prolongation of the expiratory phase. There is a point of tenderness over the left sixth and seventh ribs in the posterior axillary line, and a chest CT scan is obtained (see Figure 19-B). The most likely diagnosis is:

A. Metastatic tumor of unknown primary site.
B. Sarcoidosis.
C. Langerhans cell histiocytosis.
D. Idiopathic pulmonary fibrosis.

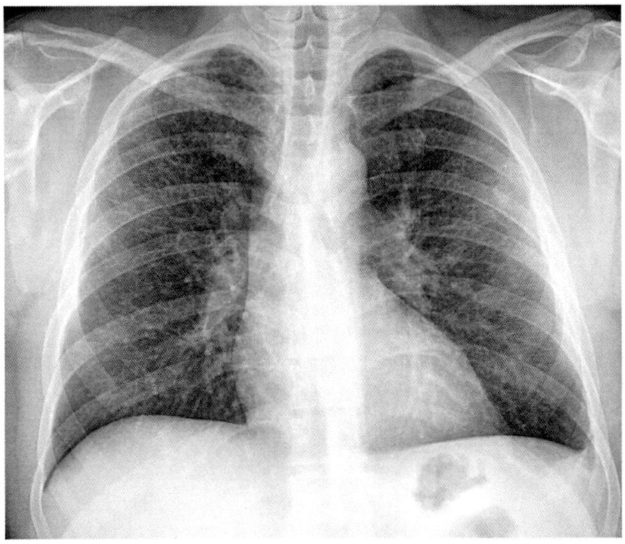

Figure 19-A

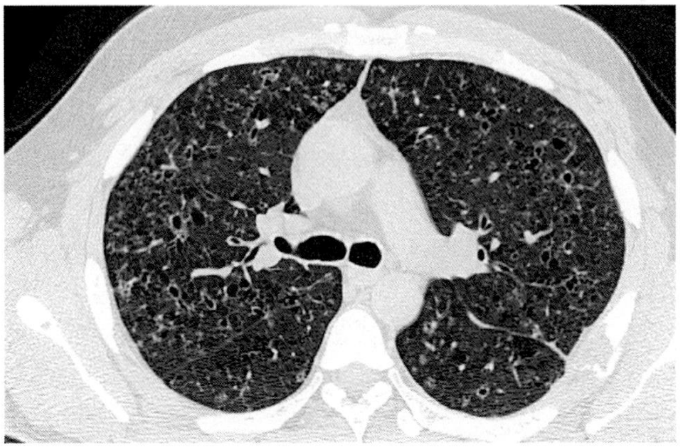

Figure 19-B

20. Which of the following is shown to occur in localities that adopt laws that eliminate smoking in indoor workplaces and public spaces?

A. Reduced incidence of lung cancer.
B Reduced incidence of nasopharyngeal carcinoma.
C. Reduced hospitalization rates for acute myocardial infarction.
D. Economic losses in bars and restaurants.

21. A 58-year-old woman was seen because of persistent cough and a progressive lung infiltrate. She was initially assessed 2 years earlier when she had reported a 4-month history of cough, which produced several teaspoons of green sputum daily. Two antibiotic courses were not helpful. Pulmonary function studies and methacholine challenge test results were normal. A short course of corticosteroids and two further antibiotic courses did not improve her symptoms. Physical examination indicated coarse bibasal crepitations. Bronchodilators, inhaled corticosteroids, and a leukotriene

receptor antagonist did not change her symptoms. Although several sputum sample results were negative, occasional samples produced *Pseudomonas aeruginosa*. A CT scan demonstrated mild cylindrical bronchiectasis in the right lower lobe segmental bronchus with ill-defined nodular and confluent densities. Bronchoscopy results indicated purulent secretions, but culture results were negative. The following test results were either normal or negative: sweat chloride, quantitative immunoglobulins, HIV serology, IgG subclass determination, rheumatoid factor, anti-DNA antibodies, and antineutrophil cytoplasmic antibody (ANCA) levels. A 24-h pH electrode study indicated no active reflux. Her cough did not improve with a course of omeprazole. A CT scan (see Figures 21-A and 21-B) showed progression of lung infiltrates. A lung biopsy also was performed (see Figures 21-C and 21-D). The most likely diagnosis is:

A. Cystic fibrosis.
B. Rheumatoid lung with bronchiolitis.
C. Lymphocytic interstitial pneumonia (LIP).
D. Idiopathic pulmonary fibrosis (IPF).

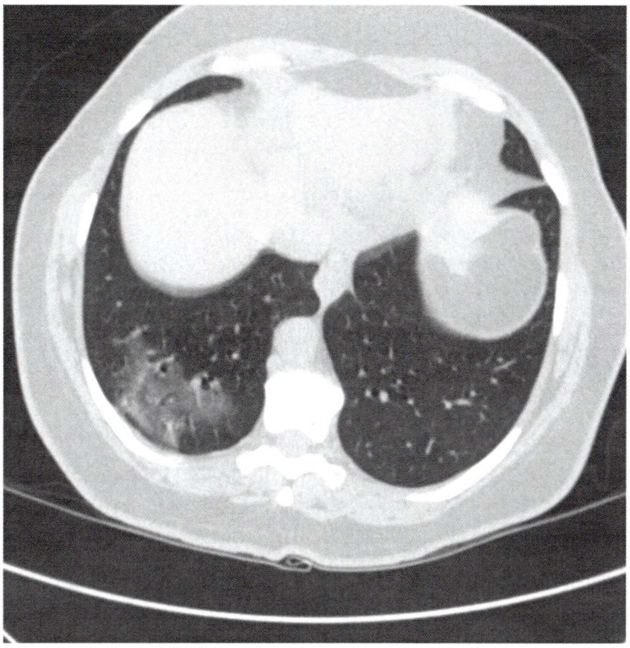

Figure 21-A

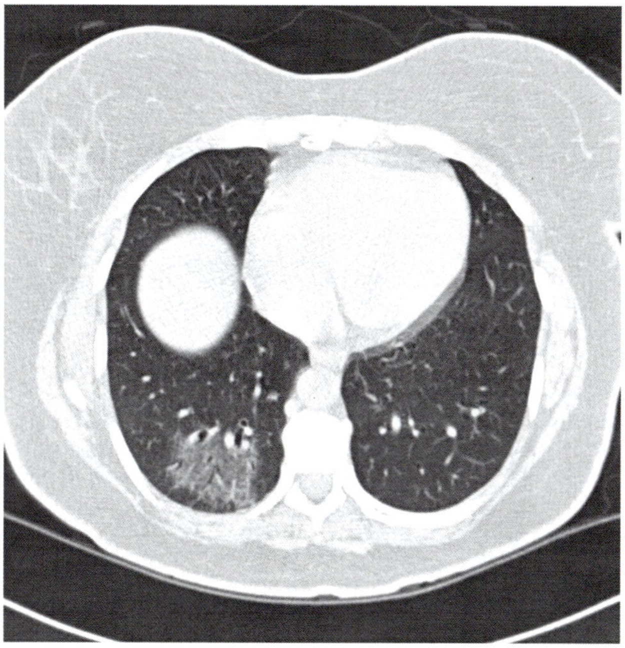

Figure 21-B

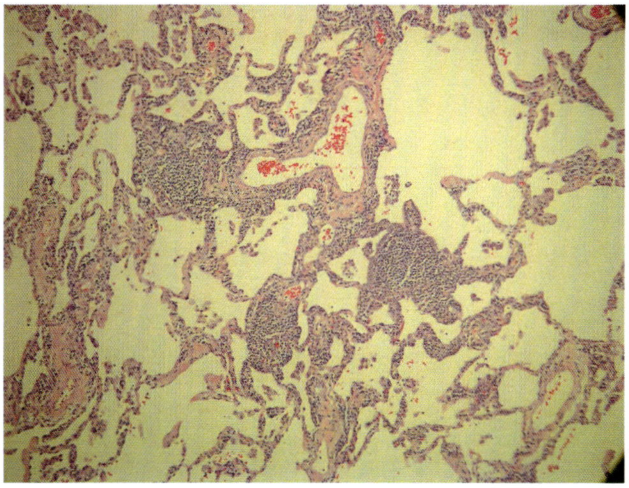

Figure 21-C
Hematoxylin-eosin

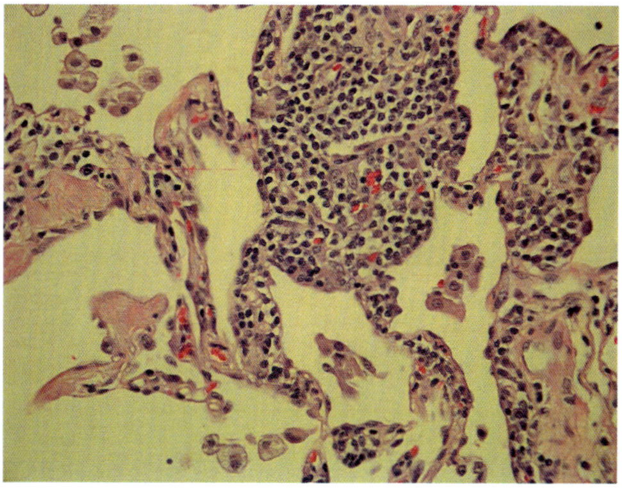

Figure 21-D
Hematoxylin-eosin

22. A 47-year-old man comes for evaluation of worsening dyspnea. He was diagnosed with sarcoidosis on transbronchial biopsy after having bilateral hilar adenopathy 8 years ago. Initially, he was not treated, but over the past 18 months, he has noted progressive cough and dyspnea on exertion that began to limit his activities. Because of worsening symptoms, progressive radiographic changes, and worsening pulmonary function tests, he was started on oral prednisone therapy 7 months ago. There was no response, either symptomatically or physiologically, to a 2-month trial of oral steroids, so therapy with methotrexate was initiated 5 months ago.

Within 3 months of initiation of methotrexate therapy, his cough improved and his dyspnea diminished. However, 6 weeks prior to his current visit, he noted significant worsening of his dyspnea that seemed to start following an upper respiratory tract infection. The symptoms were progressive, and he recently became dyspneic when walking 100 yards or climbing a half flight of stairs. Physical examination was remarkable for a respiratory rate of 20/min and a pulse rate of 90/min. His jugular venous pressure (JVP) was elevated, and there was trace pitting edema around his ankles, but the remainder of the physical examination was normal. Representative images from a CT scan performed at the initiation of methotrexate are shown in Figures 22-A and 22-B and at his current presentation in Figures 22-C and 22-D. His pulmonary function test results are shown in Table 22-1.

Table 22-1. Pulmonary Function Test Results

	Before Methotrexate*	After Methotrexate*
FEV_1, L	2.5 (71)	2.8 (80)
FVC, L	4.5 (98)	4.6 (101)
FEV_1/FVC, %	55	60
TLC, L	5.5 (81)	5.7 (85)
DLCO, L	21.7 (73)	20.6 (68)

*Corrected for hemoglobin. Values in parentheses are % predicted.

TLC = total lung capacity; DLCO = carbon monoxide diffusing capacity of the lung.

Based on the information provided, what would be your next step?

A. Initiate therapy with low-molecular-weight heparin.
B. Discontinue the methotrexate and pulse with methylprednisolone.
C. Initiate therapy with trimethoprim-sulfamethoxazole while arranging for bronchoscopy.
D. Diurese patient aggressively while arranging an echocardiogram.

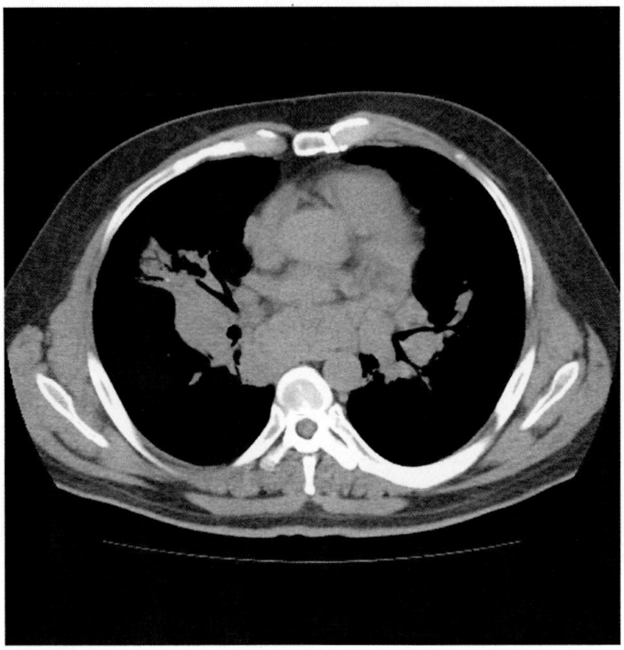

Figure 22-A

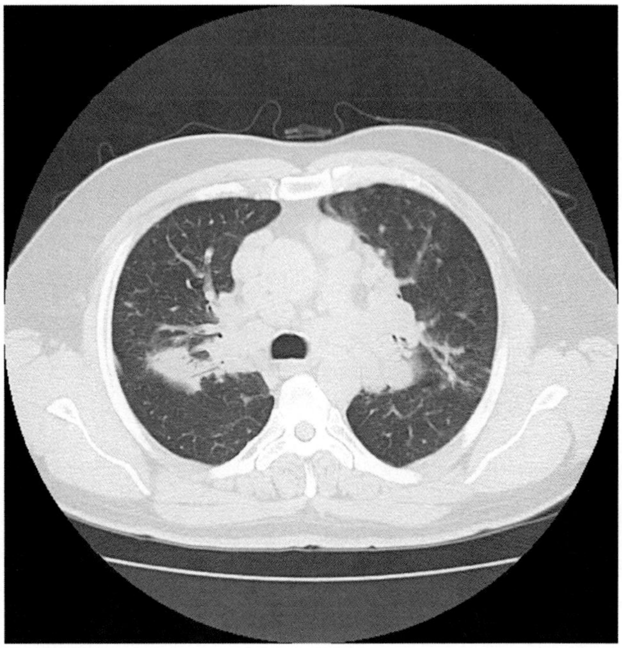

Figure 22-B

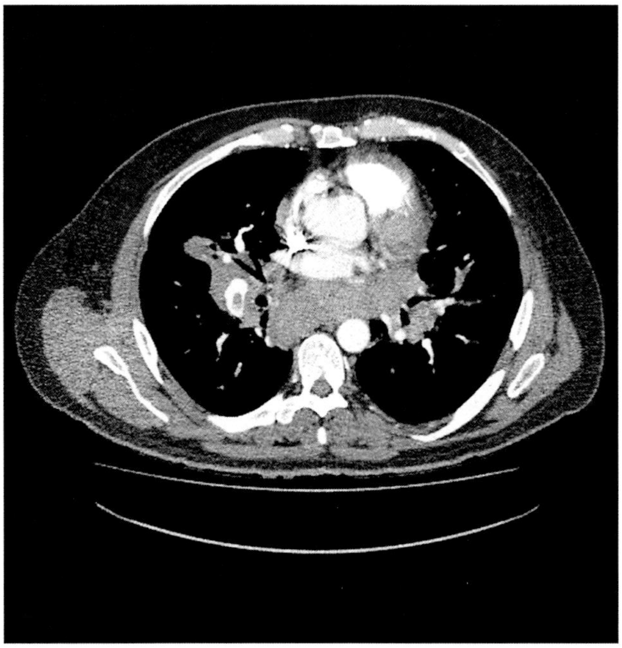

Figure 22-C

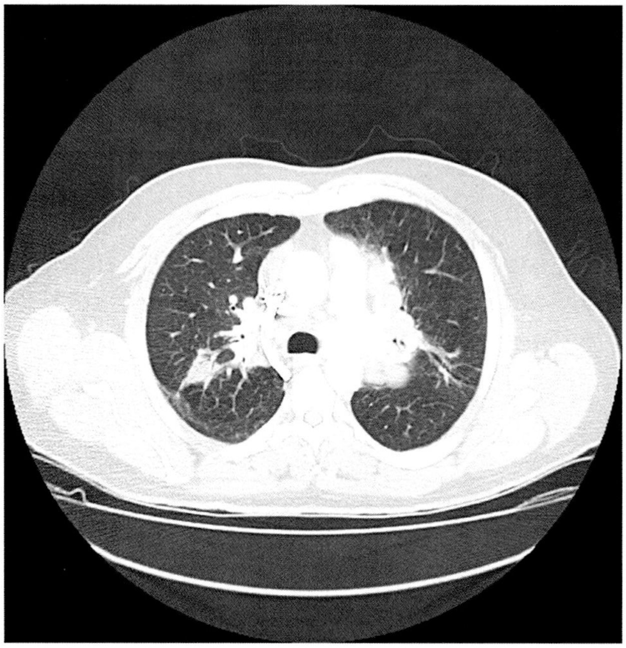

Figure 22-D

23. A 65-year-old woman is admitted for upper GI bleeding thought to be related to recent nonsteroidal antiinflammatory use for chronic right knee pain. A portable chest radiograph is obtained as part of her admission evaluation (see Figure 23-A) and shows airway wall abnormalities. This prompted a CT of the chest (see Figures 23-B, 23-C, and 23-D) after stabilization of her GI bleeding. Upper GI endoscopy shows diffuse gastritis. The patient has no current or past respiratory complaints or recurrent respiratory infections. She is a lifelong nonsmoker and denies any other health problems except coronary artery disease with bypass surgery 3 years ago and osteoarthritis in both knees. You perform a bronchoscopy and note a beaded (nodular) appearance to the anterior and lateral trachea and mainstem bronchi; the posterior membranous area of the airways is spared (see Figure 23-E). You note a grating sensation when you pass the bronchoscope tip over the nodular lesions.

Which of the following best describes the most likely cause of this patient's radiographic and bronchoscopic findings?

A. Most commonly diagnosed in patients <25 years of age.
B. Patients are most commonly symptomatic with cough and sputum production.
C. Commonly associated with systemic amyloidosis.
D. Usually does not require biopsy for diagnostic confirmation.

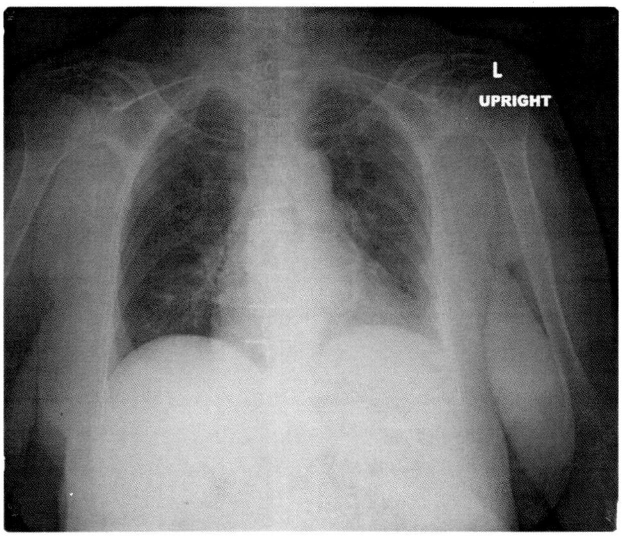

Figure 23-A

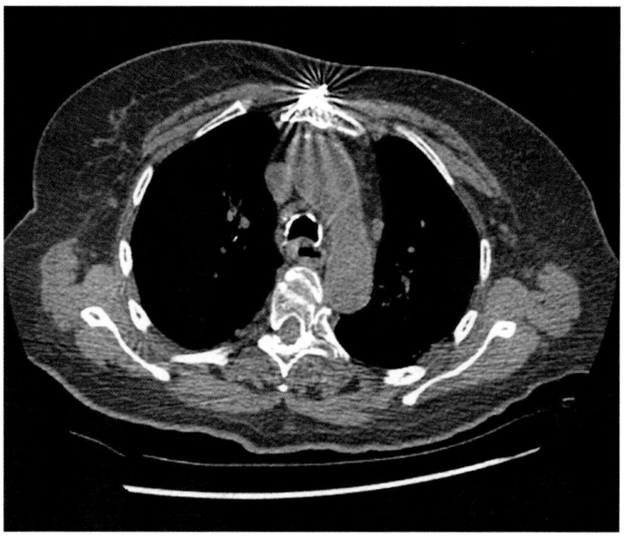

Figure 23-B

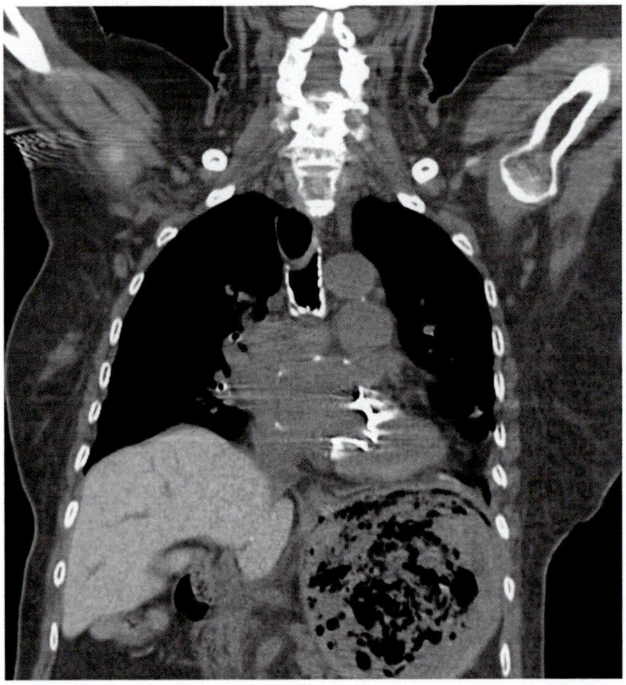

Figure 23-C

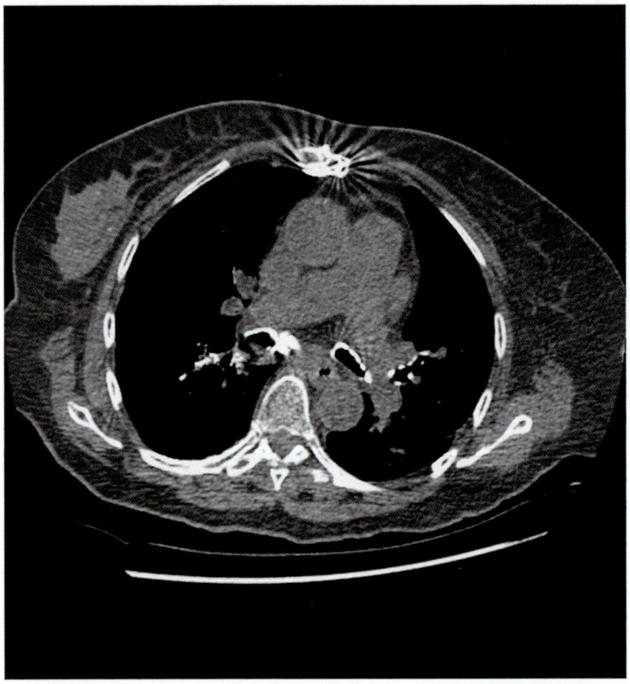

Figure 23-D

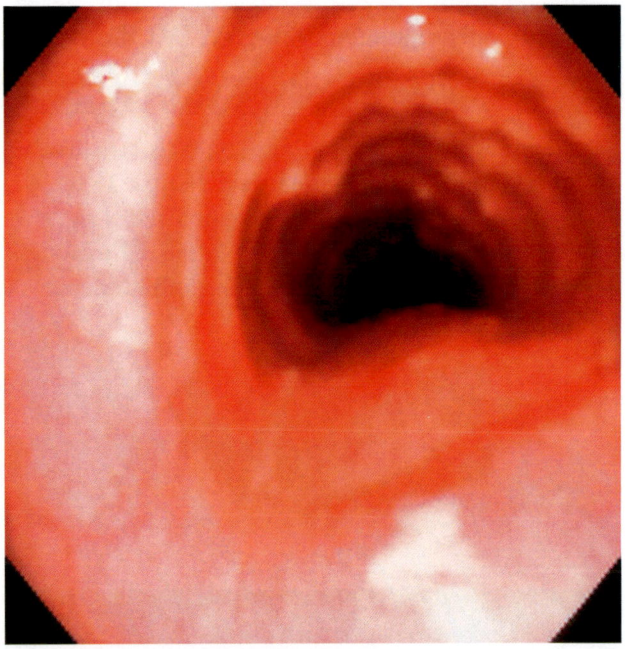

Figure 23-E

24. A 65-year-old man with COPD (60 pack-year smoker) has dyspnea while walking up a flight of stairs. He uses nebulized albuterol every 4 h and prior to bedtime. His wife notes that he snores. He awakens feeling relatively refreshed but naps every afternoon. His BMI is 30 kg/m^2. He has a prolonged expiratory phase with wheezes noted bilaterally. His heart and abdominal examinations are normal. He has 1+ pedal edema.

Pulmonary function tests reveal an FEV_1 of 0.72 L (21% of predicted), FVC of 2.88 L (64% of predicted), and FEV_1/FVC ratio of 25%. Resting room air arterial blood gas findings show a pH of 7.41, $Paco_2$ of 46 mm Hg, and Pao_2 of 58 mm Hg. Chest radiograph shows hyperinflation. An echocardiogram was unable to assess pulmonary artery pressure. A complete polysomnography revealed the following:

Total sleep time	345 min
Sleep efficiency	75%
Apnea-hypopnea index (AHI)	15/h (primarily obstructive apneas)
REM AHI	38/h
Lowest Spo_2*	63% (occurring during REM sleep)
Periodic limb movement index	4

* Oxygen saturation as measured by pulse oximetry.

Which of the following is likely to be present in this patient during sleep?

A. Diaphragmatic hypotonia.
B. Reduced airway resistance.
C. Pulmonary hypertension.
D. Increased respiratory rate.

25. A 64-year-old man with a history of hypertension and IV drug abuse and ongoing heroin and methamphetamine use is seen by his primary care physician who notes progressive dyspnea and "dizziness." The dizziness is most prominent upon standing from a seated position. His review of systems is notable for weight loss totaling 20 lbs and dyspnea on exertion over the past 2 years. He has not experienced any fevers, chills, or sweats. His past history is notable for a severe motor vehicle accident in which he was ejected from the automobile. He underwent multiple surgeries including a left chest tube thoracostomy.

On physical examination, he is afebrile and normotensive but hypoxic at rest with a room air Spo_2 of 89%. Bibasilar crackles are present, and prior thoracotomy and exploratory laparotomy incisions are present but well healed. The results of routine chemistry assessments and a hemogram were unremarkable. A chest radiograph demonstrated an abnormality. He was referred to the ED, and a CT angiography revealed an enhancing abnormality in the right lower lobe (see Figures 25-A and 25-B). An arterial blood gas with shunt study was obtained, demonstrating a shunt fraction of 12% (normal <5%). The next recommended intervention should be:

A. Serial observation.
B. Bronchoscopy with transbronchial biopsy.
C. Pulmonary angiogram.
D. Surgical consultation for resection of the lesion.

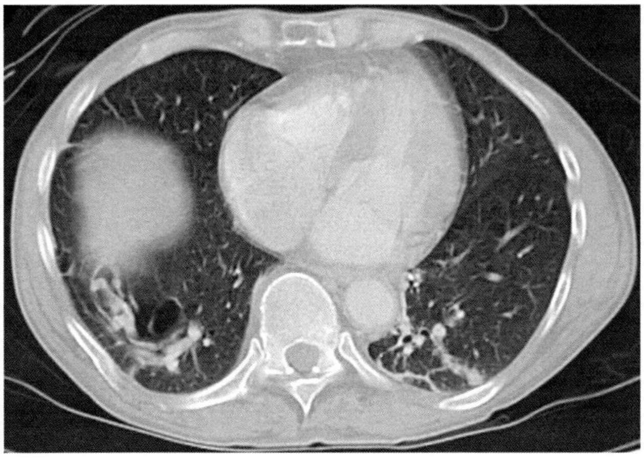

Figure 25-A

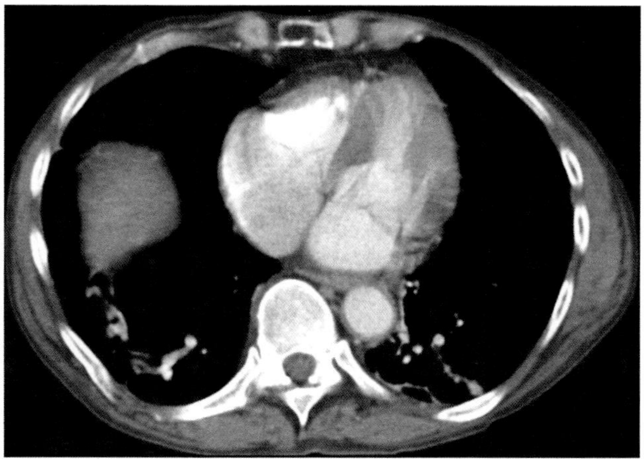

Figure 25-B

26. A 55-year-old man is intubated for an exacerbation of COPD. This is his third such episode in the past 9 months. After admission, corticosteroid therapy is initiated, as well as ceftriaxone for a right middle lobe infiltrate. Central venous catheterization is performed. On ICU day 5, he continues to receive mechanical ventilation support, and he has a temperature spike to 39.5°C. Blood, sputum, and urine cultures are ordered, and ceftriaxone is stopped. The patient then empirically receives piperacillin/tazobactam, 4.5 g IV q6h, and vancomycin, 1.25 g/day IV. However, during the subsequent 24-h period, the patient continues to have high fevers and becomes hemodynamically unstable. Sputum and blood culture results are positive for only one organism, *Enterobacter cloacae.* In addition to proper isolation and discontinuation of the catheter, and based on the susceptibility profile in Table 26.1, what antimicrobial regimen should be initiated for this patient, assuming normal renal function?

Table 26.1. Susceptibility Profile of Patient*

Aztreonam	R
Ampicillin	R
Ampicillin/sulbactam	R
Amikacin	S
Ceftazidime	R
Cefoxitin	R
Ceftriaxone	R
Cefepime	S
Ciprofloxacin	R
Gentamicin	S
Levofloxacin	S
Meropenem	S
Piperacillin/tazobactam	S
Ticarcillin	R
Tobramycin	S

*R = resistant; S = sensitive.

A. Discontinue vancomycin and continue with piperacillin/tazobactam.
B. Discontinue both vancomycin and piperacillin/tazobactam and initiate tobramycin.
C. Discontinue both vancomycin and piperacillin/tazobactam. Initiate meropenem.
D. Discontinue piperacillin/tazobactam. Continue vancomycin and initiate meropenem.

27. A 45-year-old night shift worker is referred for evaluation of frequent bouts of severe sleepiness and difficulty concentrating while at work. He works from 11:00 PM to 7:00 AM five days a week. Over the past 3 years, he has been experiencing irresistible bouts of sleepiness while at work and has, on several occasions, taken a nap in the workers' lounge during work breaks. He has fallen asleep twice while driving home from work in the morning.

His past medical history is unremarkable. He reports no witnessed apneas or symptoms suggestive of restless legs. He denies alcohol use. A review of his systems is unremarkable.

Because of complaints of nightly snoring and occasional awakenings with "gasping," he undergoes a polysomnography that reveals an apnea-hypopnea index of 4.6 events per hour. No periodic limb movements are noted.

Which of the following is the best recommendation to reduce the patient's sleepiness during shift work?

A. Expose to bright lights in the workplace.
B. Increase levels of physical activity during night shift work.
C. Take frequent breaks from work.
D. Use hypnotic agents to improve daytime sleep following night shift work.

28. A 51-year-old woman is referred for an abnormal chest radiograph obtained during an evaluation for chronic cough. The patient reports a cough for the past 8 weeks. The cough is nonproductive. She does not report hemoptysis, chest pain, fevers, chills, sweats, or weight loss. She is a 50 pack-year smoker. On physical examination, she has no adenopathy. Lungs reveal decreased breath sounds. Laboratory examination is notable for a hemoglobin concentration of 13 g/dL (130 g/L) with normocytic indices. Her chest radiograph and chest CT reveal a 3.5-cm right upper lobe mass with right hilar adenopathy. There are no enlarged mediastinal nodes, and images through the liver and adrenal glands are normal. PET scan demonstrates uptake in the mass and ipsilateral hilar node. The remainder of the staging evaluation results are negative. She undergoes bronchoscopy that reveals an endobronchial lesion in the anterior segment of the right upper lobe, and histologic findings of the endobronchial specimen are shown in Figure 28-A. The next best step in her management is:

A. Chemotherapy and radiation.
B. Radiation alone.
C. Chemotherapy alone.
D. Surgical evaluation.

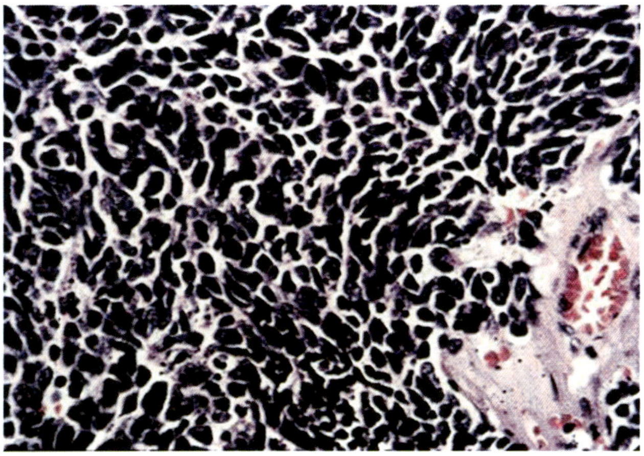

Figure 28-A
Hematoxylin-eosin

29. A 66-year-old patient is receiving controlled mechanical ventilatory support for an acute exacerbation of his COPD. He is receiving a tidal volume of 6 mL/kg ideal body weight (IBW), a set rate of 16/min without additional patient-triggered breaths, an Fio_2 of 0.4, and a PEEP of 3 cm H_2O. His pH is 7.25, his $Paco_2$ is 64 mm Hg, and his Pao_2 is 84 mm Hg. However, his plateau pressure is 36 cm H_2O, and an expiratory pause maneuver reveals a total PEEP of 18 cm H_2O. His BP also has been decreasing over the last 2 h, necessitating the initiation of vasopressors. You are concerned about both the air trapping and the respiratory acidosis and elect to increase the minute ventilation while holding the inspiratory:expiratory time ratio constant. This approach is likely to:

A. Not affect air trapping, but the increased minute ventilation (MV) will improve pH and, thus, improve cardiac function.
B. Reduce air trapping and improve pH; both effects will improve cardiac function.
C. Worsen air trapping, which will further impair cardiac function and possibly raise $Paco_2$ through increased dead space.
D. Not affect air trapping, but the increased MV will produce higher peak airway pressures, which could further impair cardiac function and increase the risk of ventilator-induced lung injury.

30. A 31-year-old woman at 15 weeks' gestation, first pregnancy, develops worsening dyspnea on exertion and bilateral ankle edema. The physical examination reveals that she is in no respiratory distress at rest but becomes dyspneic and manifests a fall in oxygen saturation to 86% on room air after ambulating 30 m. Jugular venous pressure is 11 cm above the angle of Louis, and cardiac examination reveals a prominent P2, as well as a III/VI tricuspid regurgitant murmur. Pedal edema with 2+ pitting is noted bilaterally.

Echocardiography findings show right ventricular hypertrophy, with an estimated pulmonary artery systolic pressure of 68 mm Hg. Other than tricuspid regurgitation, no valve abnormalities are noted, and the left ventricle appears normal. Extensive further evaluation is negative for pulmonary thromboembolic disease, left-sided cardiac disease, significant respiratory disease, connective tissue disease, left-to-right shunt, sleep-disordered breathing, liver disease, and HIV infection. Results of right-sided heart catheterization are shown in Table 30-1.

Table 30-1. Right-Sided Heart Catheterization Results

	Baseline	**After Inhalation of Nitric Oxide (20 ppm) for 10 min**
Central venous pressure	6 mm Hg	5 mm Hg
Pulmonary artery pressure	62/36 mm Hg (mean 45 mm Hg)	58/34 mm Hg (mean 42 mm Hg)
Pulmonary artery occlusion pressure	13 mm Hg	12 mm Hg
Cardiac index	2.6 L/min/m^2	2.5 L/min/m^2

The diagnosis of idiopathic pulmonary arterial hypertension is made. In addition to diuretics and supplemental oxygen, what agent is appropriate for therapy?

A. Bosentan.
B. Warfarin.
C. Epoprostenol.
D. Nifedipine.

31. A 37-year-old woman receives a diagnosis of acute pulmonary embolism (PE). Upon questioning, she states that she completed a 14-h transcontinental flight 2 days earlier. She does not have other medical problems and has never had a prior thrombotic event. She does not smoke tobacco. Her only medication is a low-dose oral contraceptive. There is no family history of thrombosis. Initial laboratory testing reveals that the patient is heterozygous for the factor V Leiden mutation. The patient chooses to stop the oral contraceptive and use an alternative method of birth control. How long should she be treated with a vitamin K antagonist?

A. 3 months.
B. 6 months.
C. 12 months.
D. Indefinitely.

32. A 35-year-old woman is referred for bronchoprovocation challenge testing because of a history of wheezing, normal spirometric findings, and no response to inhaled bronchodilators. She is 140 cm (64 inches) tall and weighs 58 kg (127.6 lbs). She has a 3-year history of intermittent wheezing, with worsening during the spring and with exercise. She rarely has nocturnal episodes. She averages three episodes per month, and her symptoms limit normal activity. She uses an albuterol metered-dose inhaler at least four times daily, with additional use during symptomatic wheezing. She has a 2 pack-year smoking history but stopped as a teenager; she has a boyfriend who currently smokes. She works in retail sales and has no pets.

On the day of testing, she has no symptoms. She has not used her albuterol in the last 24 h. The best results of baseline spirometry testing, as well as the results of bronchoprovocation testing, first with inhalation of normal saline and then initial inhalation of a methacholine dose of 0.5 mg/mL at level 1 and 1.0 mg/mL at level 2, are shown in Table 32-1. She reports that her "chest feels funny" after methacholine administration, but no audible wheezing is heard. The nebulizer was set at the appropriate pressure, and the methacholine was administered for >2 min. Good efforts for each maneuver are reported.

Table 32-1. Baseline Spirometry and Methacholine Challenge Testing Results

	Baseline	**Normal Saline**	**Methacholine, 0.5 mg/mL**			**Methacholine, 1.0 mg/mL**		
Maneuver			1	2	3	1	2	3
Time after methacholine, s			30	55	90	35	95	140
FEV_1, L	3.30	3.22	2.95	3.15	3.05	2.41	2.70	2.90
FVC, L	4.02							
FEV_1/FVC, %	82							
Change from baseline, %	—	−2.4	−10.6	−4.5	−7.5	−27.3	−18.1	−12.1

Which of the following is true about the methacholine testing results?

A. The methacholine was administered by nebulization incorrectly, increasing the drop in the FEV_1 at the 1.0-mg/mL dose.
B. The third maneuver at the 1.0-mg/mL dose was performed past the recommended period for FEV_1 testing after methacholine administration and, thus, should not be recorded.
C. Methacholine challenge testing should move to the next level of dosing (2 mg/mL).
D. The methacholine challenge testing should be terminated and recorded as a positive result because maneuver 1 at the 1.0-mg/mL dosing level resulted in a $>20\%$ decline in FEV_1 from baseline.

33. A 65-year-old woman is admitted to the ED after having progressive dyspnea, chest pain, and syncope at home. She has a history of hypertension and, 12 months earlier, suffered an ischemic stroke resulting in residual left leg paresis. While in the ED, she received a therapeutic dose of low-molecular-weight heparin, and a CT angiogram was performed. Representative images are displayed in Figures 33-A and 33-B. The CT angiogram and a transthoracic echocardiogram both reveal moderate-to-severe right ventricular dilatation and reduced systolic function. Shortly after admission to the ICU, she briefly lost consciousness, and her BP fell from

100/60 to 70/40 mm Hg. Following administration of 1 L of normal saline IV over 30 min, her BP is 80/45 mm Hg, and a repeat transthoracic echocardiogram reveals severe right ventricular dilatation and depressed right ventricular function.

Which of the following interventions, all of which are available at your hospital, would be most appropriate at this time?

A. Administer alteplase via a peripheral vein over 2 h.
B. Administer streptokinase via a peripheral vein over 24 h.
C. Place a pulmonary artery catheter and administer alteplase within the main pulmonary artery over 1 h.
D. Perform catheter embolectomy.

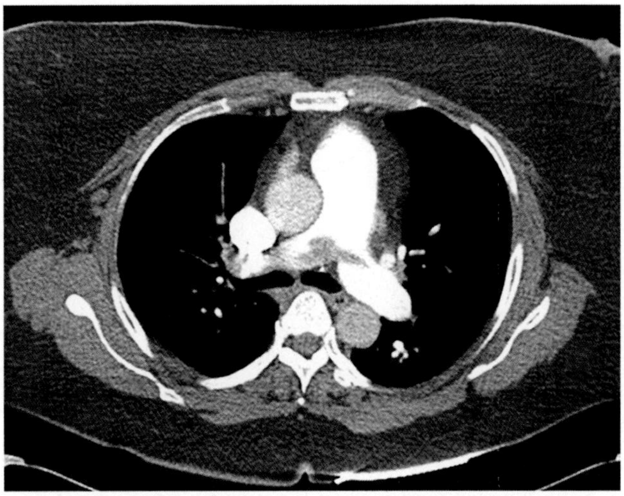

Figure 33-A

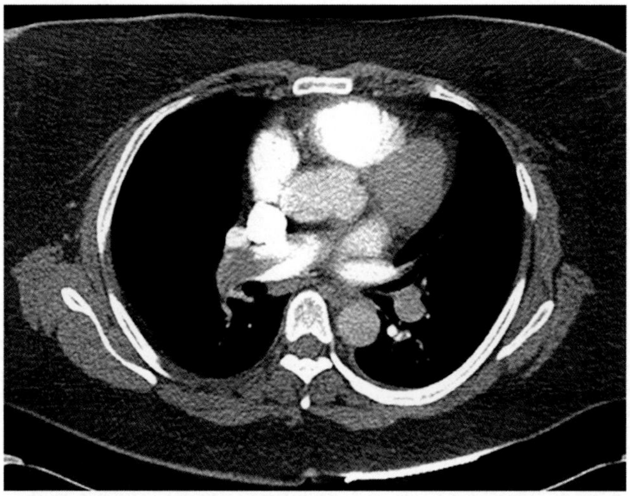

Figure 33-B

34. A 38-year-old woman with a history of alcohol-related cirrhosis is admitted with a chief complaint of the gradual onset of shortness of breath. Past medical history is otherwise unremarkable. There is no history of GI bleeding or of cardiac or renal disease. Medications include spironolactone and lactulose. She continues to drink 0.5 to 1 L of vodka per day. On physical examination, she is icteric with a BP of 100/70 mm Hg, pulse of 90/min, and respiratory rate of 17/min. She is afebrile. Her lung examination reveals decreased breath sounds throughout the right hemithorax with clear breath sounds on the left. Cardiovascular examination is normal. Abdominal examination is notable for tense ascites. Neurologic examination reveals no asterixis.

Laboratory test results reveal a hematocrit of 32% (0.32), hemoglobin of 10.8 g/dL (108 g/L), WBC count of 6,000/µL (6×10^9/L) with a normal differential, and normal electrolytes with the exception of sodium of 132 mEq/L (132 mmol/L) and glucose of 110 mg/dL (6.1 mmol/L). Laboratory tests also reveal an LDH of 200 U/L (3.3 µkat/L), total protein of 4.8 g/dL (48 g/L), albumin of 2.5 g/dL (25 g/L), and prothrombin time of 16 s. Her arterial blood gas measurements while breathing 2 L of oxygen via nasal cannula show a Pao_2 of 68 mm Hg, $Paco_2$ of 28 mm Hg, and pH of 7.48. Her chest radiograph is shown in Figure 34-A. The patient undergoes a diagnostic and therapeutic thoracentesis with removal of 1 L of fluid each day for the next 2 days. Analysis reveals the following values: WBC count of 100/µL (0.1×10^9/L) with 70% neutrophils and 30% lymphocytes, glucose of 100 mg/dL (5.6 mmol/L), LDH of 80 U/L (1.3 µkat/L), total protein of 1.1 g/dL (11 g/L), and pH of 7.46. A large-volume paracentesis is consistent with

a transudate. There is reaccumulation of the pleural and ascitic fluid, and she continues to be refractory to aggressive diuresis. The best next step in this patient's management would be:

A. Transjugular intrahepatic portosystemic shunt (TIPS).
B. Pleural-peritoneal shunt.
C. Chest tube insertion for chemical pleurodesis.
D. Repeated large-volume paracentesis.

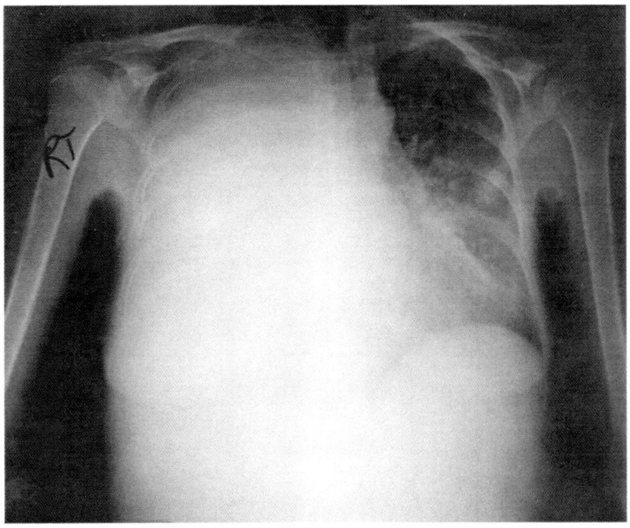

Figure 34-A

35. A 22-year-old man presents to the ED with a 3-day history of cough and hemoptysis. He was quite well until 3 days previously, when he began to feel unwell and had a cough initially productive of yellow sputum. He developed chest pain with coughing and deep inspiration. He then had fever, chills, night sweats, and noticeable hemoptysis, coughing up to a teaspoon of bright red blood. He also complained of anorexia but had noticed no weight loss. There was no history of drug abuse, TB, or TB exposure. He had recently returned home from a vacation in Tampa, FL. He has a cat at home but no other pets.

On examination, his temperature was 36.1°C, BP was 130/60 mm Hg, heart rate was 80/min, and respiratory rate was 18/min. There was no significant cervical, supraclavicular, or axillary lymphadenopathy. There were enlarged lymph nodes in both inguinal regions. The chest was clear, and the rest of the examination was normal. Laboratory tests indicated normal CBC and blood chemistries, except that the LDH level was 1,582 U/L (26.42 μkat/L). Urinalysis results were normal. A chest radiograph and CT scan are shown in Figures 35-A and 35-B. The next step in his investigation should be:

A. Perform bronchoscopy with BAL.
B. HIV serology.
C. Needle aspiration biopsy of a lung lesion.
D. Repeat the physical examination.

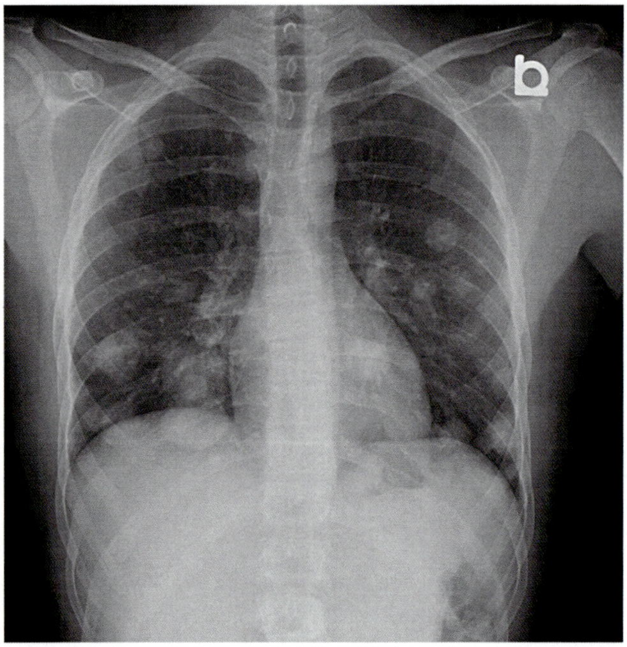

Figure 35-A

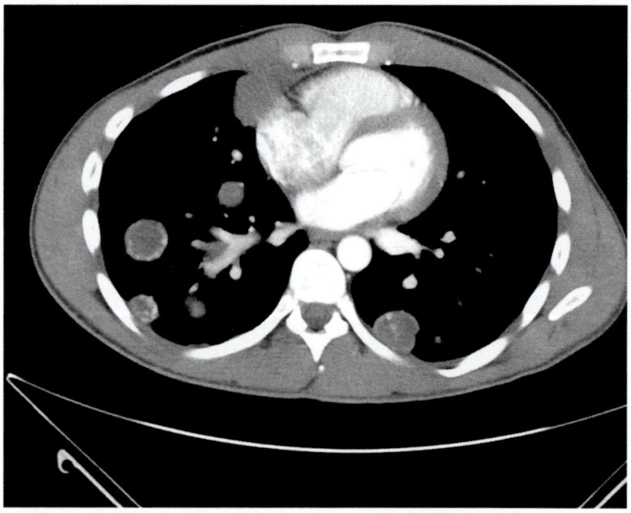

Figure 35-B

36. Which of the following statements is true regarding the polysomnogram shown in Figure 36-A?

A. Administration of positive airway pressure therapy is the treatment of choice for this patient.
B. Positive airway pressure is indicated if the apnea-hypopnea index is > 5/h, regardless of symptoms.
C. Patient preference and device utilization are likely to be greater with bilevel positive airway pressure compared with conventional continuous positive airway pressure (CPAP).
D. Autotitrating positive airway pressure is preferred over conventional CPAP if the patient has concurrent congestive heart failure.

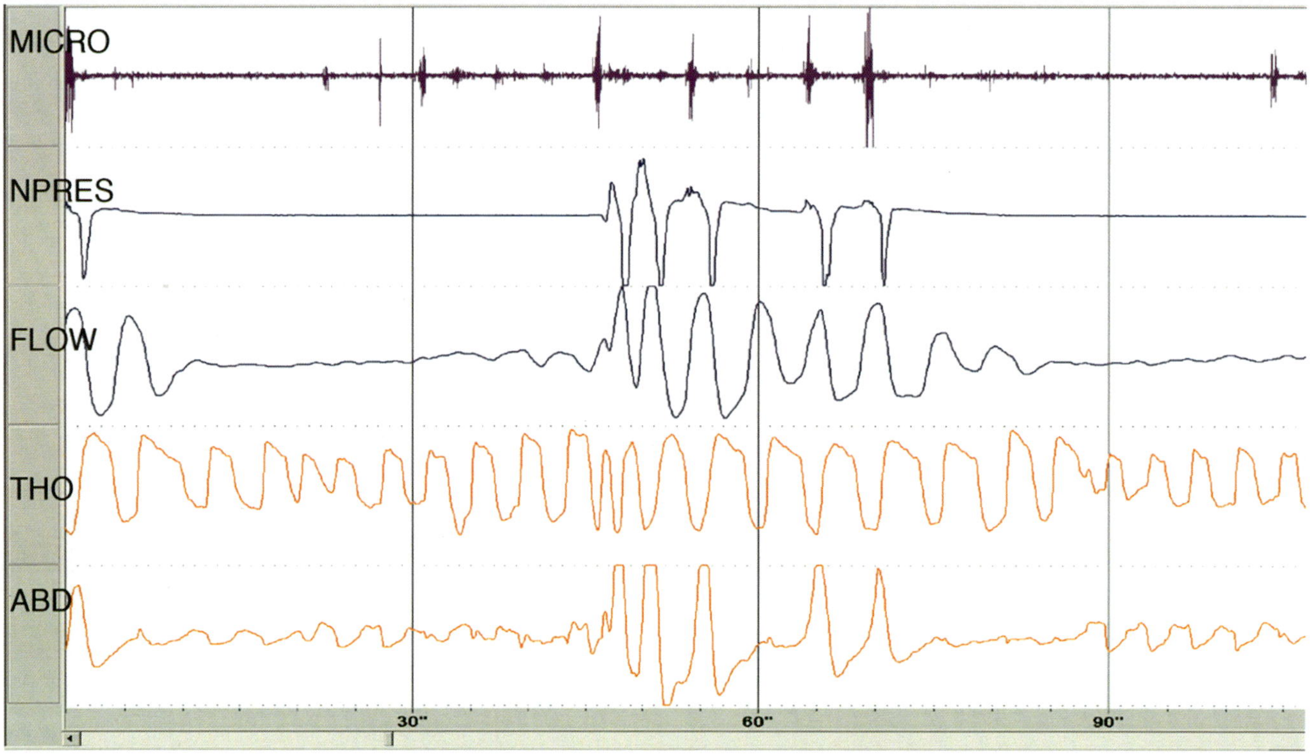

Figure 36-A

37. You are asked to evaluate a 52-year-old person with diabetes who is admitted with 2 days of fever, cough, and diarrhea. On admission, the pulse rate is 132/min, the BP is 80/60 mm Hg, and the respiratory rate is 32/min. The mucous membranes are dry, and there are crackles throughout the right lower chest posteriorly. The following laboratory study results are reported:

pH	7.32
$Paco_2$	32 mm Hg
Pao_2 (room air)	60 mm Hg
Sodium	140 mEq/L (140 mmol/L)
Potassium	4.4 mEq/L (4.4 mmol/L)
Chloride	100 mEq/L (100 mmol/L)
Bicarbonate	16 mEq/L (16 mmol/L)

What is the correct interpretation of these data?

A. Inconsistent and uninterpretable data.
B. Anion gap metabolic acidosis and nonanion gap metabolic acidosis.
C. Anion gap metabolic acidosis with appropriate respiratory compensation.
D. Anion gap metabolic acidosis, metabolic alkalosis, and respiratory alkalosis.

38. A 32-year-old woman with known sickle cell disease who was treated chronically with hydroxyurea was admitted with a sickle cell crisis. She had multiple previous admissions for sickle crises. On this occasion, she was treated with IV hydration, oxygen, and analgesia. Despite this treatment, she developed progressive dyspnea, and azithromycin and ceftriaxone were administered, followed by further hydration and bronchodilators. Physical examination indicated that she was in mild respiratory distress. Vital signs indicated a BP of 110/90 mm Hg, pulse of 105 beats/min, respiratory rate of 40/min, and temperature of 38°C. Bibasal crepitations were audible. Arterial blood gases drawn while the patient was breathing 100% oxygen via face mask indicated a pH of 7.41, $Paco_2$ of 42 mm Hg, and Pao_2 of 76 mm Hg. The hemoglobin level was 7.2 g/dL (72 g/L). The hemoglobin level increased to 9.1 g/dL (91 g/L) and the WBC count increased to 11,600/µL (11.6×10^9/L), with a slight left shift after 2 U packed RBCs were transfused. Hemoglobin electrophoresis indicated 97% hemoglobin S prior to transfusion. Chest radiographs (posteroanterior and lateral) are shown in Figures 38-A and 38-B. She was transferred to the ICU. At this point, what would you recommend?

A. Exchange transfusion.
B. Full anticoagulation with heparin.
C. Corticosteroid therapy.
D. Change antibiotics to moxifloxacin.

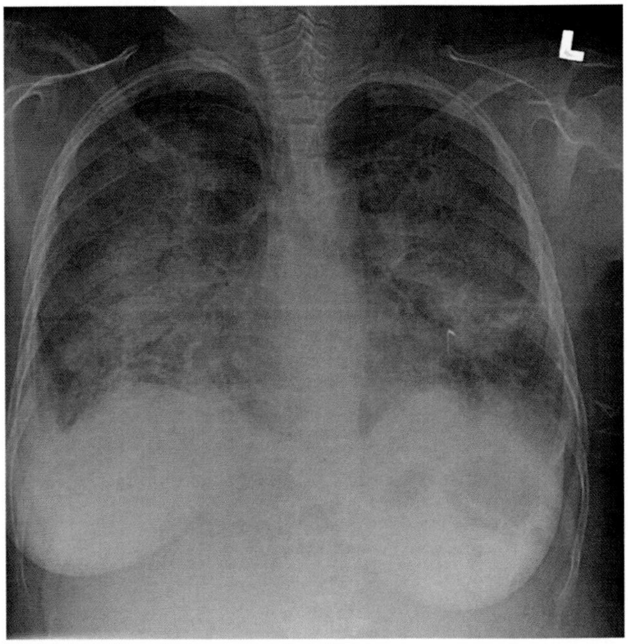

Figure 38-A

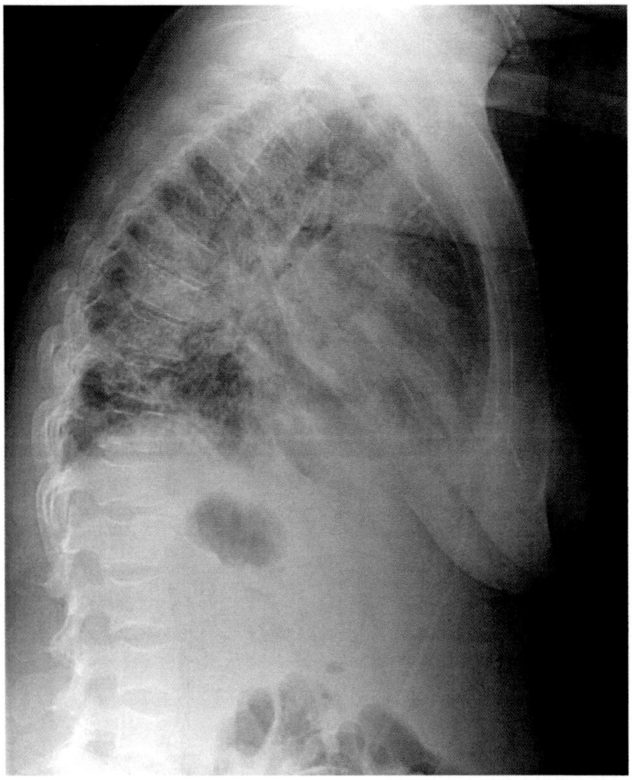

Figure 38-B

39. A 47-year-old man is referred for evaluation of dyspnea on exertion and abnormal pulmonary function tests. He reports a lifelong history of chest infections, requiring antibiotics every year or two and culminating in drainage of a right-sided empyema 2 years previously. He is a lifelong nonsmoker and a retired construction worker who denies exposure to silicates or asbestos and who had no history of travel. He grew up in a rural area, and his bedroom was above what had previously been a chicken coop. There is no family history of lung disease. His physical examination is remarkable for a well-healed right thoracotomy scar and decreased breath sounds on the right side, particularly over the middle lobe area.

Pulmonary function test results are as follows:

	Before Bronchodilator*
FEV_1, L	1.9 (69)
FVC, L	3.5 (88)
FEV_1/FVC, %	56
TLC, L	5.7 (88)
RV/TLC, L	44 (110)
DLCO, L	19.3 (71)

*Values in parentheses are % predicted. TLC = total lung capacity; RV = residual volume; DLCO = diffusing capacity of the lung for carbon monoxide.

Representative images from his CT scan are shown in Figures 39-A, 39-B, and 39-C; from his perfusion scan in Figure 39-D; and from his ventilation scan in Figure 39-E.

Which of the following is the most likely cause of these findings?

A. Silicosis.
B. Histoplasmosis.
C. Sarcoidosis.
D. Lymphoma.

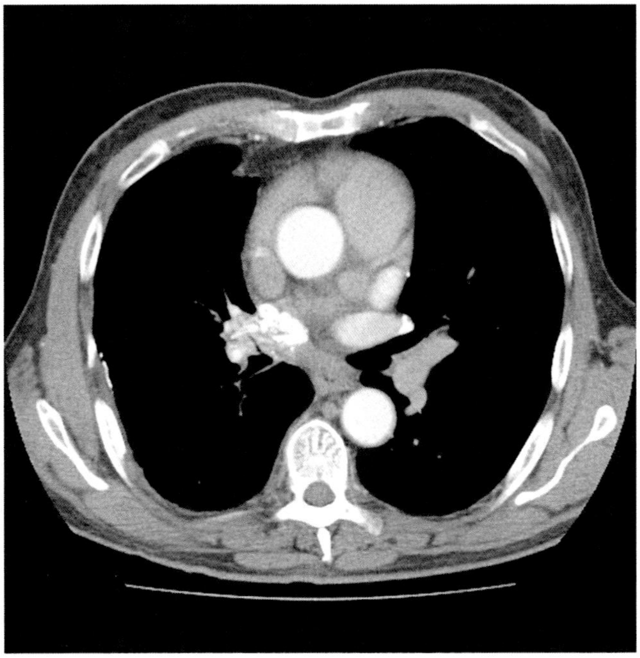

Figure 39-A

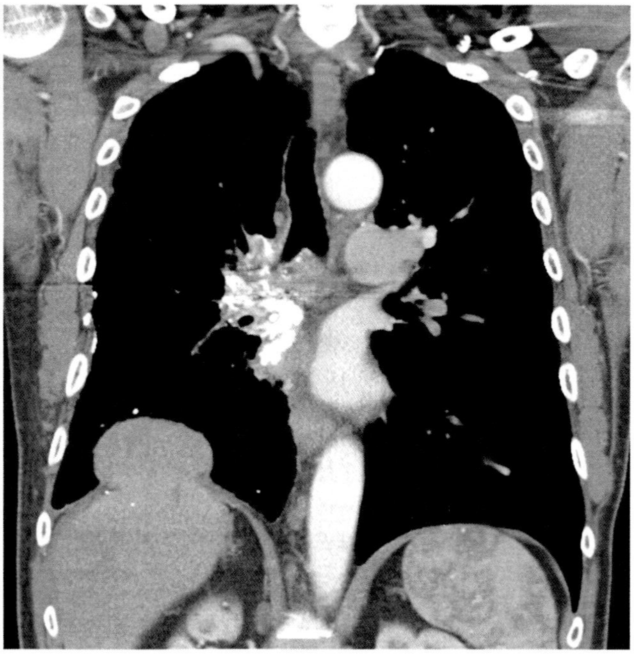

Figure 39-B

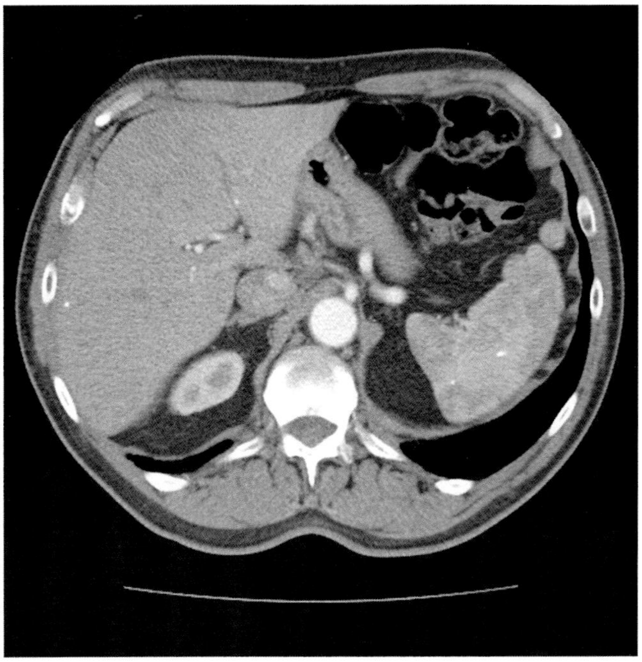

Figure 39-C

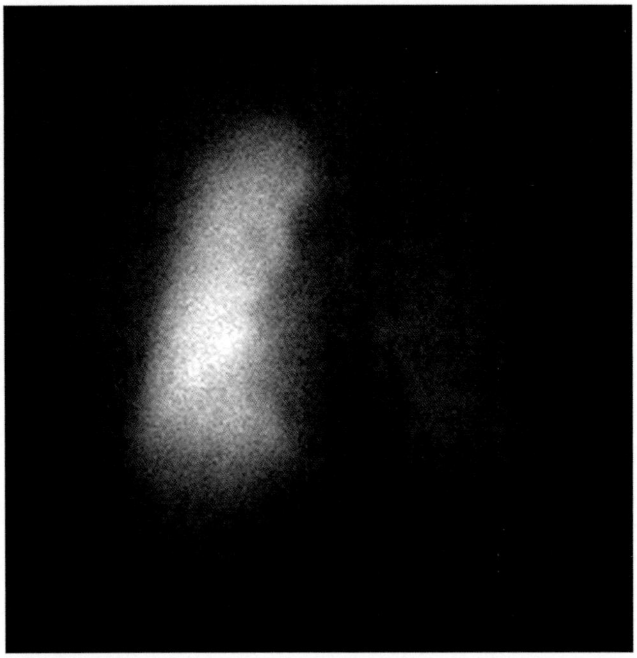

Figure 39-D
Posterior view

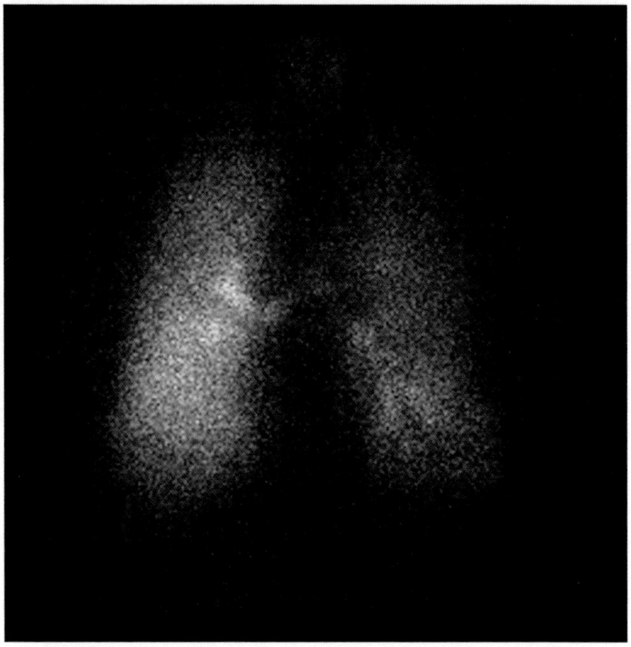

Figure 39-E
Posterior view

40. A 25-year-old healthy man was bitten on the side of the neck by a rattlesnake. He was immediately taken to the local hospital, which was < 10 min away. Upon arrival to the hospital he was awake, alert, and oriented. His BP was 80/50 mm Hg, pulse was 96/min, and respiratory rate was 24/min. The bite mark on the lateral neck was characterized by two marks within close proximity. The area was mildly erythematous. Over the ensuing 10 min, the area of erythema doubled in size. He denied any symptoms other than a metallic taste in his mouth. In addition to administration of IV fluids, the next immediate intervention should be:

A. Administration of antivenin.
B. IV diphenhydramine.
C. Endotracheal intubation.
D. Excision of the bite down to the fascia.

41. A 56-year-old man with deforming rheumatoid arthritis (RA) controlled on biweekly subcutaneous etanercept seeks treatment by his primary care physician for persistent right axillary chest pain and generalized malaise. A cardiac evaluation is performed, including a cardiac catheterization, which is unremarkable for significant coronary artery disease. His symptoms persist over the next 2 months and are accompanied by progressive breathlessness and a non-productive cough with routine activity. Given his progressive symptoms, chest radiography and a high-resolution CT scan are performed (see Figure 41-A). Which of the following is the next appropriate step in his management?

A. Perform flexible bronchoscopy and BAL.
B. Empiric treatment for a community-acquired pneumonia.
C. Initiation of corticosteroid therapy for organizing pneumonia.
D. Video-assisted thoracoscopic surgical lung biopsy.

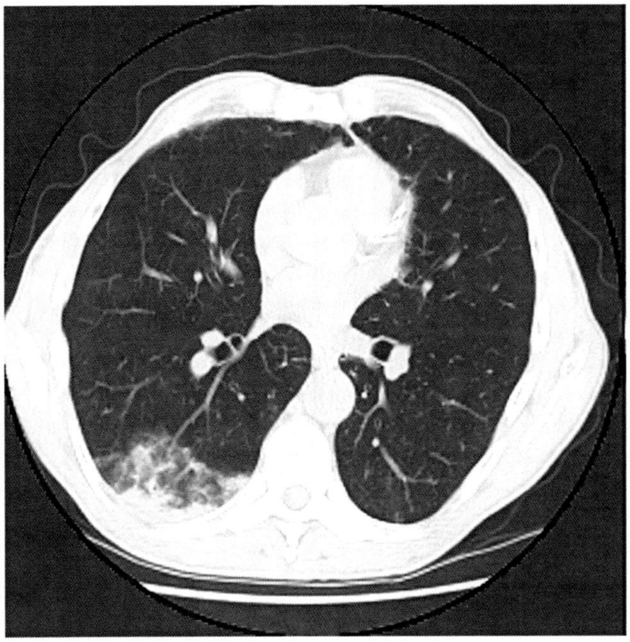

Figure 41-A

42. A 55-year-old woman is referred for progressive shortness of breath. She was born and raised in Japan. She has worked for 25 years as a business consultant, traveling extensively to urban centers around the world, but has recently been transferred permanently to Chicago. She has had long-standing symptoms of sinus congestion and typically receives a course of antibiotics once a year for what was thought to be acute sinusitis. Her shortness of breath was slowly progressive and noticed for the past 2 years. Spirometry indicated moderately severe obstruction and wheezing, which was treated with short- and long-acting inhaled β-agonists and inhaled corticosteroids, all with little benefit.

She is a lifelong nonsmoker and has no industrial or pet exposures. Her long-standing symptoms and poor response to asthma treatment resulted in chest imaging by CT scan, which is shown in Figure 42-A. A bronchoscopy with BAL was performed, and results of bacteria, fungi, and mycobacteria cultures were negative. A lung biopsy with video-assisted thoracoscopic surgery was performed and revealed neutrophilic intraluminal cellular debris (see Figure 42-B), thickening of the walls of the respiratory bronchioles, and lipid-laden or "foamy" macrophage infiltrates of the airway walls (see Figure 42-C, arrows).

Which of the following statements about treatment of this disorder is correct?

A. Macrolide antibiotics should be used in management regardless of culture results.
B. Despite a lack of positive culture results, multidrug treatment to prevent atypical mycobacterial infection should be given indefinitely.
C. High-dose immunosuppression with prednisone and cyclophosphamide should be started and continued until all imaging abnormalities are reversed.
D. IV immunoglobulin should be given.

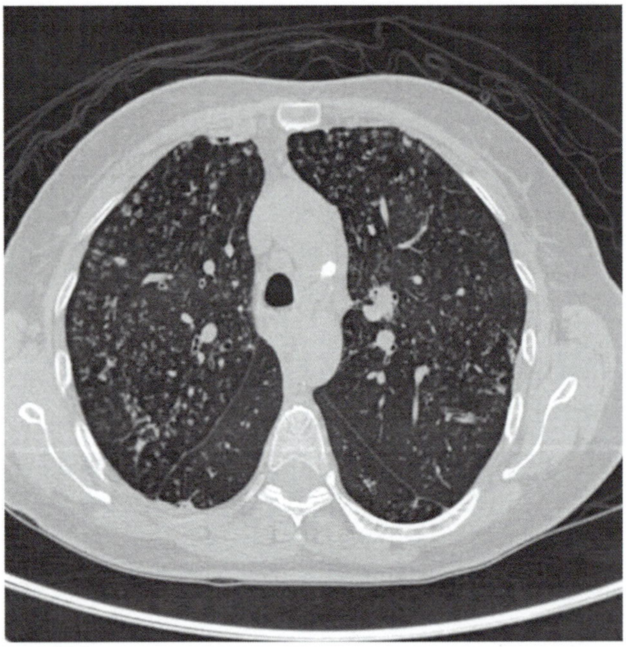

Figure 42-A

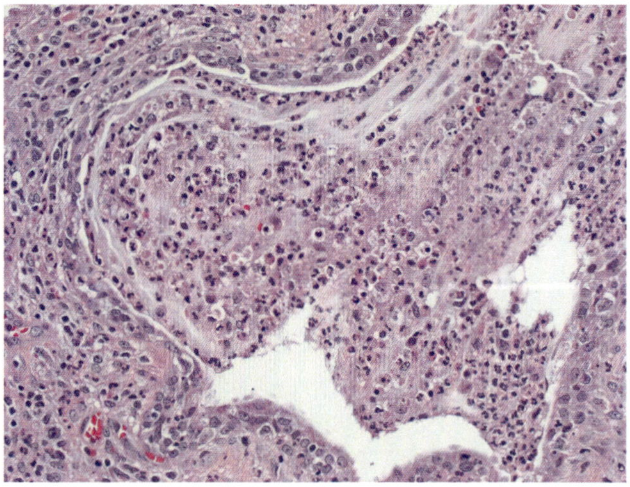

Figure 42-B
Hematoxylin-eosin

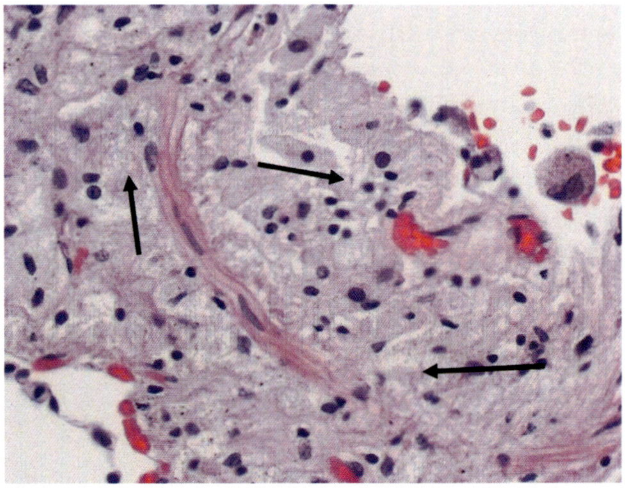

Figure 42-C
Hematoxylin-eosin

43. Which of the following statements best describes the effect of alcohol on sleep?

A. It is sedating at both rising and falling phases of blood alcohol levels.
B. Latency to stage rapid eye movement (REM) from sleep onset is decreased during acute alcohol ingestion.
C. REM sleep decreases during alcohol withdrawal.
D. Sleep disturbances persist for several years following cessation of alcohol use.

44. A 30-year-old woman G2P1Ab0 at 9 weeks' gestation is referred for evaluation of a purified protein derivative of 12 mm of induration and a chest radiograph, with abdominal shielding, that revealed upper lobe fibrocavitary changes. She reports fever, cough, and night sweats for the past 3 weeks. She does not report shortness of breath, weight loss, or hemoptysis. Her past medical history is unremarkable. Two sputum specimens sent from her employee health clinic are now reported to be acid-fast bacillus–positive, with a positive DNA probe for *Mycobacterium tuberculosis.* She has never been a smoker and is employed as a retail worker. Her physical examination and other laboratory studies are unremarkable. Results of HIV testing are negative. The best initial treatment for this patient is:

A. Begin isoniazid, rifampin, pyrazinamide, and moxifloxacin.
B. Begin isoniazid, rifampin, and ethambutol.
C. Defer treatment until after the first trimester.
D. Begin isoniazid and rifampin.

45. A 76-year-old postoperative patient is receiving volume control ventilation with a tidal volume of 6 mL/kg ideal body weight, a set rate of 16/min (no additional spontaneous breaths), an inspired oxygen fraction of 0.4, and an applied PEEP of 10 cm H_2O. His plateau pressure is 18 cm H_2O. He has an esophageal pressure catheter in place and shows an end-inspiratory pressure of 5 cm H_2O. During an extubation attempt, he has a large aspiration event and is promptly reintubated. A chest radiograph shows new bilateral infiltrates. His respiratory system pressures are now likely to show:

A. Increased plateau and increased esophageal pressures.
B. Increased plateau but unchanged esophageal pressures.
C. Increased plateau and lower esophageal pressures.
D. Unchanged plateau but increased esophageal pressures.

46. A 74-year-old woman is referred for evaluation of a left pleural effusion. Approximately 10 days earlier, she underwent uneventful placement of a permanent DDD pacemaker for symptomatic bradycardia due to sick sinus syndrome. A postprocedure chest radiograph showed the pacemaker leads in good position, and no pneumothorax or pleural effusions were seen. Her past medical history is notable only for hypertension, for which she takes benazepril, and gout, for which she takes allopurinol. The effusion was discovered after she developed progressive dyspnea, and her primary care physician's clinical and radiographic findings suggested a moderate-sized pleural effusion on the left side.

Physical examination findings are notable only for diminished breath sounds and dullness to percussion approximately halfway up the left hemithorax. Posteroanterior, lateral, and left lateral decubitus radiographs confirm a moderate, free-flowing, left-sided pleural effusion without evidence of loculation or pleural thickening. Venipuncture and thoracentesis are performed, with the following findings:

Blood	
Total protein	6.9 g/dL (69 g/L)
LDH	134 U/L (2.24 µkat/L)
Glucose	104 mg/dL (5.77 mmol/L)
Triglycerides	143 mg/dL (1.61 mmol/L)
Total cholesterol	226 mg/dL (5.84 mmol/L)
Amylase	64 U/L (1.07 µkat/L)
Pleural fluid	
Appearance	Turbid
pH	7.44
Total protein	4.3 g/dL (43 g/L)
LDH	92 U/L (1.54 µkat/L)
Glucose	90 mg/dL (5.02 mmol/L)
Triglycerides	116 mg/dL (1.31 mmol/L)
Total cholesterol	41 mg/dL (1.06 mmol/L)

Which of the following is the most likely explanation for the patient's pleural effusion?

A. Chylothorax.
B. Empyema.
C. Heart failure.
D. Pulmonary embolism.

47. You are asked to see in consultation a 56-year-old woman with a history of pneumothoraces. She had a left pneumothorax at the age of 26 years, managed by chest tube insertion; a right pneumothorax at age 50 years, managed with chest tube insertion; and a recurrent left pneumothorax at age 55 years, managed surgically. She is a lifelong nonsmoker and has no other history of respiratory illness. She has a younger sister who has had two prior pneumothoraces. She is currently asymptomatic and otherwise healthy and specifically denies chest pain, shortness of breath, activity limitation, cough, or hemoptysis. Results of physical examination are normal.

Pulmonary function test results are shown in Table 47-1.

Table 47-1. Pulmonary Function Test Results*

Variable	Predicted	Observed	% Predicted
FEV_1, L	2.27	2.21	97
FVC, L	2.93	3.05	96
FEV_1/FVC	0.74	0.75	101
TLC, L	4.26	4.72	90
FRC, L	2.61	2.22	95
RV, L	1.73	1.54	89
DLCO, $mL \cdot min^{-1} \cdot mm\ Hg^{-1}$	24.5	20.6	84

*TLC = total lung capacity; FRC = functional residual capacity; RV = residual volume; DLCO = diffusing capacity of the lung for carbon monoxide.

The patient's chest radiograph (see Figure 47-A) and a representative section from the CT scan of the chest (see Figure 47-B) are shown. What would be your next investigation for confirming a diagnosis in this patient?

A. Referral for genetic testing.
B. CT scan of the head.
C. α_1-Antitrypsin level.
D. Thoracoscopic lung biopsy.

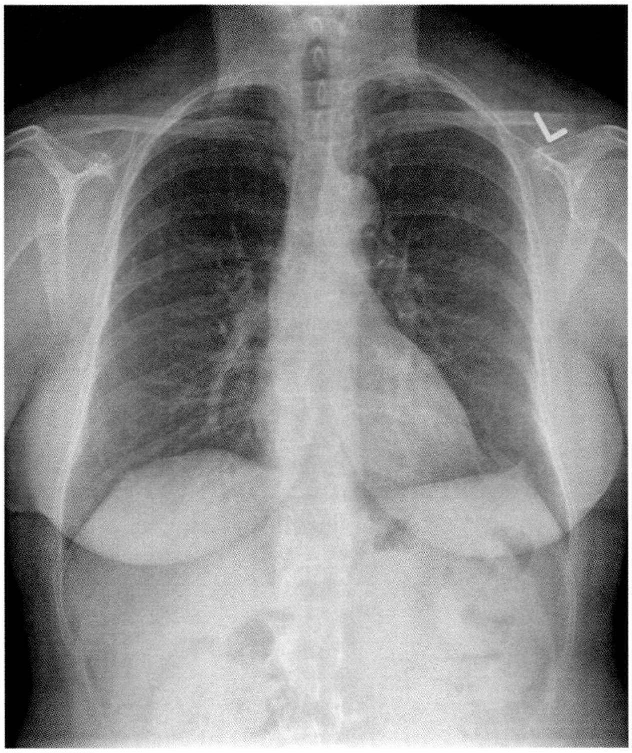

Figure 47-A

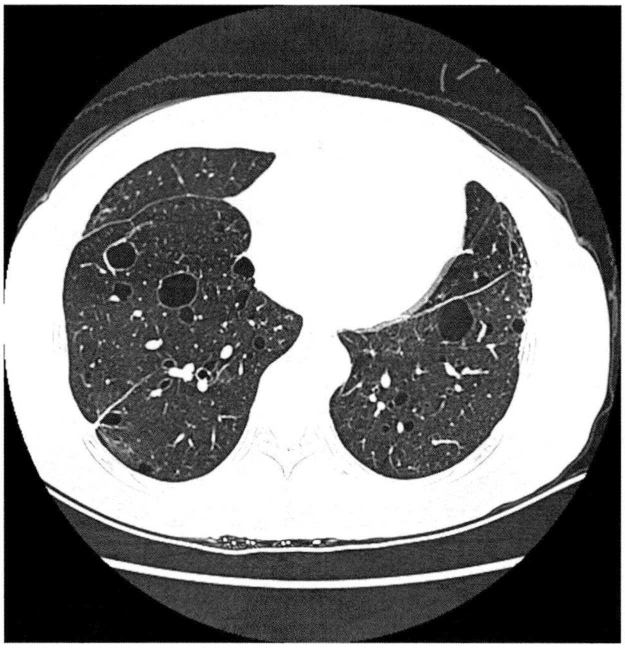

Figure 47-B

48. A 48-year-old nonsmoking woman with hypertension and diabetes underwent an electron-beam CT for cardiac screening. A possible right lung nodule is seen. A follow-up contrast-enhanced spiral CT of the chest confirms a $2.4 \times 1.5 \times 2$-cm lobular nodule in the inferior aspect of the right middle lobe. Two consecutive images are shown in Figures 48-A and 48-B. No other abnormalities are seen. The patient denies any personal or family history of epistaxis, hemoptysis, or GI bleeding. The results of physical examination are unremarkable. Spirometry is normal. Arterial blood gas results on room air and after breathing 100% oxygen for 20 min are shown in Table 48-1.

Table 48-1. Arterial Blood Gas Results

	Room Air	**100% Oxygen**
pH	7.39	7.43
$Paco_2$	36.1 mm Hg	33.8 mm Hg
Pao_2	89 mm Hg	510 mm Hg

The next step in the management of this patient is to:

A. Initiate low-dose estradiol therapy.
B. Initiate interferon therapy.
C. Refer for surgical resection.
D. Refer for embolotherapy.

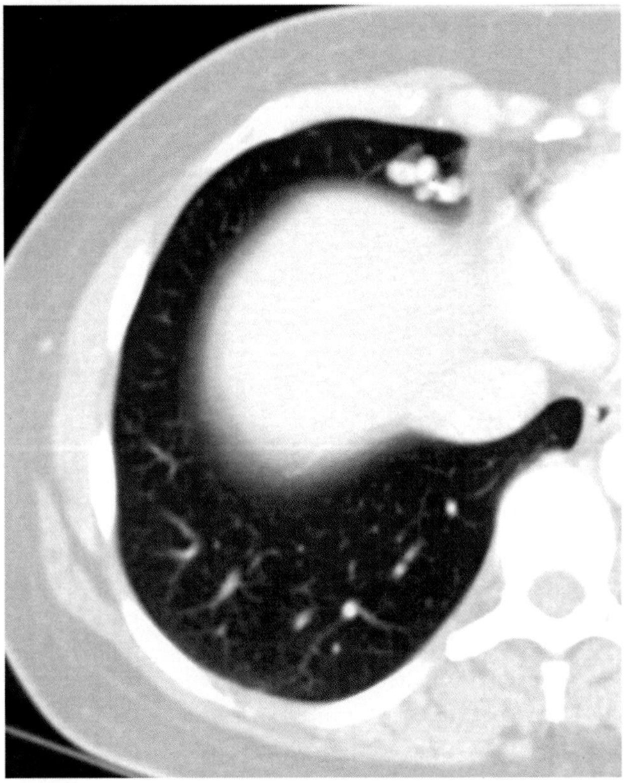

Figure 48-A

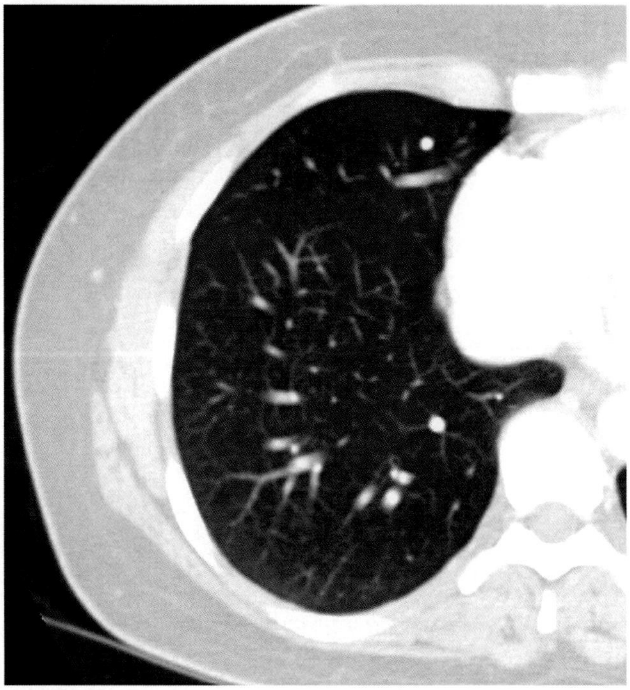

Figure 48-B

49. A 28-year-old woman comes to the ED with acute respiratory distress. She works at a local factory that produces agricultural pesticides. Yesterday, at the factory, a container line ruptured, resulting in a gas leak inside the plant. Three workers, including the patient, were exposed to the gas, as well as some unknown liquid. The patient developed some mild eye and throat irritation and was seen at another local hospital where she was decontaminated and sent home. Later that night, her coughing increased and she had shortness of breath, fatigue, and some pink-tinged sputum production. She has no history of an illness prior to this event and no history of pulmonary symptoms.

On arrival in the ED, her heart rate was 136/min, BP was 175/100 mm Hg, respiratory rate was 34/min, and she had an oxygen saturation level of 86% on room air. She could barely speak one- to two-word sentences and was using accessory muscles of respiration. The ED physician rapidly intubated her for impending hypoxic respiratory failure. Her chest radiograph taken immediately after intubation is shown in Figure 49-A.

What is the cause of this patient's respiratory failure?

A. Organophosphates.
B. Isocyanate.
C. Pyrethrin.
D. Phosgene.

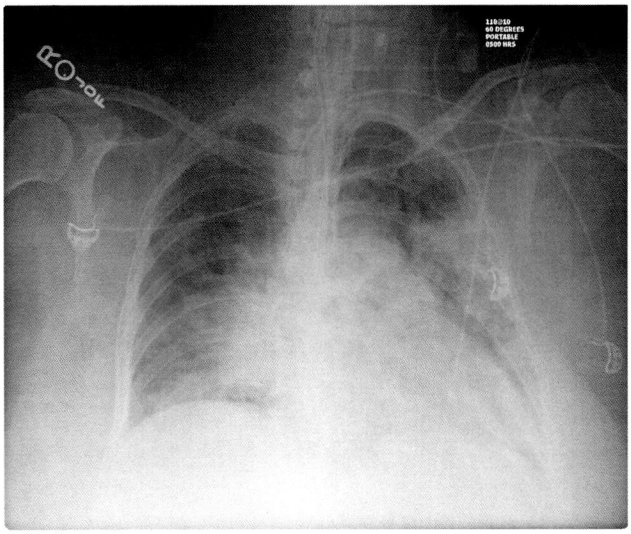

Figure 49-A

50. A 30-year-old woman with status asthmaticus has been endotracheally intubated and is supported by mechanical ventilation. She has had a progressive decline in her BP over the past 30 min, to 80/40 mm Hg, as well as decreasing oxygen saturation, which is 91%. Her heart rate is 126/min. Examination of her chest reveals hyperinflation and faint breath sounds with inspiratory and expiratory wheezes bilaterally. The breath sounds are more faint than previously noted, but equal bilaterally. Minimal secretions are recovered with tracheal suction. She is deeply sedated as a result of receiving continuous IV sedation and analgesia with midazolam and fentanyl. Her current ventilator settings include pressure-targeted assist-control ventilation with set rate of 20, inspiratory pressure of 25 cm H_2O, inspiratory time of 1 s, PEEP of 5 cm H_2O, and Fio_2 of 0.5. Her total respiratory rate is 20/min, and the expired tidal volumes have decreased from about 500 to 350 mL with no change in ventilator settings. A chest radiograph performed immediately after intubation 3 h earlier showed the endotracheal tube (ET) to be in good position and revealed bilateral hyperinflation with clear lung fields. Arterial blood gas tests revealed the following: Pao_2 of 70 mm Hg, $Paco_2$ of 60 mm Hg, and pH of 7.24.

Among the following options, the best is:

A. Deep tracheal suction with saline lavage and then increase the inspiratory pressure to 30 cm H_2O.
B. Deep tracheal suction with saline lavage and then change to volume-assist control mode with set tidal volume of 500 mL.
C. Briefly disconnect the ET from ventilator tubing and then reduce the set rate to 12/min.
D. Briefly disconnect the ET from ventilator tubing and then increase the inspiratory pressure to 30 cm H_2O.

51. What is most likely explanation for the abnormality in the chest radiograph shown in Figure 51-A?

A. Left pleural effusion.
B. Left lower lobe atelectasis.
C. Left lower lobe resection.
D. Left lower lobe pneumonia.

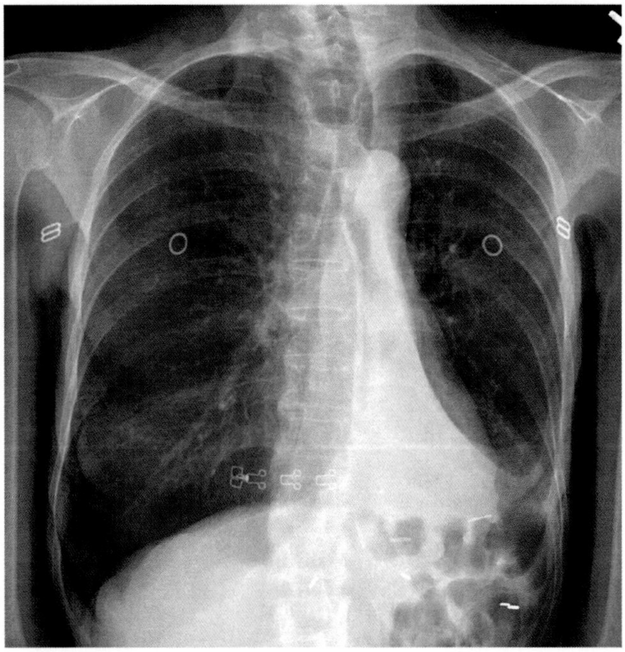

Figure 51-A

52. A 50-year-old woman presents with a 2-week history of increasing shortness of breath and dry cough. She also has had fatigue and one episode of chills but no documented fever. She becomes dyspneic after walking only a few steps. She was treated with a 1-week course of oral antibiotics with no improvement. She is a lifelong nonsmoker.

She has a 10-year history of rheumatoid arthritis for which she currently is treated with leflunomide 20 mg daily, prednisone 5 mg twice daily, and acetaminophen as needed (prn). This combination has kept her joint disease under good control, and she has not experienced any extraarticular manifestations to date. She was treated with methotrexate approximately 5 years ago, with very little improvement in her joint symptoms.

On examination, she is afebrile, with BP of 130/80 mm Hg, pulse of 110/min, and respiratory rate of 25/min. Oxygen saturation while breathing room air is 86% and improves to 93% with 2 L/min of supplemental oxygen. Aside from some joint changes consistent with her arthritis, physical examination is remarkable only for some diffuse wheezing with forced expiration. Spirometry reveals FEV_1 of 1.34 L (62% of predicted), FVC of 1.54 L (57% of predicted), and FEV_1/FVC of 86%. Total lung capacity is 3.70 L (75% of predicted), and DLCO is 58% of predicted. A bronchoscopy with BAL reveals a lymphocytosis, a low CD4/CD8 ratio, and negative culture results. A representative image from a CT scan is shown in Figure 52-A, and pathologic findings from a bronchoscopic biopsy specimen are shown in Figure 52-B.

Which of the following is the most likely diagnosis?

A. Bronchiolitis obliterans.
B. Organizing pneumonia.
C. Delayed methotrexate toxicity.
D. Sarcoidosis.

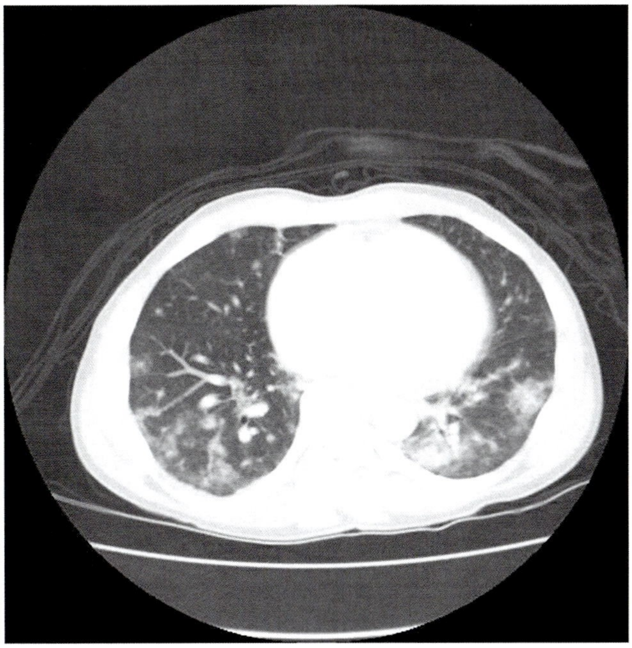

Figure 52-A

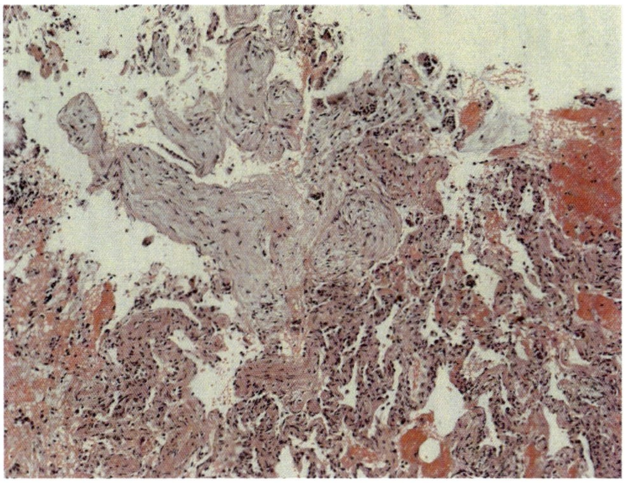

Figure 52-B
Hematoxylin-eosin

53. A 52-year-old man has a history of asthma since age 40 that has progressively worsened, and he is admitted for aspirin desensitization. Recently, he has developed recurrent sinusitis and nasal polyposis; he required sinus surgery at the age of 44 years. The patient also has a history of allergic rhinitis. Dysphonia and wheezing while taking aspirin have occurred since the age of 40 years. The patient has a history of an anaphylactoid reaction requiring intubation 2 years ago following aspirin ingestion. Prior to admission, the patient became more adherent to taking asthma medication, with improvement in his asthma symptoms and morning peak expiratory flow values. His medications include an inhaled and nasal corticosteroid, inhaled long-acting β_2-agonist, and montelukast.

Upon admission, all of his asthma medications are continued, and oral ranitidine is begun. Aspirin titration is begun the morning of admission, with a 30-mg dose followed by gradually increasing doses of aspirin given every 3 h. Peak expiratory flow rates are checked prior to the first dose of aspirin, before each subsequent dose, and any time the patient develops any respiratory complaints. The patient is checked every hour for subjective symptoms (wheezing, dyspnea, nasal congestion, dizziness, nausea) and for skin reactions. Shortly after the third dose of aspirin (provocative dose), the patient complains of patchy itching and mild increased dyspnea. The nurse notes several areas of urticaria on the patient's arms and back. Peak flow values have decreased 25% from baseline. His vital signs are stable and include a respiratory rate of 16/min, temperature of 98.0°F (37.0°C), pulse of 95/min (slightly elevated from a baseline of 80/min), and BP of 107/64 mm Hg. Oxygen saturation is 97% while breathing room air. In addition to ordering an inhaled β_2-agonist, which of following is the best next step in his treatment?

A. Abandon all desensitization efforts.
B. Immediate IV diphenhydramine and corticosteroids; hold aspirin overnight; restart the provocative aspirin dose.
C. Immediate IV diphenhydramine, epinephrine, ranitidine, and corticosteroids; abandon further desensitization efforts.
D. Immediate intubation, given the patient's prior history of an anaphylactoid reaction.

54. A 59-year-old woman is referred because of a slowly enlarging solitary pulmonary nodule noted on chest CT scan. The patient denies respiratory symptoms. She smoked one pack of cigarettes per day for 25 years but stopped smoking 20 years ago. She denies occupational exposure to toxins. Her past medical history is notable for a diagnosis of Cushing syndrome made 7 years ago. Evaluation at that time showed a normal-appearing pituitary on CT scan and a normal adrenocorticotropic hormone gradient between the petrosal sinus and peripheral blood. Therapeutic bilateral adrenalectomy had confirmed adrenal hyperplasia. At that time, a chest CT scan had been reportedly unremarkable, but 3 years ago, an 8-mm nodule was noted on a chest CT scan. The most recent chest CT scan shows that the nodule has grown larger (see Figure 54-A). A fine needle aspirate of the nodule is performed (see Figure 54-B), and the sample is stained for adrenocorticotropic hormone (see Figure 54-C). Of the following therapies, which one would be most appropriate for this patient?

A. Combined chemoradiotherapy.
B. Segmental resection.
C. Segmental resection with mediastinal lymph node sampling.
D. Curative intent radiotherapy.

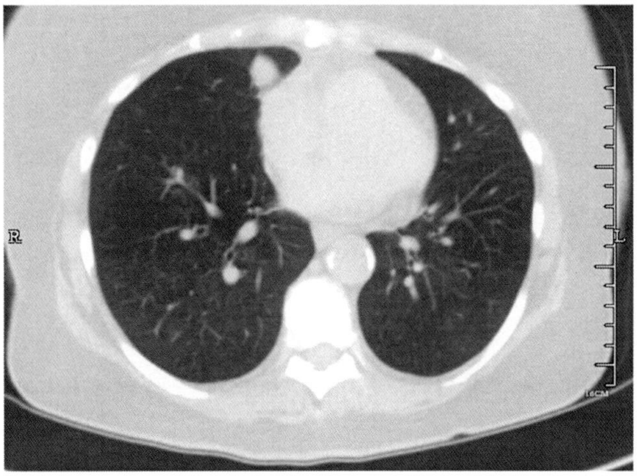

Figure 54-A

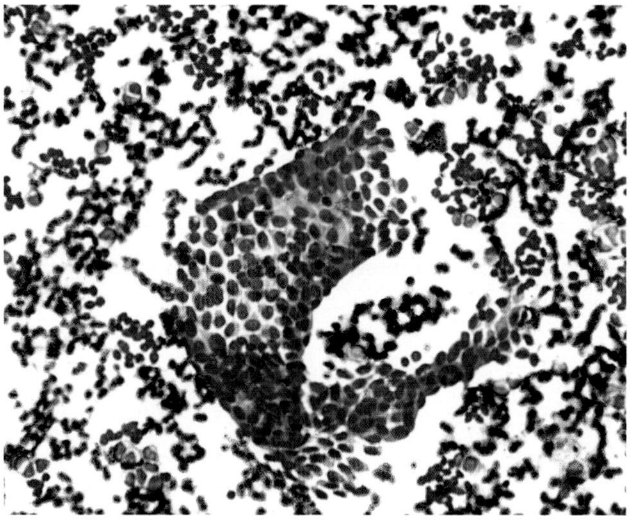

Figure 54-B
Wright-Giemsa

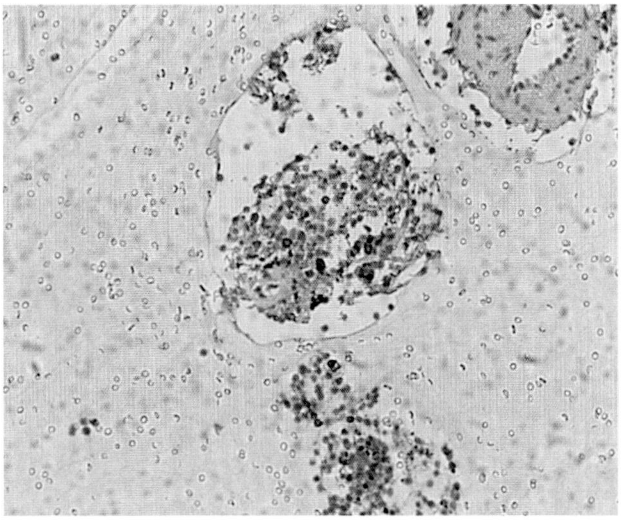

Figure 54-C
Immunoperoxidase

55. In order to evaluate whether a silver-coated endotracheal tube would reduce the incidence of ventilator-associated pneumonia (VAP) compared with a standard tube, a multicenter randomized controlled study was conducted, and $>$2,000 patients who were expected to receive mechanical ventilation support for $>$24 h were enrolled. After patients were excluded because they were intubated for $<$24 h, the results are shown in Table 55-1.

Table 55-1. Incidence of VAP With Silver-Coated vs Uncoated Tube

	No Pneumonia (n = 1,416)	Pneumonia (n = 93)
Silver-coated tube (n = 766)	37	729
Uncoated tube (n = 743)	56	687

Assuming that the groups who did and did not develop pneumonia were similar at the time of enrollment in the study and that the diagnosis of pneumonia was made by an investigator who did not know which tube the patients received, how many patients must receive a silver-coated tube to prevent one case of ventilator-associated pneumonia?

A. 3 patients.
B. 16 patients.
C. 37 patients.
D. 76 patients.

56. Which of the following statements regarding the seven-valent conjugate pneumococcal vaccine administered to children is correct?

A. It has led to an increase in the amount of invasive pneumococcal disease among HIV-infected adults.
B. It is associated with a 25% reduction in invasive pneumococcal disease in normal and immunocompromised children and adults.
C. It has led to a decrease in the number of penicillin-resistant pneumococcal strains among adults $\geq$65 years.
D. There has been no change in invasive pneumococcal disease caused by nonvaccine serotypes among children.

57. A 49-year-old woman is assessed regarding progressive dyspnea. She has a 15-year history of rheumatoid arthritis (RA) currently treated with weekly intramuscular methotrexate (for the past 6 years) and ketoprofen. She noted the insidious onset of dyspnea on exertion approximately 5 years previously, which has progressed slowly. Currently, she can climb one flight of stairs or walk two city blocks before noticing chest tightness and dyspnea. She also has a nonproductive cough made worse on exposure to cold air or exertion. She had been treated with various combinations of inhaled steroids, long-acting β-agonists, and leukotriene receptor antagonists with no significant relief. She is a lifelong nonsmoker. Physical examination is unremarkable aside from some joint changes consistent with her known rheumatoid arthritis. Representative images from her CT scan are shown in Figures 57-A and 57-B. Her pulmonary function tests are shown in Table 57-1.

Table 57-1. Pulmonary Function Test Results

	Before Bronchodilator*	After Bronchodilator*
FEV_1, L	1.34 (50)	1.37 (51)
FVC, L	2.80 (85)	2.81 (85)
FEV_1/FVC, %	48	49
TLC, L	4.93 (99)	
RV/TLC, L	41 (117)	
DLCO, L	19.6 (95)	

*Values in parentheses are % predicted. TLC = total lung capacity; RV = residual capacity; DLCO = diffusing capacity of the lung for carbon monoxide.

The most likely cause of her lung disease is:

A. Lung toxicity attributable to methotrexate therapy.
B. Interstitial lung disease attributable to her rheumatoid arthritis.
C. Emphysema.
D. Bronchiolitis obliterans attributable to her rheumatoid arthritis.

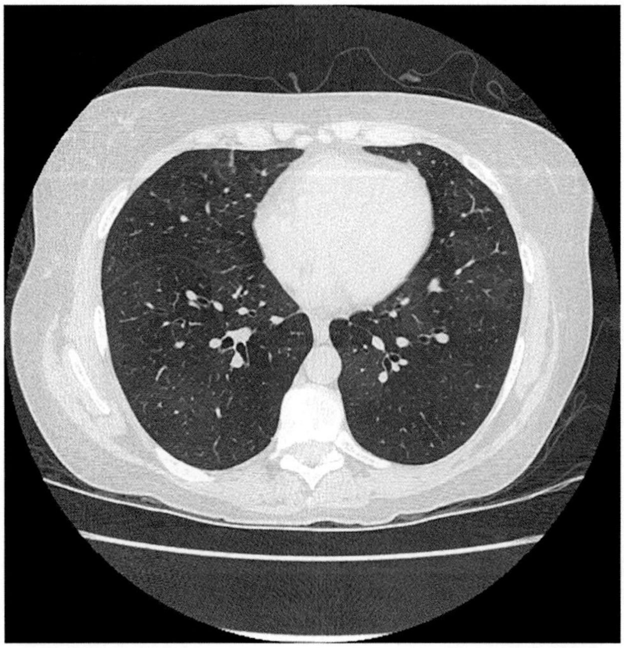

Figure 57-A

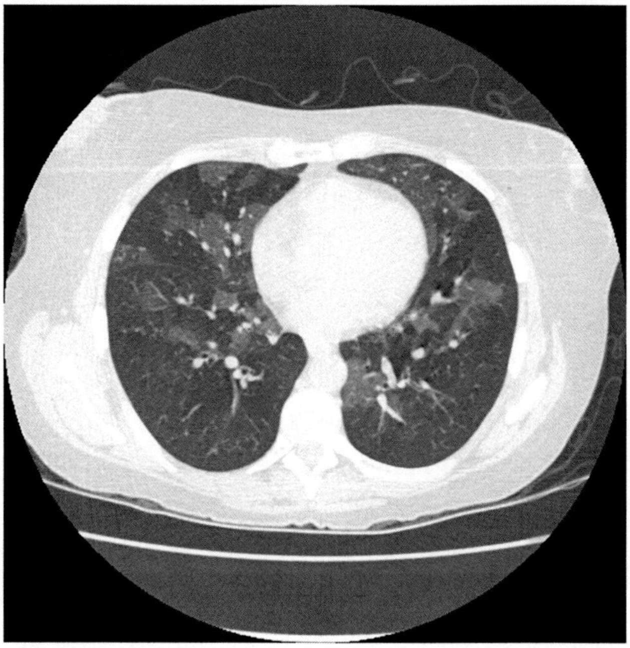

Figure 57-B

58. A 58-year-old man with a recent diagnosis of a malignant right pleural effusion, due to adenocarcinoma of the lung, has had significantly increased shortness of breath over the last 2 weeks. His chest radiograph shows considerable increase in the right-sided pleural effusion compared with a radiograph 3 weeks ago obtained after a therapeutic thoracentesis. A therapeutic thoracentesis incorporating pleural manometry is performed. A small-bore catheter is used to perform the thoracentesis and is left in place in anticipation of performing pleurodesis to prevent effusion reoccurrence. The following three possible pleural elastance curves are shown in Figure 58-A.

Which pleural elastance curve is most compatible with a subsequent successful pleurodesis procedure?

A. Curve A.
B. Curve B.
C. Curve C.
D. None of the curves predict success.

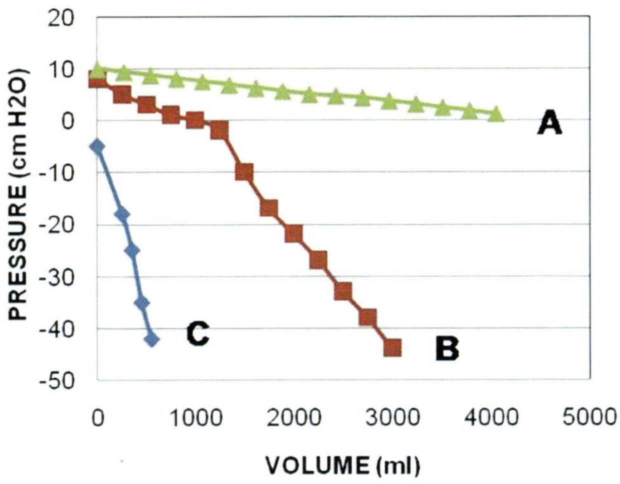

Figure 58-A

59. A 32-year-old, multiparous woman during her third trimester (week 28) of her fourth pregnancy is seen with a weight gain of 5 lbs over the past 3 days. She also has a mild headache and mild right upper quadrant pain. Her BP is 140/90 mm Hg, pulse is 110/min, respiratory rate is 18/min, and oxygen saturation on room air is 95%. Her chest was clear to auscultation and percussion, her heart examination revealed a soft systolic murmur, and she had bilateral lower extremity pedal edema. Laboratory testing revealed the following values: a hemoglobin of 8 g/dL (80 g/L), a hematocrit of 32%, a platelet count of $75 \times 10^3/\mu L$ ($75 \times 10^9/L$), BUN of 31 mg/dL (11.1 mmol/L), creatinine of 1.3 mg/dL (114.9 µmol/L), aspartate aminotransferase of 125 U/L (2.1 µkat/L), and alanine aminotransferase of 240 U/L (4 µkat/L). She receives 2 U of packed RBCs, and a repeat hemoglobin level is 12 g/dL (120 g/L). One hour later, she is noted to have a BP of 90/60 mm Hg and a pulse rate of 125/min. The next most appropriate step is to:

A. Infuse magnesium sulfate.
B. Transfuse platelets.
C. Obtain CT scan of the abdomen.
D. Perform an emergency Cesarean section.

60. A 56-year-old woman arrives at your office for an evaluation of progressive dyspnea, fatigue, intermittent double vision, and hoarseness most notable with prolonged conversations. Her symptoms began 6 months ago and have slowly worsened. Three weeks ago, she suffered a "cold" marked by rhinorrhea and a sore throat. Her previous symptoms significantly worsened after her cold such that she is now dyspneic with activities of daily living. She has not experienced any fevers, chills, sweats, or myalgias but does note that she has been hypersomnolent with intermittent "jerks or spasms" in her hands and legs. She also has had difficulty swallowing liquids and solids. She does not take any medications for her symptoms.

Physical examination was remarkable for intermittent, spontaneous myoclonus, decreased short-term memory and hypersomnolence, and horizontal nystagmus. She was able to answer detailed questions, although tangentially. Her voice was hoarse and weak in amplitude. Rapid, shallow respirations were present. Lung fields were clear but markedly diminished, without identifiable excursion of the diaphragm. Reflexes were intact, as was motor strength, both proximally and distally. Rapid, alternating movements were normal without fatigue.

An arterial blood gas measurement obtained while she was receiving nasal oxygen at 2 L/min supplemental oxygen revealed a Pao_2 of 43 mm Hg, $Paco_2$ of 105 mm Hg, and pH of 7.29. What is the most appropriate next management step at this point?

A. Institution of noninvasive mechanical ventilation.
B. Administration of levothyroxine.
C. IV administration of "pulse-dose" corticosteroids.
D. Intubation following paralysis with succinylcholine.

61. A 36-year-old woman is admitted to the ICU for treatment of pneumococcal sepsis and severe acute hypoxemic respiratory failure. She is intubated, fluid-resuscitated, and treated for septic shock. Her medications include heparin 5,000 U SC q8h, famotidine 20 mg IV q12h, ceftriaxone 1 g/day IV, moxifloxacin 400 mg/day IV, fentanyl 50 μg/h infusion, and lorazepam 10 mg/h infusion.

On day 7, she develops acute renal failure as reflected by a doubling of the serum creatinine to 2.0 mg/dL (177 μmol/L) with anuria. Other laboratory findings are as follows:

Sodium	138 mEq/L (138 mmol/L)
Potassium	5.2 mEq/L (5.2 mmol/L)
Chloride	103 mEq/L (103 mmol/L)
Bicarbonate	14 mEq/L (14 mmol/L)
Glucose	180 mg/dL (9.99 mmol/L)
BUN	28 mg/dL (10 mmol/L)
Serum osmolality	348 mOsm/kg (348 mmol/kg)

Which of her medications is the most likely cause of the acute renal failure?

A. Famotidine.
B. Ceftriaxone.
C. Moxifloxacin.
D. Lorazepam.

62. A 28-year-old woman is referred for persistent insomnia and unusual sleep-related behavior. She relates a 10-year history of gradually worsening insomnia, with both difficulty falling asleep and frequent prolonged nighttime awakenings. She has tried melatonin and several over-the-counter antihistamine agents in the past but reports that they were generally ineffective. A year ago, she enrolled in a class involving a therapist-guided cognitive behavioral therapy; this, too, provided minimal benefit.

She admits to snoring but denies any witnessed apneas. There is no report of sleep paralysis or cataplexy. She occasionally feels a vague uncomfortable sensation in her feet and calves at night. Two months ago, she tripped over a chair as she was "sleep walking" across her bedroom. On another occasion, she kicked her husband and hit him with the back of her hand while she was asleep. She has no recollection of doing these things. Her visit today is prompted by her husband's report of her walking "aimlessly" in her kitchen two nights ago as she was holding a knife and eating leftovers from dinner. When confronted, she merely walked past him and returned to bed still wielding the steak knife.

She describes a childhood history of sleepwalking that persisted until late adolescence. Three months ago, she was prescribed zolpidem, which she takes regularly for her insomnia. Review of systems reveals sleep talking and several recent episodes of enuresis. She drinks alcohol nightly with dinner and occasionally at bedtime, as well, to help her to sleep. She prefers drinking tea occasionally with her breakfast but does not drink coffee. She quit smoking 5 years ago.

Which of the following would be the most appropriate first step in the management of this patient?

A. Trial of low-dose clonazepam.
B. Electroencephalography.
C. Advise on sleep extension.
D. Discontinue zolpidem.

63. A 43-year-old woman with a diagnosis of systemic lupus erythematosus (SLE) has progressive shortness of breath over a 4-month period. She does not have chest pain, cough, fever, or chills. She has a history of a lupus anticoagulant, has been taking warfarin with variable compliance, and is receiving no other therapy. On physical examination, she is in no distress when at rest. Her vital signs are stable with the exception of a respiratory rate of 18/min. Lungs are clear without crackles or wheezes. Cardiovascular examination reveals normal heart sounds without a murmur, and there is no increase in the second heart sound. Results of pulmonary function tests are shown in Table 63.1.

Table 63.1. Pulmonary Function Test Results*

FEV_1	1.8 L (55% of predicted)
FVC	2.3 L (58% of predicted)
FEV_1/FVC	0.78
TLC	3.8 L (68% of predicted)
RV	100% of predicted
DLCO	11 $mL \cdot min^{-1} \cdot mm\ Hg^{-1}$ (77% of predicted)
DLCO adjusted for alveolar volume	102% of predicted

*TLC = total lung capacity; RV = residual volume; DLCO = diffusing capacity of the lung for carbon monoxide.

A chest radiograph shows small lung volumes without infiltrates or pleural effusions. A high-resolution CT scan shows no evidence of interstitial disease or pleural effusion.

What is the next best test for the further evaluation of this patient?

A. Perform bronchoscopy with transbronchial biopsy.
B. Order a ventilation-perfusion scan.
C. Measure maximal expiratory and inspiratory pressures.
D. Order an echocardiogram.

64. A 59-year-old patient with severe COPD and no known cardiac disease is being evaluated for pulmonary rehabilitation. An exercise test is performed and shows the following response at a symptom-limited maximum load:

Oxygen consumption ($\dot{V}O_2$) = 42% of predicted
SpO_2 = 93%
Exercise ventilation/maximal voluntary ventilation = 0.60
Heart rate = 105% of predicted with a normal 12-lead ECG

Based on these results, your evaluation of the patient would be:

A. Poor exercise rehabilitation candidate because heart rate is excessive.
B. Poor exercise rehabilitation candidate because exercise ventilation is too low.
C. Poor exercise rehabilitation candidate because $\dot{V}O_2$/heart rate (O_2 pulse) is too low.
D. Excellent exercise rehabilitation candidate.

65. A 28-year-old medical resident seeks evaluation because she is 22 weeks pregnant, and an HIV-positive inpatient under her care 4 weeks ago was diagnosed with smear-positive TB last week. The patient had not been moved to

respiratory isolation when he was under her care, and she also had a number of prior encounters with him, during which time she did not wear a mask. She has been feeling fatigued, but otherwise well, and denies fever, cough, hemoptysis, night sweats, or weight loss. Results of physical examination are unremarkable except for a soft systolic flow murmur and a gravid uterus that is appropriate size for dates.

Her last negative purified protein derivative test (PPD; 0-mm induration) was 8 months ago. A 5-tuberculin unit (TU) tuberculin skin test is placed on her left forearm and develops 7 mm of induration at 72 h. A posteroanterior chest radiograph is performed with fetal shielding and is normal.

What course of action is most appropriate at this point?

A. Begin treatment with isoniazid.
B. Begin treatment with isoniazid, rifampin, pyrazinamide, and ethambutol.
C. Perform a 250-TU tuberculin skin test now.
D. Repeat a 5-TU tuberculin skin test in 8 to 12 weeks.

66. A 38-year-old man is referred to you for management of α_1-antitrypsin (A1AT) deficiency. The patient's 48-year-old brother had a diagnosis of COPD (FEV_1 = 55% of predicted, FEV_1/FVC = 0.44) associated with A1AT deficiency (A1AT level = 0.11 g/L [normal values = 1.5 to 3.5 g/L]). During family screening genetic testing, the patient's A1AT level was measured as 0.40 g/L. A repeat level was 0.38 g/L, and his A1AT phenotype was reported as PI*ZZ. The patient has no respiratory or abdominal symptoms. He is a nonsmoker and drinks approximately one glass of wine per week. He takes no medications and is employed as an accountant. He has recently received both the influenza and pneumococcal vaccinations. Results of physical examination are normal. Sao_2 on room air is 99%. Results of a chest film and CT scan of the chest are normal, and liver enzymes values and function tests are also normal.

Pulmonary function tests are shown in Table 66-1.

Table 66-1. Pulmonary Function Test Results*

Variable	Predicted	Observed	% Predicted
FEV_1, L	4.06	5.14	127
FVC, L	5.32	6.60	124
FEV_1/FVC	0.76	0.78	103
TLC, L	7.23	8.55	118
FRC, L	4.10	4.54	111
RV, L	2.07	1.98	96
DLCO, $mL \cdot min^{-1} \cdot mm\ Hg^{-1}$	40.2	39.7	99

*TLC = total lung capacity; FRC = functional residual capacity; RV = residual volume; DLCO = diffusing capacity of the lung for carbon monoxide.

What would you do next in the management of this patient with PI*ZZ A1AT deficiency?

A. Initiate augmentation therapy with weekly IV A1AT replacement therapy.
B. Initiate regular maintenance bronchodilator therapy with tiotropium.
C. Initiate augmentation therapy with nebulized A1AT replacement therapy.
D. Arrange follow-up assessment and pulmonary function testing in 6 months.

67. A 65-year-old man has dyspnea on exertion 4 months after coronary artery bypass grafting (CABG). He denies fever, orthopnea, paroxysmal nocturnal dyspnea, chest pain, edema, or weight gain. He had a chest radiograph 6 weeks after surgery that revealed a small effusion on the right side. An echocardiogram done at about the same time revealed an ejection fraction of 52%. On physical examination, the patient is afebrile with a BP of 124/88 mm Hg, pulse rate of 85/min, and respiratory rate of 16/min. He has no jugular venous distension. Heart sounds are regular without an S3 or murmur. Breath sounds are reduced on the right but otherwise are clear. There is no pleural or cardiac rub. There is no hepatomegaly or hepatojugular reflux. There is a well-healed vein harvest scar on the left lower extremity, with mild pitting edema below the knee. The right lower extremity is normal without edema. A chest radiograph taken today in the pulmonary clinic is shown (see Figure 67-A). An ECG is without any acute changes. A thoracentesis reveals a nonbloody, exudative, lymphocyte-predominate effusion. A portion of his postthoracentesis chest radiograph is shown (see Figure 67-B).

The next step in the management of the patient is to:

A. Repeat thoracentesis with pleural manometry.
B. Place a chest tube for complete drainage.
C. Refer for pericardiectomy.
D. Initiate aspirin therapy.

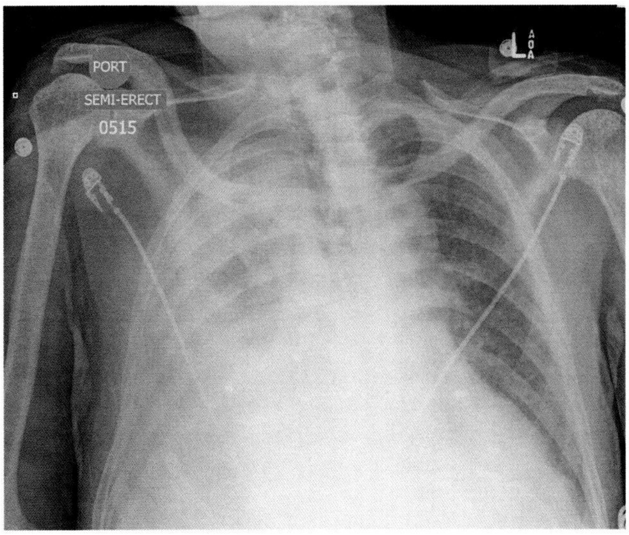

Figure 67-A

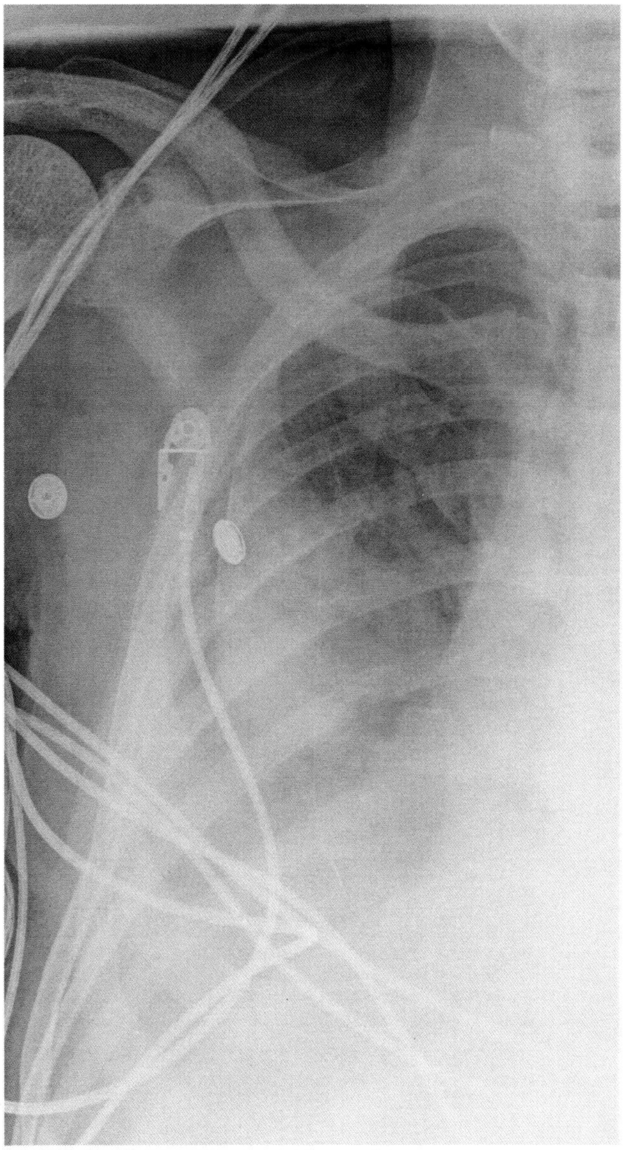

Figure 67-B

68. Two of your patients supported by mechanical ventilation are undergoing spontaneous breathing trials using automatic tube compensation (ATC). You observe that the positive airway pressure is averaging about 10 cm H_2O with each breath for patient A, and 4 cm H_2O with each breath for patient B.

Which of the following differences in settings and respiration is most likely to explain the higher airway pressure for patient A?

A. The percent tube compensation is set at 40% for patient A and 100% for patient B.
B. Patient A has a tracheostomy tube, and patient B has an endotracheal tube with identical internal diameter (ID).
C. Patient A has a tube with an ID of 8.0 mm, whereas the ID of patient B's tube is 6.0 mm.
D. Patient A is generating flow rates of 80 L/min vs 40 L/min by patient B.

69. A 29-year-old woman presents with chronic right lower quadrant and pelvic pain, noting menorrhagia and dysmenorrhea 1 week prior to her menses. A year ago, she underwent a total abdominal hysterectomy and right salpingo-oophorectomy for a right ovarian mass noted on ultrasound. Postoperatively she had ongoing pelvic pain. A CT scan of her abdomen showed no abnormalities but did reveal a right-lower-lobe cavitary nodule. A single nodule was confirmed by chest CT scan. She denies pulmonary symptoms other than two recent episodes of coughing up bright red blood, each about a month apart.

On physical examination, she is afebrile with BP of 110/70 mm Hg, pulse of 82/min, and respiratory rate of 12/min. Her lung and heart examinations are normal, and she is tender to palpation of her right lower quadrant but has no rebound or guarding. Her gynecologic examination reveals no masses. Her laboratory tests reveal a normal WBC count, normal serum chemistries, normal liver function tests, and normal urinalysis. Her serum pregnancy test is negative. What is the most likely diagnosis in this patient?

A. TB.
B. Wegener granulomatosis.
C. Thoracic endometriosis.
D. Choriocarcinoma.

70. A 75-year-old man is referred for management of obstructive sleep apnea. The patient brings with him a copy of the results of his polysomnography that was done 2 months ago for evaluation of his snoring and witnessed apneas. He denies daytime sleepiness, and his Epworth sleepiness scale score during the visit is 6. Past medical history is significant for occasional insomnia and possible depression, for which he started to receive a selective serotonin reuptake inhibitor. Surgeries included a childhood tonsillectomy and right knee replacement. He denies smoking or the use of alcohol, coffee, tea, or soda.

On physical examination, the patient is noted to be edentulous and mildly overweight. Other pertinent findings include a long thin uvula and a marked overbite. Lung, cardiac, and neurologic examinations are normal. The patient's sleep study data are as follows:

Polysomnographic data	**Baseline data**
Total recording time, 431 min	Total apnea-hypopnea index (AHI), 26.0 events/h
Total sleep time, 288 min	Supine AHI, 45.2 events/h
Sleep efficiency, 67%	Nonsupine AHI, 3.5 events/h
Sleep latency, 58 min	Nonrapid eye movement AHI, 25.1 events/h
	Rapid eye movement AHI, 32.0 events/h Periodic limb movement index, 4.9 events/h Lowest oxygen desaturation, 86%
CPAP titration data Pressure (cm H_2O), AHI (events/h): 5, 18.2/h; 7, 11.7/h; 11, 3.2/h	

The patient reports that he was unable to tolerate the prescribed continuous positive airway pressure and is not interested in using this device in the future. A surgeon he previously consulted suggested that he is not a good candidate for uvulopalatopharyngoplasty, given his upper airway anatomy. What is the most appropriate recommendation at this time?

A. Positional therapy with avoidance of a supine sleep position.
B. Increase the dose of his selective serotonin reuptake inhibitor.
C. Referral to a dental sleep specialist for a mandibular advancer.
D. Prescribe nocturnal oxygen supplementation at 2 L/min via nasal cannula.

71. A 45-year-old married man presents to the ED with cough and dyspnea. He had a recent flu-like illness followed by sudden onset of fever, weakness, and worsening cough. He has a 10 pack-year smoking history and has type 2 diabetes mellitus controlled with oral hypoglycemic agents. The pulse was 100/min, respiratory rate was 24/min, BP was 150/80 mm Hg, temperature was 38.5°C, and Sao_2 was 93%. The chest examination indicates left-sided crackles. Laboratory investigations indicate a WBC count of 13,800/µL (13.8×10^9/L) with a left shift and BUN of 11.8 mg/dL (4.2 mmol/L). Posteroanterior and lateral chest radiographs are shown in Figures 71-A and 71-B. You are asked to see the patient in consultation for further management. Based on this patient's level of illness, you should do which of the following?

A. Admit the patient to the hospital and initiate antibiotic therapy.
B. Start antibiotic therapy in the ED and send the patient home with appropriate follow-up.
C. Arrange a chest CT scan.
D. Obtain sputum culture and blood culture, and base a therapeutic decision on the results.

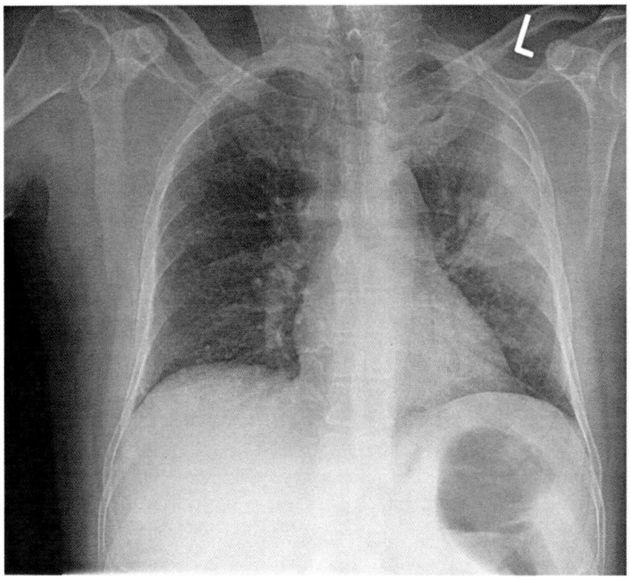

Figure 71-A

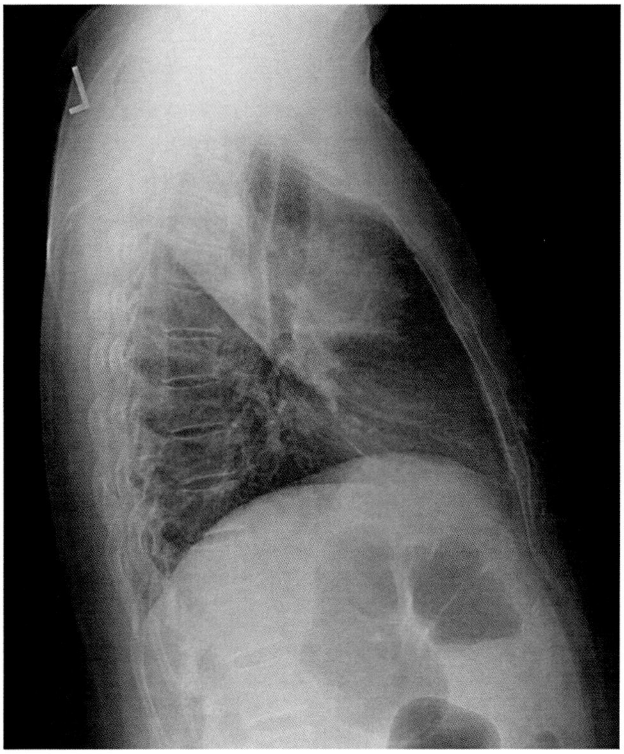
Figure 71-B

72. Figure 72-A is a thoracic ultrasound image taken with the transducer in the midaxillary line in a longitudinal plane, with the head of the patient at the left of the figure. What does it show?

A. Lung mass.
B. Pleural effusion.
C. Pleural effusion with ascites.
D. Complex septated pleural effusion.

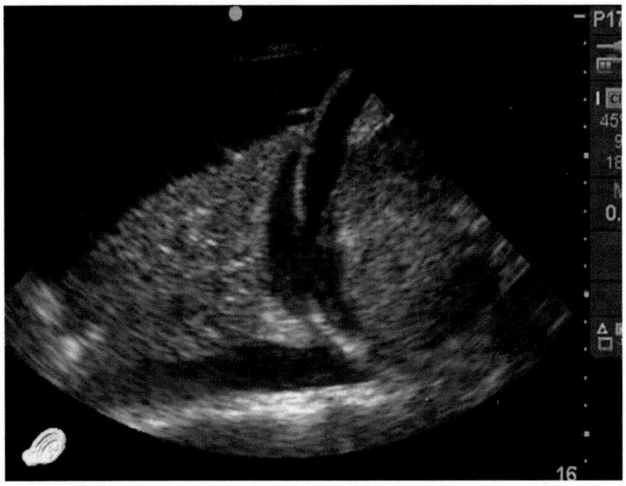

Figure 72-A

73. A 72-year-old man was referred for assessment of dyspnea. He had smoked a pack of cigarettes daily for 25 years but stopped 20 years earlier. He owned his own construction company and had been exposed to asbestos during the course of his working career. He had been well until he was the driver of a car involved in a motor vehicle accident 2 years ago. He suffered a severe head injury with a depressed fractured skull and loss of consciousness, multiple right-sided rib injuries, a lung contusion, and a dislocated jaw. He required neurosurgical intervention, but the chest wall injuries resolved spontaneously, and no chest tubes were placed. Since that time, he has complained of intermittent right-sided chest discomfort and exertional dyspnea. He can walk one or two blocks on a level plain before having to stop and catch his breath. Prior to the accident, he was quite active. He denied cough, sputum production, or hemoptysis. Physical examination indicated indrawing of the right chest with inspiration. There was poor air entry bilaterally. Pulmonary function studies indicated moderate airflow obstruction (FEV_1 of 58% predicted), hyperinflation (total lung capacity, 134% predicted), and air trapping but normal lung diffusion. A chest radiograph is shown in Figure 73-A. At this point, what would you arrange?

A. Pulmonary exercise study.
B. Thoracic surgery consultation.
C. CT angiogram.
D. Methacholine challenge study.

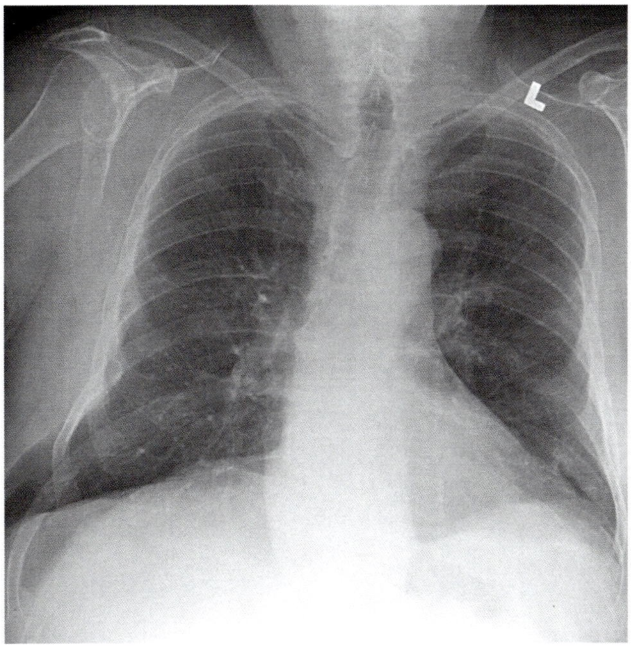

Figure 73-A

74. A 27-year-old man with cystic fibrosis undergoes bilateral lung transplantation and is discharged from the hospital. His discharge medications include trimethoprim-sulfamethoxazole three times weekly, valganciclovir daily, cyclosporine twice daily, prednisone daily, azathioprine daily, cotazyme with meals, hydromorphine orally three times daily and 4 to 6 mg po q3h prn, and domperidone with meals. He returns for a follow-up visit 3 months later and undergoes transbronchial biopsies to monitor for rejection (see Figures 74-A and 74-B). He is asymptomatic from a respiratory standpoint, although he still complains of postoperative sternotomy pain. His physical examination is unremarkable. Results of his chest radiograph and CBC are normal. Spirometry is unchanged from 2 months previously and shows no airflow obstruction.

What would you recommend based on the transbronchial biopsy results?

A. Increasing the dose of antirejection medications.
B. Consideration of fundoplication to prevent aspiration.
C. Referral for counseling.
D. Addition of broad-spectrum antibiotics.

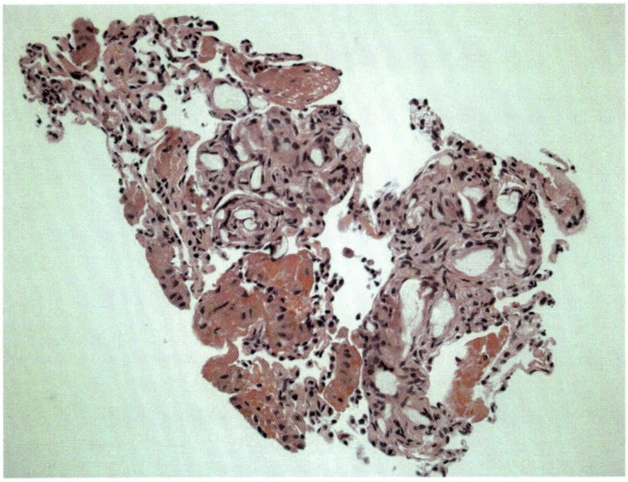

Figure 74-A
Hematoxylin-eosin

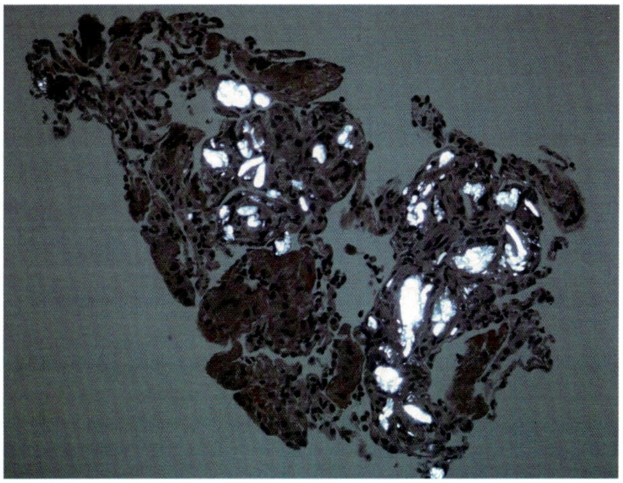

Figure 74-B
Hematoxylin-eosin

75. A 44-year-old man is intubated due to a lorazepam overdose. The patient's past medical history is significant for AIDS diagnosed 1 year earlier; the patient is nonadherent with his antiretroviral therapy. He also has a history of hepatitis C and latent syphilis. You are consulted because of new chest radiographic changes (see Figure 75-A) compared with a radiograph 2 months earlier. Sputum staining for acid-fast bacilli (AFB) and fungi is negative in triplicate. Bronchoscopy with BAL and bronchial washings are negative for AFB and fungi. Culture results from the sputum and bronchoscopy samples are pending. Because of pancytopenia, a bone marrow biopsy is performed (see Figure 75-B).

Which of the following statements about the patient's disease is correct?

A. CD4 count is likely > 300 cells/μL (> 0.30×10^9/L).
B. Blood culture results are rarely diagnostic.
C. Transbronchial biopsies aid diagnosis in > 50% of cases.
D. Skin testing specific to the disease is frequently positive.

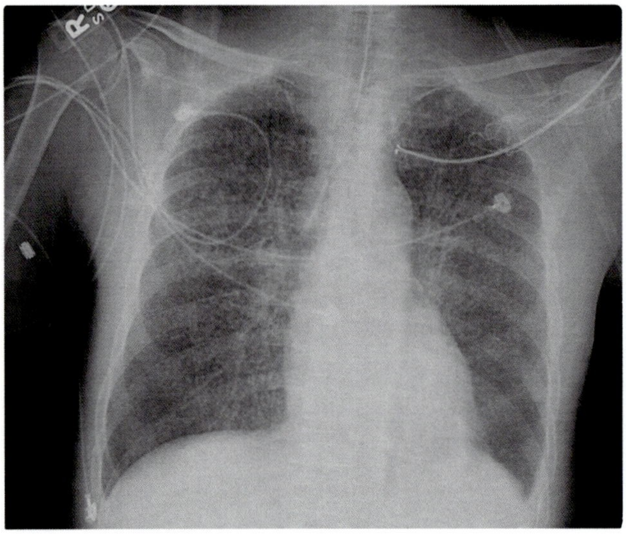

Figure 75-A

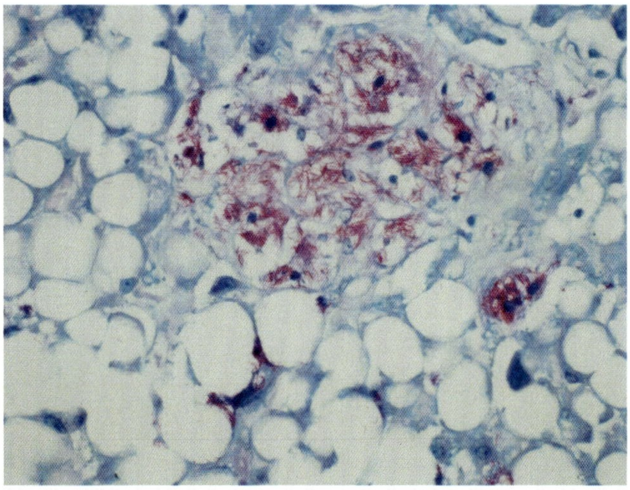

Figure 75-B
Ziehl-Nielsen

76. A 54-year-old woman (BMI of 38 kg/m^2) complains of daytime sleepiness that has been present for 10 years. She snores, and her husband has witnessed her "stop breathing" during sleep. Her Epworth sleepiness scale score was 16 (normal < 8). An overnight polysomnogram shows evidence of obstructive sleep apnea, with an apnea-hypopnea index of 36 and associated oxygen desaturation to a low of 54% during rapid eye movement (REM) sleep. Continuous positive airway pressure (CPAP) is adequately titrated in the sleep laboratory. Eight weeks later, she feels better but still complains of daytime sleepiness that affects her daytime functioning. Her Epworth sleepiness scale score is now 12. She is using CPAP every night for ≥ 6 h. This is documented objectively by the download from her machine. A follow-up polysomnogram while using CPAP at 10 cm H_2O pressure support is performed. She slept for 7 h during this study. An apnea-hypopnea index of 4 is noted. Results of a urine drug screen are normal. The day following this CPAP study, a multiple sleep latency test (MSLT) is performed, and the results are shown in Table 76-1.

Table 76-1. Results of MSLT

	Sleep Latency, min	REM Sleep During Nap
Nap 1	7	No
Nap 2	6	No
Nap 3	5	No
Nap 4	4	No
Nap 5	5	No

What intervention should be done next?

A. Prescribe modafinil.
B. Prescribe methylphenidate.
C. Titrate with bilevel positive airway pressure.
D. Refer for an oral appliance.

77. A 64-year-old woman with bladder carcinoma complains of shortness of breath and chest pressure during a follow-up visit with her primary care physician. These symptoms have been present for 48 h, and she describes the chest tightness as nonradiating, right-sided in location, and not associated with diaphoresis or nausea. A review of systems was significant for anorexia and a 10-lb weight loss over 2 months and orthostasis over the past 2 to 3 weeks. She underwent radical cystectomy for bladder carcinoma 6 months prior to her symptoms.

Physical examination reveals her to be afebrile with a pulse of 111 beats/min, a BP of 112/69 mm Hg, and a respiratory rate of 18/min. Room air oxygen saturation is 91% at rest but decreases to 78% with ambulation of 50 feet. Jugular venous distention is present to the level of the mandible. The precordium is hyperdynamic, but no murmurs, rubs, or adventitious heart sounds are detected. Through auscultation, it is determined that the lung fields are clear. Hepatojugular reflux and lower extremity edema are not present.

Laboratory studies were notable for a d-dimer of 4.2 µg/mL (22.9 nmol/L) and a brain naturetic peptide of 1,230 pg/mL (1,230 ng/L). An ECG was obtained (see Figure 77-A), and results were abnormal. Serial assessments of troponin did not reveal myocardial injury. A chest radiograph suggested prominent pulmonary vascular marking and fullness of the aortopulmonary window (see Figure 77-B). CT angiography, lower extremity ultrasonography, and a pulmonary angiogram were performed but did not reveal any abnormalities suggestive of thromboembolic disease. Transthoracic echocardiography revealed a moderately enlarged right ventricle that was hypokinetic with septal bowing. Early transit of contrast within the left atrium suggested an intraatrial shunt. Over the next 2 days, she experienced progressive hypoxemia and died secondary to a pulseless electrical activity cardiac arrest. What diagnostic study could have been performed to confirm a diagnosis before she died?

A. Testing for HIV.
B. Coronary angiography.
C. Ventilation/perfusion scintigraphy.
D. Pulmonary artery balloon catheter occlusion and aspiration for cytologic examination.

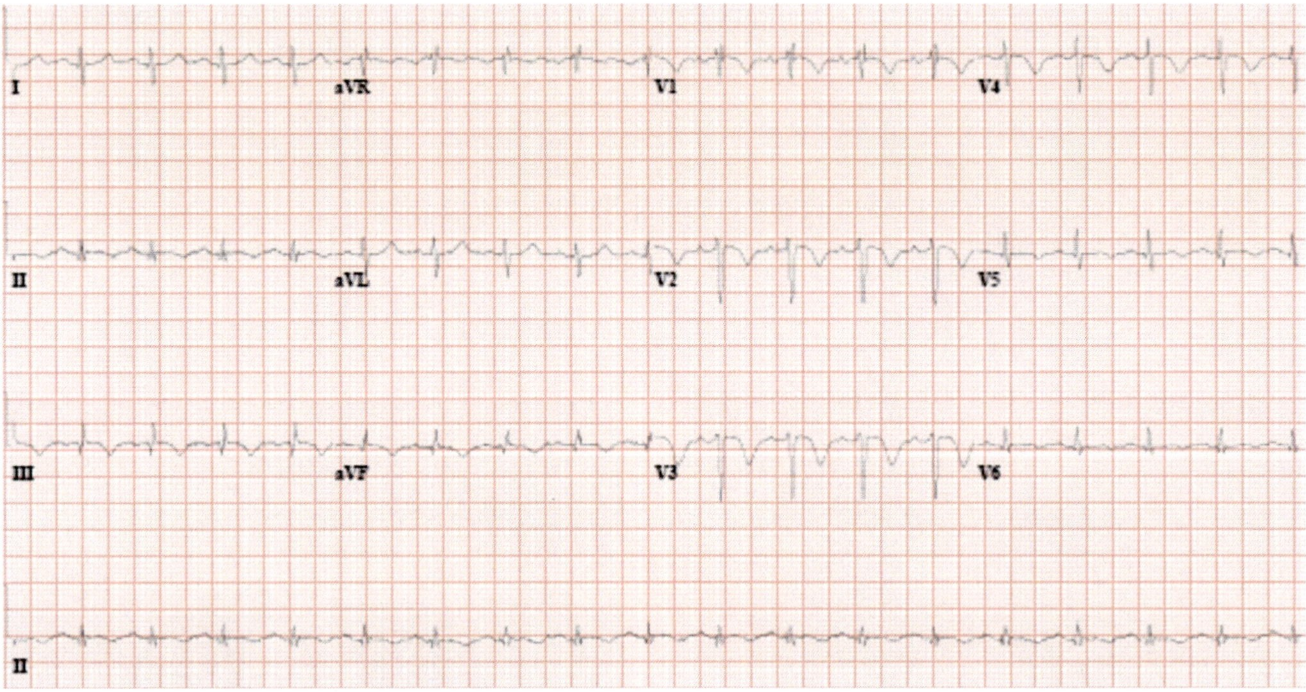

Figure 77-A

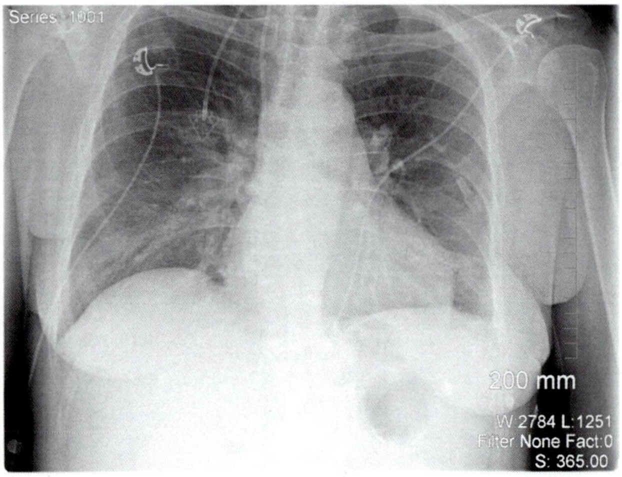

Figure 77-B

78. A 52-year-old woman is being evaluated for recurrent hemoptysis. She is a lifelong nonsmoker with no history of TB or other lung infections. She has never been hospitalized and has no known chronic medical conditions. For 6 months, she has experienced a number of episodes of sudden expectoration of a teaspoon or less of blood, which was not heralded or accompanied by other symptoms. She did not seek care until 6 weeks ago when she suddenly began coughing up large amounts of frank blood, and she was admitted to a local hospital. Flexible bronchoscopy was performed urgently, and the bleeding was noted to be arising from the left lung, but no airway abnormality was noted within the left mainstem bronchus. Other visualization was limited. The bleeding abated spontaneously. A chest radiograph at this time (see Figure 78-A, arrows) revealed calcified granulomas in the left lower lobe and calcified hilar lymph nodes. The estimated blood loss was 300 mL over 24 h.

When her condition stabilized, pulmonary function tests were performed and revealed an FEV_1, FVC, and DLCO > 90% of predicted. A chest CT with contrast was done (see Figure 78-B, arrow), which revealed a bronchiectactic airway in the left lung with an intraluminal calcified mass. There was no evidence of pulmonary embolus.

Prior to your evaluation, the patient has another episode of hemoptysis of at least 700 mL over 24 h, and once again, the bleeding spontaneously resolves. The results of laboratory testing reveal normal coagulation parameters.

The most appropriate recommendation for treatment at this point is:

A. Repeat bronchoscopy with instillation of amphotericin in the involved airway segment.
B. Refer for surgical resection.
C. Systemic treatment with itraconazole for 3 months.
D. Rigid bronchoscopy.

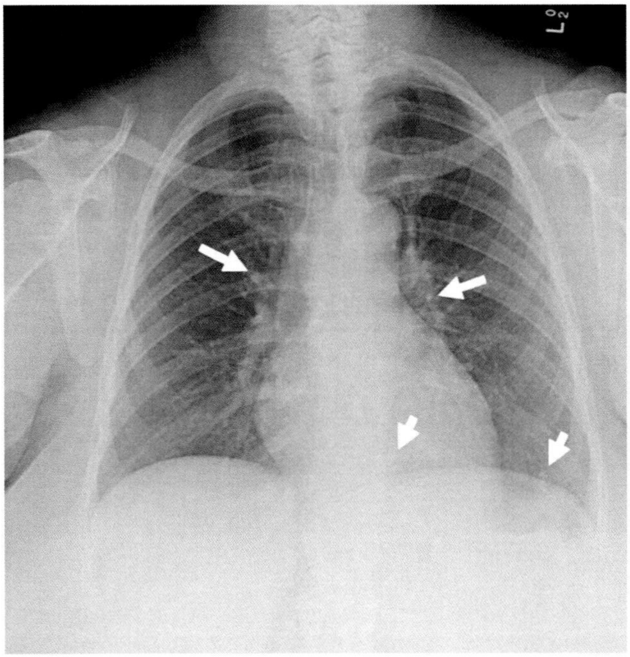

Figure 78-A

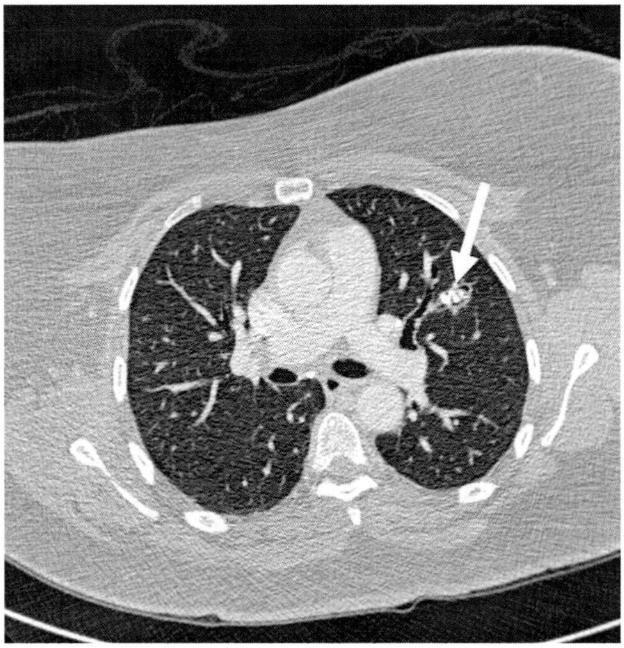

Figure 78-B

79. Which of the following is a consequence of sleep deprivation (SD)?

A. Increase in serum levels of leptin and decrease in ghrelin.
B. Hypoactive gag and deep tendon reflexes.
C. Decreased febrile response to endotoxin and antibody titers to influenza vaccination.
D. Increase in growth hormone secretion and prolactin.

80. A 54-year-old man underwent a right single-lung transplant for COPD 3 years ago. His initial postoperative course was uncomplicated. He was cytomegalovirus (CMV)-negative prior to the transplant and received a graft from a CMV-positive donor. He had an episode of acute rejection at 4 months after transplantation. He has had gradual onset of shortness of breath and progressive dyspnea on exertion. His current medications include prednisone, mycophenolate mofetil, tacrolimus, valganciclovir, and trimethoprim-sulfamethoxazole. The results of a lung examination reveal clear breath sounds on the right and decreased breath sounds on the left. His best posttransplant baseline pulmonary function test (PFT) results were FEV_1 of 1.9 L and FVC of 2.4 L, and his current PFT results are FEV_1 of 1.4 L and FVC of 2.3 L. His chest radiograph (see Figure 80-A) is unchanged from baseline. The laboratory examination is unremarkable, and his tacrolimus level is 9 ng/mL (therapeutic level = 8 to 12 ng/mL). The patient undergoes bronchoscopy with transbronchial biopsy. The histologic findings are shown in Figure 80-B. The most likely diagnosis for this patient is:

A. Acute rejection.
B. CMV pneumonia.
C. Drug toxicity.
D. Bronchiolitis obliterans (BO).

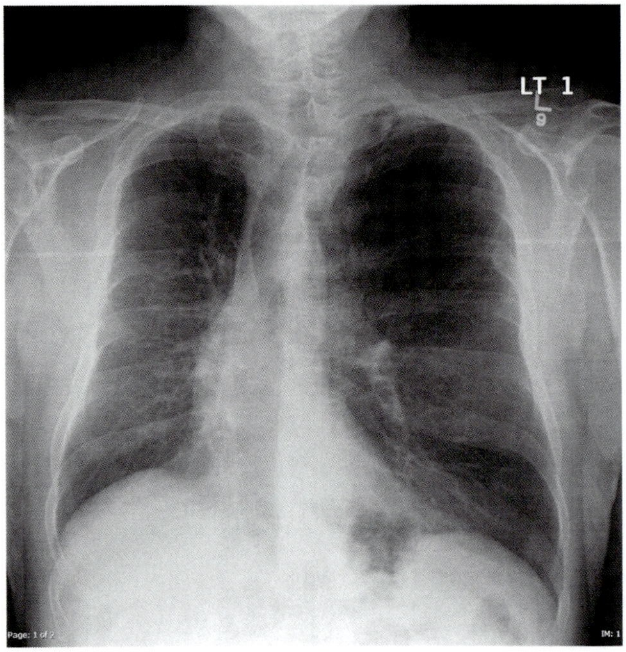

Figure 80-A

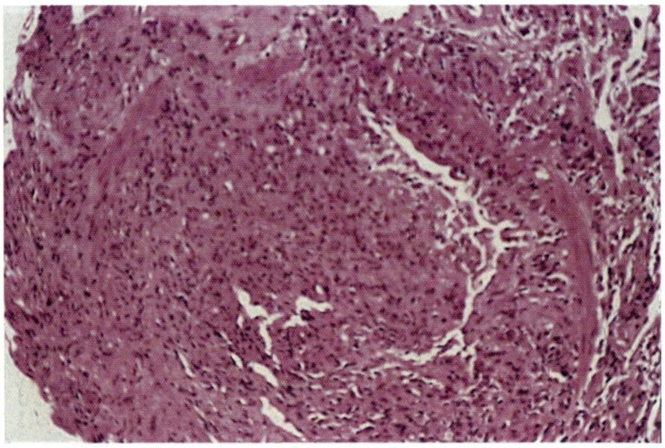

Figure 80-B
Hematoxylin-eosin

81. A 58-year-old patient with ARDS is supported by volume assist-control ventilation. She is receiving a tidal volume of 6 mL/kg ideal body weight, an FIO_2 of 0.7, and a PEEP of 5 cm H_2O. Her arterial blood gas levels are acceptable, and plateau pressure is 25 cm H_2O. In an effort to reduce FIO_2 exposure, you increase PEEP to 12 cm H_2O. This improves her oxygenation and allows a reduction in FIO_2.

Based on several large randomized clinical trials, this change will also:

A. Reduce plateau pressures and improve mortality.
B. Reduce plateau pressures and not affect mortality.
C. Increase plateau pressures and improve mortality.
D. Increase plateau pressures and not affect mortality.

82. A 71-year-old woman with type 2 diabetes mellitus was admitted to the hospital for community-acquired pneumonia 3 days ago with fever, productive cough, listlessness, and consolidation of the right middle lobe. Cultures and Gram stain of sputum and blood culture results were negative.

She has been treated with IV ceftriaxone and azithromycin and has improved clinically. Her normal alertness has returned, glycemic control is adequate, and she is eating and drinking normally. Her fever curve is improving (she has been afebrile for approximately 28 h), and her physical examination findings are notable for a heart rate of 84/min, respiratory rate of 20/min, BP of 128/86 mm Hg, and room air oxygen saturation of 93%. Auscultation of the lateral segment of the right middle lobe reveals crackles, bronchial breath sounds, and egophony, all slightly improved since admission.

Her chest radiograph shows no change in the opacification of the right middle lobe that was noted on her admission film, and her WBC count has decreased from 19,700/µL (19.7×10^9/L) with 6% band forms on admission to 13,500/µL (13.5×10^9/L) without band forms. She lives with her daughter and her daughter's family, who are eager for her to return home and who can assist with her care.

How should her pneumonia be managed at this point?

A. Inpatient IV antibiotics for ≥7 days.
B. Start an oral antibiotic and overlap with the IV antibiotic for 24 h and then discharge if she is stable.
C. Switch to an oral antibiotic and discharge now.
D. Switch to an oral antibiotic now, observe for 24 to 48 h, and discharge if she is stable.

83. You are asked to assess a 48-year-old obstetrical nurse in the ED because of possible TB. She is currently on vacation, has not worked for the past 2 weeks, and has a 3-day history of cough and fever (up to 38.9°C). For the past 24 h, her cough has become productive of very small amounts of yellow-green sputum. There is no hemoptysis. She is a lifetime nonsmoker, consumes one to two drinks of alcohol per week, and has been otherwise healthy. She denies any weight loss, rash, arthralgias, visual disturbances, hematuria, loss of consciousness, or chest pain and has no known drug allergies. She lives with her husband and four children aged 8 to 16 years, and they are currently asymptomatic. Her employment-screening tuberculin skin test result 1 year ago was 0 mm. She has never traveled or worked outside the United States and has had no known recent contact with patients who have TB. Physical examination findings are as follows: temperature of 38.6°C, respiratory rate of 14/min, pulse rate of 92/min, BP of 125/76 mm Hg, and oxygen saturation of 97% while breathing room air. The remainder of the examination is notable for decreased breath sounds and crackles over the right superior chest at the back. Her CBC results are normal except for a WBC count of 11,500/µL (11.5×10^9/L) with a left shift. She is unable to produce sputum for culture and sensitivity tests or for an acid-fast bacilli smear and culture. A chest radiograph was obtained (see Figures 83-A and 83-B). The referring ED physician thinks she might have TB.

In addition to a tuberculin skin test, how would you manage this patient's treatment?

A. Begin therapy with clarithromycin for 1 week, discharge from the ED, and arrange a follow-up visit in 1 week.
B. Initiate respiratory isolation and begin therapy with isoniazid, rifampin, pyrazinamide, and ethambutol.
C. Initiate respiratory isolation and withhold antituberculous therapy pending further results.
D. Initiate respiratory isolation and arrange for bronchoscopy first thing in the morning.

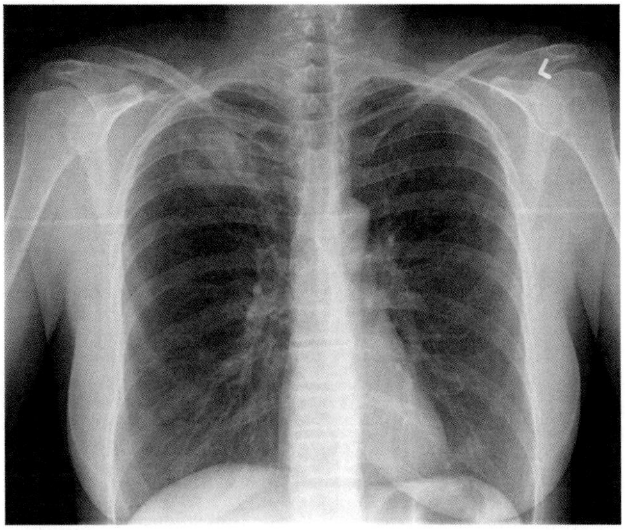

Figure 83-A

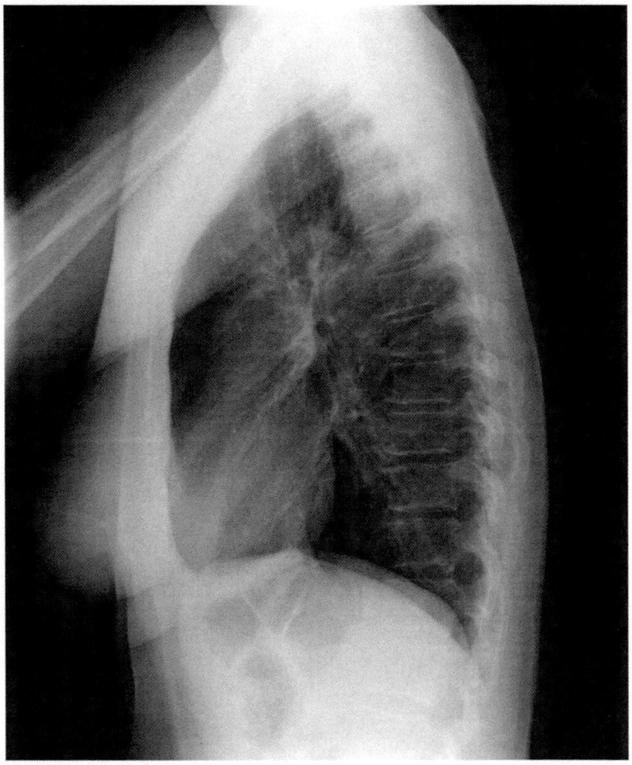

Figure 83-B

84. A 45-year-old man has a 2-day history of headache, fever, and generalized weakness. He also complains of mild shortness of breath and right-sided pleuritic chest pain. He underwent a cadaveric kidney transplant 5 years ago. His medications include 5 mg of tacrolimus twice a day and 10 mg of prednisone daily. On neurologic examination, he is confused and incoherent. Cranial nerves are normal. The results of a strength examination reveal an inability to overcome minimal resistance that is more prominent on the right side. Deep tendon reflexes are exaggerated. Pulmonary examination findings reveal decreased breath sounds and egophany in the right lower lung field. Chest radiograph shows a right lower lobe peripheral consolidation with cavitation. MRI of the brain with the administration of gadolinium shows multiple enhancing lesions in both cerebral hemispheres. Lumbar puncture is performed and reveals 1,100 nucleated cells/µL, with 88% neutrophils; a protein level of 212 mg/dL; and a glucose level of 47 mg/dL (2.6 mmol/L). Bronchoscopy with BAL and a transbronchial biopsy are performed. A smear of the lung tissue is shown (see Figure 84-A).

The next step in the management of this patient is to begin therapy with:

A. Isoniazid, rifampin, ethambutol, and pyrazinamide.
B. Penicillin.
C. Trimethoprim-sulfamethoxazole.
D. Pyrimethamine and sulfadiazine.

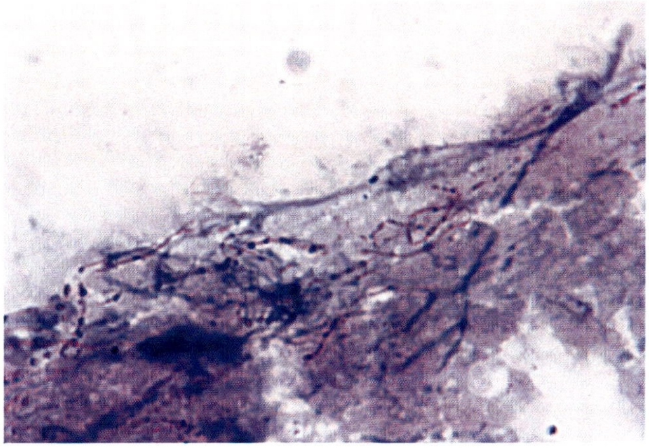

Figure 84-A
Modified Kinyoun acid-fast

85. Which of the following is true regarding nonmassive pleural effusions in patients supported by mechanical ventilation who have been in the medical ICU for longer than 24 h?

A. A majority are benign and do not impact mortality.
B. More than 80% develop during the patient's ICU stay.
C. A thoracentesis will improve pulmonary resistance and compliance for patients receiving mechanical ventilation.
D. Mechanical ventilation with a larger tidal volume (> 8 mL/kg) is more likely to lead to an effusion when compared with lower tidal volume ventilation (< 6 mL/kg).

86. A 59-year-old man complains of cough, hoarseness, and increasing wheezing. These symptoms had been present for 6 months but have been progressing recently. Two days ago, he coughed up a small amount of blood. He had a history of asthma dating back to childhood, but over the past few years, his disease had been very well controlled with fluticasone, 250 µg bid, and an occasional puff of albuterol (salbutamol). He is a nonsmoker, claims to be compliant with his medications, and has no other medical problems aside from occasional heartburn, for which he takes over-the-counter medications.

Physical examination reveals a well-nourished man breathing comfortably at 16/min, with no use of accessory muscles. He has dysphonia without stridor, and there is no evidence for oral candidiasis or nasal polyps. Chest, cardiac, and abdominal examinations are unremarkable.

Spirometry reveals FEV_1 of 3.10 L (90% of predicted), FVC of 4.24 L (97% of predicted), and FEV_1/FVC of 0.73. The inspiratory loop is normal. A chest radiograph is normal. Because of the new complaint of hemoptysis, a bronchoscopy is performed revealing the abnormality shown in Figure 86-A.

What should you do next?

A. Start treatment with a proton pump inhibitor.
B. Stop the inhaled steroid therapy.
C. Start treatment with acyclovir.
D. Arrange laser therapy of the lesions.

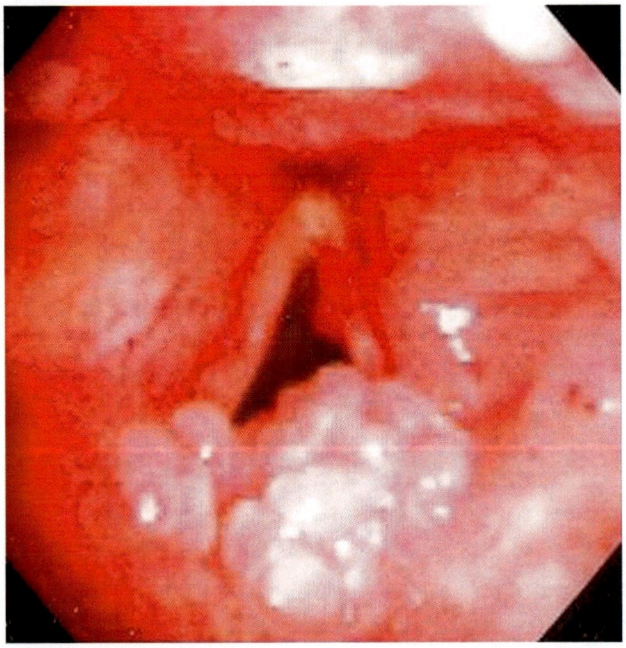

Figure 86-A

87. A 64-year-old woman is referred for evaluation of an enlarging left upper lobe nodule noted on serial chest CT scans (see Figure 87-A for a representative image). The patient smoked two packs of cigarettes per day for 25 years but stopped 5 years ago. Chronic bronchitis was diagnosed about 10 years ago, and airflow obstruction was noted 5 years ago. Her weight has been stable. Lymphadenopathy, skin nodules, neurologic abnormalities, organomegaly, and bone tenderness are not detected. The CT scan shows extensive upper lobe emphysema, with relative sparing of the lower lobes and no mediastinal lymphadenopathy. A PET scan confirms increased uptake in the lung nodule with no increased uptake elsewhere. Bronchoscopy does not reveal endobronchial abnormalities, but cytologic study of washings from the left upper lobe are interpreted as showing adenocarcinoma. CBC and liver function test results are normal. Postbronchodilator spirometry shows an FEV_1 of 0.8 L (29% of predicted). The D_{LCO} is 7.3 $mL \cdot min^{-1} \cdot mm\ Hg^{-1}$ (26% of predicted). Cycle ergometry shows a maximal exercise capacity of 23 W.

Which of the following treatments should be recommended for this patient?

A. Surgical resection with lung volume reduction surgery.
B. Radiotherapy for curative intent.
C. Radiotherapy deferred until symptoms develop.
D. Radiofrequency ablation.

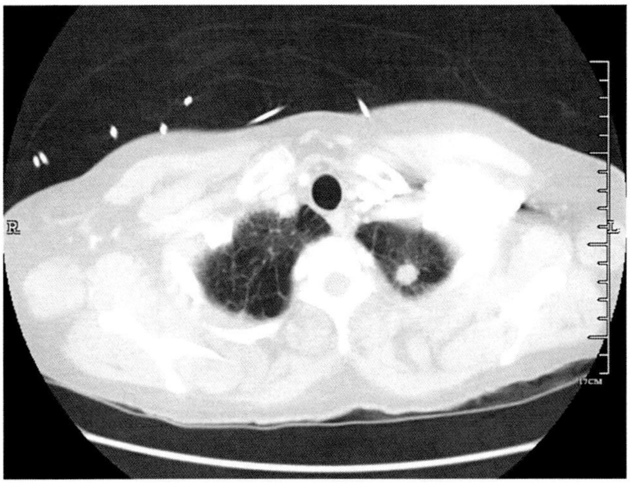

Figure 87-A

88. A 42-year-old woman is referred from the rheumatology clinic for evaluation of dyspnea on exertion. She had an unambiguous diagnosis of systemic lupus erythematosus made 8 years earlier. Since then, she has been treated with hydroxychloroquine and prednisone, the latter adjusted between 20 and 40 mg daily, titrated for intermittent symptoms of pleuritis and her serologic findings.

For the past 6 months, in addition to occasional pleurisy, she has noted progressive shortness of breath, and she is now unable to climb one flight of stairs without stopping to rest. An echocardiogram was performed that revealed a small pericardial effusion, as in the past, with no evidence of tamponade physiology and no evidence of impaired ventricular function or pulmonary hypertension. A cardiac stress test did not reveal evidence of ischemia, and a ventilation-perfusion scan did not have perfusion abnormalities. An antiphospholipid antibody panel is negative. A recent hemoglobin measurement is 10.1 g/dL (101 g/L) at baseline, and there is no elevation of serum muscle enzyme levels.

A chest radiograph shows low lung volumes and atelectasis (see Figure 88-A), and a representative image of a high-resolution CT scan of the chest is shown in Figure 88-B. Pulmonary function testing is performed and shows total lung capacity of 50% of predicted, residual volume of 72% of predicted, FEV_1 of 50% of predicted, and FVC of 39% of predicted. The DLCO is 56% of predicted, unadjusted for lung volume. The flow-volume loops indicate good effort, negative inspiratory pressure is –100 cm H_2O, and the positive expiratory pressure is 90 cm H_2O.

On examination, the patient is not obese, has normal vital signs, and has a normal cardiac examination. Lung excursion is diminished, but no abnormalities on auscultation are appreciated. There is no skin rash, and moderate small joint tenderness is present.

Which of the following would be the most appropriate assessment and recommendation to the referring physician?

A. Taper and then stop corticosteroids to treat likely steroid-induced myopathy.
B. Proceed to right heart catheterization and to endomyocardial biopsy to assess for pulmonary hypertension and cardiomyopathy producing diastolic dysfunction.
C. Assume this clinical presentation is consistent with "shrinking lung syndrome," and continue to treat with immunosuppressives, with a consideration for escalating treatment.
D. Perform coronary angiography to exclude occult disease undetected by noninvasive stress testing.

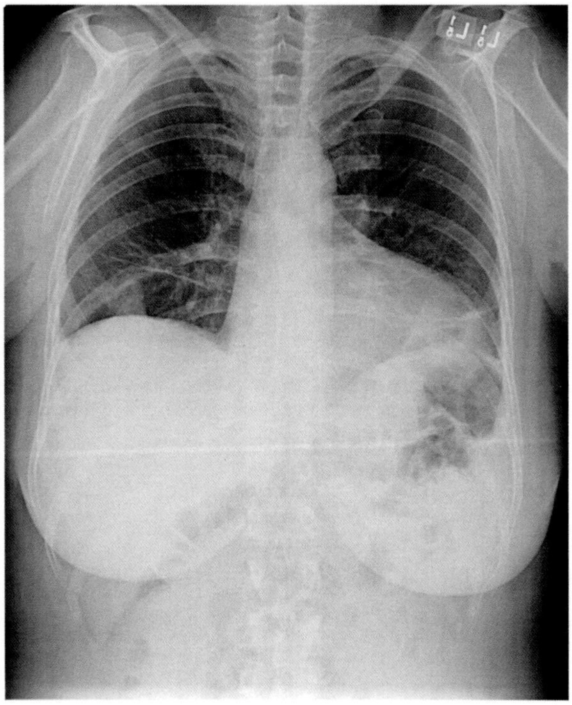

Figure 88-A

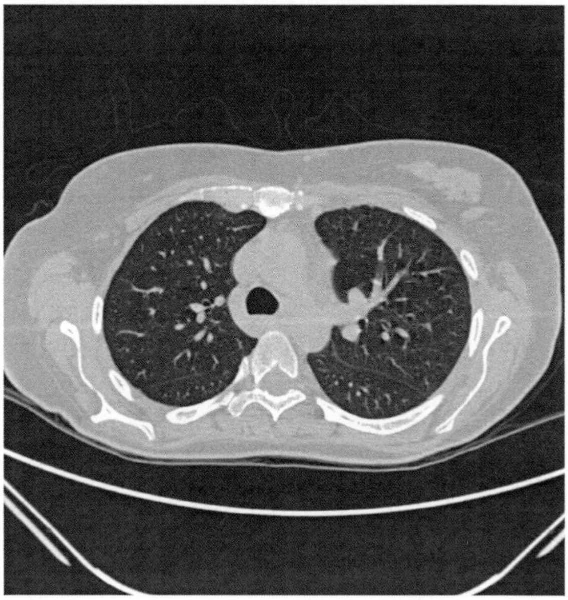

Figure 88-B

89. A 48-year-old woman with chronic asthma, chronic rhinosinus disease, aspirin sensitivity, and a past history of bilateral nasal polypectomies on three separate occasions over the past 9 years (the last time 1 year ago) complains of worsening bilateral nasal stuffiness, complete loss of sense of smell and taste, and frontal headaches. One week ago, she finished a 6-week, slowly tapering course of oral prednisone that began with 50 mg/day for 3 days. At this time, she has avoided nonsteroidal antiinflammatory drugs and takes acetaminophen 1,000 mg bid as needed for headaches, oral montelukast 10 mg/day, inhaled albuterol by metered-dose inhaler 180 μg as needed up to qid, inhaled fluticasone (250 μg)/salmeterol (50 μg) bid, and intranasal mometasone 100 μg once a day. With the exception of postnasal discharge, the physical examination is normal. Peak expiratory flow is 350 L/min. The results of nasopharyngoscopy are shown in Figure 89-A.

Which of the following recommendations has the best chance of providing the patient with long-term relief of her nasal problem?

A. Doubling the dose of intranasal mometasone.
B. Nasal polypectomy followed by aspirin desensitization and treatment.
C. Nasal polypectomy followed by complete absence of exposure to all pain medications.
D. Nasal polypectomy followed by doubling the dose of oral montelukast.

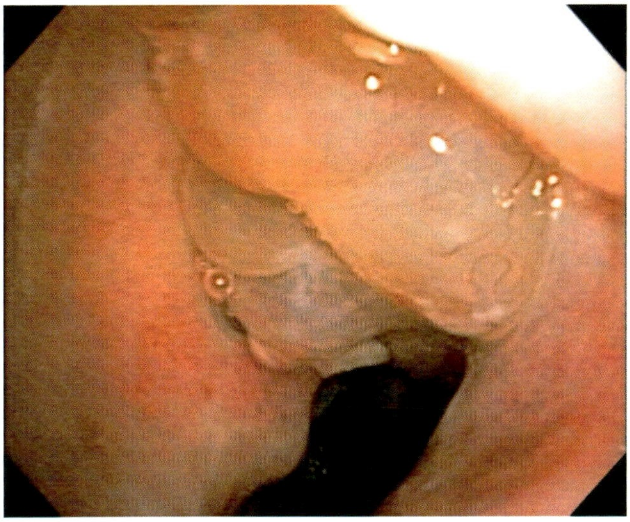

Figure 89-A

90. Which of the following images shows the most desirable anatomy for placement of a central venous catheter?

A. Figure 90-A.
B. Figure 90-B.
C. Figure 90-C.
D. Figure 90-D.

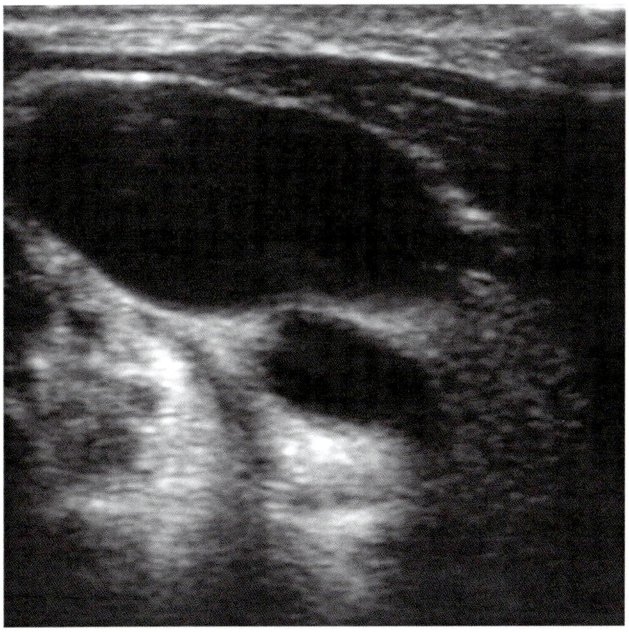

Figure 90-A

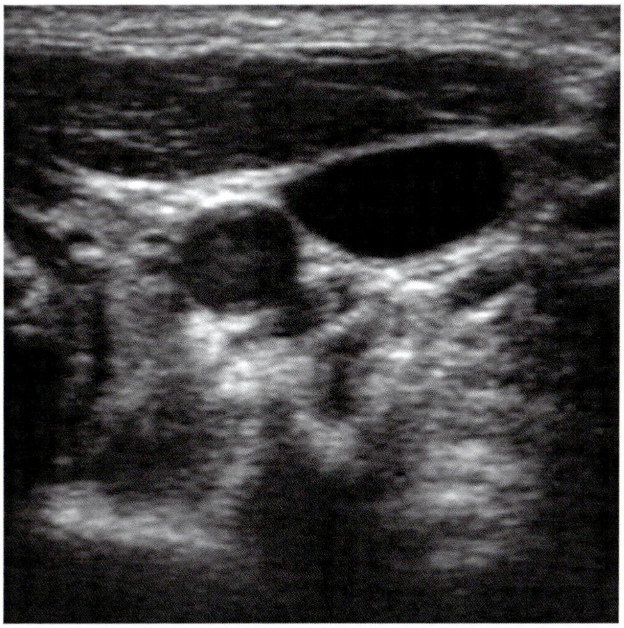

Figure 90-B

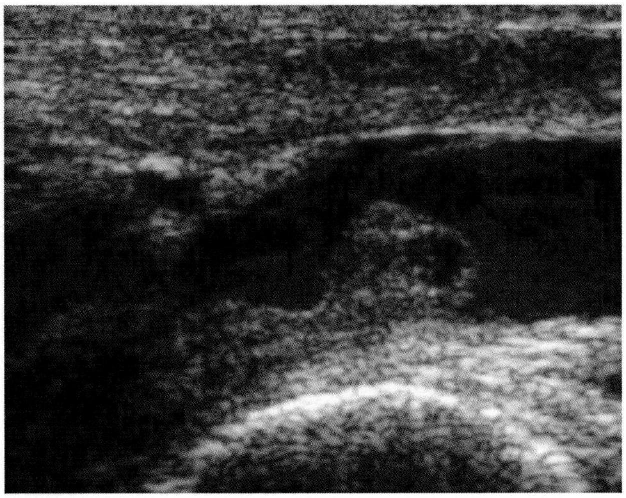

Figure 90-C

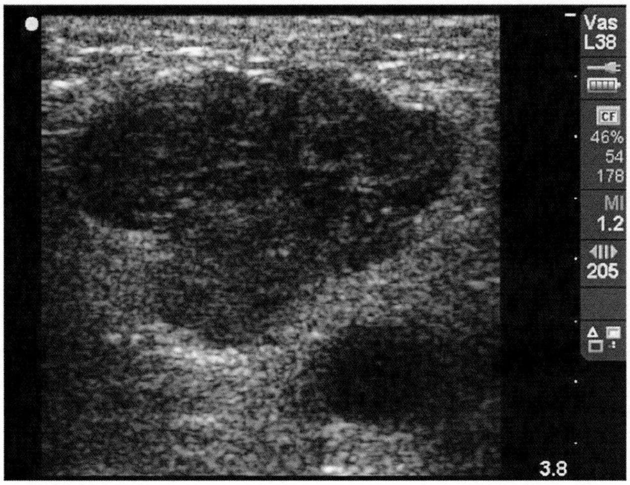

Figure 90-D

91. A 62-year-old man has had ARDS secondary to pancreatitis for the past 2 weeks. He has persistent hypoxemia despite prolonged mechanical ventilation with substantial amounts of PEEP. On an FIO_2 of 0.7 and PEEP of 20 cm H_2O, his current arterial blood gas findings indicate a PaO_2 of 58 mm Hg, $PaCO_2$ of 55 mm Hg, and pH of 7.34. You contemplate therapy using prone positioning.

With this therapy, you would anticipate:

A. Reduced ICU and hospital mortality.
B. Increased risk of ventilator-associated pneumonia.
C. Improved oxygenation.
D. Fewer pressure ulcers.

92. A 55-year-old man is referred for evaluation of an abnormal CT scan. He has a 3- to 4-year history of intermittent fevers, occurring in 4- to 6-week cycles, with temperatures as high as 39.4°C. He underwent a thorough investigation during a hospitalization for fever of unknown origin 2 years previously, and at that time, CT scans of the chest, abdomen, and pelvis were normal, and HIV testing and other infectious serologic results were negative. His family physician had recently ordered a new CT scan, and representative images are shown in Figures 92-A and 92-B. (The density seen in the right lung in Figure 92-B is the tip of the diaphragm.)

He has no traditional HIV risk factors, no significant occupational risk factors or hobbies, and is a nonsmoker. His past medical history is remarkable for Barrett esophagus and a recent diagnosis of psoriasis. His physical examination reveals psoriatic lesions on his elbows and nail pitting. His chest is clear. Bronchoscopy and BAL do not reveal any infectious pathogens, and flow cytometry reveals a normal cell profile. An open lung biopsy is performed, and the results are shown in Figures 92-C and 92-D. Figure 92-C shows a bronchiole demonstrating acute and chronic inflammation; Figure 92-D is of a bronchiole showing partial luminal obstruction by subepithelial fibrosis, consistent with a component of constrictive bronchiolitis.

The most likely cause of his abnormal CT scan is:

A. Recurrent aspiration.
B. Sarcoidosis.
C. Vasculitis.
D. Cryptogenic organizing pneumonia.

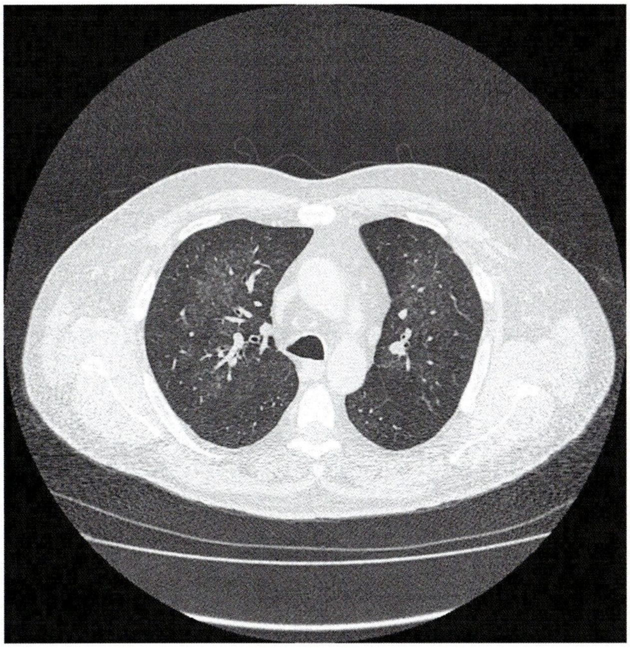

Figure 92-A

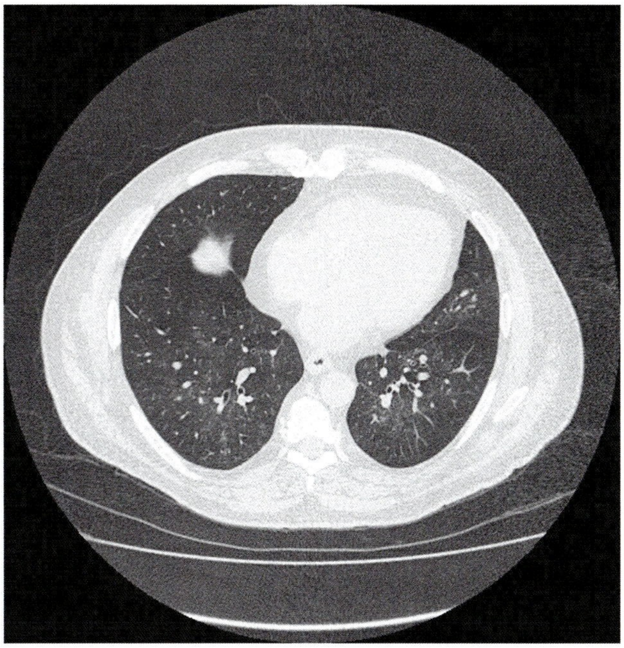

Figure 92-B

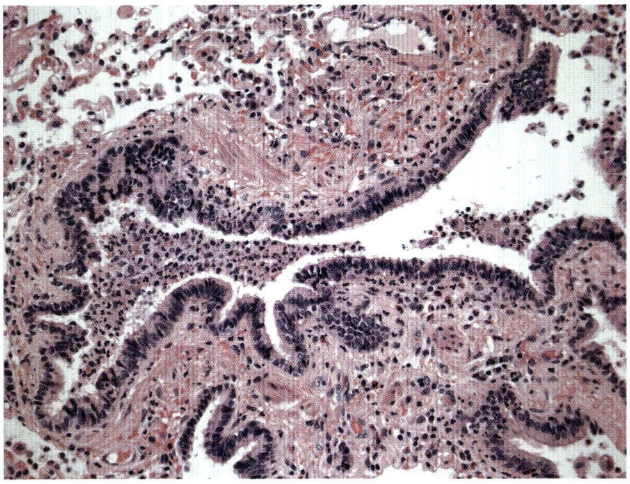

Figure 92-C
Hematoxylin-eosin

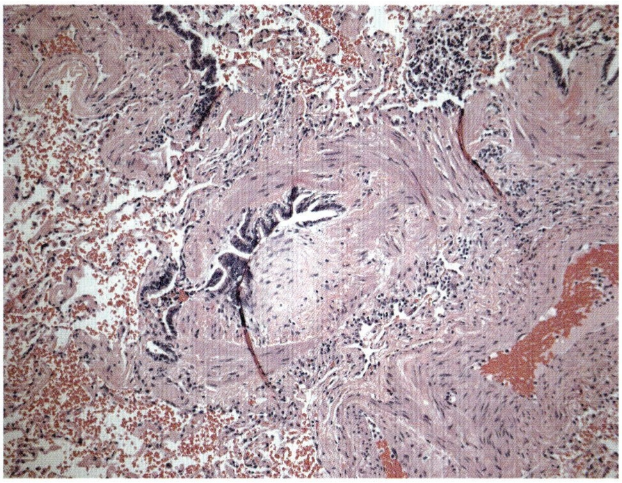

Figure 92-D
Hematoxylin-eosin

93. A 30-year-old woman with a 2-year history of breast cancer and a known prior small right-sided malignant pleural effusion is admitted because of severe dyspnea worsening over the prior 4 weeks. Her admission chest radiograph is shown (see Figure 93-A). A consultant places a chest tube (see Figure 93-B), with rapid removal of > 2.2 L of pleural fluid and a new patient complaint of mild cough. Despite the cough, the patient has initial partial relief of her dyspnea. Over the next 2 h, the patient develops more dyspnea, requiring an increase in her oxygen supplementation from 2 L/min of oxygen by nasal cannula to a nonrebreather mask with an FIO_2 of 1.0 to maintain her oxygen saturation > 90%. A repeat chest radiograph is shown (see Figure 93-C).

Which of the following factors is *most* likely associated with the cause of this patient's worsening dyspnea, declining oxygenation, and acute chest radiograph changes?

A. Patient's age.
B. Volume of fluid removed.
C. Absolute change in pleural pressure.
D. Cough development during fluid removal.

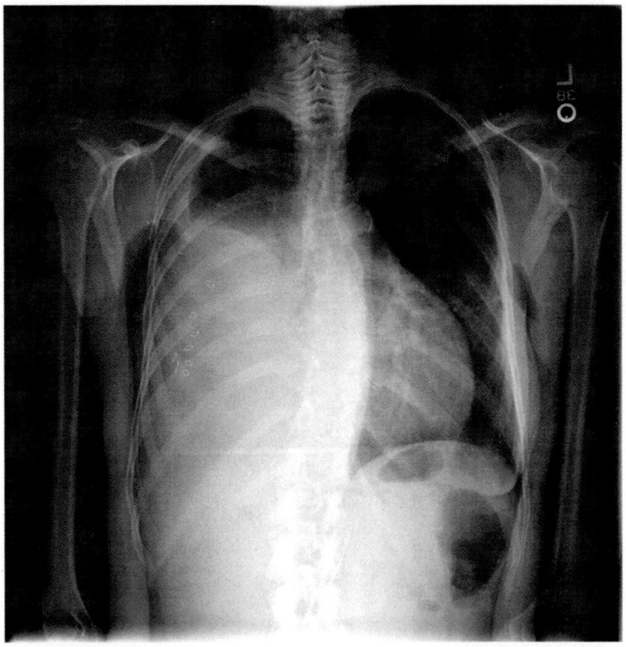

Figure 93-A

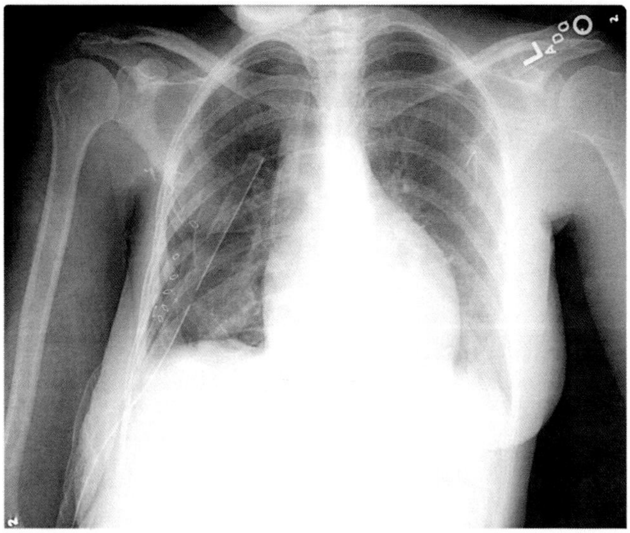

Figure 93-B

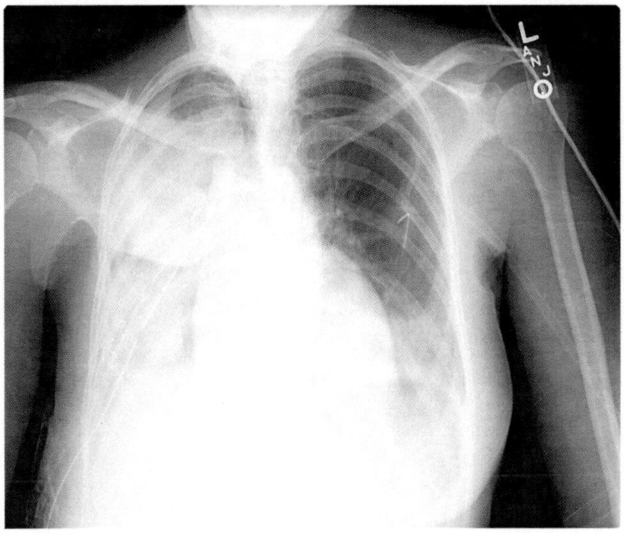

Figure 93-C

94. A 66-year-old woman is seen for evaluation 3 months after being hospitalized for acute nitrofurantoin pulmonary toxicity. She was intubated and supported by mechanical ventilation for 3 days but responded to therapy with corticosteroids and returned to her baseline activity of hiking 10 miles a day. She recently has noted progressive dyspnea on exertion, coincident with tapering of her corticosteroids. Results of a CT scan of the chest, 6-min walk test, and physical examination were normal. Spirometry was performed.

Which diagnosis is most consistent with the flow-volume loop shown in Figure 94-A?

A. Vocal cord dysfunction.
B. Restrictive lung disease from chronic nitrofurantoin lung toxicity.
C. Constrictive bronchiolitis.
D. Fixed, large airway obstruction.

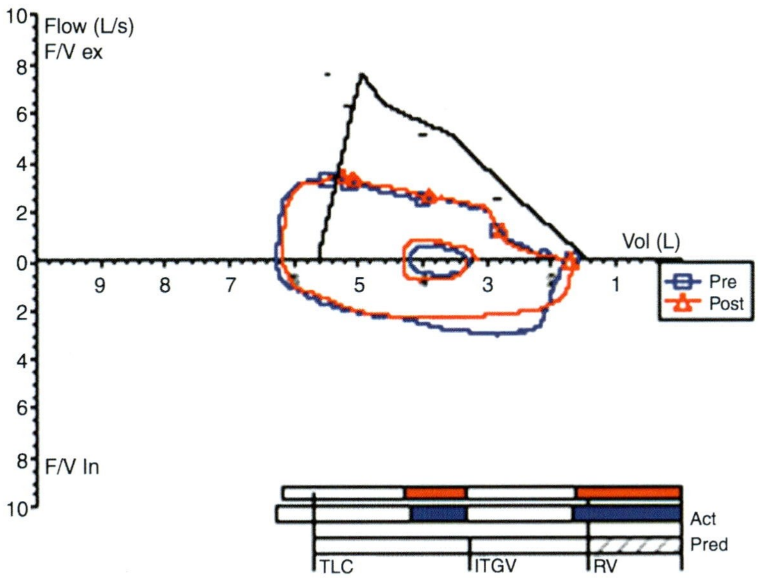

Figure 94-A

95. A 45-year-old man with ciliary dyskinesia and associated situs inversus undergoes bilateral lung transplant for severe bronchiectasis and progressive chronic ventilatory failure. The transplant surgical course goes well. The patient is discharged from the ICU on the third hospital day and from the hospital on the ninth postoperative day.

He now returns for a routine 2-week postoperative visit. He is continuing to gradually increase his activity and is pleased with the improvement in lung function he notes. His physical examination is not remarkable, and his surgical wounds appear to be healing well. A surveillance chest radiograph is obtained that shows small bilateral apical pneumothoraces (see Figure 95-A, arrows).

The patient is admitted to the hospital, and a right-sided chest tube is placed. A small but continuous air leak is present.

In light of these findings, the proper management at this point is:

A. Follow the patient clinically with chest radiographs daily until resolution.
B. Increase immunosuppressive medications.
C. Place a contralateral chest tube.
D. Perform bronchoscopy with central airway inspection.

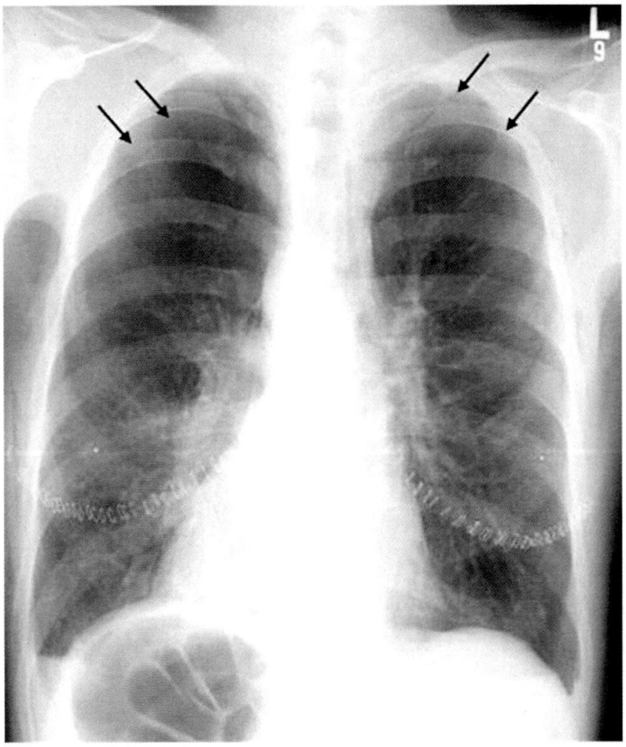

Figure 95-A

96. A 52-year-old man is referred for evaluation of an abnormal chest radiograph noted on a preemployment examination. His past medical history is negative. He does not report shortness of breath, cough, hemoptysis, weight loss, fevers, chills, or sweats. He had a purified protein derivative (PPD) test as part of the new employment evaluation, and it was nonreactive. His social history is notable for a 60 pack-year history of tobacco use, and he still smokes one or two packs of cigarettes per day. He is employed in construction. He does not recall ever having a prior chest radiograph. Physical examination and laboratory results are unremarkable. His posteroanterior chest radiograph, lateral chest radiograph, and CT are shown in Figures 96-A, 96-B, and 96-C. The remainder of the parenchyma is normal, and there is no hilar or mediastinal adenopathy.

The most likely diagnosis is:

A. Bronchogenic carcinoma.
B. Granuloma.
C. Hamartoma.
D. Lipoma.

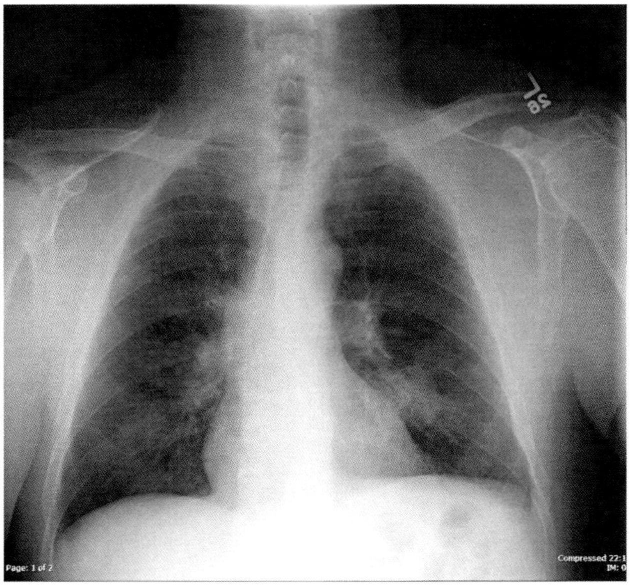

Figure 96-A

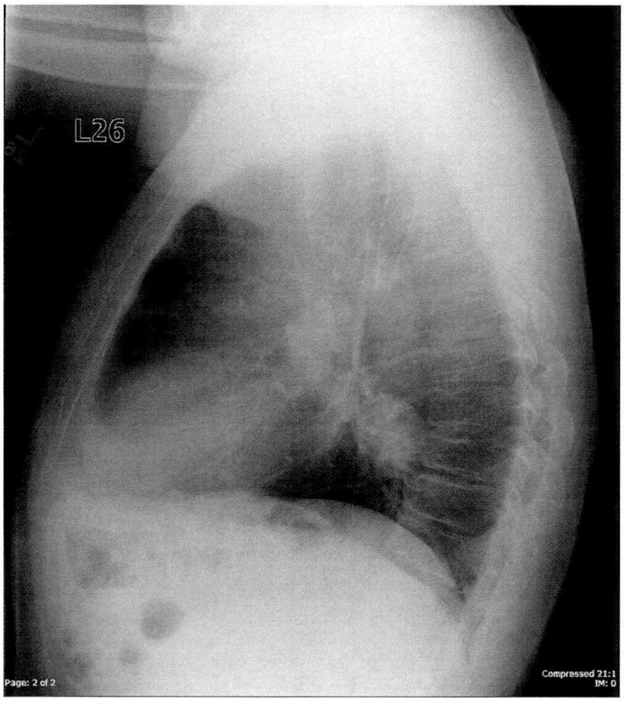

Figure 96-B

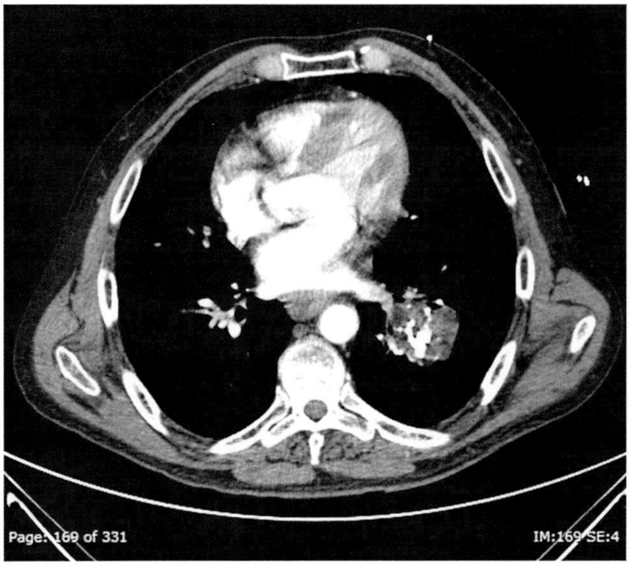

Figure 96-C

97. A 50-year-old patient with severe ARDS from sepsis is receiving pressure-assist control ventilation. An inspiratory pressure of 22 cm H_2O results in a tidal volume of 6 mL/kg ideal body weight. He requires an F_{IO_2} of 0.8 and a PEEP of 12 cm H_2O to produce a Pa_{O_2} of 57 mm Hg. You elect to try to improve gas exchange and lower the F_{IO_2} exposure by heavily sedating the patient and using a recruitment maneuver (RM) of 40 cm H_2O continuous positive airway pressure (CPAP) for 40 s. At the end of the maneuver, the Pa_{O_2} has risen to 106 mm Hg.

The duration of this improvement depends most importantly on:

A. The subsequent increase in PEEP setting.
B. The reduction in F_{IO_2} that can be done.
C. Routinely performing repeated 40-cm H_2O RMs every 3 to 6 h.
D. Immediately repeating the RM with 50 cm H_2O.

98. A 71-year-old woman is referred to you for treatment of interstitial lung disease (ILD) associated with progressive systemic sclerosis. She has had long-standing and progressive Raynaud phenomenon and gastroesophageal reflux disease and was recently evaluated by her internist and a rheumatologist who diagnosed progressive systemic sclerosis on the basis of characteristic skin thickening, esophageal changes, digital telangiectasias, and the presence of antibodies against DNA topoisomerase I (Scl-70) and RNA polymerase III.

She is referred because of dyspnea on exertion, which has been progressive over the past 6 months and which she notes is most prominent on hills or stairs. She remains independent in activities of daily living but now needs to walk more slowly than most people her age. Her only medication is benazepril, and she is a lifetime nonsmoker who denies significant industrial exposures.

Her physical examination results are notable for a respiratory rate of 18/min, room air oxygen saturation of 93%, and bibasilar inspiratory crackles without evidence of consolidation. Diffuse skin thickening is noted, along with telangiectasias that are most prominent on the distal upper extremities. No peripheral edema is present.

Spirometry is notable for a FVC of 63% predicted, without airflow obstruction. A high-resolution CT scan of the chest reveals multiple basilar predominant areas of ground-glass attenuation consistent with active alveolitis.

Which therapy is most appropriate to prescribe for her pulmonary process?

A. Azathioprine.
B. Cyclophosphamide.
C. Cyclosporine.
D. Prednisone.

99. You are asked to assess a 66-year-old retired teacher with COPD whose chief complaint is worsening activity limitation. He has a previous 45 pack-year smoking history, having quit 6 years ago when the diagnosis of COPD was first established. He feels he has done very well over the years; however, in the past 6 months he has had to stop and catch his breath after walking approximately one-half block. He denies any associated chest pain, palpitations, lightheadedness, syncope, sweating, abdominal pain, cough, or hemoptysis. He states he is otherwise in good health and denies prior COPD exacerbations. His medications are tiotropium and combination inhaled fluticasone/salmeterol, as well as salbutamol as needed. Physical examination findings are remarkable for decreased breath sounds to both lung fields. His ECG results are normal, and a chest radiograph shows only hyperinflation. Spirometry reveals an FEV_1 of 1.54 L (49% predicted), FVC of 3.91 L (85% predicted), and an FEV_1/FVC of 0.39. Cardiopulmonary exercise test results are shown in Table 99-1 and in Figures 99-A and 99-B.

Table 99-1. Cardiopulmonary Exercise Test Results*

Variable	Rest	End-Exercise	Predicted Maximum	% Predicted
Workload (W)	—	79	194	41
$\dot{V}O_2$ (L/min)	0.343	1.228	2.571	48
$\dot{V}E$ (L/min)	13.3	36.3	53.9	67
SpO_2	96	94		
HR	76	105	167	63
BP (mm Hg)	130/85	155/85		
Modified Borg: dyspnea	0	4		
Modified Borg: leg fatigue	0	5		

* $\dot{V}O_2$ = oxygen consumption; $\dot{V}E$ = expired volume per unit time; SpO_2 = oxygen saturation as measured by pulse oximetry; HR = heart rate.

There were no arrhythmias or significant ST segment or T-wave changes. The patient reported discontinuing exercise because of a combination of leg fatigue and shortness of breath.

Based on the results of the exercise test, what would you do next with this patient?

A. Arrange for a complete cardiology assessment, including an echocardiogram to assess pulmonary artery pressures.
B. Prescribe a regular exercise program or refer him to a pulmonary rehabilitation program.
C. Prescribe theophylline, checking serum levels in 1 week to ensure they are therapeutic.
D. Prescribe supplemental oxygen with exertion, as needed.

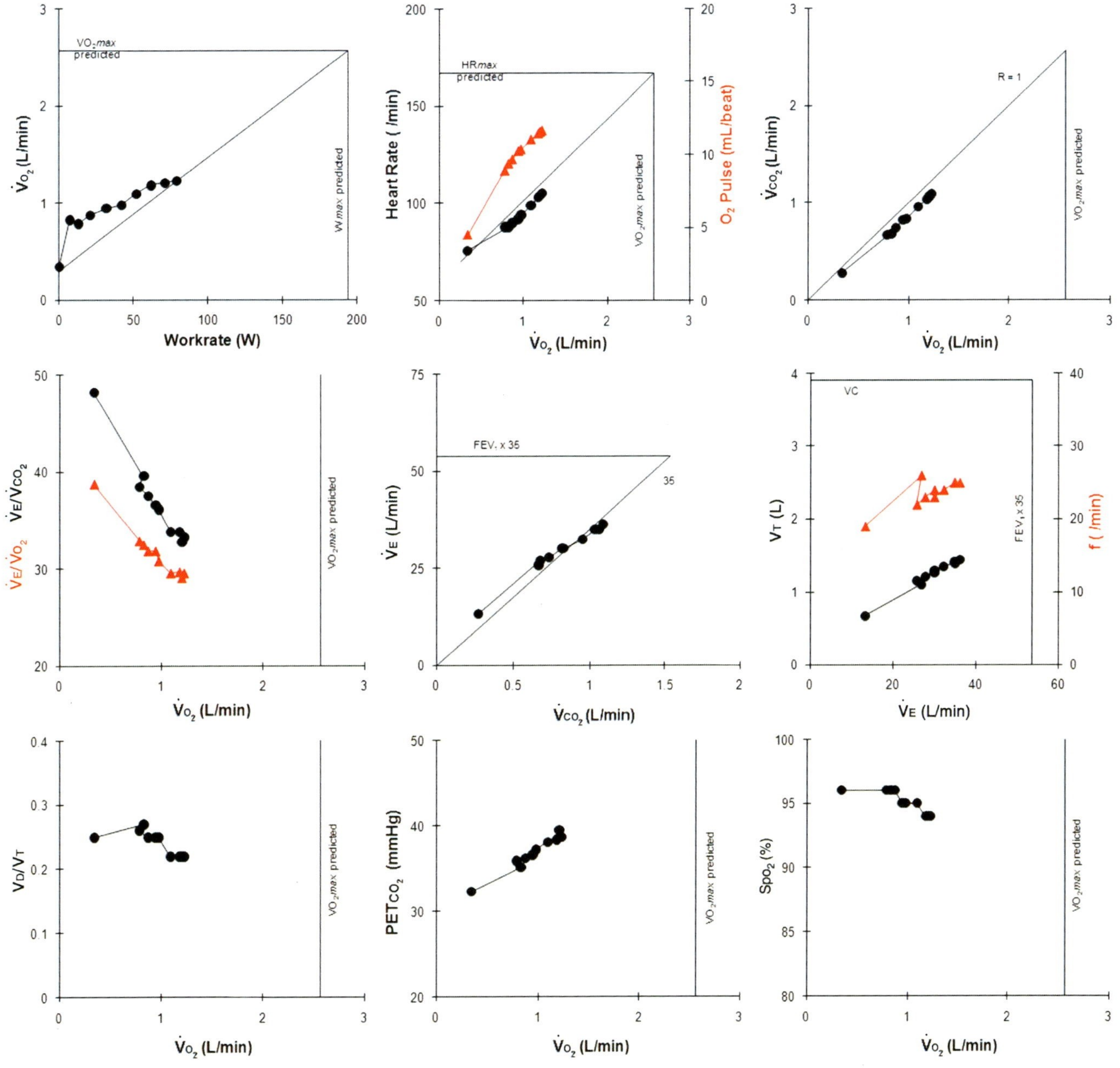

Figure 99-A

$\dot{V}o_2$ = oxygen consumption; $\dot{V}co_2$ = carbon dioxide output; HRmax = predicted maximal heart rate; $\dot{V}$E = expired volume per unit time; VT = tidal volume; f = respiratory frequency; VD/VT = dead space ventilation; $PETco_2$ = end-tidal CO_2; Spo_2 = oxygen saturation as measured by pulse oximetry.

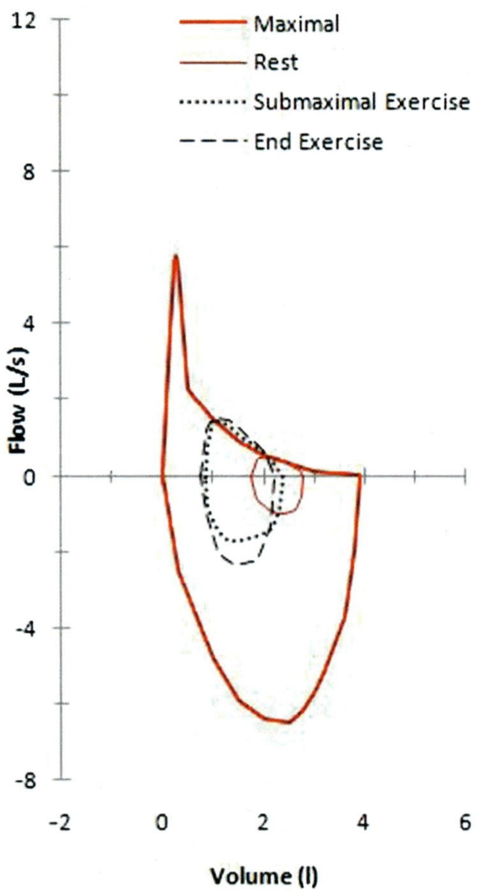

Figure 99-B

100. A 19-year-old woman with cystic fibrosis is evaluated for a several-month history of increased daily sputum production. She has not had any fevers, but does note some mild increase in her baseline level of dyspnea. Her medical regimen, in addition to home chest physiotherapy, includes inhaled bronchodilators, recombinant human deoxyribonuclease I (rhDNase I; dornase alfa), and inhaled tobramycin (secondary to documented chronic Pseudomonas infection). On physical examination, she is a thin, young woman who appears well. She is afebrile. Pulmonary examination reveals diffuse expiratory wheezing, but the remainder of her examination is unremarkable. Her spirometry today reveals moderate obstruction without a significant bronchodilator effect that is essentially unchanged from measurements done 3 months ago. At this point, you should consider adding which of the following to her medical regimen?

A. Systemic glucocorticoids.
B. Inhaled glucocorticoids.
C. Ibuprofen.
D. Azithromycin.

101. A 45-year-old teacher is admitted to the ICU with respiratory failure. He has no past medical history and was feeling well until 2 weeks prior to admission when he developed a fever, malaise, aches, and a sore throat. He did not seek medical attention but missed 3 days of school while taking ibuprofen and "some herbs." Three days prior to admission, he developed fatigue, fever, and shortness of breath. On the day of admission, his shortness of breath worsened, and he drove himself to the ED.

He has no recent travel, pets, or hobbies, and he lives alone. He does not smoke tobacco and drinks one glass of wine on the weekends. He teaches kindergarten at the local elementary school. Prior to the December holiday break, a few

of the children had impetigo, but more recently, some children have been missing from his class because of a febrile illness. None of his friends or colleagues is ill.

On arrival in the ED, he is in acute respiratory distress. His temperature is 38.8°C, pulse rate is 135/min, BP is 95/55 mm Hg, and respiratory rate is 42/min. His weight is 127 kg. His Spo_2 is 92% on room air, and he is only able to speak in one- to two-word sentences. Given his respiratory distress, he is rapidly intubated and given a single dose of ceftriaxone, 2 g, and vancomycin, 1g, IV. A chest radiograph and CT scan of his chest are shown in Figures 101-A and 101-B. His WBC count is 23,500/µL (23.5 × 10^9/L), hematocrit concentration is 31%, and platelet count is 85 × 10^3/µL (85 × 10^9/L). His serum bicarbonate concentration is 11 mEq/L (11 mmol/L), and creatinine concentration is 1.1 mg/dL (87.3 µmol/L). He is admitted to the ICU.

Which of the following antibiotics would you administer in the ICU?

A. Nafcillin.
B. Continue with vancomycin and ceftriaxone.
C. Ceftriaxone and azithromycin.
D. Linezolid and ceftriaxone.

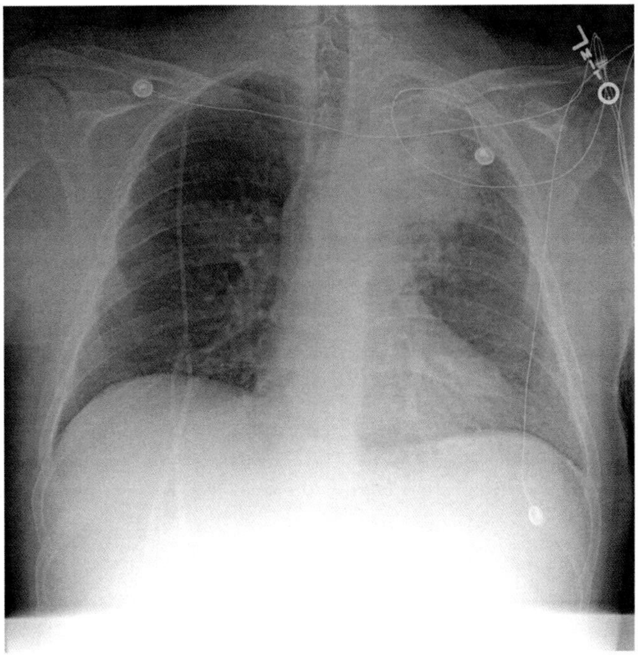

Figure 101-A

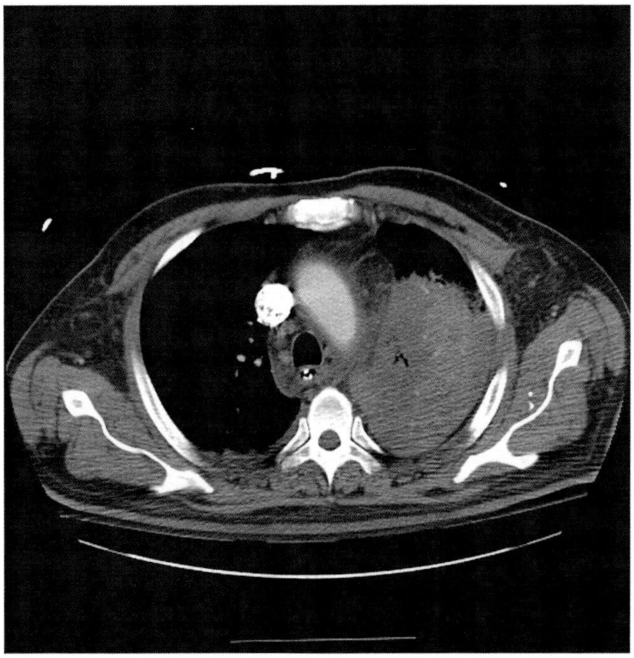

Figure 101-B

102. Figure 102-A represents a display of ECG (red), airflow (blue), and airway pressure (black) tracings during 50 s of positive pressure ventilation.

Which of the following forms of patient ventilator asynchrony is demonstrated in Figure 102-A?

A. Double triggering.
B. Autotriggering.
C. Ineffective triggering.
D. Flow asynchrony.

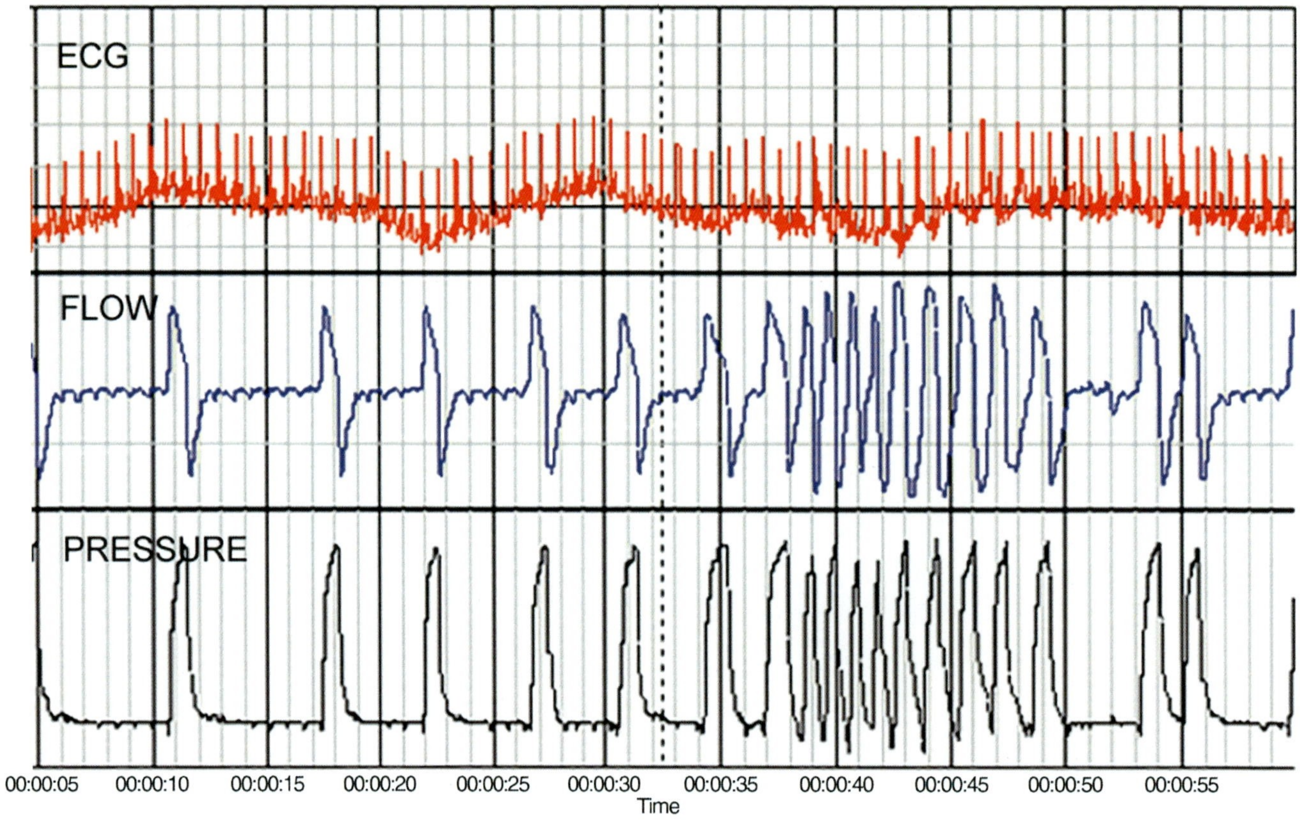

Figure 102-A

103. A 65-year-old man is referred for the gradual onset of shortness of breath over the prior 2 years. He has a 45 pack-year history of tobacco use. You obtain pulmonary function tests that reveal mild-moderate obstruction, and after discussion of the results, the patient seeks your assistance in initiating smoking cessation. In order to obtain the highest likelihood of successful smoking cessation, you should recommend which of the following?

A. Nicotine replacement therapy and behavioral therapy.
B. Bupropion and behavioral therapy.
C. Varenicline and behavioral therapy.
D. Behavioral therapy alone.

104. The diagnosis of significant airflow obstruction is often based on the spirometric FEV_1/FVC ratio. Recommended cutoffs for diagnosing obstruction include a fixed value (*eg*, 0.70) or, alternatively, using values outside a 95% CI for predicted FEV_1/FVC ratios (below the "lower limit of normal"). Compared with the 95% confidence intervals approach, the fixed ratio approach corresponds to which of the following?

A. It is virtually identical in diagnosing obstruction in most subjects.
B. It will overdiagnose obstruction in older subjects and underdiagnose obstruction in younger subjects.
C. It will underdiagnose obstruction in older subjects and overdiagnose obstruction in younger subjects.
D. It will overdiagnose obstruction in all subjects.

105. A 41-year-old man with refractory acute lymphoblastic leukemia undergoes high-dose chemotherapy in preparation for stem cell transplantation. He experiences prolonged neutropenia and develops fevers that continue despite several days of therapy with IV vancomycin, cefepime, and levofloxacin. Empiric voriconazole is added, but the fevers persist. Chest radiographs reveal a new hazy density and volume loss in the left midlung field. Bronchoscopy is performed, and a lesion is found

at the secondary carina on the left (see Figure 105-A). A biopsy of this lesion is done, and the histologic specimen is shown in Figure 105-B. What is the most appropriate management step at this point?

A. Continue the voriconazole.
B. Switch to posaconazole.
C. Switch to liposomal amphotericin B.
D. Switch to itraconazole.

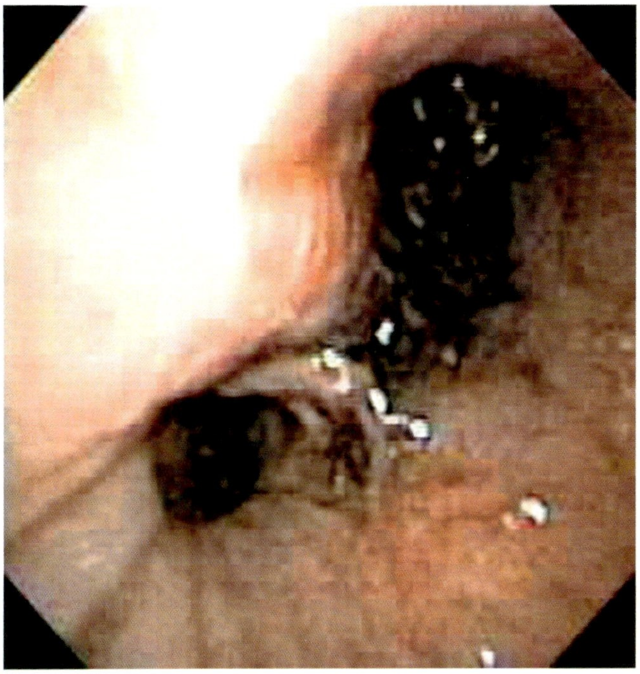

Figure 105-A

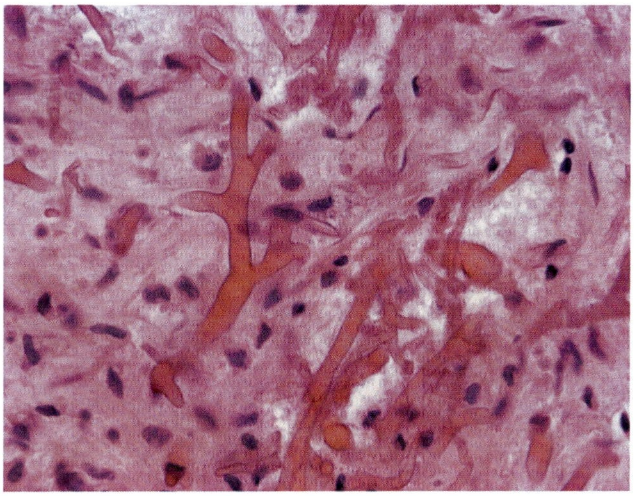

Figure 105-B
Hematoxylin-eosin

106. Which of the following is true about lung cancer in patients with HIV infection?

A. Lung cancer is the most common non–AIDS-defining malignancy.
B. The risk of lung cancer increases with declining CD4+ cell counts.
C. The incidence of lung cancer in patients with HIV has declined worldwide as the use of combination antiretroviral therapy (ART) has increased.
D. Squamous cell carcinoma is the most common cell type.

107. In which of the following clinical scenarios of patients with *Streptococcus pneumoniae* respiratory tract infections would *in vitro* bacterial resistance be expected to predict clinical failure if discordant therapy (an antibiotic is given to which *in vitro* susceptibility testing suggests the organism is resistant) is prescribed?

A. A 27-year-old man is treated for pneumococcal bacteremic pneumonia with clarithromycin. A sputum culture produces a macrolide-resistant strain (erythromycin minimum inhibitory concentration required to inhibit the growth of 90% of organisms [MIC_{90}] = 2 μg/mL).
B. A 35-year-old woman is treated for pneumococcal pneumonia as an outpatient with amoxicillin 3 g/day. Sputum culture results indicate a penicillin-resistant strain (penicillin MIC_{90} = 2 μg/mL).
C. A 74-year-old woman is admitted to the hospital for treatment of multilobar pneumococcal pneumonia. Administration of ceftriaxone 2 g/day is begun. Blood culture results reveal a penicillin-resistant strain (penicillin MIC_{90} = 4 μg/mL).
D. A 68-year-old man is treated with moxifloxacin 400 mg/day for an acute exacerbation of COPD. Sputum culture results show a quinolone-resistant strain (levofloxacin MIC_{90} = 2 μg/mL).

108. A 52-year-old man is referred for evaluation of cough and an abnormal CT scan. He was born in Michigan, has not traveled recently, and works as an accountant. He was previously well except for long-standing chronic hepatitis C infection presumably contracted following a transfusion consequent to a motor vehicle accident in his 20s. Because of a rising viral titer, therapy was initiated with pegylated interferon alpha and ribavirin 6 months previously. He initially reported malaise but after 2 months of therapy, he felt well. Over the preceding 2 months, he noted the insidious onset of a dry cough and some mild dyspnea if he climbed two flights of stairs quickly. He denied use of IV drugs and was HIV negative. A chest radiograph was reported as abnormal, leading to the performance of a CT scan. Representative images are shown in Figures 108-A and 108-B.

Physical examination was unremarkable, and pulmonary function testing revealed no abnormalities. Bronchoscopy revealed normal-appearing airways, and a transbronchial biopsy revealed the changes shown in Figure 108-C.

What would you suggest at the present time?

A. Initiate therapy with prednisone.
B. Discontinue interferon/ribavirin therapy.
C. Refer the patient to an oncologist.
D. Initiate therapy with four antituberculous agents.

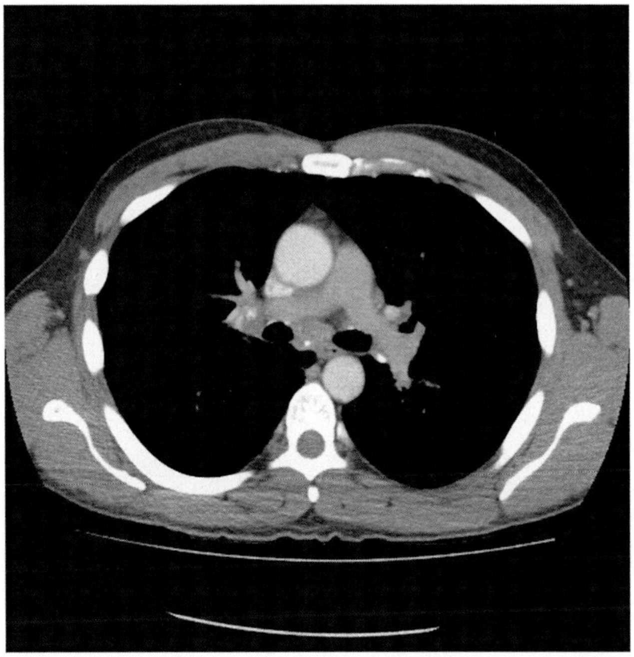

Figure 108-A

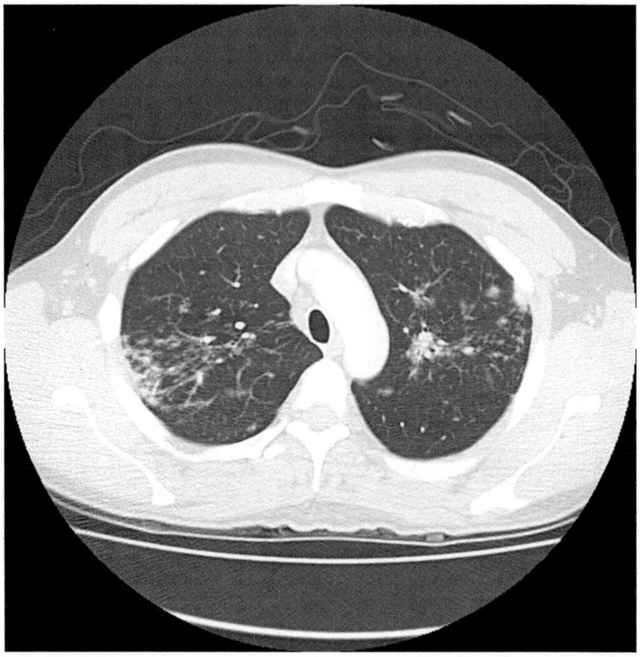

Figure 108-B

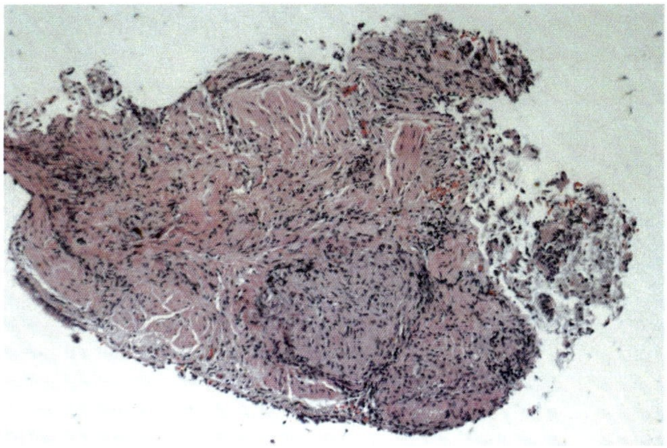

Figure 108-C
Hematoxylin-eosin

109. A 32-year-old man has had a chronic cough productive of thick purulent sputum, without hemoptysis, since he was a teenager. He denies any new or changed symptoms over the last month, has had bronchitis treated many times by antibiotics, and is a lifelong nonsmoker. Multiple physicians have seen the patient, and nondiagnostic evaluations include sweat chloride testing, gene testing for cystic fibrosis (CF), ciliary structure assessment, γ-globulin and HIV testing, serum α_1-antitrypsin level, and rheumatoid factor testing. Evaluation for allergic bronchopulmonary aspergillosis is negative. He has no history compatible with inflammatory bowel disease, chronic aspiration, or gastroesophageal reflux. Lung function testing shows moderate obstruction. The most recent chest radiograph (see Figure 109-A) and high-resolution CT scan of the chest (see Figures 109-B and 109-C) are unchanged from those taken a month ago. You are asked by the consulting physician to suggest ongoing treatment.

Which of the following is the most appropriate therapy for this patient?

A. Inhaled tobramycin.
B. Chest physiotherapy.
C. Recombinant human DNase.
D. Chronic oral corticosteroids.

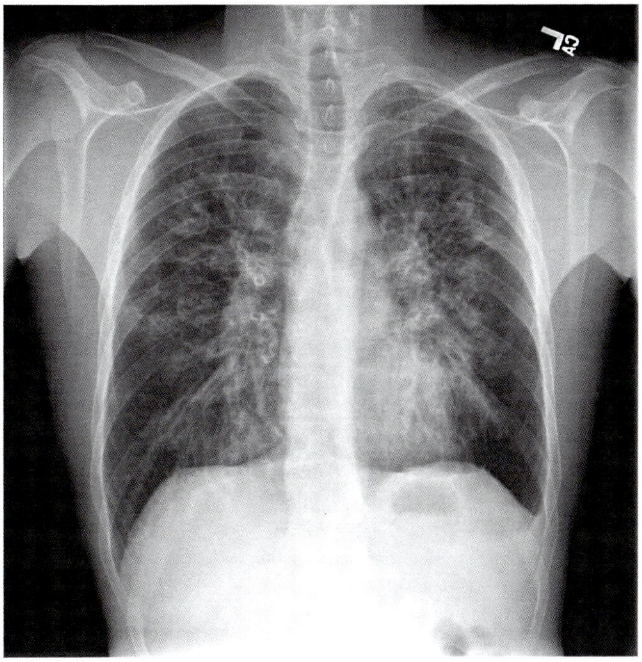

Figure 109-A

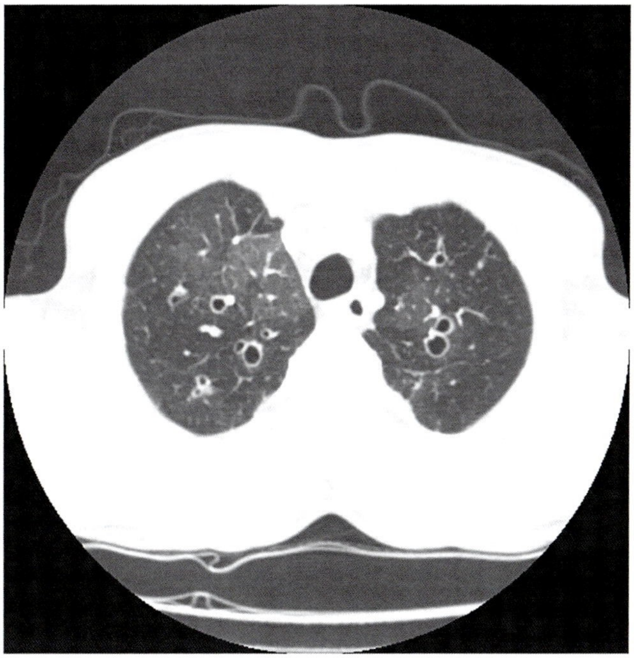

Figure 109-B

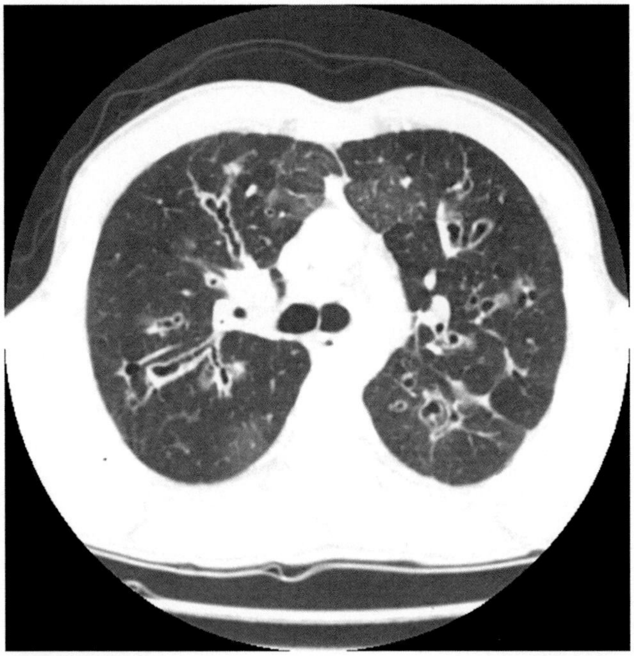

Figure 109-C

110. A 62-year-old man with chronic pancreatitis and diabetes mellitus is admitted to the ED with abdominal pain and vomiting for the last week. He was taking sodium bicarbonate for his abdominal pain. He was afebrile with a pulse of 100/min (120/min sitting), respiratory rate of 22/min, and BP of 126/90 mm Hg (supine) and 98/60 mm Hg (sitting). His mucus membranes were dry. He has mild abdominal distention and epigastric tenderness but no other abnormal physical findings. A nasogastric tube is placed. Two hundred milliliters of bilious-colored gastric fluid are removed, and the tube is set to low, intermittent suction. Laboratory data revealed the following concentrations: sodium of 140 mEq/L (140 mmol/L), potassium of 3.0 mEq/L (3.0 mmol/L), chloride of 68 mEq/L (68 mmol/L), bicarbonate of 41 mEq/L (41 mmol/L), creatinine of 2.3 mg/dL (203 μmol/L), and glucose of 108 mg/dL (6 mmol/L). Urine chloride concentration was 9 mmol/L. Results of liver function tests and amylase were normal. Arterial blood gases on room air revealed a pH of 7.74, $Paco_2$ of 23 mm Hg, and Pao_2 of 85 mm Hg. ECG, chest and abdominal radiographs, and urine analysis were normal. Saline is administered intravenously.

Which of the following should be administered *next*?

A. Hydrochloric acid.
B. H2 blocker.
C. Acetazolamide.
D. Potassium chloride.

111. A 39-year-old woman is admitted with a massive pulmonary embolus and associated shock. Prior medical history is noncontributory. CT with contrast of the chest reveals a significant saddle embolus. Doppler ultrasounds of both lower extremities are significant for thrombus in the popliteal vein. A heparin infusion titrated to a goal-activated partial thromboplastin time (aPTT) of two to three times normal is initiated, and she receives one dose of alteplase, 90 mg IV. The patient is intubated for hypoxia and respiratory failure. On day 6, the patient develops a new fever. Blood, sputum, and urine culture results are negative. Doppler ultrasounds of both lower extremities are ordered and demonstrate a new thrombus in the common iliac vein. On day 7, there is an acute decrease in platelet count from $256 \times 10^3/\mu L$ ($256 \times 10^9/L$) to $98 \times 10^3/\mu L$ ($98 \times 10^9/L$). The heparin infusion is discontinued, and an enzyme-linked immunosorbent assay (ELISA) heparin-induced thrombocytopenia PF4 assay is ordered. Serum chemistry concentrations are significant: an elevated BUN of 47 mg/dL (16.9 mmol/L) and a creatinine of 2.1 mg/dL (186 μmol/L). CBC and liver function test results are normal except for the aforementioned platelet count.

Which heparin alternative anticoagulant therapy should be given?

A. Fondaparinux.
B. Lepirudin.
C. Argatroban.
D. Enoxaparin.

112. A 33-year-old man undergoes a polysomnographic study for suspected obstructive sleep apnea. He describes a 5-year history of nightly loud snoring, witnessed apneas, morning headaches, and fatigue. His past medical history is unremarkable, and he takes no medications. His BMI is 36 kg/m^2, and neck circumference is 48 cm. Examination of the oropharynx reveals a Mallampati score class of 3 (soft and hard palate and base of the uvula are visible). Polysomnographic data (see Table 112-1) and CPAP titration data (see Table 112-2) are shown below.

Table 112-1. Polysomnographic Data*

Sleep Architecture	
Total recording time	389 min
Total sleep time	301 min
Sleep efficiency	77%
Sleep latency	22 min
Baseline Diagnostic Data	
Total AHI	63.2 events/h
OAI	15.1 events/h
OHI	44.2 events/h
CAI	3.9 events/h
Periodic limb movement index	2.1 events/h
Lowest oxygen desaturation	83%

*AHI = apnea-hypopnea index; OAI = obstructive apnea index; OHI = obstructive hypopnea index; CAI = central apnea index.

Table 112-2. CPAP Titration Data

Pressure, cm H_2O	**OAI**	**OHI**	**CAI**	**AHI**
5	13.7	43.1	1.5	58.3
7	2.0	36.7	6.0	44.7
9	1.1	12.4	32.4	45.9
11	0	4.3	35.2	39.5
13	0	4.1	38.6	42.7

Which of the following is the most appropriate next step in the management of this patient?

A. Prescribe autotitrating positive airway pressure (APAP) therapy with upper and lower limits of 5 and 11 cm H_2O, respectively.
B. Schedule a repeat polysomnography with adaptive servoventilation titration.
C. Have the patient take zolpidem, 5 mg, during a repeat CPAP titration sleep study.
D. Prescribe low-dose nocturnal oxygen therapy.

113. Which of the following pulmonary function measurements is significantly decreased during pregnancy?

A. FEV_1.
B. Functional residual capacity.
C. Vital capacity.
D. Tidal volume.

114. A 56-year-old man is referred for pulmonary function testing. Spirometry demonstrates moderate obstruction (FEV_1 = 58% predicted). A nitrogen washout determination of functional residual capacity (FRC) and lung volumes is performed. These reveal an FRC of 190% predicted and a residual volume (RV) of 201% predicted. The nitrogen washout tracing is shown in Figure 114-A. Your interpretation of these results is:

A. Normal lung volumes and good gas mixing.
B. Significant air trapping with poor gas mixing.
C. Significant air trapping with good gas mixing.
D. Uninterpretable values because of system leak.

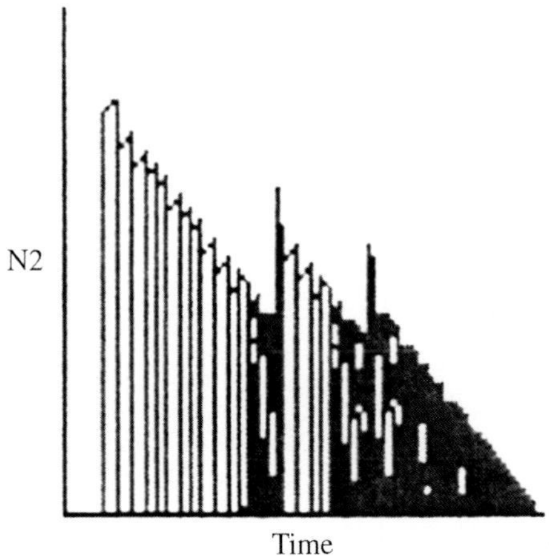

Figure 114-A

115. An asymptomatic 42-year-old nonsmoking man is referred after a chest radiograph was obtained 2 weeks ago during a respiratory infection. The patient's respiratory symptoms have since resolved without treatment, and the radiograph was negative for pulmonary infiltrates. However, a 2-cm smooth, noncalcified, homogeneous mass was noted in the left superior paravertebral region of the posterior mediastinum (see Figure 115-A).

What is the most likely diagnosis?

A. Ganglioneuroma.
B. Lymphoma.
C. Parathyroid adenoma.
D. Teratoma.

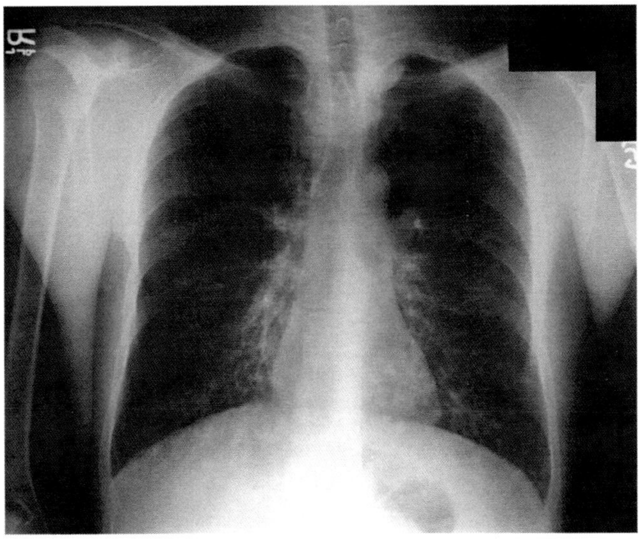

Figure 115-A

116. An 18-year-old woman is referred for examination of unexplained dyspnea. She has noted progressive shortness of breath for approximately 1 year and received a diagnosis of asthma from her family physician a few months ago. She did not note any symptomatic benefit with the use of salbutamol and budesonide inhalers. Her symptoms have precluded her from participating in gym class. She denies any cough, sputum production, hemoptysis, or illicit drug use and is currently not taking any medications. Results of physical examination are normal. Her CBC results are normal. Spirometry reveals an FEV_1 of 2.97 L (102% predicted), FVC of 3.29 L (107% predicted), and an FEV_1/FVC of 0.90. The provocative concentration of substance causing 20% fall (PC_{20}) from a methacholine challenge test was 24.3 mg/mL. The results from cardiopulmonary exercise testing are shown in Table 116-1 and in Figures 116-A and 116-B.

Table 116-1. Cardiopulmonary Exercise Test Results*

Variable	Rest	End-Exercise	Predicted Maximum	% Predicted
Workload (W)	—	65	137	47
$\dot{V}O_2$ (L/min)	0.203	1.315	1.790	73
$\dot{V}E$ (L/min)	9.6	35.5	103.9	34
SpO_2	99	98		
HR	86	148	197	75
BP (mm Hg)	110/65	130/75		
Modified Borg: dyspnea	1	9		
Modified Borg: leg fatigue	0	3		

* $\dot{V}O_2$ = oxygen consumption; $\dot{V}E$ = expired volume per unit time; SpO_2 = oxygen saturation as measured by pulse oximetry; HR = heart rate.

Repeated spirometry for 30 min following exercise did not reveal any reduction in flows. The patient reported discontinuing exercise because of severe shortness of breath. What would you do next in the management of this patient?

A. Order a chest CT scan.
B. Order testing for anticentromere antibodies (ACA), anti-DNA topoisomerase I (Scl-70) antibodies, and U3-RNP (fibrillarin) antibodies.
C. Empirically anticoagulate pending d-dimer, ventilation-perfusion ($\dot{V}/\dot{Q}$) scan, and leg Doppler ultrasounds (if the $\dot{V}/\dot{Q}$ scan results were normal or indeterminate).
D. Inform the patient of the diagnosis of primary hyperventilation syndrome and explore possible contributing factors.

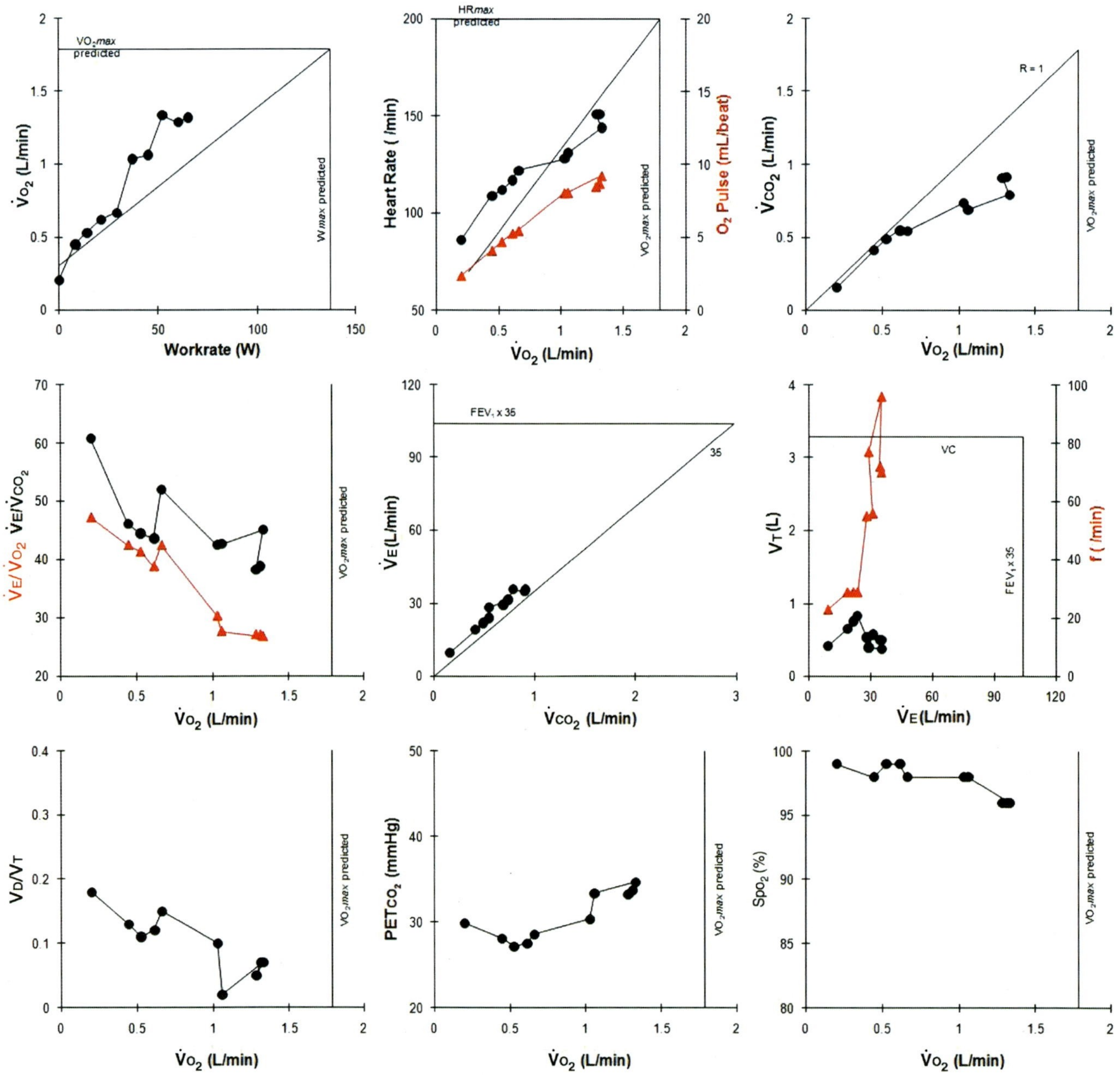

Figure 116-A

$\dot{V}O_2$ = oxygen consumption; $\dot{V}CO_2$ = carbon dioxide output; HRmax = predicted maximal heart rate; $\dot{V}E$ = expired volume per unit time; VT = tidal volume; f = respiratory frequency; VD/VT = dead space ventilation; $PETCO_2$ = end-tidal CO_2; SpO_2 = oxygen saturation as measured by pulse oximetry.

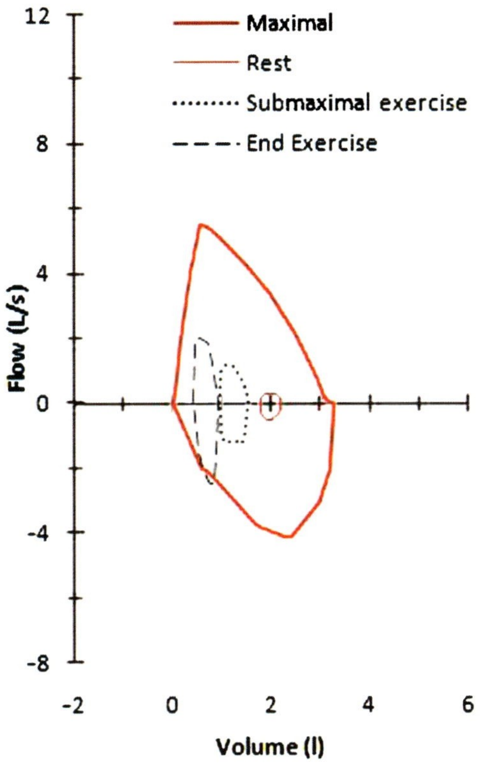

Figure 116-B

117. A 39-year-old man with asthma has an increased need for his inhaled bronchodilator, despite an increase in his inhaled corticosteroids 4 weeks ago. He reports increased cough and sputum production but has not had any fever or hemoptysis. He also does not have any sinus congestion, postnasal drip, or reflux symptoms. His primary care doctor had ordered a chest radiograph, which was concerning because of the presence of a lung mass, so he sent the patient for a CT scan of the chest (a representative image is shown in Figure 117-A). His current medical regimen includes a fluticasone/salmeterol inhaler, 500 µg/50 µg twice daily; albuterol sulfate inhaler, two puffs every 4 h as needed; and montelukast sodium, 10 mg daily. Results of physical examination reveal diffuse expiratory wheezing and rhonchi throughout the upper lung fields, but otherwise are completely normal. Spirometry is notable for moderate obstruction, with a significant response to the bronchodilator. His FEV_1 is reduced by 300 mL compared with testing done 4 weeks ago. Results of a CBC done today are the following:

WBC	7,100/µL (7.1 × 10^9/L)
Hemoglobin	16.4 g/dL (164 g/L)
Hematocrit	46.5% (0.465)
Platelets	275 × 10^3/µL (275 × 10^9/L)
Neutrophils	51.3% (0.513)
Lymphocytes	19.1% (0.191)
Monocytes	10.8% (0.108)
Eosinophils	17.8% (0.178)
ESR*	10 mm/h
C-reactive protein	0.08 mg/L (0.76 nmol/L)

* ESR = erythrocyte sedimentation rate.

The most appropriate diagnostic test in this patient is:

A. A serum IgE level.
B. A serum antineutrophil cytoplasmic antibody level.
C. A sinus CT scan.
D. Flexible bronchoscopy.

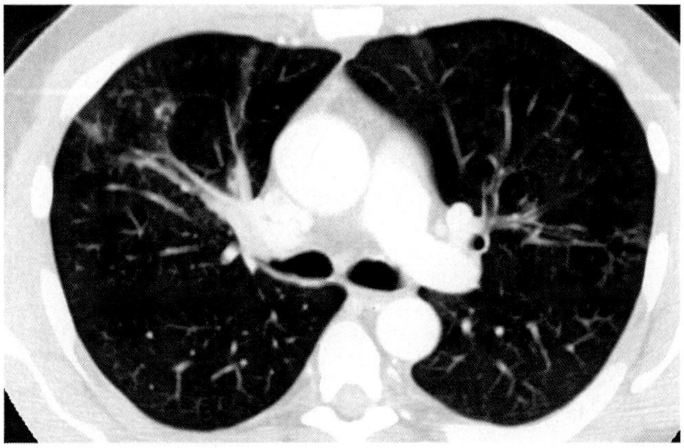

Figure 117-A

118. A nurse in your hospital's ICU has been told by the employee health service to start isoniazid therapy for a reactive tuberculin skin test (TST) measuring 11 mm at 72 h. She is 24 years old and has just started working at the hospital. She was born in India but moved to the United States at age 2 years. She had bacillus Calmette-Guérin (BCG) vaccination as a child but has not reported any contact in her work with patients known to have TB. She is married to a surgeon at your hospital, and he thinks that the test was administered incorrectly. She requested your advice as the staff pulmonologist.

Which of the following is true regarding her TST?

A. Her 11-mm reaction to the TST is from exposure to TB.
B. If her interferon-γ release assay is negative, her reactive TST is from the BCG or non-TB mycobacteria exposure.
C. Her reactivity to the TST is a booster response.
D. Her TST is 11 mm because administration was subcutaneous rather than intradermal.

119. A 30-year-old man is referred for evaluation of dyspnea on exertion and anterior chest pain after exertion. He is otherwise healthy and takes no medications. He has been active throughout adolescence and adulthood but has experienced some exercise intolerance. The findings of physical examination are that the patient is a tall, thin man. The results of a chest examination reveal pectus excavatum and normal lung auscultation, and the findings of a cardiac examination are normal. His posteroanterior and lateral view chest radiographs are displayed in Figures 119-A and 119-B.

Which of the following statements about this condition in patients with exertional dyspnea is true?

A. Pulmonary function studies typically reveal airflow obstruction with air trapping.
B. Surgical repair usually produces lasting improvement in pulmonary function.
C. Maximum exercise tests demonstrate cardiovascular limitation to exercise.
D. Compression of the left ventricle and the left ventricular outflow tract is common.

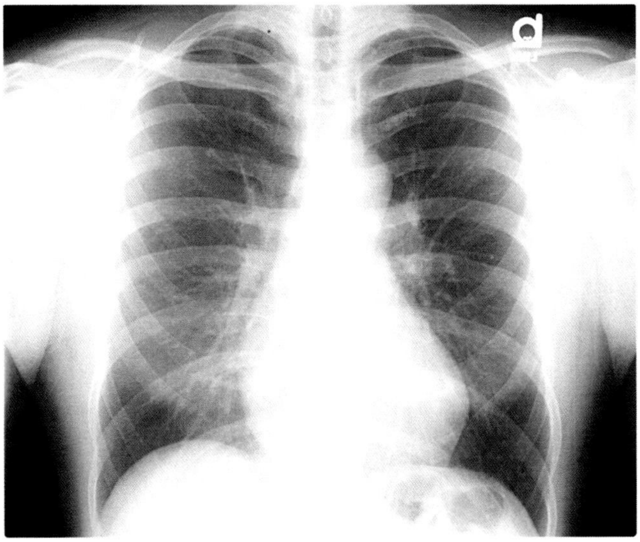

Figure 119-A

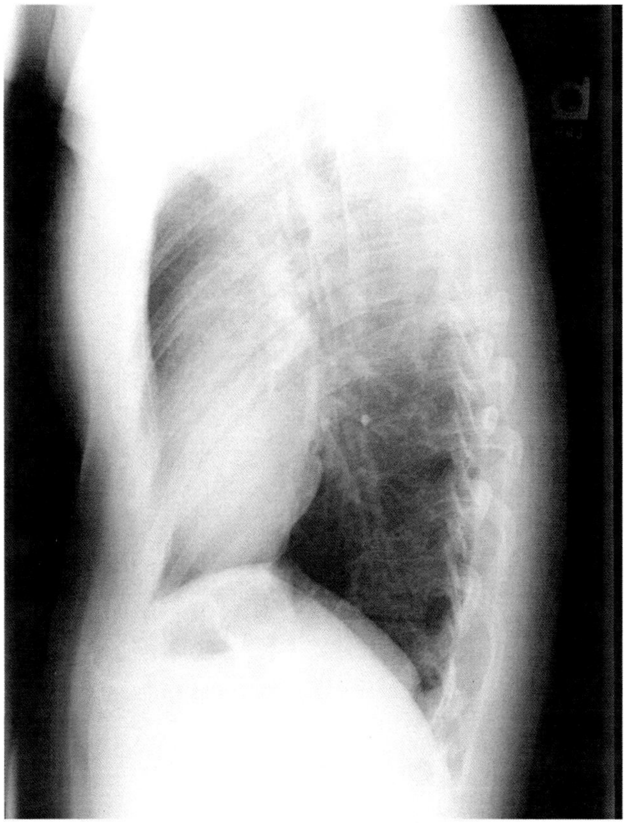

Figure 119-B

120. Which of the following increases a person's risk of developing high-altitude pulmonary edema?

A. Patent foramen ovale.
B. Asthma.
C. Increasing age.
D. Administration of salmeterol before ascent.

121. A 75-year-old woman is readmitted to hospital for the fourth time in 2 years with profound hyponatremia. Each episode was preceded by vomiting and mild diarrhea and associated with confusion, and each episode resolved following conservative management with fluid restriction. No specific cause was ever found. Her previous health was excellent other than hypertension, osteoporosis, and osteoarthritis, for which she receives diclofenac, misoprostol, etidronate, enalapril, and atenolol. Her son stated that she has had right flank discomfort for the past 3 months, during which time she lost 15 to 30 lbs (6.8 to 13.6 kg). She was born in India and lived in North America for more than 20 years. She is a nonsmoker.

Physical examination is completely normal except for profound confusion. Laboratory examination indicates normal CBC and urinalysis results. The serum sodium is 103 mEq/L (103 mmol/L), potassium is 2.5 mEq/L (2.5 mmol/L), chloride is 85 mEq/L (85 mmol/L), and bicarbonate is 26 mEq/L (26 mmol/L). Serum osmolality is markedly reduced. Urine sodium is 64 mEq/L (64 mmol/L). A chest radiograph and CT scan led to a chest MRI. The representative images are shown in Figures 121-A, 121-B, 121-C, and 121-D. A bronchoscopy shows no evidence of tumor or infection.

Which of the following is the most likely diagnosis?

A. Metastatic lung cancer.
B. Pulmonary and spinal TB.
C. Drug-induced inappropriate antidiuretic hormone syndrome.
D. Histoplasmosis.

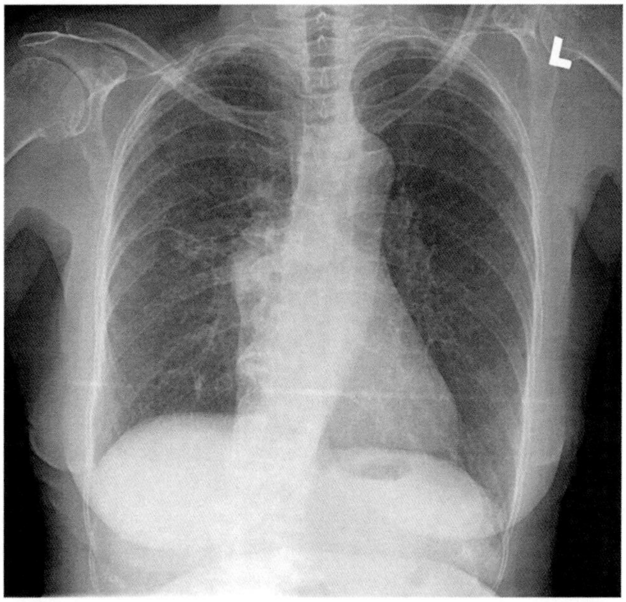

Figure 121-A

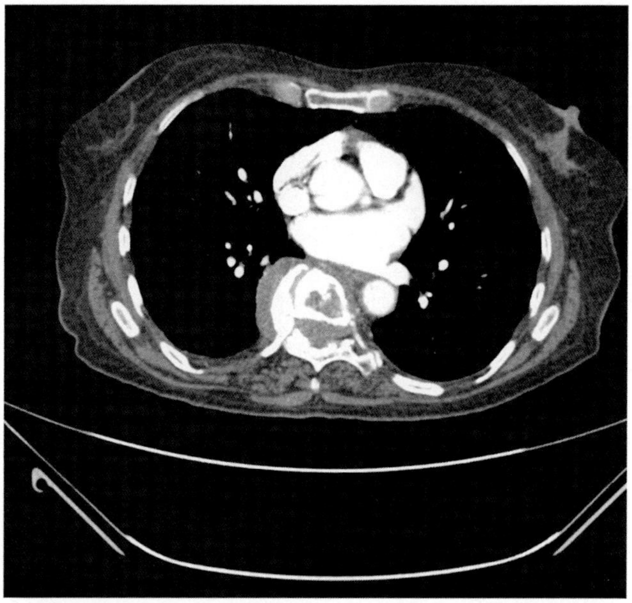

Figure 121-B

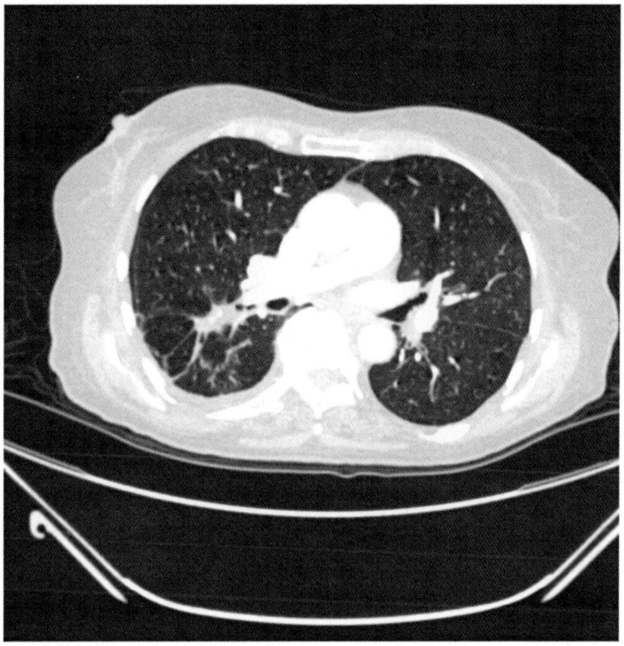

Figure 121-C

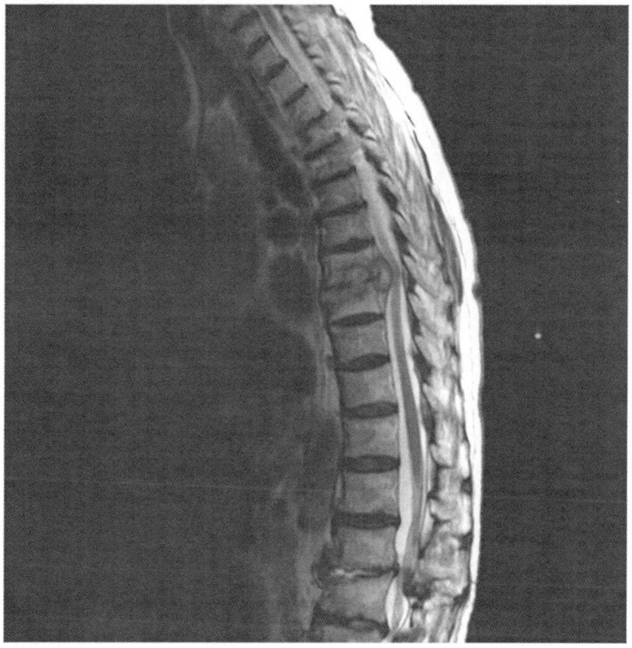

Figure 121-D

122. A 72-year-old woman with long-standing ankylosing spondylitis presents with shortness of breath for 1 year. She noted intermittent polyarthritis and chronic diarrhea for a year during which she lost 30 lbs (13.61 kg). An echocardiogram shows global left ventricular dysfunction with moderate-to-severe mitral regurgitation. Four months earlier, she had multiple subcutaneous masses in her right groin, bilateral axillae, and lower abdomen. A biopsy was performed on one of the masses and interpreted as showing panniculitis with fat necrosis, but no vasculitis was seen. No treatment was given. Five days after admission, she developed progressive shortness of breath, requiring 70% oxygen by face mask, despite diuresis. She had one episode of hemoptysis on the day before this examination.

On physical examination, the patient is tachypneic, but the rest of her vital signs are normal. Her lungs show bibasilar crackles with no wheezing. She has bilateral axillary subcutaneous masses. Her blood gas tests show a Po_2 of 63 mm Hg, Pco_2 of 34 mm Hg, and pH of 7.45 on an Fio_2 of 70% (0.70). Her WBC count is normal, sedimentation rate is elevated at 66 mm/h, and serum test result is positive for perinuclear antineutrophil cytoplasmic antibodies.

Her serum chemistries are normal. Her urine immunofixation shows lambda monoclonal light chains, and her serum immunofixation shows a monoclonal free lambda band. Her chest radiograph shows bibasilar nodular infiltrates. Bronchoscopy with transbronchial biopsy is performed, and a specimen is shown in Figure 122-A.

Which of the following statements best describes this patient's prognosis?

A. She will probably improve dramatically with treatment.
B. She has an indolent disease with good survival.
C. Patients typically die of pulmonary complications.
D. Mortality best correlates with degree of cardiac involvement.

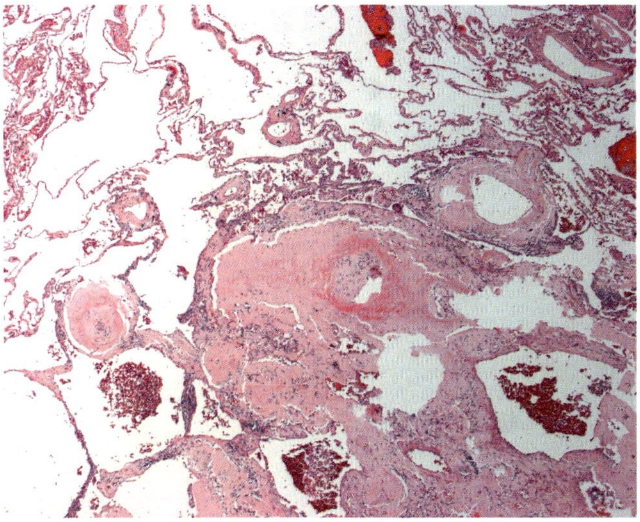

Figure 122-A
Hematoxylin-eosin

123. A 68-year-old man underwent overnight polysomnography in your sleep laboratory. He presented with complaints of dyspnea about 6 months ago. Subsequent evaluation, including echocardiography, confirmed an initial suspicion of congestive heart failure. His cardiologist was concerned about an overnight continuous pulse oximetry report that indicated the presence of significant oxygen desaturation with frequent episodes of Sao_2 reaching the low 80s. Arterial blood gas testing while the patient is awake shows a Pao_2 of 84 mm Hg and a $Paco_2$ of 32 mm Hg. This prompted the sleep study that revealed the following polysomnographic data:

Total recording time	491 min
Total sleep time	325 min
Sleep efficiency	78%
Sleep latency	3 min
AHI*	22.1 events/h
Supine AHI	21.4 events/h
Nonsupine AHI	23.6 events/h
Nonrapid eye movement AHI	22.1 events/h
Rapid eye movement AHI	0 events/h
Periodic limb movement index	0 events/h
Lowest oxygen desaturation	84%

*AHI = apnea-hypopnea index.

A sample epoch is provided in Figure 123-A.

Which of the following statements about this patient's sleep disorder is correct?

A. There is a correlation between this disorder and decreased left ventricular ejection fraction and lower awake $Paco_2$.
B. It is more common in patients with decreased hypercapnic chemoresponsiveness during wakefulness than in those with a normal $Paco_2$.
C. Positive airway pressure therapy is unlikely to offer any benefit because the upper airways are patent in this disorder.
D. Acetazolamide reverses most cases of this form of sleep-related breathing disorder.

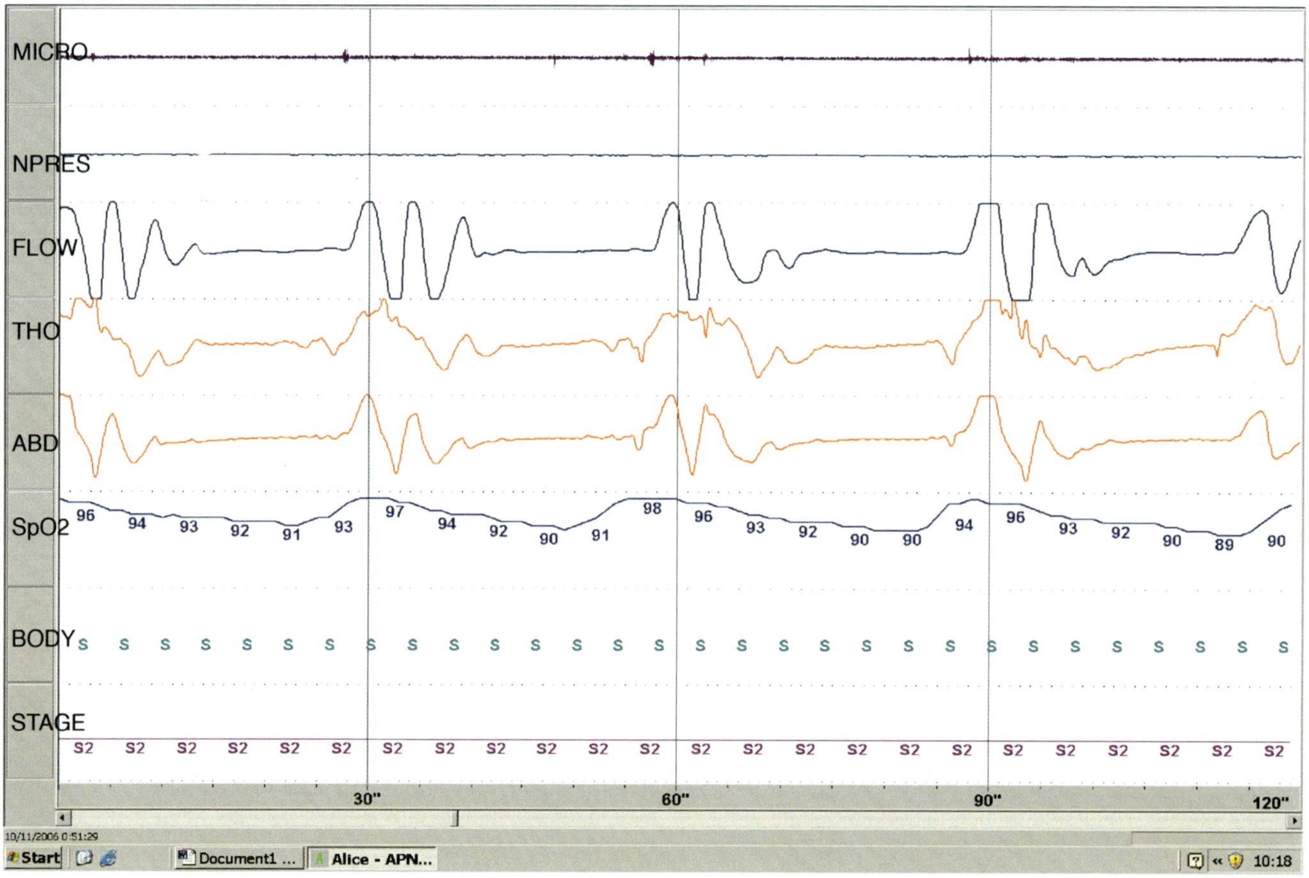

Figure 123-A
MICRO = microphone; NPRES = nasal pressure; FLOW = airflow; THO = thoracic; ABD = abdominal;
Spo_2 = oxygen saturation as measured by pulse oximetry.

124. An 84-year-old man with sarcoidosis underwent pulmonary function tests under proper testing conditions, and the following values represent the best efforts of three reproducible maneuvers:

FEV_1, L	1.16 (58% predicted)
FVC, L	1.75 (66% predicted)
FEV_1/FVC	0.66
Forced expiratory time	5.42 s
TLC,* L	4.74 (92% predicted)
VC* (slow)	1.79 (68% predicted)
RV*	2.51 (103% predicted)
FRC,* L	3.17 (98% predicted)

*TLC = total lung capacity; VC = vital capacity; RV = residual volume; FRC = functional residual capacity.

Which of the following is the correct interpretation of these tests?

A. Obstructive impairment.
B. Restrictive impairment.
C. Mixed restriction and obstruction.
D. Uninterpretable because of poor effort.

125. A 19-year-old man is referred because of episodes of voice change, severe cough, and wheezing after peanut ingestion. The results of a physical examination are normal, and results from a chest radiograph and pulmonary function test are normal. The result of an allergy skin-prick test for peanuts is positive. Peanut-specific IgE antibodies are detected in high titer.

Which of the following statements regarding this condition is true?

A. A food challenge is necessary to confirm the diagnosis in this patient.
B. The patient should be advised to avoid other nuts.
C. The patient should be offered desensitization therapy.
D. A written action plan should be offered.

126. A 52-year-old man is seen for evaluation of worsening asthma symptoms. He has a 13-year history of asthma, and he had frequent ED visits and courses of oral corticosteroids over the years, usually due to intermittent non-compliance with prescribed medications and concurrent respiratory tract infections. He currently takes a fluticasone (250 μg)/salmeterol (50 μg) combination dry powder inhaler twice daily and albuterol for breakthrough symptoms. Recently, he was using his albuterol four to six times daily and had a productive cough.

His past medical history is unremarkable. He has smoked less then a package of cigarettes daily in an on-and-off fashion for the better part of 29 years. He frequently smokes marijuana. He has an extensive family history of asthma, including a brother and an aunt who died from the disease. He works as a radiographer for a natural gas company and travels extensively for work.

Over the past year, he had two episodes of left lower lobe pneumonia, each responding promptly to antibiotic and oral corticosteroid therapy. He denied any symptoms suggestive of gastroesophageal reflux and was on no other medications.

Physical examination revealed a man with mild Cushing disease with a BP of 146/78 mm Hg with no pulsus paradoxus, a pulse rate of 84/min, and a respiratory rate of 20/min. There was mild use of accessory muscles but no intercostal indrawing. There were decreased breath sounds bilaterally with a prolonged forced expiratory time ≥6 s and a focal wheeze heard over the left lower lobe. Spirometry results are shown in Table 126-1.

Table 126-1. Spirometry Results*

	Predicted	Observed	After Bronchodilator	% Change
FEV_1, L	4.43	2.27 (51)	3.01 (68)	33
FVC, L	5.67	3.23 (57)	4.07 (72)	26
FEV_1/FVC, %	78	70	74	6

*Values in parentheses are % predicted.

His CBC results are normal, with a normal eosinophil count and serum IgE concentration. Representative images from his chest CT scan are shown in Figures 126-A and 126-B.

What would you do next?

A. Allergy skin testing.
B. Measure *Aspergillus precipitins.*
C. Double the dose of fluticasone.
D. Bronchoscopy.

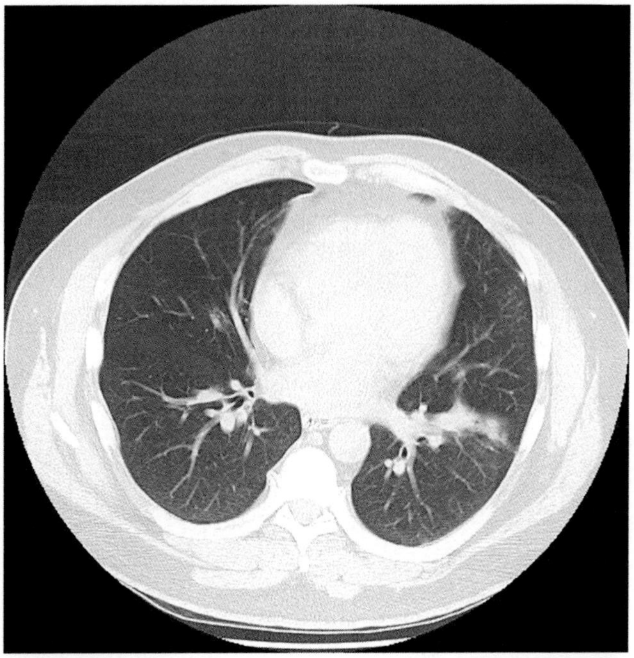

Figure 126-A

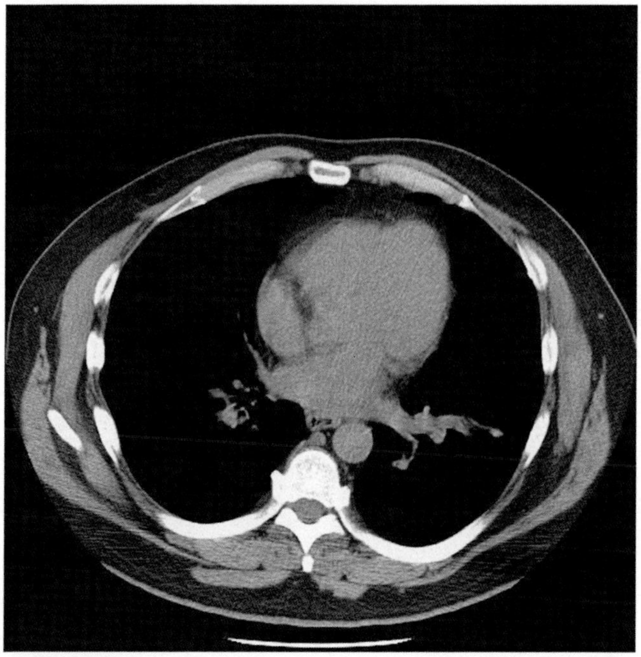

Figure 126-B

127. A 26-year-old man has a long-standing history of asthma. He is taking fluticasone proprionate (500 μg)/ salmeterol (50 μg) twice daily and montelukast nightly. Excellent adherence is reported, and he uses the inhaler in an acceptable fashion. For the last 4 months, he has reported an increase in asthma symptoms and has required two ED visits and two nonscheduled visits to his primary care physician. His morning peak flows vary significantly on a daily basis, ranging from 250 to 380 L/min. The result of a skin test was positive for tree and grass pollens and dust, and immunotherapy was started 3 months ago. His IgE level is 3,000 μg/L (3 mg/L) (normal = 0 to 1,500 μg/L [0 to 1.5 mg/L]).

The next most appropriate step is to administer:

A. Oral corticosteroid.
B. Theophylline.
C. Omalizumab.
D. Tiotropium.

128. A 23-year-old patient is noted to be hypoxic during an annual athletics physical. She is active and competes as a collegiate diver but has noted dyspnea on exertion that has been progressive over the past 2 years. In addition to her dyspnea, she reports a dry cough, mostly in the morning. She has no significant occupational, environmental, or avocational exposures. She does not use petroleum jelly for nasal lubrication and does not smoke tobacco. Physical examination is remarkable for a resting saturation of 88% on room air and bibasilar crackles on pulmonary examination. Results of routine chemistries and CBC are normal. She has normal lung volumes and flow rates, but the DLCO is 57% predicted. A chest radiograph and CT scan are obtained (see Figures 128-A and 128-B).

Which of the following is the most appropriate treatment?

A. Trimethaprim-sulfamethoxazole.
B. Corticosteroids.
C. Granulocyte-macrophage colony-stimulating factor (GM-CSF).
D. Cyclophosphamide.

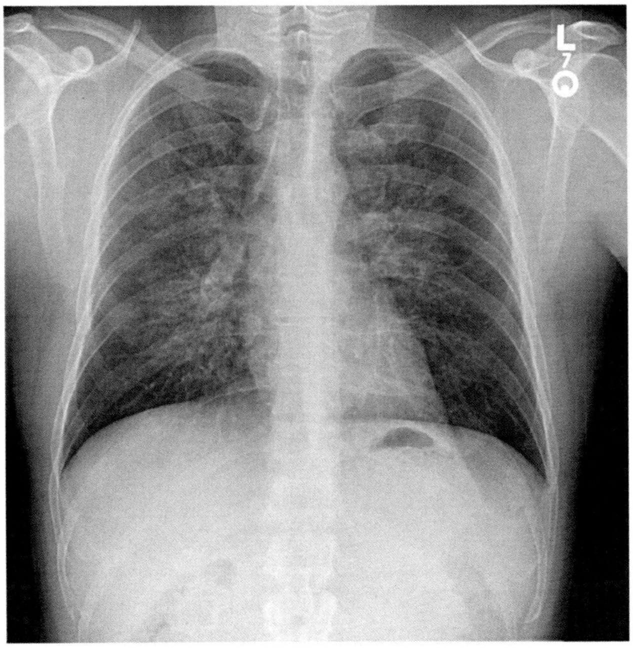

Figure 128-A

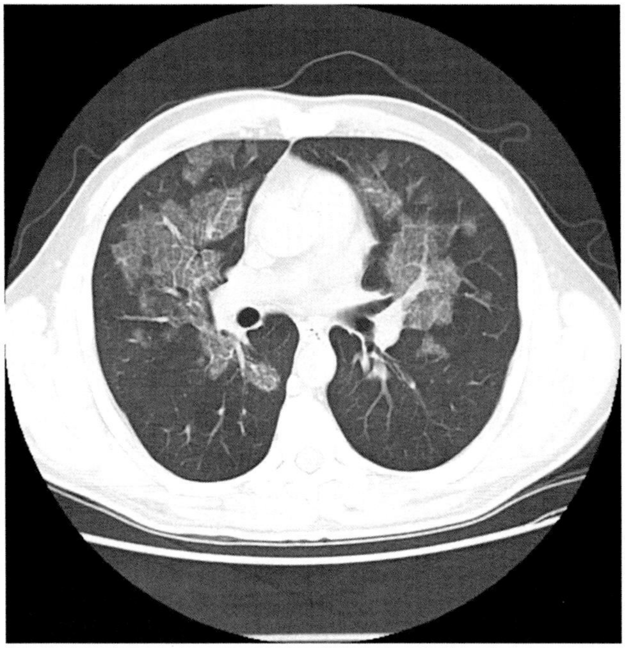

Figure 128-B

129. A 55-year-old man with advanced emphysema undergoes a left single-lung transplantation. His postoperative course is complicated by a nosocomial pneumonia that responds to empiric antibiotic treatment for 10 days, and he is discharged after a 16-day admission. His chest radiograph at 1 month following discharge shows hyperinflation of the right lung and no infiltrate in the allograft.

He now arrives for his 12-week postoperative clinic visit and reports that he feels generally well, but he has observed a 15% decline in home spirometry measurements over the last 4 days. He has not noted fevers, chills, cough, hemoptysis, or sputum production. His physical examination is remarkable for diminished breath sounds in the right lung.

A chest radiograph is obtained and is shown in Figure 129-A.

Given this presentation and the findings on chest radiograph, the most likely diagnosis is:

A. Staphylococcal pneumonia.
B. Acute rejection of the allograft.
C. Cytomegalovirus (CMV) pneumonitis.
D. Cardiogenic pulmonary edema.

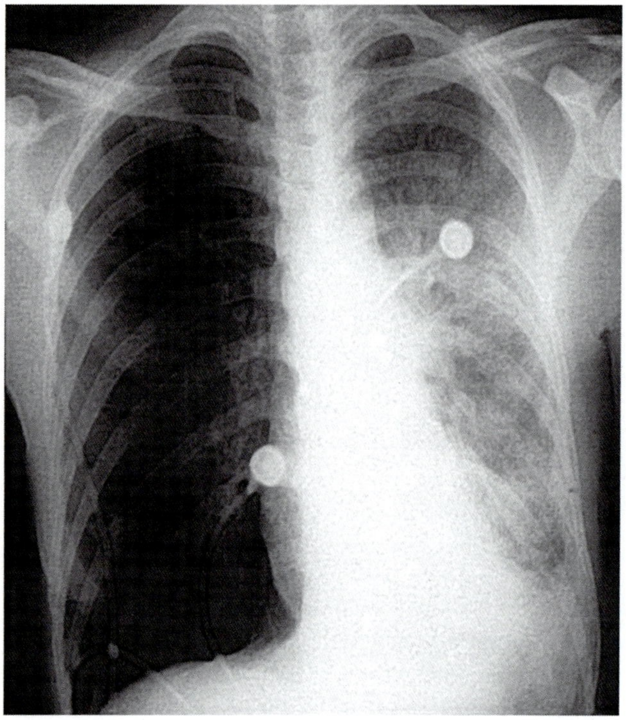

Figure 129-A

130. According to the 2007 American Academy of Sleep Medicine rules for the scoring of sleep, what sleep stage does this 30-s epoch (see Figure 130-A) represent?

A. Stage N1.
B. Stage N2.
C. Stage N3.
D. Stage R.

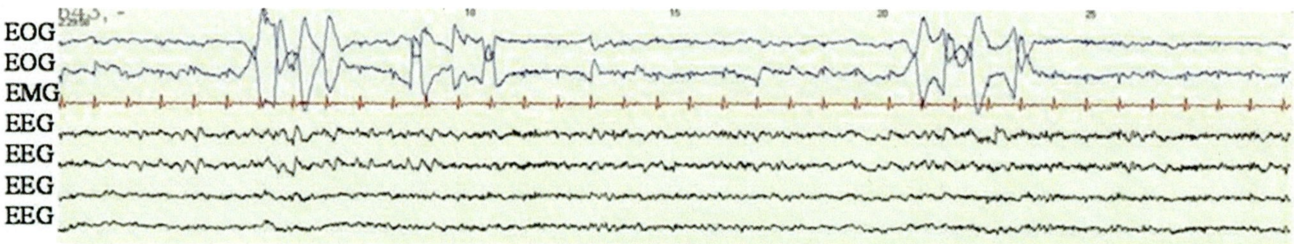

Figure 130-A

131. Which of the following patients, assessed following rehabilitation, would be the best candidate for lung volume reduction surgery (LVRS)?

A. A 60-year-old man with upper lobe emphysema and an exercise capacity of 30 W following rehabilitation. FEV_1 is 30% predicted, and DLCO is 28% predicted.
B. A 52-year-old woman with diffuse emphysema and an exercise capacity of 50 W following rehabilitation. FEV_1 is 28% predicted, and DLCO is 30% predicted.
C. A 58-year-old man with upper lobe emphysema and an exercise capacity of 60 W following rehabilitation. FEV_1 is 32% predicted, and DLCO is 40% predicted.
D. A 68-year-old man with diffuse emphysema and an exercise capacity of 30 W following rehabilitation. FEV_1 is 18% predicted, and DLCO is 15% predicted.

132. A 66-year-old man has received mechanical ventilatory support for an acute exacerbation of COPD. His lung function has now improved, and he has just passed a spontaneous breathing trial. Extubation is performed, but over the next hour, he becomes tachypneic, tachycardic, hypoxemic (Spo_2 of 84%), and anxious. His $Paco_2$ also has risen 12 mm Hg. His breath sounds are normal. He has a satisfactory cough and is able to follow commands.

What is the next step?

A. Reintubation and mechanical ventilation.
B. Noninvasive ventilation.
C. Increase the Fio_2 for 60 min and double the bronchodilator dose.
D. Steroids should be given to reduce laryngeal edema.

133. A 64-year-old woman with significant COPD (baseline FEV_1 of 810 mL, 31% predicted) is admitted to her local hospital with an acute exacerbation characterized by a 2-day history of increased cough and sputum production and a change in her sputum character to more yellow and thick, accompanied by worsened dyspnea. She has approximately one or two exacerbations per year (the most recent was approximately 8 months ago), has never been intubated, and is not treated chronically with oral glucocorticoids. When admitted, her physical examination findings are notable for diffuse expiratory wheezes without focal consolidation, and a chest radiograph does not show significant changes from her baseline films.

She is treated as an inpatient for 72 h with oral moxifloxacin, supplemental oxygen, inhaled albuterol and ipratropium, and IV methylprednisolone and is clinically improved.

How long should the patient receive a total course of glucocorticoids (IV plus oral)?

A. 3 days.
B. 5 days.
C. 2 weeks.
D. 8 weeks.

134. A 31-year-old woman is referred to you for assessment of an abnormal chest radiograph. An initial chest radiograph was ordered 6 months ago because of her planned travel to South Africa and revealed a 2-cm right lung nodule. Results of a chest radiograph 4 years prior were normal. A repeat chest radiograph performed today shows persistence of the lesion, which now measures 2.3 cm. She denies shortness of breath, cough, sputum production, hemoptysis, or chest pain. She notes no fevers, chills, night sweats, weight loss, or loss of appetite. A recent tuberculin skin test

result was 0 mm. She has no other health problems, is taking no medications, is a lifelong nonsmoker, and is currently asymptomatic. She is heterosexual and has had one male partner since becoming sexually active. She was last HIV-tested 1 month ago (3 years after this relationship ended) and was HIV-negative. She is a health-care volunteer who works as an administrator in rural HIV clinics. In the past 4 years, she has worked in Indonesia (4 months), Costa Rica (2 months), South Africa (9 months), and Mozambique (10 months). She has been healthy during these travels except for an episode of diarrhea 2 years ago while in Mozambique that resolved with supportive care. Physical examination results are normal. Stool for ova and parasites was recently sent for testing, and results are negative. Her chest radiograph from this visit is shown (see Figure 134-A). Representative images from a CT scan of the chest perfomed today are also shown (see Figures 134-B and 134-C). The lesion measures 2.3 × 2.3 cm, and the density is 43 Hounsfield units. No other lung nodules are evident, and the lung parenchyma is otherwise normal. There are no pleural effusions or enlarged lymph nodes. The mediastinum and cardiac structures are normal, and no lesions in the liver or spleen are seen.

What would you recommend?

A. A repeat CT scan in 3 months.
B. A transthoracic needle biopsy.
C. A PET scan.
D. Serologic tests for Paragonimus, Echinococcus, and Strongyloides; stool samples for Paragonimus sp.

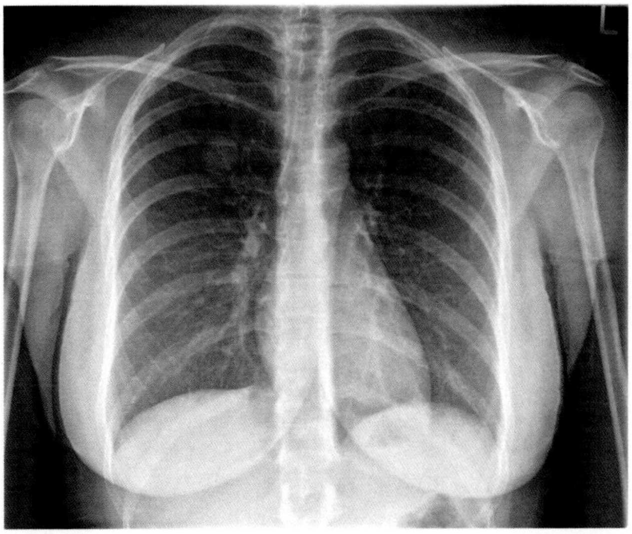

Figure 134-A

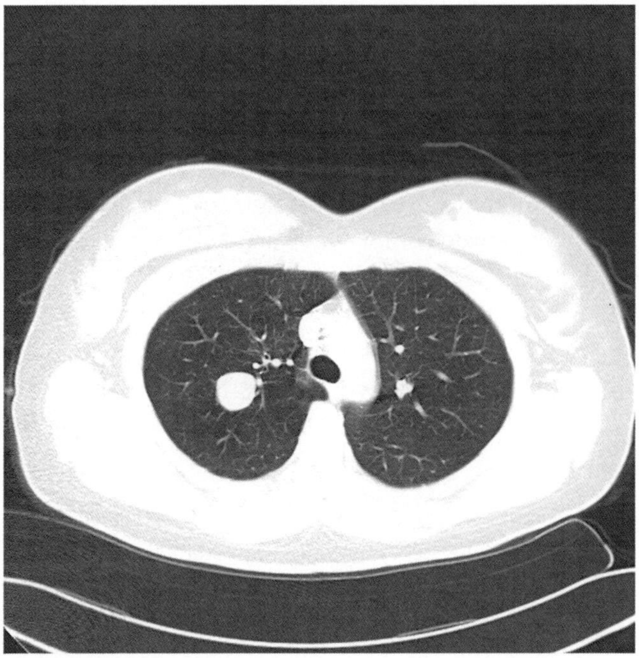

Figure 134-B

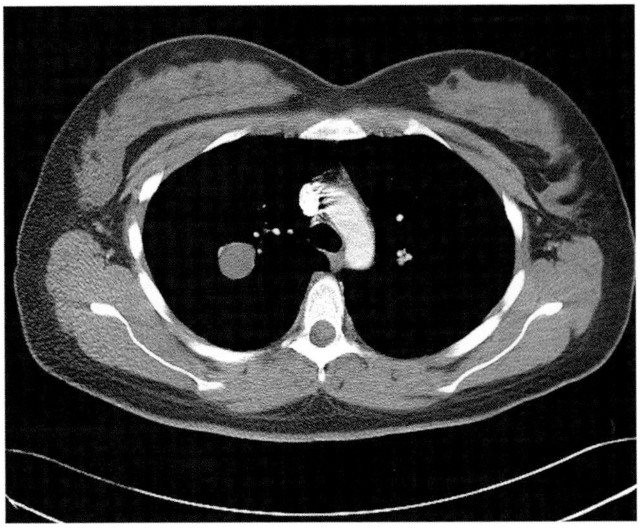

Figure 134-C

135. A 41-year-old woman with metastatic ovarian cancer is admitted with new-onset gait instability and headaches. A representative image from her brain MRI done on admission is shown (see Figure 135-A), revealing a heterogeneous cerebellar mass consistent with metastasis. On day 2 in the hospital, she develops acute onset of severe dyspnea and hypoxemia. A spiral CT angiogram is performed, and a representative image is shown (see Figure 135-B). She is placed on 100% oxygen via face mask, and her hypoxemia improves, with an oxygen saturation of 91%. She becomes hypotensive with a BP of 80/50 mm Hg. Two liters of normal saline are given, and her BP remains low at 85/53 mm Hg. A bedside echocardiogram confirms moderate right ventricular dysfunction.

In addition to the oxygen, fluids, and vasopressors as needed, current American College of Chest Physicians guidelines recommend which of the following as the next step?

A. Administer IV unfractionated heparin (UFH).
B. Administer recombinant tissue plasminogen activator.
C. Place an inferior vena cava filter.
D. Perform catheter fragmentation and extraction of the embolus.

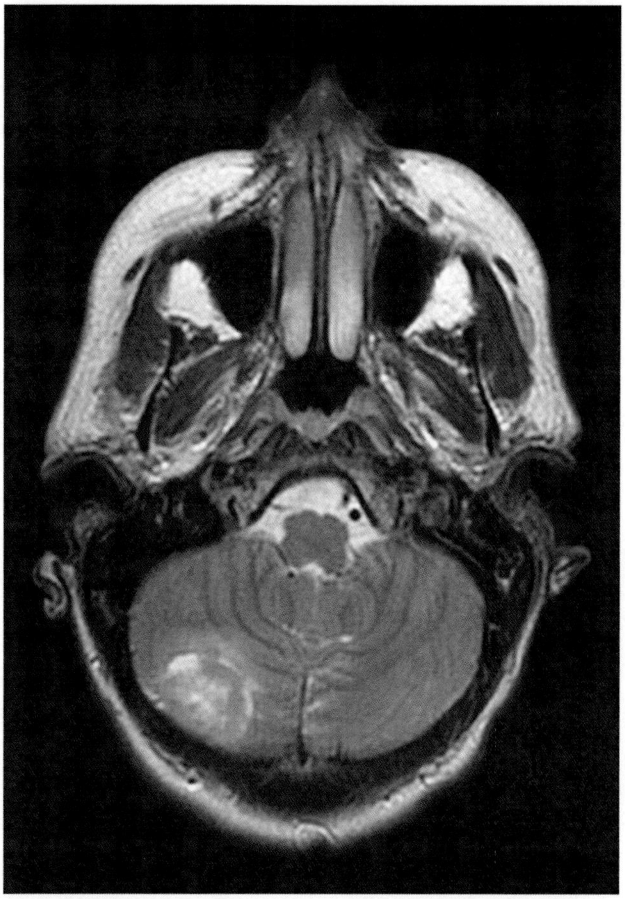

Figure 135-A

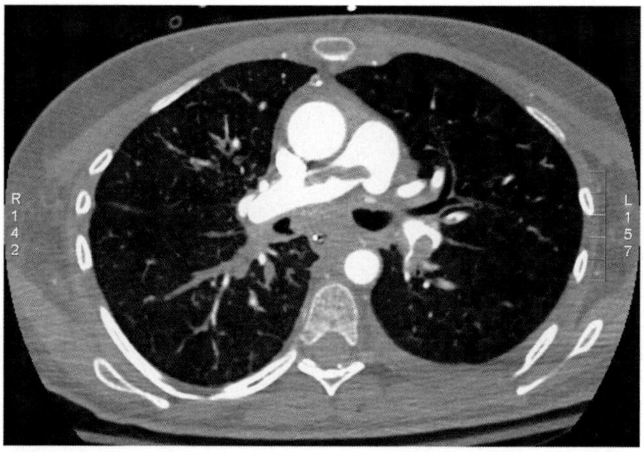

Figure 135-B

136. Which of the following is true regarding reactive airways dysfunction syndrome (RADS)?

A. A history of atopy is common in patients with RADS.
B. BAL reveals a predominance of lymphocytes and eosinophils.
C. Symptoms usually persist for months after exposure and can persist for years.
D. Reexposure to the offending agent at low levels in a clinical setting will reproduce symptoms.

137. Opioid analgesics are commonly used in the management of patients supported by mechanical ventilation.

Which of the following statements regarding opioid analgesic medications is true?

A. Remifentanil is metabolized via tissue esterases to active metabolites.
B. Morphine sulfate is metabolized in the liver to active metabolites that accumulate in renal failure.
C. Fentanyl has high lipophilicity and a delayed onset of action.
D. Hydromorphone is associated with prolonged QT syndrome and tachyarrhythmias.

138. A 30-year-old man is brought to the ED by his roommate because of agitation. He was at a party with friends who took him home when he became unruly and agitated. There is no past medical history. Examination shows a disheveled man who is constantly coughing. There are burn marks on the fingers of both hands. His temperature is 38°C, BP is 190/110 mm Hg, heart rate is 110/min and regular, respiratory rate is 32/min, and Spo_2 is 78% while breathing room air. There are diffuse crackles heard over both lungs, and the patient is expectorating black-colored

sputum. A chest radiograph is obtained (see Figure 138-A). WBC count is 22,000/µL (22 × 10^9/L) with 87% segmented neutrophils, 8% band forms, and 5% lymphocytes. The hemoglobin level is 12 g/dL (120 g/L), with a normal platelet count. Serum electrolytes are unremarkable. A chest CT scan is shown in Figure 138-B. Blood cultures are obtained, and the patient begins treatment of IV levofloxacin, 750 mg once daily. He is given 35% oxygen via face mask, and his Spo_2 rises to 91%.

Which of the following tests will most likely diagnose this patient's illness?

A. Chest CT scan with pulmonary embolus protocol.
B. Urine toxicology screen.
C. Bronchoscopy.
D. Gram stain.

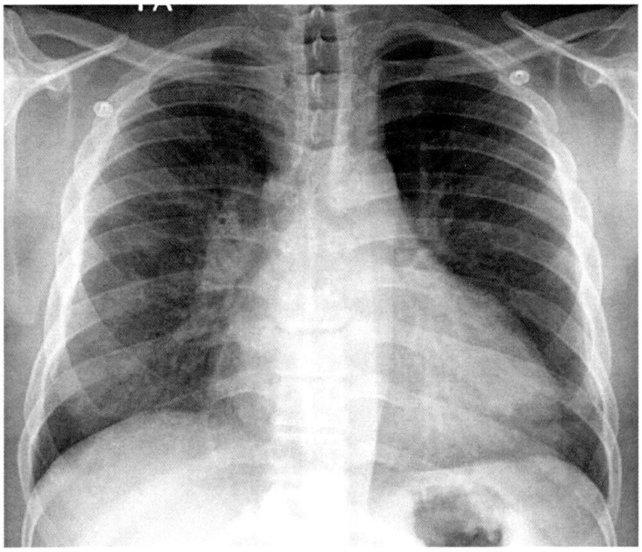

Figure 138-A

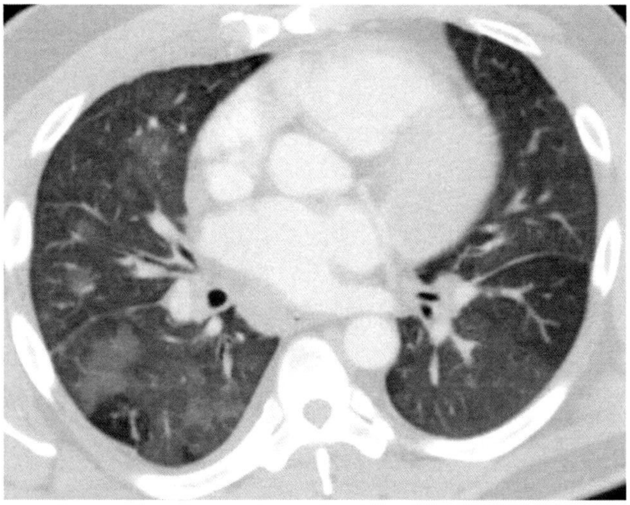

Figure 138-B

139. A 55-year-old man is scheduled for flexible bronchoscopy with transbronchial biopsy to assess diffuse lung disease. His medical history is remarkable for coronary artery disease including a non-ST segment myocardial infarction 12 weeks ago and mild hypertension. He is a former smoker, but quit 12 weeks ago. His medications include daily aspirin, clopidogrel, atorvastatin, hydrochlorothiazide, and metoprolol.

Which of the following should you recommend?

A. Discontinue aspirin for 7 days before performing bronchoscopy.
B. Discontinue clopidogrel for 7 days before performing bronchoscopy.
C. Eliminate all topical lidocaine anesthetic from the procedure.
D. Delay performing bronchoscopy until 6 months after the myocardial infarction.

140. A 46-year-old man is seen because of 4 months of increasing cough. He has HIV infection, and his CD4+ lymphocyte count 3 months ago was 240 cells/µL (0.24 × 10^9/L) and has been stable for several years with combination antiretroviral therapy. He smokes two packs of cigarettes daily and stopped using IV drugs 10 years ago. He denies fever, chills, and night sweats, but lost 18 lbs (8 kg) since the onset of the illness.

A chest radiograph and representative CT scan images are shown in Figures 140-A, 140-B, and 140-C.

What is the most likely diagnosis?

A. *Pneumocystis jiroveci* pneumonia.
B. Kaposi sarcoma.
C. Aspergillosis.
D. Adenocarcinoma.

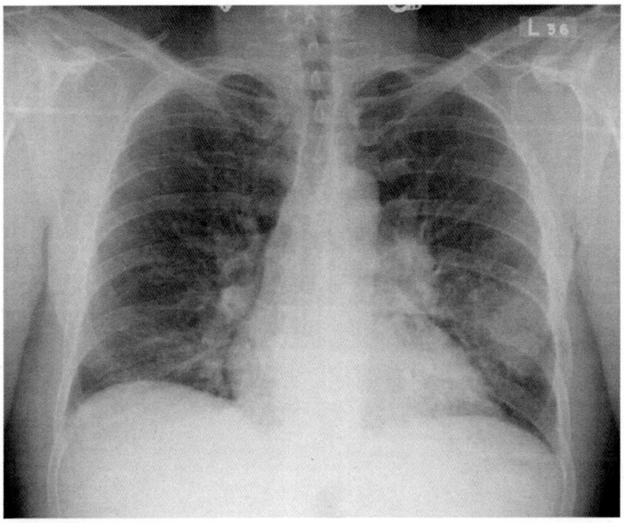

Figure 140-A

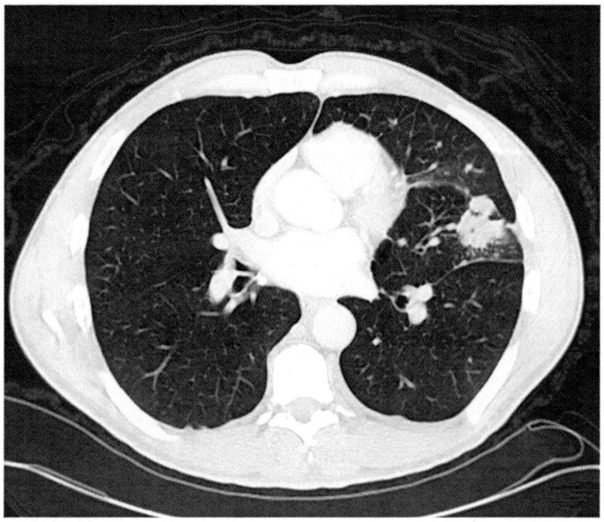

Figure 140-B

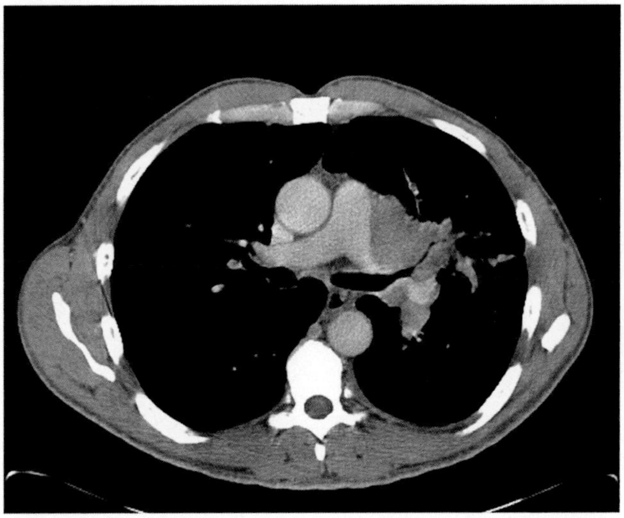

Figure 140-C

141. Which of the following is true about measurements of pulmonary function with aging?

A. Lung static recoil increases.
B. The chest wall becomes more compliant.
C. Residual volume (RV) increases.
D. Total lung capacity (TLC) decreases.

142. A 57-year-old man underwent bilateral lung transplantation for treatment of chronic thromboembolic pulmonary hypertension. The donor was cytomegalovirus (CMV) antibody-negative, and the recipient was CMV

antibody-positive. His postoperative course was complicated by hemolysis, acute renal failure, and initial weaning difficulties, but he improved and was discharged to a rehabilitation facility 2 months postoperatively. Subsequent to that, he remained well with no new pulmonary complaints. His medications included trimethoprim-sulfamethoxazole three times weekly, cyclosporine twice daily, 20 mg prednisone daily, mycophenolate mofetil twice daily, valganciclovir daily (planned for 3 months), and low-molecular-weight heparin.

He underwent routine surveillance transbronchial biopsies to monitor for rejection at 1 and 2 months after discharge, and no abnormalities were noted. Monthly monitoring of his blood for CMV pp65 antigen remained negative postoperatively. A routine surveillance transbronchial biopsy done 4 months after discharge is shown in Figure 142-A. A representative image from a CT scan done at the same time is shown in Figure 142-B. The patient feels good except for mild, occasional cough and sputum, and results of a physical exam are normal.

The abnormalities demonstrated are most likely due to:

A. Posttransplant lymphoproliferative disease.
B. Early lung transplant rejection.
C. Cytomegalovirus infection.
D. *Pneumocystis jirovecii* infection.

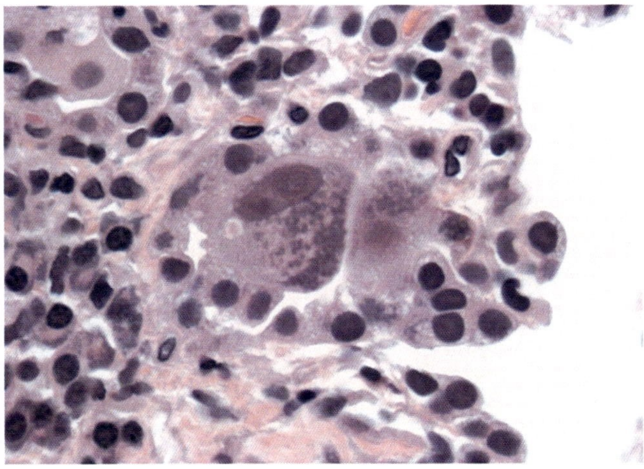

Figure 142-A
Hematoxylin-eosin

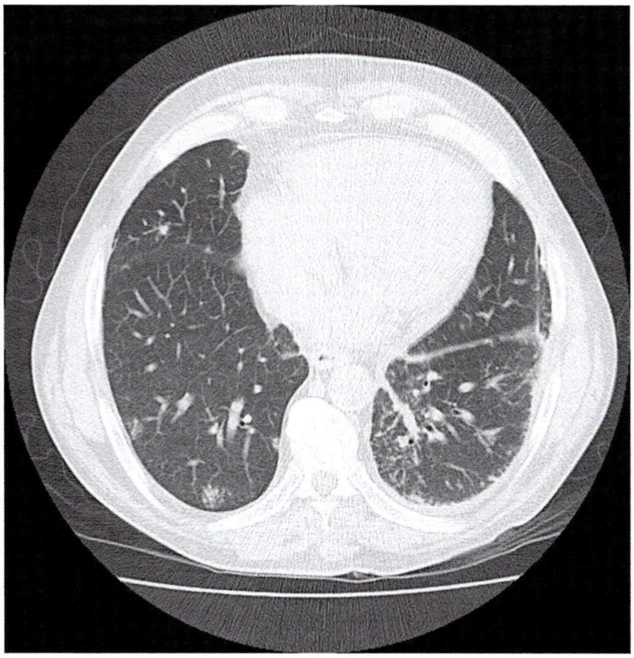

Figure 142-B

143. A 41-year-old woman is referred to you with a persistent, nonproductive cough for the last 3 months accompanied by a gradual increase in dyspnea on exertion. She has been treated with several courses of different oral antibiotics without appreciable improvement. The patient's history is notable for an allogeneic bone marrow transplantation performed 11 months ago for chronic myelogenous leukemia. For the last 5 months, she has been treated for chronic graft-vs-host disease (GVHD), manifested by skin and GI complications and treated by alterations in her corticosteroid regimen. Her pretransplantation pulmonary function test results are normal; her current tests show an FEV_1 of 1.13 L (46% of predicted), FVC of 2.11 L (71% of predicted), and FEV_1/FVC of 54% without bronchodilator response. Physical examination is notable for a normal lung examination. Her chest radiograph and representative high-resolution CT scan (inspiratory and expiratory images) are both interpreted as normal. The patient undergoes a nondiagnostic bronchoscopy with BAL and transbronchial biopsies (all culture and stain results were negative).

Her hematologist requests more information, and the patient undergoes an open lung biopsy (see Figure 143-A, low power; and Figure 143-B, high power).

Which of the following best describes this patient's disorder?

A. More commonly found in autologous compared with allogeneic bone marrow transplantation patients.
B. Choice of transplantation conditioning regimen influences the risk of developing this disorder.
C. Usually occurs within the first 15 days after transplantation.
D. Associated mortality rate is < 5%.

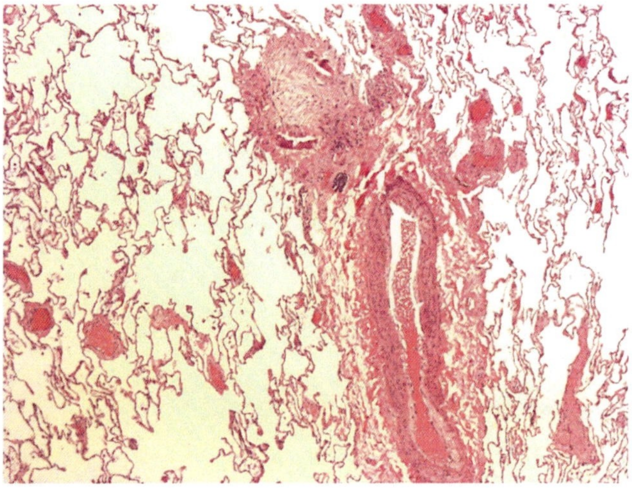

Figure 143-A
Hematoxylin-eosin

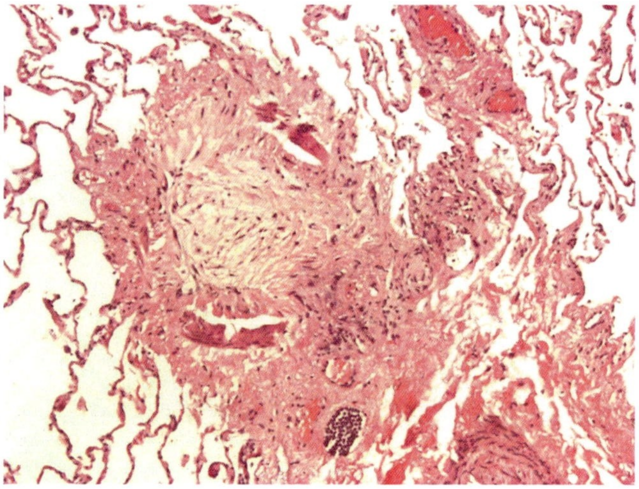

Figure 143-B
Hematoxylin-eosin

144. A 68-year-old woman is brought to the ED after collapsing during church services where she was singing. Upon the arrival of emergency medical services, she was hypotensive with a systolic BP of 60 mm Hg and a heart rate of 55/min. She was orally intubated and brought to the ED for evaluation. Prior to the episode of syncope, the patient screamed out in pain and grabbed her chest and then her back. Pertinent past history was significant for long-standing hypertension that was well controlled with medication and chronic kidney disease with a baseline creatinine level of 3.2 mg/dL (244 μmol/L). You are asked to see the patient, given her presentation and abnormal chest radiograph. A chest radiograph report from 3 months ago showed "no acute disease." Among the choices offered, which of the following is the most appropriate next step?

A. Transesophageal echocardiography (TEE).
B. CT angiography.
C. MRI with angiography.
D. D-dimer.

145. A 45-year-old man with a history of Duke stage B colon cancer treated with a complete resection has an abnormal chest radiograph 6 months later. He has never been a smoker. Results of a physical examination reveal a well-healed abdominal incision, a nontender abdomen, and no palpable adenopathy. Laboratory examination findings reveal normal CBC values and a carcinoembryonic antigen concentration of 2.8 ng/mL (2.8 μg/L; normal ≤ 3 μg/L). Pulmonary function is within normal limits. The result of an abdominal CT is unremarkable. A high-resolution CT scan confirms the presence of a single left midlung field nodule that is 1.3 cm in diameter (see Figures 145-A and 145-B). There is no adenopathy. A PET scan demonstrates uptake only in the areas of the lesion noted on chest CT. Percutaneous lung biopsy results reveal adenocarcinoma, and immunohistochemical findings confirm that it is

consistent with the primary colon carcinoma. The tumor does not change in size with additional chemotherapy. The patient is now being considered for metastasectomy. Which of the following would portend a less favorable prognosis after metastasectomy in this patient?

A. The carcinoembryonic antigen level.
B. The disease-free interval.
C. The location of the nodule.
D. The size of the nodule.

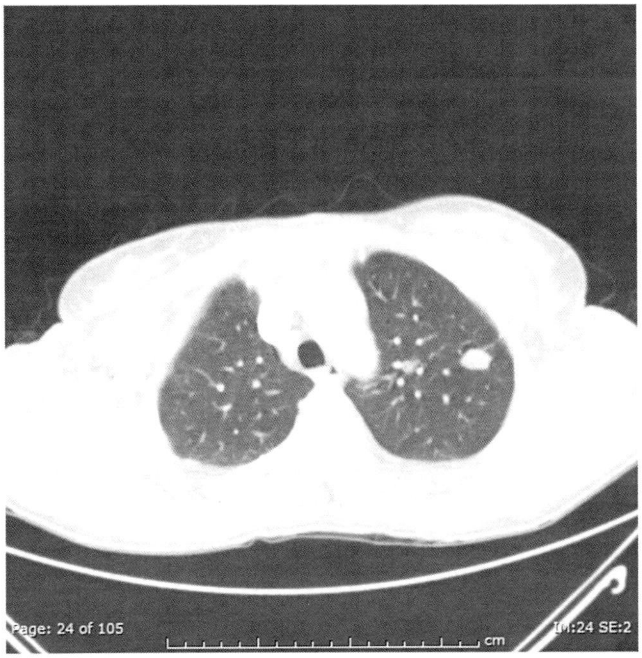

Figure 145-A

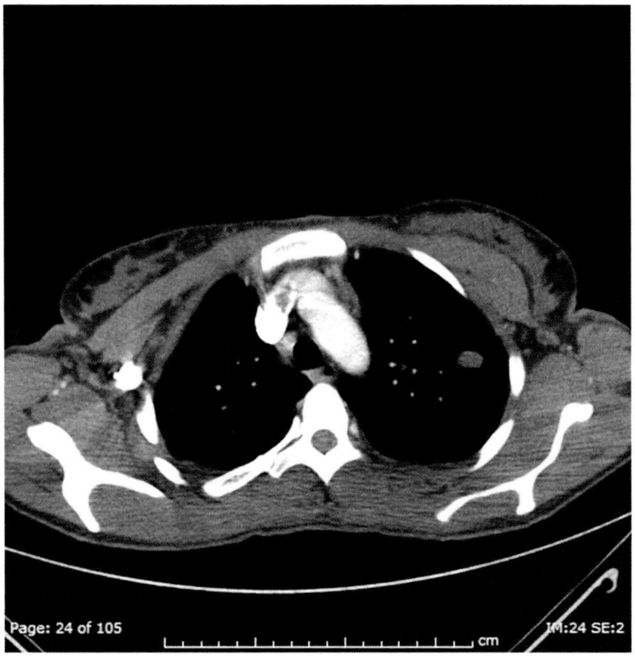

Figure 145-B

146. A 65-year-old patient with COPD has an FEV_1 of 28% predicted. In addition to this spirometry data, the recently described BODE score provides useful survival prediction data in this type of patient. What additional data are required to calculate this BODE score?

A. $Pa{O_2}$, $Pa{CO_2}$, and 6-min walk distance (6MWD).
B. Arterial pH, dyspnea score, and 6MWD.
C. Dyspnea score, BMI, and 6MWD.
D. Arterial pH, BMI, and residual volume.

147. A 24-year-old woman has had long-standing mild, persistent asthma for which she has been using approximately four puffs (44 µg/puff) per day of inhaled fluticasone and approximately two to four puffs of albuterol per week with good results. However, approximately 6 months ago, she and her husband bought and moved into a new house, which they are living in and slowly renovating. Although the main triggers to her asthma are believed to be cats and ragweed, she has noted a deterioration in her asthma since they moved in, despite multiple steps to limit her potential exposure to dust and mold during the renovations. She has continued her fluticasone at the same dose but is now using two puffs of albuterol four to six times per day. She awakens because of asthma symptoms approximately once per week, and although she has not curtailed her regular activities, she reports feeling "more winded than usual."

Physical examination results are notable only for rare scattered wheezes on exhalation. FEV_1 is 2.99 L (74% predicted), and FVC is 4.69 (98% predicted); the flow-volume loop shows mild expiratory coving.

Assuming that no additional opportunities for trigger avoidance are identified, what is the most appropriate next step in her pharmacologic management?

A. Add a long-acting β-agonist to her current dose of inhaled fluticasone.
B. Add montelukast to her current dose of inhaled fluticasone.
C. Add omalizumab therapy to her current dose of inhaled fluticasone.
D. Change her dose of inhaled fluticasone to four puffs bid of the 220 μg/puff preparation.

148. A 48-year-old male office worker received a diagnosis of pulmonary alveolar proteinosis 9 years ago secondary to sandblasting because of a 10-day history of increasing shortness of breath and nonproductive cough. He notes worsening chest heaviness, low-grade fevers (38.1°C), and lassitude. His symptoms are getting progressively worse. He underwent bilateral whole-lung lavage 8 years ago and has been well until the past 10 days, with no activity limitation and only occasional chest heaviness and infrequent cough. He played recreational hockey three times a week during the past 8 years. He denies hemoptysis, chills, or chest pain. His only medication is lisinopril for hypertension. Physical examination results are notable for a pulse of 82/min, BP of 135/75 mm Hg, respiratory rate of 20/min, temperature of 37.9°C, and an oxygen saturation of 94% on room air. Breath sounds are slightly reduced, and a few late-inspiratory crackles are present in both mid- and lower-lung fields. There are no signs of consolidation. His CBC results are normal except for a WBC count of 12,900/μL (12.9×10^9/L) (normal count is 4,500 to 11,000/μL [4.5 to 11.0×10^9/L]), with a normal differential count. He is unable to produce sputum for testing. Spirometry reveals an FEV_1 of 3.54 L (105% predicted), FVC of 4.16 L (93% predicted), and FEV_1/FVC of 0.85. The total lung capacity is 5.54 L (91% predicted), and the DLCO is 21.4 $mL \cdot min^{-1} \cdot mm\ Hg^{-1}$ (63% predicted). These results are unchanged from prior testing 6 months previously except for a previous DLCO of 74% predicted. His prior chest radiographs are not immediately available (you have requested them), but a chest radiograph from this visit is shown in Figures 148-A and 148-B.

What would you do next in the management of this patient?

A. Arrange for diagnostic bronchoscopy.
B. Start granulocyte-macrophage colony-stimulating factor (GM-CSF) therapy.
C. Arrange for therapeutic whole-lung lavage.
D. Begin IV methylprednisolone.

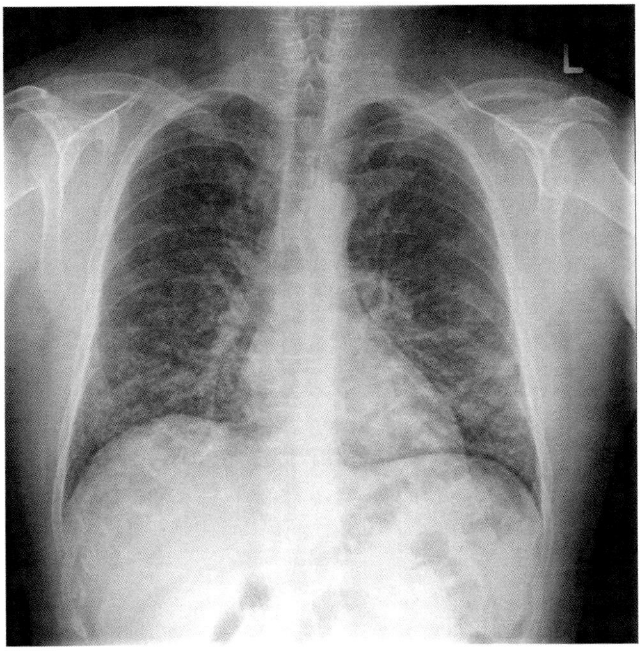

Figure 148-A

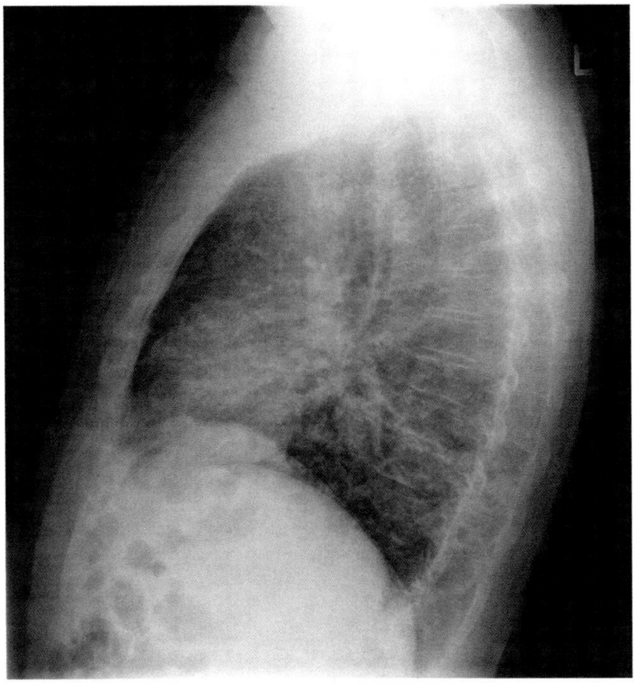

Figure 148-B

149. As opposed to patients who have typical pulmonary sarcoidosis, patients who have the nodular (nummular, alveolar) form:

A. Are more frequently young, white men.
B. More frequently have extrapulmonary involvement.
C. Less frequently display hilar adenopathy.
D. Have a better overall prognosis.

150. You are asked by the local health officer to attend a meeting regarding asbestos exposure in a community with several closed gold mines, as well as two active strip mines. Recent studies from a graduate student doing environmental sampling in the area detected low levels of asbestos in the local park, elementary school playground, and the center of town.

Which of the following is true regarding the community's risk of malignancy?

A. It is increased for malignant mesothelioma.
B. It is increased for bronchogenic carcinoma.
C. It is increased for laryngeal carcinoma.
D. There is no increased risk with low-level exposure to asbestos from industrial emissions.

151. A 24-year-old man with diabetes and chronic kidney disease is admitted with altered mental status and hyperglycemia. Laboratory tests revealed the following:

Arterial pH	7.10
Pco_2	35 mm Hg
Serum bicarbonate	12 mEq/L (12 mmol/L)
Sodium	140 mEq/L (140 mmol/L)
Chloride	112 mEq/L (112 mmol/L)
Potassium	3.5 mEq/L (3.5 mmol/L)
Phosphorus	4.0 mEq/L (1.3 mmol/L)
Albumin	2.5 g/dL (25 g/L)

Additional testing reveals absence of ethanol in the blood, the presence of ketones in the urine, and a positive urinary test result for opioids.

Which acid-base abnormality is present?

A. Anion gap metabolic acidosis + non-anion gap metabolic acidosis + respiratory acidosis.
B. Anion gap metabolic acidosis + non-anion gap metabolic acidosis + respiratory alkalosis.
C. Non-anion gap metabolic acidosis + chronic respiratory acidosis.
D. Metabolic acidosis only.

152. A 63-year-old man presents to the ED with fevers, weight loss, and malaise for 2 to 3 weeks. He has a history of myelodysplastic syndrome, which was diagnosed 3 years ago. He is currently taking prednisone, 20 mg daily. A chest CT scan is obtained, and representative images are shown in Figures 152-A and 152-B. An acid-fast stain of BAL fluid is negative. Thoracentesis reveals an exudate with no acid-fast bacilli noted. Mediastinoscopy is performed, and samples are acquired (see Figures 152-C and 152-D). DNA probes of growth in liquid culture medium confirm the presence of *Mycobacterium kansasii*.

Which of the following treatment regimens would you recommend?

A. Rifampin, ethambutol, and clarithromycin, each administered three times weekly.
B. Isoniazid, rifampin, and ethambutol.
C. Isoniazid, rifampin, ethambutol, and pyrazinamide.
D. Isoniazid, rifampin, ethambutol, and streptomycin three times weekly.

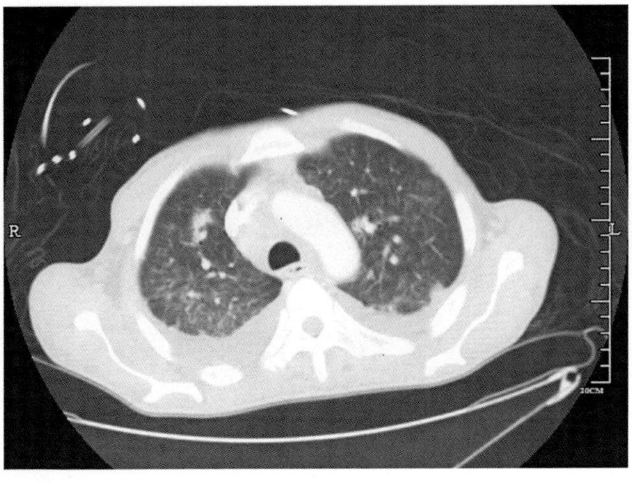

Figure 152-A

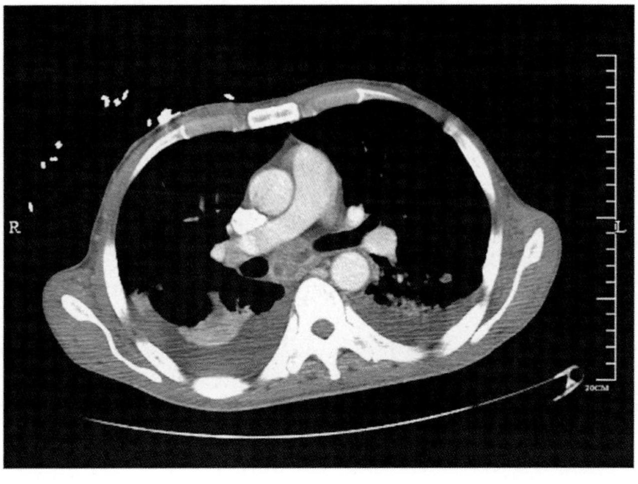

Figure 152-B

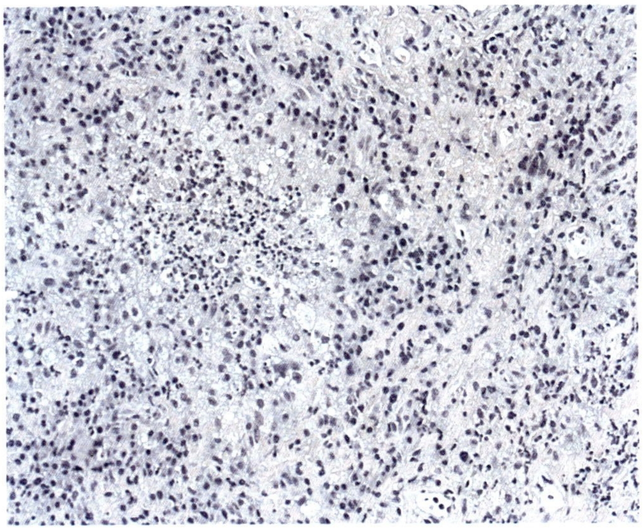

Figure 152-C

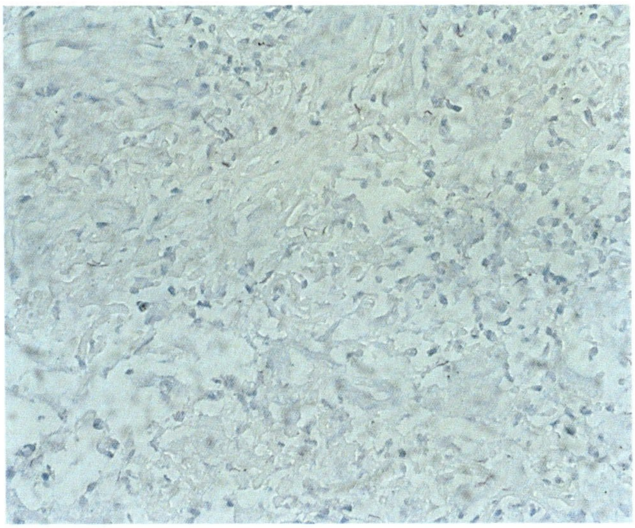

Figure 152-D

153. Which of the following patients would be most appropriate to undergo lung transplantation now?

A. A 32-year-old woman with cystic fibrosis. She has an FEV_1 of 0.9 L (25% predicted) and has required frequent hospitalizations for exacerbations with a recent sputum culture growing *Burkholderia cepacia* genomovar 3.
B. A 63-year-old man with tobacco-related COPD who stopped smoking 12 months ago. He has an FEV_1 of 0.8 L (20% predicted), a BODE score of 8, and no other significant medical history. He is being treated with prednisone, 20 mg po qd.
C. A 35-year-old woman with pulmonary hypertension and New York Heart Association class 3 symptoms. She is being treated with sildenafil.
D. A 69-year-old woman with usual interstitial pneumonitis. Her vital capacity is 58% of predicted. She is being treated with corticosteroids and azathioprine. She has a T score at the spine of -3 on bone densitometry.

154. A 19-year-old nonsmoking man complains of a history of cough, intermittently productive of yellow sputum, over the past several years. He does not have shortness of breath or chest pain and has never had hemoptysis or pneumonia, but he has had several sinus infections in the past. He is a marathon runner and has not noted a change in his exercise tolerance. He has no other medical history and is not taking any medications. He is not currently sexually active and has not had children.

On examination, he is appears well and is afebrile. There is no sinus tenderness. His heart sounds are normal but distant. He has scattered rhonchi on the right. There is no cyanosis or clubbing. Screening spirometry reveals FVC of 4.80 L (86% of predicted), FEV_1 of 3.61 L (77% of predicted), and FEV_1/FVC of 0.75. There is no significant response to inhaled bronchodilator. A high-resolution CT scan is obtained, and representative images are shown in Figures 154-A and 154-B.

Which of the following tests will most likely confirm the suspected diagnosis?

A. A sweat chloride test.
B. Assessment of sperm motility.
C. Quantitative immunoglobulins.
D. α_1-Antitrypsin level.

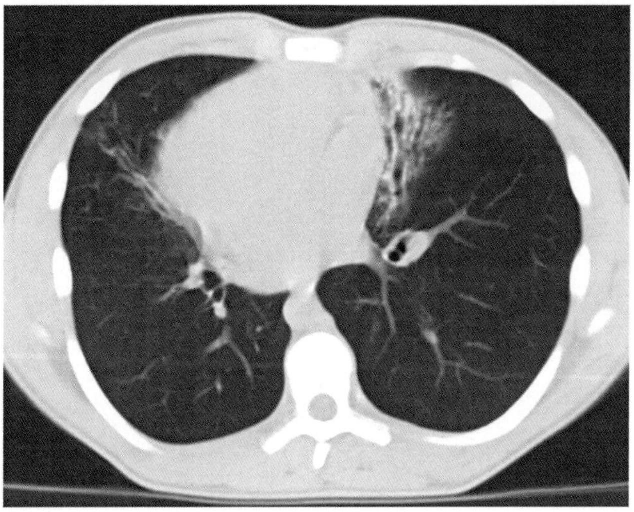

Figure 154-A

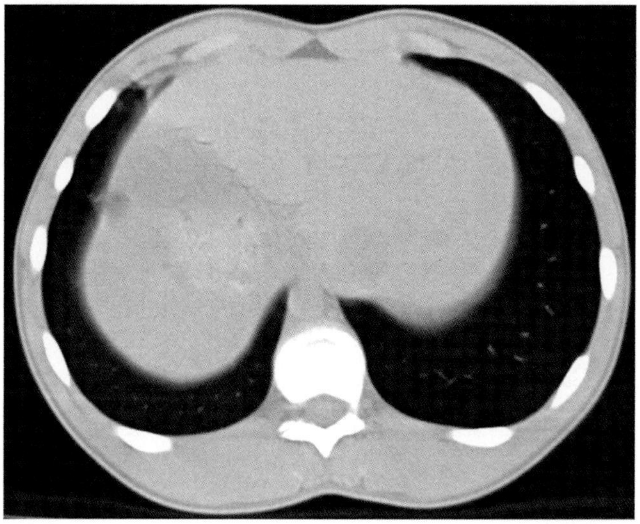

Figure 154-B

155. Addition of which of the following drugs is most likely to increase the serum theophylline concentration in a patient on a stable maintenance regimen?

A. Omeprazole.
B. Low-molecular-weight heparin.
C. Prednisone.
D. Clarithromycin.

156. A 46-year-old man is admitted with pain in his left posterior chest and a cough of 3 months' duration. He has a 25 pack-year smoking history. He has no fever, chills, weight loss, or sputum production. The salient abnormal CT images are shown in Figures 156-A and 156-B; there are no other radiographic abnormalities. Which of the following is the most likely diagnosis?

A. TB.
B. Lymphoma.
C. Small-cell carcinoma of the lung.
D. Malignant thymoma.

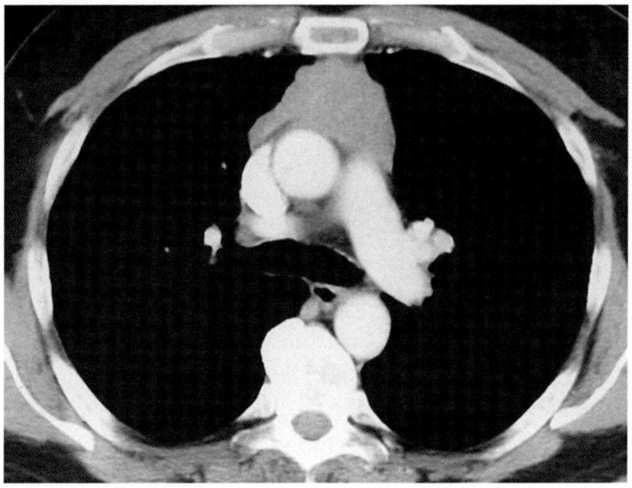

Figure 156-A

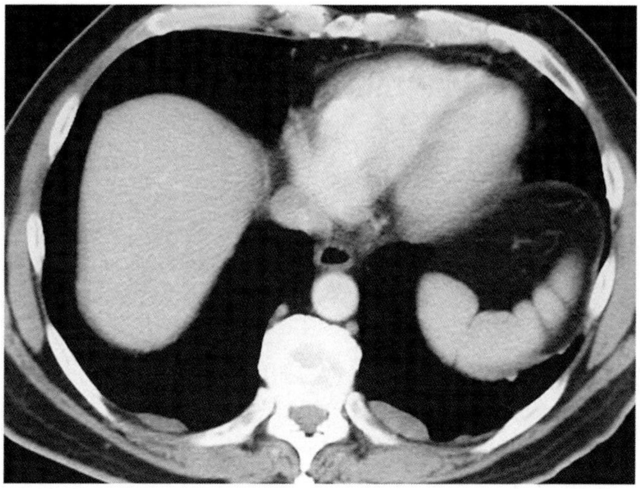

Figure 156-B

157. A 72-year-old woman was admitted to the hospital for management of pneumonia. She was well until 1 week prior to admission when she developed fever and flu-like symptoms. She denied cough, sputum production, hemoptysis, chest pain, or dyspnea. She arrived at the ED because of persistence of the flu-like symptoms. Physical examination revealed that she was febrile with a temperature of 38.4°C, BP of 147/82 mm Hg, irregular pulse of 147/min, and crackles audible in the left anterior chest. The hemoglobin level was 15.5 g/dL (155 g/L), WBC count was 10,500/μL (10.5 × 10^9/L) with a left shift, and platelet count was normal. Other routine chemistry results were normal except for a serum sodium concentration of 129 mEq/L (129 mmol/L). The admission chest radiograph and a CT taken the following day are shown (see Figures 157-A and 157-B). She was admitted to the ICU. The Legionella sp urinary antigen test result was positive. At this point, you would treat her with:

A. Clarithromycin + rifampin.
B. Levofloxacin.
C. Ceftriaxone.
D. Clarithromycin.

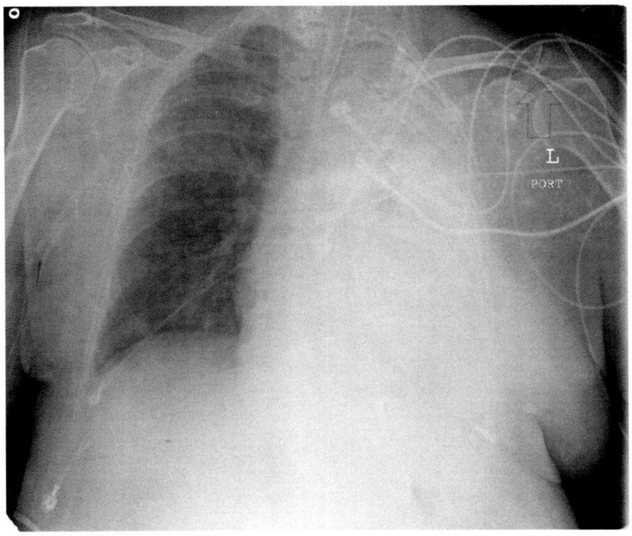

Figure 157-A

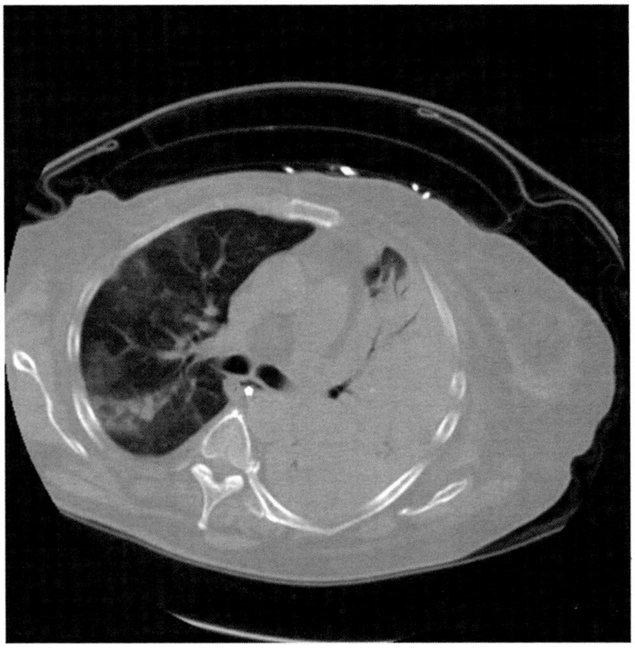
Figure 157-B

158. You are asked to assess a 23-year-old man regarding fever and progressive pulmonary infiltrates. He received a diagnosis of acute lymphoblastic leukemia in the Philippines 20 months previously and was treated with chemotherapy, leading to a remission. He subsequently received consolidative therapy with vincristine, dexamethasone, 6-mercaptopurine, and methotrexate. Routine testing of cerebrospinal fluid 6 months previously had revealed asymptomatic CNS involvement for which he was receiving intrathecal methotrexate and cytarabine therapy. After a second remission, he was switched to vinblastine, dexamethasone, doxorubicin, and L-asparaginase. However, 1 month earlier, he was again found to have peripheral blasts and was switched to etoposide therapy because there were no human leukocyte antigen–matched donors found. Six days after his initial 5-day infusion, he came to the ED with hypotension, dyspnea, a temperature of 39.5°C, and neutropenia. His blood culture results were positive for *Pseudomonas aeruginosa,* and therapy with piperacillin/tazobactam and tobramycin was started.

After a few days of therapy, he remained febrile, with a hemoglobin concentration of 8.1 g/dL (81 g/L) that had been stable for 2 months, WBC count of 33,000/μL (33.0 × 10^9/L), and a platelet count of 8 × 10^3/μL (8 × 10^9/L). His WBC differential included 300/μL (0.3 × 10^9/L) neutrophils, 3,000/μL (3.0 × 10^9/L) lymphocytes, and 28,380/μL (28.38 × 10^9/L) blasts. Representative images from his CT scan are shown in Figures 158-A and 158-B. Bronchoscopy revealed mucosal pallor and cough petechiae but was otherwise unremarkable, and the BAL return was clear. BAL results are shown in Figure 158-C. Papanicolaou and Gomori methenamine silver stain results were negative.

What is the most likely explanation for his pulmonary infiltrates?

A. Leukemic infiltrates.
B. Alveolar hemorrhage.
C. Fungal infection.
D. Chemotherapy-induced pneumonitis.

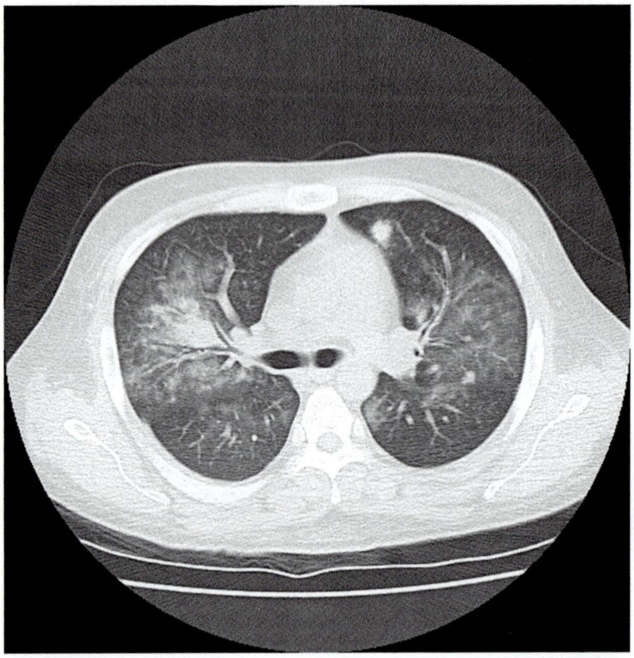

Figure 158-A

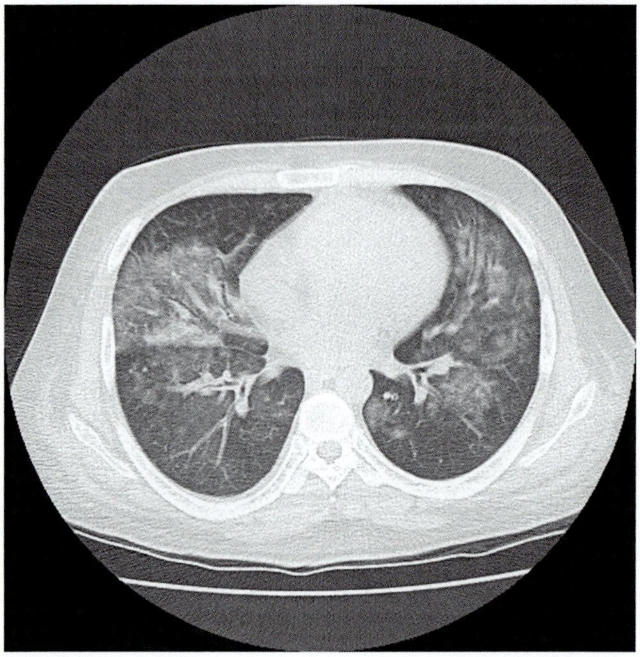

Figure 158-B

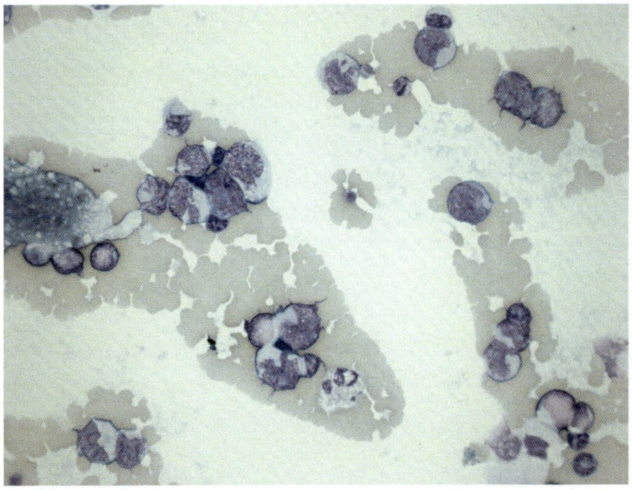

Figure 158-C
Romanowsky

159. You are asked to evaluate a 39-year-old man because of an abnormal CT of the chest obtained by his primary care physician at the patient's request to "look for cancer" (see Figure 159-A). The patient has a 20 pack-year smoking history and has no pulmonary symptoms. Physical examination is unremarkable. CBC and serum chemistry results are normal. A CT-directed core needle biopsy of the lesion (see Figure 159-A) is reported to show a tumor composed of spindle cells and hyaline collagen in a "patternless pattern." The spindle cells do not show mitotic activity. A representative area is shown in Figure 159-B. The lesion is CD34+ and keratin-negative, and immunohistochemical characteristics include vimentin.

Which of the following best describes this type of lesion?

A. Smoking increases the risk of developing this lesion.
B. Asbestos exposure plays an integral role in pathogenesis.
C. Distant metastases are unlikely.
D. Hypertrophic pulmonary osteoarthropathy is rare.

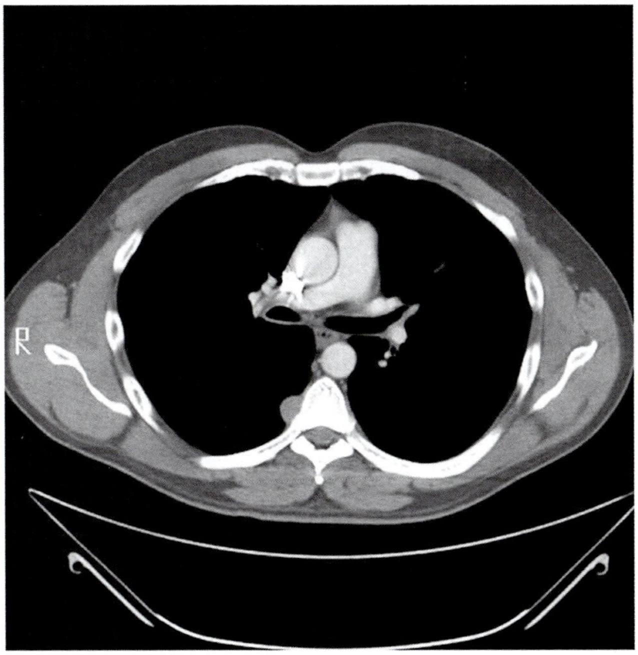

Figure 159-A

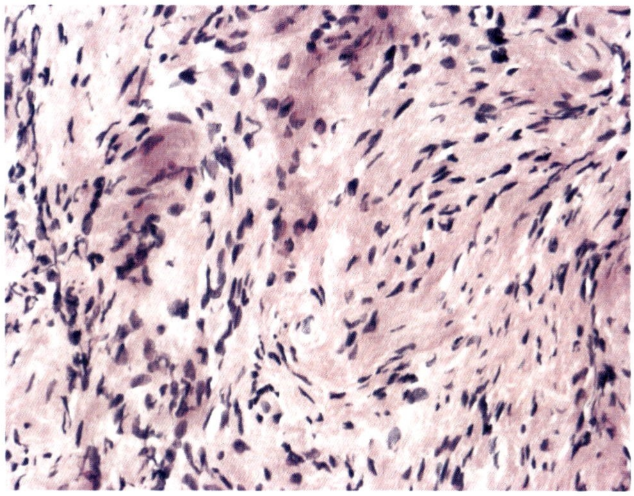

Figure 159-B
Hematoxylin-eosin

160. A 52-year-old man undergoes a total hip arthroplasty with the use of general anesthesia and endotracheal intubation. He is otherwise healthy and has no medical illnesses. He is extubated following surgery but develops stridor and begins to use his accessory muscles. With a decrease in his oxygen saturation to 65% despite the use of oxygen administered by full face mask, he is intubated. A chest radiograph reveals diffuse pulmonary edema with a "bat wing" appearance. An ECG reveals a sinus tachycardia. His BP is 120/60 mm Hg. His oxyhemoglobin saturation improved to 95% following intubation. In addition to providing mechanical ventilatory support with an F_{IO_2} of 60% and a PEEP of 5 cm H_2O, which of the following should be performed next?

A. CT angiogram.
B. Administer antibiotics.
C. Continue current therapy.
D. Increase PEEP.

161. A 60-year-old woman arrives at your office seeking advice for the management of a solitary pulmonary nodule and her risk of having lung cancer. She came to the ED 2 weeks ago with acute chest pain that ultimately proved to be a result of costochondritis, but during her evaluation, a chest CT with contrast was performed. This study revealed a left lower lobe lobulated nodule adjacent to the aorta that measured 21 mm in its greatest dimension (see Figure 161-A). This study also identified centrilobular emphysema throughout all lobes. No lymphadenopathy or extrapulmonary abnormalities were seen. No calcification was detected in the nodule.

The patient has no prior medical or surgical history. She has never had chest imaging prior to this event. She has smoked one pack of cigarettes daily for the past 40 years. Her symptoms of chest pain have resolved, and apart from

this, she has had no respiratory symptoms, weight loss, fevers, or sweats. She was born and raised in New York City. For the past 30 years, she has owned and operated a chain of stores and has spent her time divided between Chicago and Phoenix. A purified protein derivative test was done during her ED evaluation, and the result was negative. There is no personal or family history of cancer.

After the CT scan findings were obtained, an ^{18}F-fluorodeoxyglucose PET scan was performed, which demonstrated no increased uptake of the nodule relative to surrounding tissue. In view of the CT and PET findings coupled with the patient's demographics, which of the following statements concerning her risk of lung cancer is true?

A. Despite the relatively large size of the nodule and her long smoking history, the negative PET scan result makes the likelihood of lung cancer quite low and likely $<5\%$.
B. The location of the nodule in a lower lobe makes the risk of lung cancer higher than if the abnormality had been located in an upper lobe.
C. Given her smoking history and the large nodule, the risk of lung cancer remains at least 50% despite the PET scan findings.
D. If PET scanning is repeated in 6 months and the metabolic activity of the nodule is unchanged, the risk of malignancy is essentially zero.

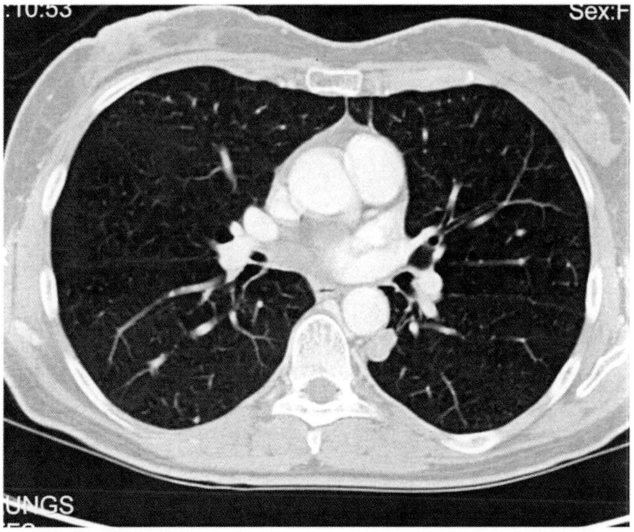

Figure 161-A

162. A 63-year-old man returns for follow-up for a previously diagnosed severe obstructive sleep apnea. His apnea-hypopnea index (AHI) during polysomnography was 62 events/h. Continuous positive airway pressure (CPAP) at a setting of 17 cm H_2O reduces the AHI to 6 events/h and normalizes oxygen saturation during sleep. Medical history includes hypertension and erectile dysfunction. He takes diphenhydramine for chronic postnasal discharge. Physical examination reveals a BMI of 34 kg/m^2. He has retrognathia, relative macroglossia, and a low-lying palate.

The patient is prescribed CPAP, and data on adherence downloaded from his device reveal the following:

Days, total	20 d
Days of device usage	7 d
Days without device usage	13 d
Percentage of days with device usage	35%
Average usage (days used)	1 h, 8 min
Percentage of days with usage ≥ 4 h	14%

Which of the following interventions would improve this patient's adherence to positive airway pressure (PAP) therapy?

A. Provision of heated humidification.
B. Addition of pressure relief technology to the PAP device.
C. Use of autotitrating positive airway pressure (APAP) devices.
D. Use of bilevel positive airway pressure therapy (BPAP).

163. A 68-year-old man is referred for chest pain and an abnormal chest radiograph. The patient reports the gradual onset of left-sided, constant, dull chest pain over 8 to 10 weeks. He reports marked shortness of breath and dyspnea with the chest pain but had resisted seeking medical care until now. He does not report fever, chills, or sweats but has noted a 12-lb weight loss. He also noted a dry cough without hemoptysis. His past medical history is unremarkable. He is a current smoker with a 50 pack-year history of tobacco use and has been self-employed as owner of a brake shop for 40 years. The findings of a physical examination are that he is in mild respiratory distress and has decreased breath sounds on the left, with decreased chest wall excursion. The results of a laboratory examination are notable for a hematocrit of 33% (0.33) and a platelet count of $550 \times 10^3/\mu L$ ($550 \times 10^9/L$). Room air saturation is 87%. His chest CT is shown in Figure 163-A. Which of the following statements regarding the most likely diagnosis is correct?

A. Tobacco is a likely contributing factor.
B. Calretinin staining of the tissue will be positive.
C. Hypoglycemia is present in 30% of patients.
D. Median survival with this process is 36 months.

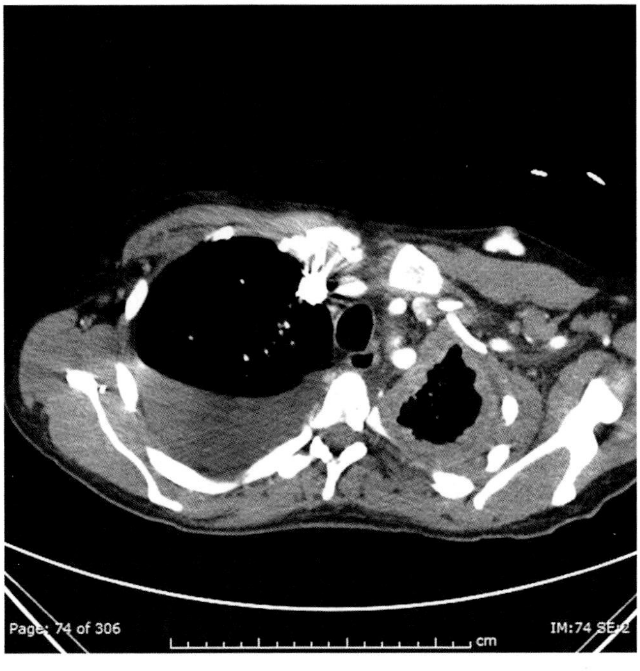

Figure 163-A

164. A severely obese patient (BMI of 53 kg/m^2) is supported by mechanical ventilation following knee replacement surgery complicated by aspiration. The portable chest radiograph shows small lung volumes and bibasilar opacities. The ventilator settings are volume-assist control, with a tidal volume of 530 mL (8 mL/kg ideal body weight), an FIO_2 of 1.0, and a PEEP setting of 12 cm H_2O. The blood gas results are PaO_2 of 52 mm Hg, $PaCO_2$ of 64 mm Hg, and a pH of 7.18. The plateau pressure is 38 cm H_2O. Which adjustment to the ventilator should be made to address the hypoxemia and still maintain optimal lung protection from ventilator-induced lung injury?

A. Increase PEEP and accept higher plateau pressure.
B. Increase PEEP and reduce tidal volume to limit plateau pressure from rising further.
C. Increase tidal volume and reduce PEEP to limit plateau pressure from rising further.
D. Reduce tidal volume and PEEP to reduce plateau pressure and increase the set rate.

165. Which of the following sedatives can cause reversible suppression of the adrenal cortex?

A. Etomidate.
B. Ketamine.
C. Midazolam.
D. Propofol.

166. You are asked to see a 29-year-old woman with hereditary hemorrhagic telangiectasia (HHT) who is contemplating pregnancy. The diagnosis was made 7 years previously after she was referred for nosebleeds. She has had documented pulmonary atrioventricular (AV) malformations, twice treated with angiography and coils, the last time 3 years ago. Results of a cerebral MRI were normal at the time of initial diagnosis. She is currently asymptomatic and specifically denies hemoptysis, shortness of breath, activity limitation, or headaches. Her only medication is iron supplementation for chronic anemia, although she does receive prophylactic treatment with an antibiotic for dental procedures. She has four sisters and one brother who all have HHT. She is awaiting assessment by an obstetrician. Physical examination is notable for a room air oxygen saturation of 98% and scattered mucocutaneous telangiectasias. Her CBC results are normal. Spirometry reveals an FEV_1 of 3.59 L (116% predicted), FVC of 4.65 L (118% predicted), and an FEV_1/FVC of 0.75. The total lung capacity is 6.14 L (115% predicted), and the DLCO is 21.3 $mL \cdot min^{-1} \cdot mm\ Hg^{-1}$ (72% predicted). A chest radiograph is shown (see Figures 166-A and 166-B).

A physiologic shunt study reveals a shunt fraction of 5.8%. A CT scan of the chest does not reveal any new AV malformations or feeding vessels and is unchanged from a study conducted 18 months ago. How would you advise this patient?

A. Pregnancy is contraindicated in patients with HHT.
B. She should undergo a cerebral MRI prior to getting pregnant.
C. Continuous antibiotic prophylaxis should be offered to prevent intrauterine infection.
D. This would be a low-risk pregnancy, and no unique precautions would be required.

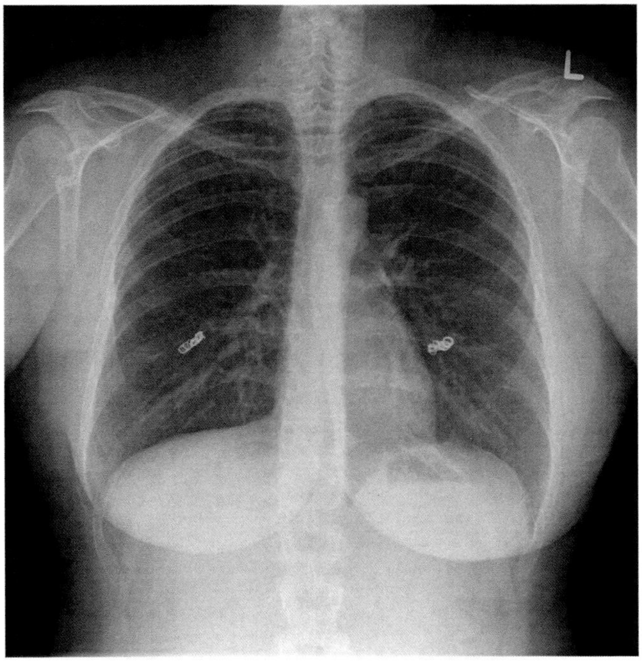

Figure 166-A

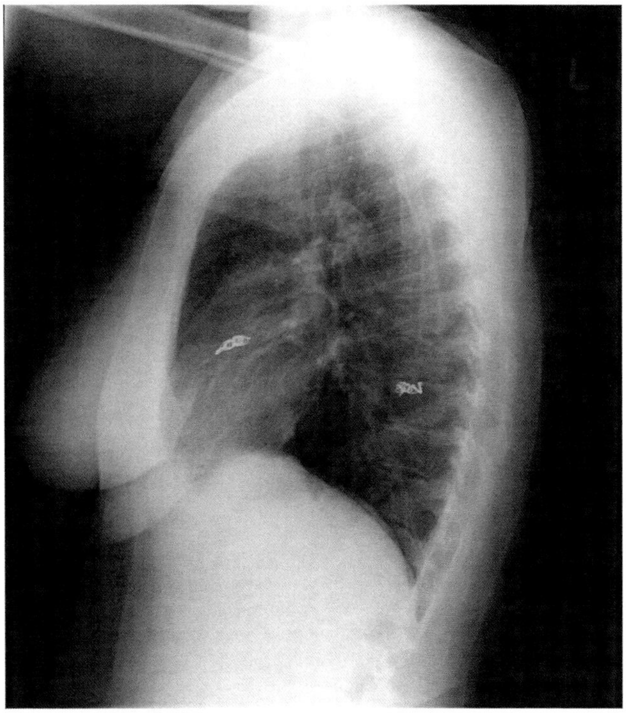

Figure 166-B

167. A 76-year-old woman with a history of hypertension and hyperlipidemia complains of a several-month history of progressive fatigue and dyspnea on exertion. She states that she has also had a cough productive of yellow-green sputum, that has often been blood-streaked, over the past 3 weeks. She reports mild night sweats and a 15-lb weight loss over 3 months but has not had any fevers. She is a lifelong nonsmoker with no history of lung disease. She does not drink alcohol. Medications include irbesartan, 150 mg twice daily; metoprolol, 100 mg twice daily; and simvastatin, 10 mg daily. The results of physical examination reveal a thin, elderly woman with moderate kyphoscoliosis. She is afebrile. Pulmonary examination findings show mild rhonchi in the upper lung fields, but otherwise, results are normal. The results of the rest of the physical examination are normal. Chest radiograph reveals a hazy infiltrate in the right midlung. Follow-up chest CT reveals scattered bilateral nodular densities, particularly in the right middle lobe and lingular regions (see Figure 167-A). Sputum samples are sent to the laboratory on 3 successive days, and all three eventually grow *Mycobacterium avium* complex (MAC). The recommended treatment would be:

A. Clarithromycin, ethambutol, and rifampin daily.
B. Clarithromycin, ethambutol, rifampin, and amikacin daily.
C. Clarithromycin, ethambutol, and rifampin three times weekly.
D. Clarithromycin, ethambutol, rifampin, and amikacin three times weekly.

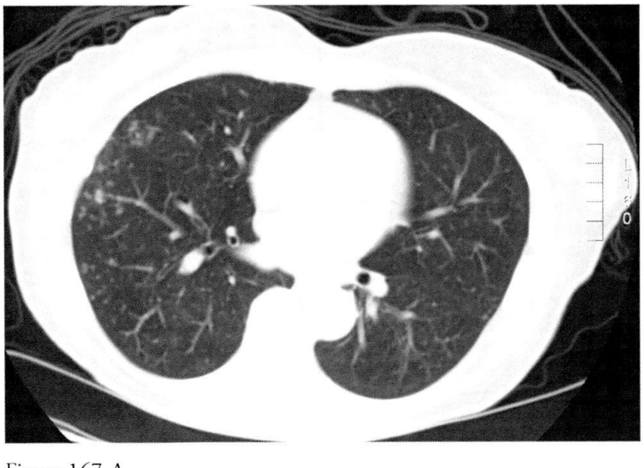

Figure 167-A

168. A 47-year-old man is admitted to the hospital after a narcotics overdose and is intubated in the ED. The results of his chest radiograph are shown in Figure 168-A. He has had a 2-month duration of fevers, chills, night sweats, and a 9-kg weight loss. He emigrated from Cambodia to the United States 11 months ago and is working as a migrant farm worker. He does not speak English and lives with his wife, four children, mother-in-law, sister-in-law, and four nieces and nephews in a small house near a farm. He has a 30 pack-year history of tobacco use and does not use recreational drugs. He has no history of TB, and his tuberculin skin test was nonreactive at the refugee camp in Cambodia prior to immigration.

An acid-fast smear of an induced sputum sample yields a positive result for multiple acid-fast bacilli (AFB). He is started on isoniazid, rifampin, pyrazinamide, and ethambutol. After 2 weeks of therapy, he is discharged and sent home, with county public health management of his TB therapy.

Eight weeks later, he returns under direct admission by order of the county health officer. He had been receiving directly observed therapy (DOT) 3 days a week, but compliance has been difficult to obtain because of his work on the farm and interference from his large family. Without a translator in his local dialect, management of some depression symptoms, nausea, and fatigue also has been difficult. His AFB culture grew *Mycobacterium tuberculosis,* and susceptibility testing results showed that his strain was resistant to isoniazid, rifampin, ciprofloxacin, and the aminoglycosides (amikacin). He is maintained on therapy with pyrazinamide and ethambutol, and cycloserine, paraaminosalicylic acid (PAS), clofazimine, and ethionamide are added.

Which of the following is the best course of treatment?

A. Six-drug therapy for 12 months.
B. Six-drug therapy for 6 months and two-drug therapy for 12 months, followed by surgical resection of the cavity.
C. Six-drug therapy for 3 months followed by surgical resection of the cavity with postoperative therapy for 18 months.
D. Surgical therapy now followed by six-drug therapy for 18 months.

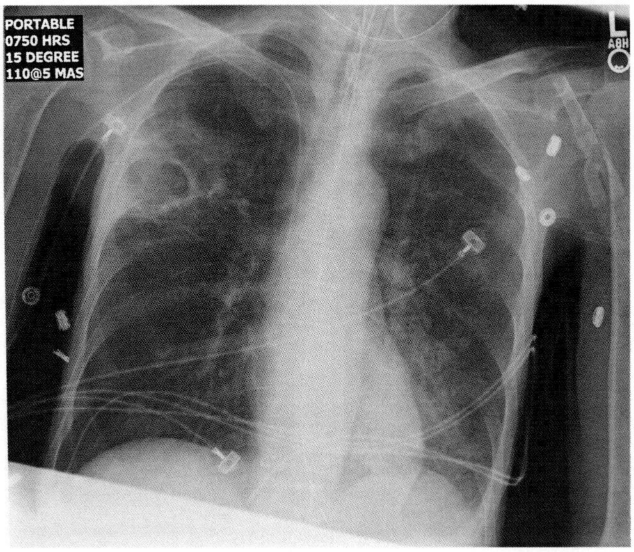

Figure 168-A

169. A 74-year-old man is admitted to the ICU after having a stroke. He is comatose. You note that he has an unusual respiratory pattern and retrieve a graphic record of his respirations from the bedside monitoring software, which are displayed in Figure 169-A.

Which of the following respiratory patterns is displayed in the tracing?

A. Cheyne-Stokes.
B. Cluster breathing.
C. Apneustic breathing.
D. Central neurogenic hyperventilation.

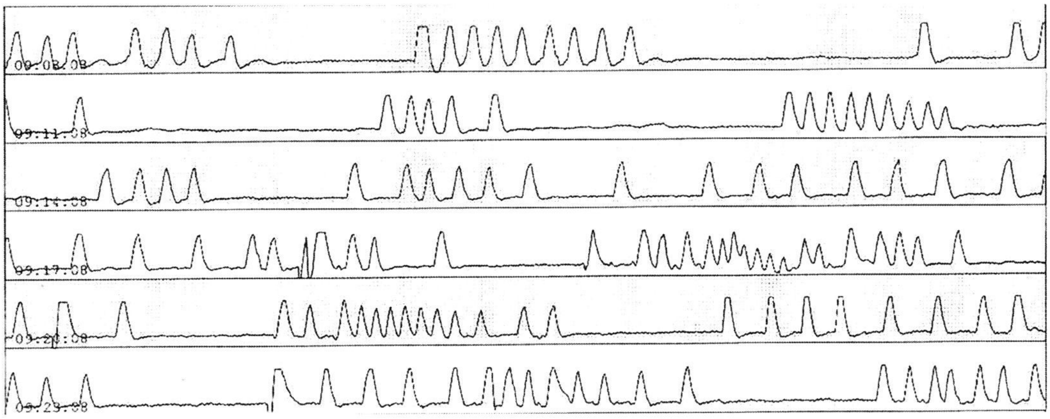

Figure 169-A

170. A 55-year-old woman is referred for evaluation of progressive exertional dyspnea. She also describes wheezing that occurs when she walks fast and states that both symptoms occur when she bends over or reaches overhead. She also states that she has been in good health and has not seen a physician in many years, although she was told she had an enlarged thyroid gland years ago. Upon questioning, she admits to recent onset of mild heat intolerance and nervousness. Physical examination is remarkable for an enlarged nodular thyroid gland and heart rate of 100/min. Lung examination is clear at rest, but faint wheezing is produced when she breathes rapidly. A radiograph of the neck is shown in Figure 170-A.

In addition to performing spirometry with a flow volume loop, which of the following should you do first?

A. Contrast CT scan of the chest.
B. Ultrasound of the cervical thyroid gland.
C. Radionuclide thyroid scan.
D. Thyroid function tests.

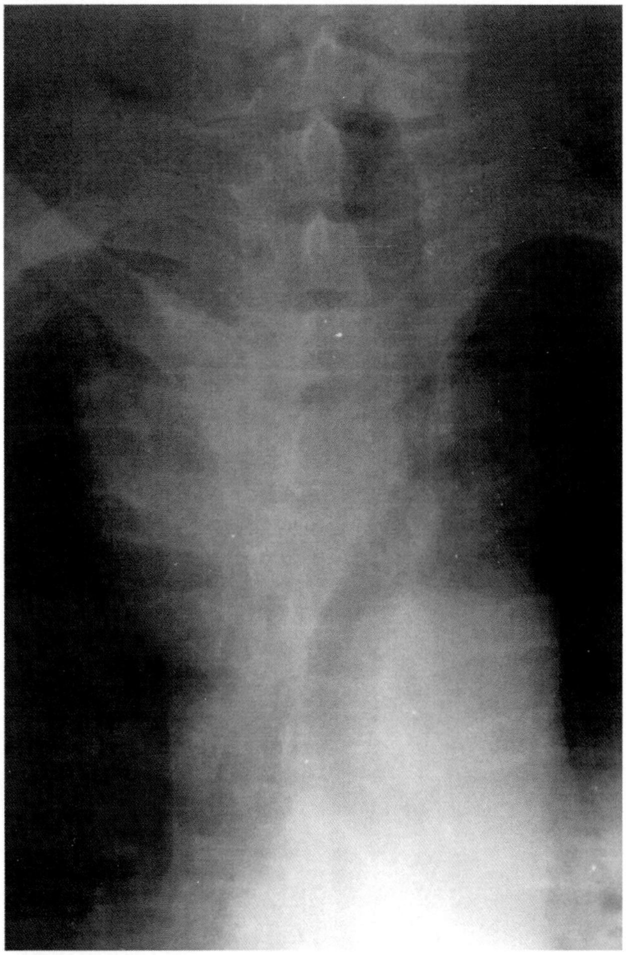

Figure 170-A

171. You are asked to consult on a 30-year-old woman with lung infiltrates. She has a 2-year history of ulcerative colitis treated with enteric-coated 5-aminosalicylic acid. One month ago, she was switched to mesalamine because of light-headedness, headaches, and nausea. Over the past 3 weeks, she noted a nonproductive cough, night sweats, and progressive exertional dyspnea. She was sent to the ED where her family physician ordered a chest radiograph that showed infiltrates.

On examination, her BP is 93/65 mm Hg, pulse is 90/min, respiratory rate is 18/min, and temperature is 36.7°C. Left basal crackles are audible. Blood work indicates a hemoglobin level of 8.5 g/dL (85 g/L) and WBC count of 10,800/μL (10.8×10^9/L), with 10% eosinophils. The sedimentation rate is 120 mm/h. Serum electrolytes, creatinine, urea, and liver function study results are normal. Urinalysis results are negative. A chest radiograph and chest CT scan are shown in Figures 171-A and 171-B.

Which of the following is the best next step?

A. Give azithromycin and ceftriaxone.
B. Initiate isoniazid, rifampin, pyrazinamide, and ethambutol pending culture results.
C. Stop mesalamine and consider prednisone therapy.
D. Arrange video-assisted thoracoscopic lung biopsy.

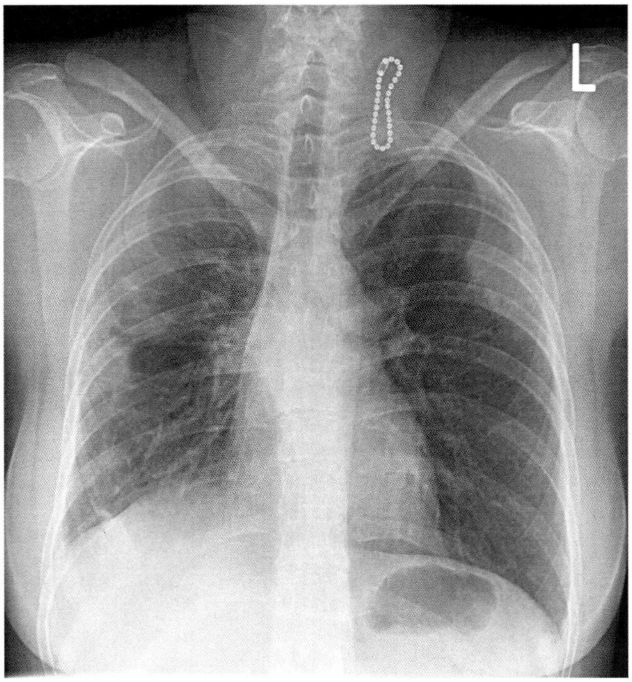

Figure 171-A

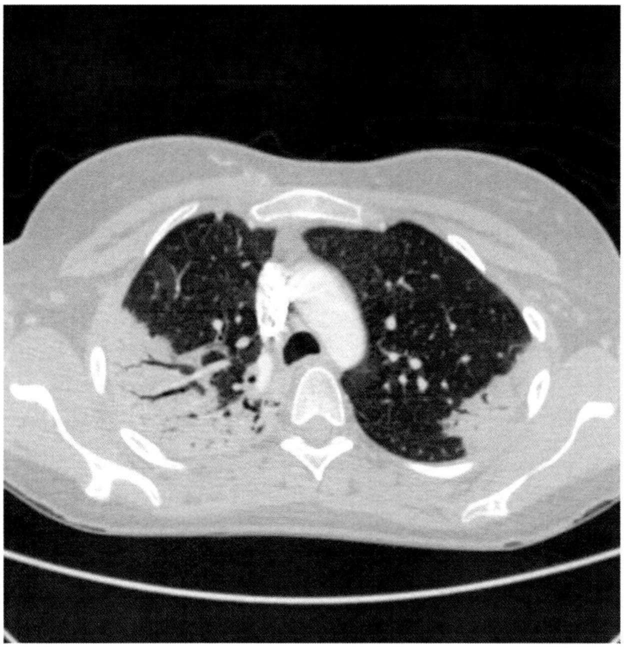

Figure 171-B

172. A 54-year-old man developed progressive dyspnea with effort and presyncope when climbing stairs. He was previously well except for having Raynaud phenomenon and symptoms suggestive of gastroesophageal reflux. He had mild telangiectasia over the chest and early sclerodactyly. He did not have clubbing or cyanosis. Respiratory rate was 28/min and resting oxygen saturation was 94% while receiving 4 L of oxygen by nasal prongs. Examination of the heart revealed an elevation in his jugular venous pulsation, right ventricular lift, loud pulmonic component of the second heart sound, and systolic murmur that increased on inspiration. Auscultation of the lungs was normal. FVC was 78% predicted, and FEV_1 was 75% predicted. DLCO was 52% predicted. Transthoracic echocardiography showed a right ventricular systolic pressure of 75 mm Hg (estimated right atrial pressure of 10 mm Hg) and moderate right ventricular dilation and dysfunction. Left ventricular function was graded as I out of IV. Ventilation-perfusion lung scan was rated as low probability for pulmonary embolism. CT scan of the chest is shown in Figures 172-A and 172-B.

The patient was taken to the cardiac catheterization laboratory for a formal hemodynamic assessment, revealing the following data:

Heart rate	88/min
Right atrial pressure, mm Hg (systolic/diastolic/mean)	22/14/16
Right ventricular pressure, mm Hg	65/8/37
Pulmonary arterial pressure, mm Hg	63/32/48
Pulmonary artery occlusion pressure, mm Hg (mean)	12
Cardiac index, $L/min/m^2$	1.3
Pulmonary vascular resistance, $dynes \cdot s \cdot cm^{-5}$	1,450
Mixed venous oxygen saturation	61%

Owing to his advanced disease, an indwelling tunneled central venous catheter was inserted, and he was started on continuous epoprostenol sodium. Two days later, he developed increasing breathlessness and worsening hypoxemia. What is the most likely diagnosis?

A. Left heart failure.
B. Worsening interstitial lung disease from scleroderma.
C. Pulmonary venoocclusive disease.
D. Lymphangitic spread of cancer.

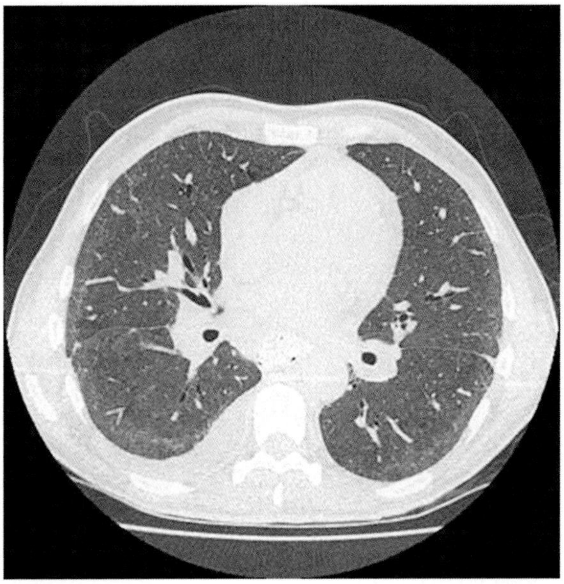

Figure 172-A

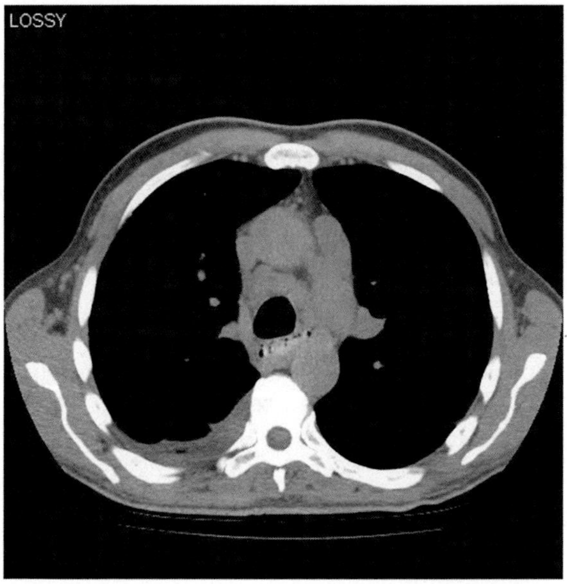

Figure 172-B

173. What is most likely explanation for the abnormality in the posteroanterior (PA) and lateral chest films shown in Figure 173-A?

A. Left pleural effusion.
B. Left upper lobe collapse.
C. Unilateral pulmonary edema.
D. Left hemidiaphragm paresis.

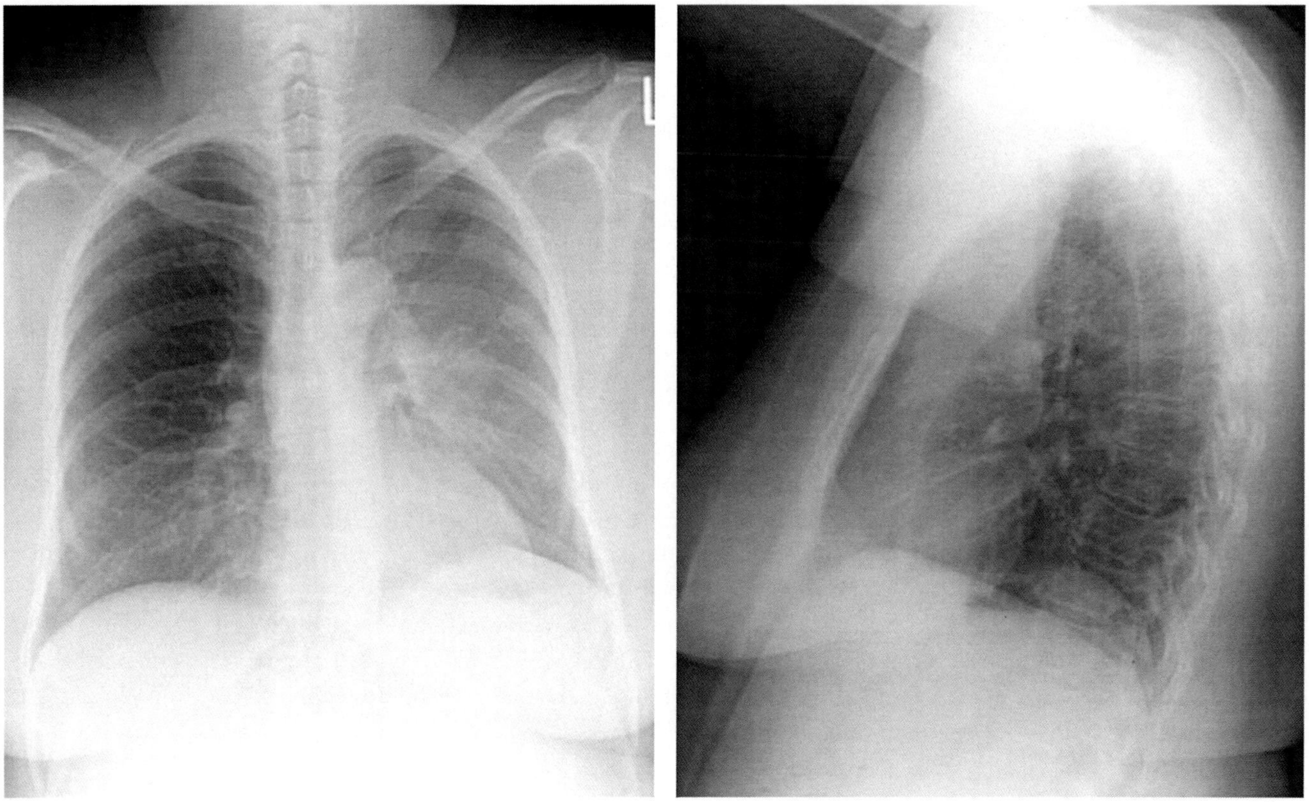

Figure 173-A

174. A 60-year-old women arrives at the ED complaining of vague chest discomfort, dyspnea, neck fullness, and increasing nontender abdominal distension that developed over the past day after a brief coughing spell precipitated by drinking water. The patient denies any history of dysphagia, noting that she was distracted while drinking water during a conversation, causing her to aspirate the water. She has no significant past medical history, takes no medications, and is a lifelong nonsmoker. Vital signs are a BP of 120/60 mm Hg, a respiratory rate of 16/min, heart rate of 90/min, temperature of 37.0°C, and room air oxygen saturation of 97%. The patient is mildly anxious and has subcutaneous crepitation of the neck, shoulders, and anterior and posterior back. Cardiac and respiratory examination results are normal. The abdomen is distended and nontender, with tympany. A chest radiograph is obtained (see Figure 174-A) prompting a CT of the chest, abdomen, and pelvis. A representative section is shown in Figure 174-B. Formal interpretation of the CT notes no esophageal abnormalities. Laboratory evaluation includes a normal WBC count (without a left shift) and normal sodium, potassium, chloride, bicarbonate, and creatinine values.

Which of the following management options should be pursued next?

A. Drainage of the pericardium.
B. Surgical exploration of the abdomen.
C. Upper GI endoscopy.
D. Observation.

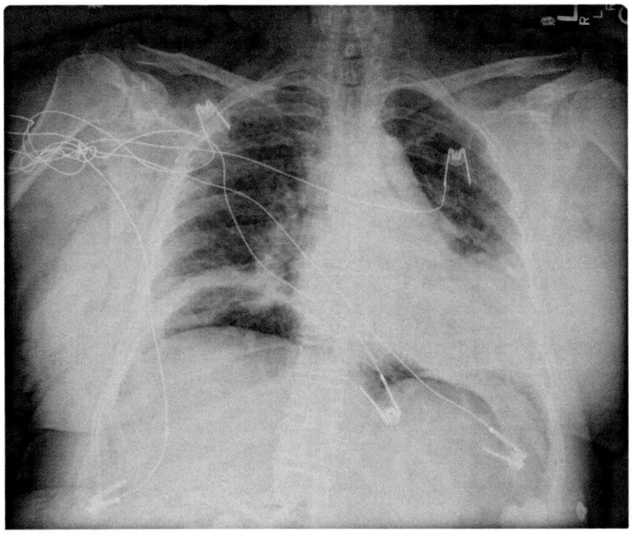

Figure 174-A

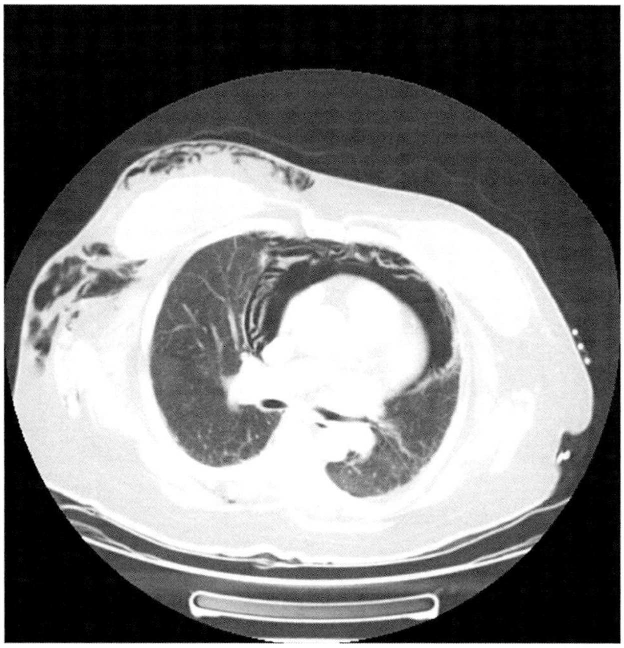

Figure 174-B

175. A 36-year-old woman is referred for an evaluation of a chronic, productive cough that has been persistent for the past 5 to 6 years. She notes purulent sputum each morning and mild dyspnea on exertion. For her symptoms, she has been repeatedly treated with antibiotics without a durable response. She was hospitalized 8 months ago, at which time she received a diagnosis of multifocal *Staphylococcus aureus* pneumonia. Her past history is notable for recurrent sinus infections and bronchitis. She was hospitalized once during adolescence for "pneumonia." Pulmonary function tests from her visit today demonstrate mild-to-moderate airflow limitation with an elevated residual volume. Based on her symptoms and radiographic abnormalities (see Figures 175-A and 175-B), a sweat chloride test is performed that shows increased levels of 85 and 78 mEq/L (85 and 78 mmol/L). The patient is interested in genetic counseling to see if additional counseling is warranted for her family members. What would be the most appropriate genetic testing in this setting?

A. *hTERT* and *hTR*.
B. ΔF508 *CFTR*.
C. Hemoglobin electrophoresis.
D. α_1-Antitrypsin.

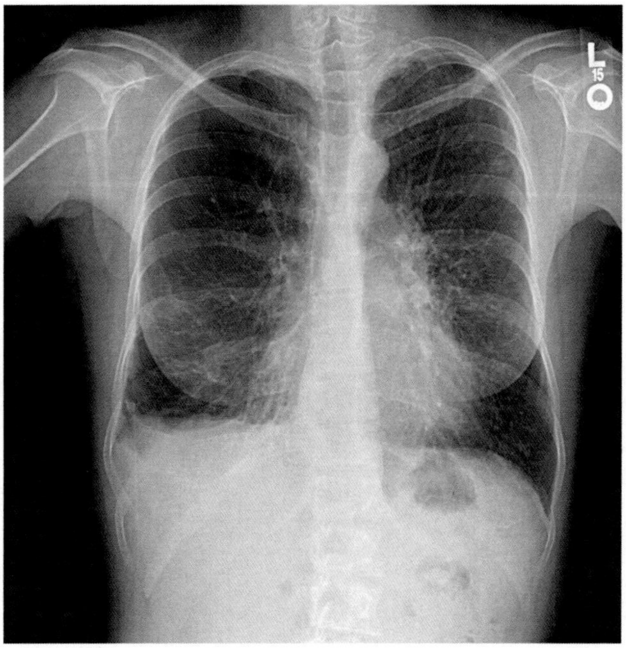

Figure 175-A

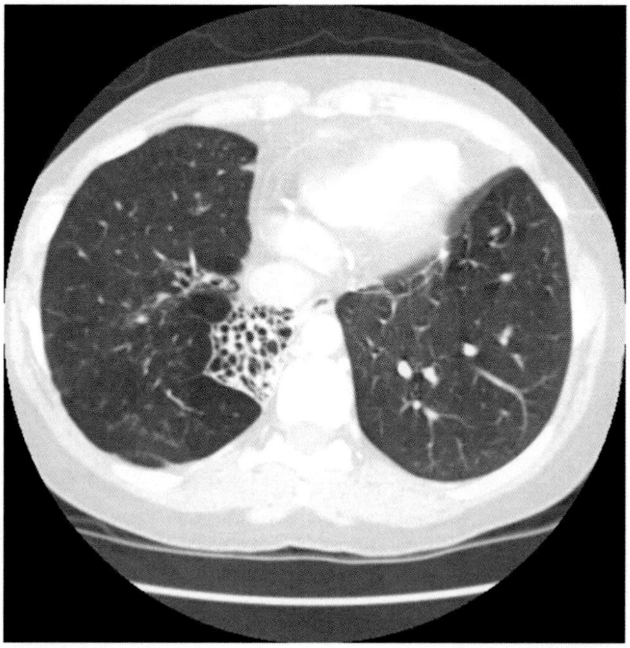

Figure 175-B

176. A patient is referred for thoracentesis. She is a 54-year-old woman with a 4-year history of cryptogenic cirrhosis characterized by intermittent episodes of hepatic encephalopathy but no evidence of ascites. In view of her progressive cirrhosis, an evaluation for liver transplantation began 6 months ago. This evaluation demonstrated a 5-cm mass of the right lobe of the liver that proved to be hepatocellular carcinoma on biopsy. Four months ago, the patient underwent chemoembolization of the hepatic tumor, which was repeated 2 months ago. By evaluation using CT scan, the tumor underwent necrosis and shrank substantially in size. A chest radiograph obtained during the hospitalization 2 months ago (see Figure 176-A) was unremarkable. In view of the salutary response to chemoembolization, the patient was placed on the liver transplant list.

Two weeks ago, the patient noted the onset of an unproductive cough and progressive shortness of breath. These symptoms were accompanied by dull aching in the right chest that was most noticeable deep to the scapula. She came to the clinic and was noted to be tachypneic when she moved about the examining room, with an Sao_2 86% on room air that improved to 94% with 3 L oxygen by nasal cannula. A chest radiograph (see Figure 176-B) was obtained, and the patient was admitted.

She has not experienced fevers, chills, leg pain, or hemoptysis. Her examination is remarkable for dullness to percussion and diminished breath sounds throughout the right posterior chest. Her abdominal examination is unremarkable.

Her admission laboratory tests are as follows:

WBC count	7,800/μL (7.8×10^9/L)
Differential count	74 PMN,* 6 bands, 20 lymphocytes
Total bilirubin	5.5 mg/dL (94.5 μmol/L)
LDH	100 U/L (1.67 μkat/L)
Platelet count	158×10^3/μL (158×10^9/L)
Albumin	2.8 g/dL (28 g/L)
INR*	1.9
Serum glucose	249 mg/dL (13.8 mmol/L)

* PMN = polymorphonuclear leukocytes; INR = international normalized ratio.

A thoracentesis is performed under ultrasound guidance, which yields 1.8 L of turbid yellow fluid with the following characteristics:

Total cell count	4,221
	(1,540 RBCs, 2,681 WBCs [94% PMNs])
pH	6.7
Amylase	50 U/L (0.83 μkat/L)
LDH	1,195 U/L (20 μkat/L)
Total bilirubin	18.4 mg/dL (315 μmol/L)
Total protein	2.6 g/dL (20 g/L)
Glucose	169 mg/dL (9.4 mmol/L)

This presentation and these findings are most consistent with:

A. Spontaneous bacterial peritonitis with ascitic fluid migrating across the diaphragm.
B. Pneumonia with empyema.
C. Pancreatic pseudocyst with communication to the pleural space.
D. Pleurobiliary fistula.

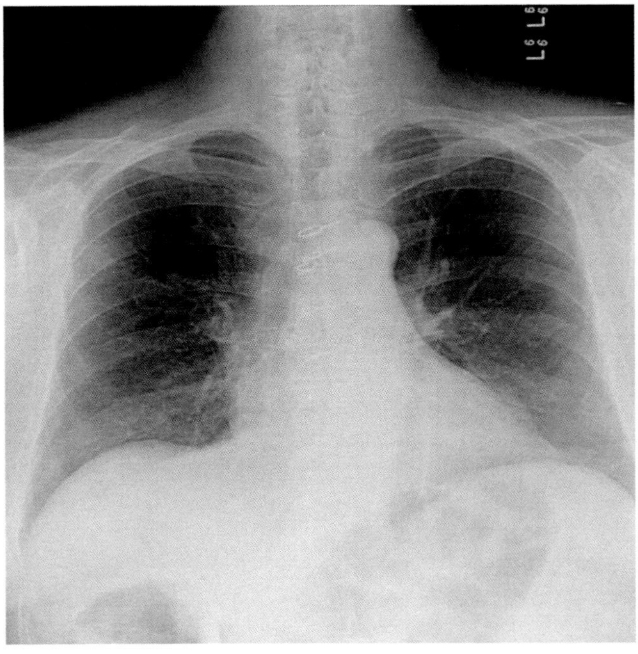

Figure 176-A

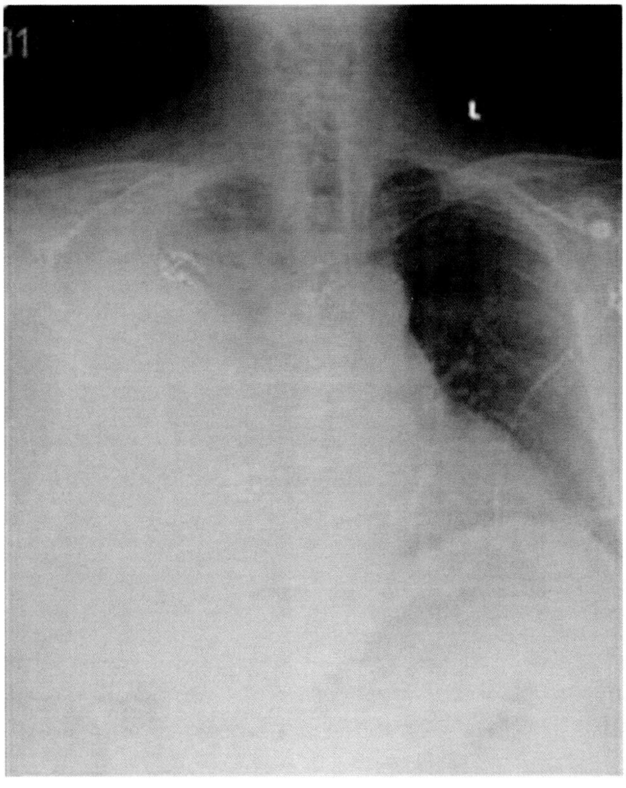

Figure 176-B

177. Which of the following patients should receive isoniazid prophylaxis for latent TB infection (LTBI)?

A. A 50-year-old man with rheumatoid arthritis with a purified protein derivative (PPD) result of 12-mm induration being evaluated for infliximab therapy. His chest radiograph is clear.
B. A 45-year-old woman who is an office worker. A PPD test placed during an executive physical shows a 12-mm induration. Her last PPD test from 5 years ago was nonreactive. She has no underlying medical problems. Her chest radiograph is clear.
C. A 53-year-old man who is an HIV-negative injection drug user and has a PPD result of 8-mm induration. His chest radiograph is clear.
D. A 60-year-old man who was a former foundry worker with a PPD result of 13-mm induration. He reports a chronic cough over the past year. A chest radiograph shows mixed upper lobe disease with areas of progressive massive fibrosis and fibrocavitary changes.

178. A 37-year-old woman is supported by mechanical ventilation for pancreatitis-related ARDS. She is receiving volume-assist control ventilation with 6-mL/kg ideal body weight (IBW) tidal volumes. However, she appears quite uncomfortable; her ventilator graphics are shown in Figure 178-A, left panel. You make a change in ventilator settings, which seems to make her more comfortable (see Figure 178-A, right panel).

What is the change?

A. Mode change to pressure-assist control ventilation.
B. Flow profile change to constant flow setting.
C. Flow profile change to sine wave flow setting.
D. Tidal volume increase to 7 mL/kg IBW.

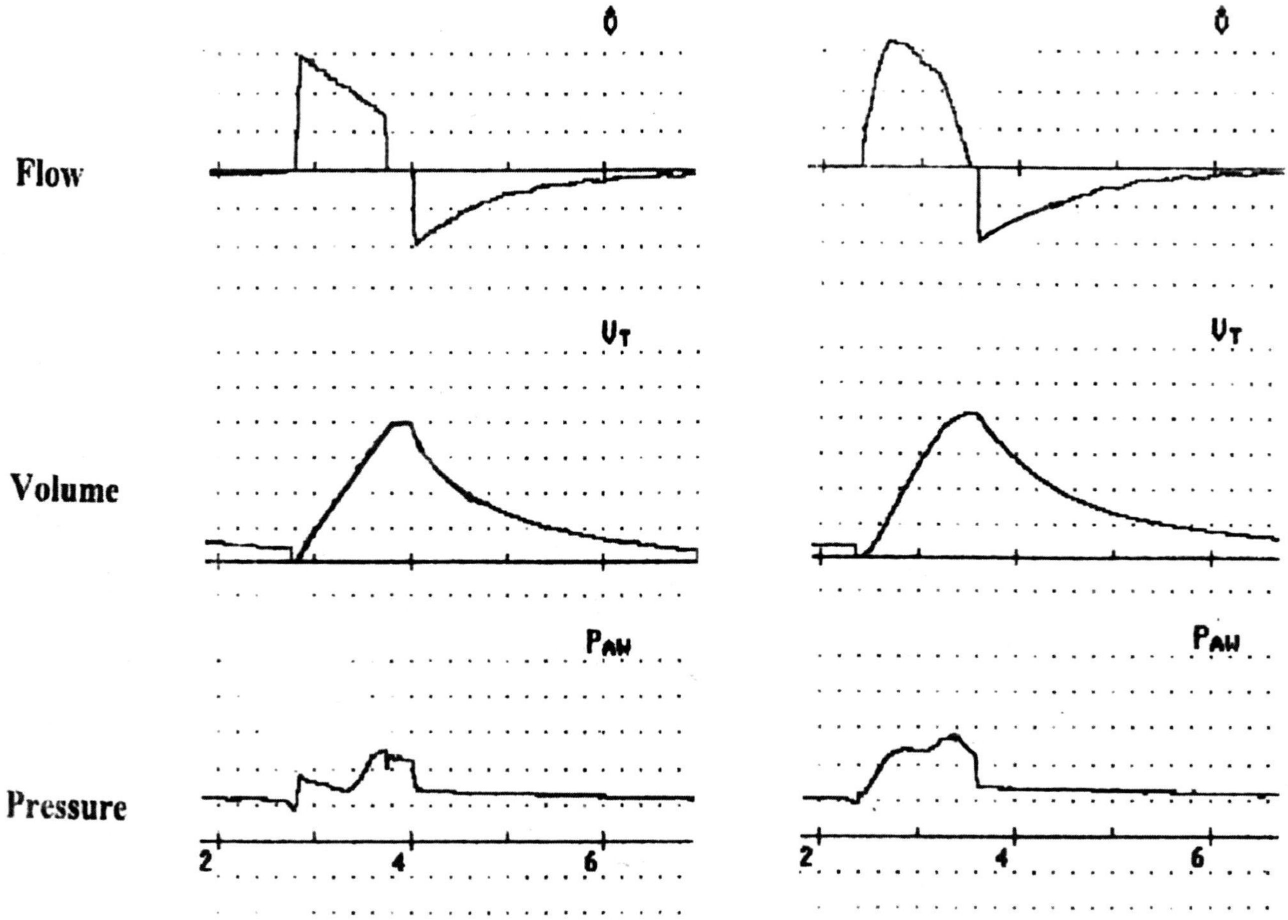

Figure 178-A

179. A 17-year-old adolescent girl is referred to you for assessment of difficult-to-control asthma. She received a diagnosis of asthma at age 15 years, and her symptoms have persisted despite therapy with albuterol, budesonide, montelukast, and, for the past 3 months, a combination inhaled corticosteroid/long-acting β_2-agonist (her current medication). She uses salbutamol about five times per day. She and her mother confirm that she is adherent. She has never been admitted to the hospital for asthma and denies sinus congestion, hay fever, acetylsalicylic acid intolerance, or dyspepsia. She is adopted. There are no pets at home, and she has no unusual hobbies. Results of her physical examination are normal, and results from a chest radiograph are normal, as well. Spirometry reveals an FEV_1 of 2.80 L (96% predicted), FVC of 3.43 L (112% predicted), and an FEV_1/FVC of 0.82. These spirometry results are after using a bronchodilator: two puffs of salbutamol 30 min prior to testing. The patient's flow-volume curve is shown in Figure 179-A.

Skin-prick sensitivity test results from a battery of common allergens are negative. What would you do next?

A. Request a dynamic (both inspiratory and expiratory) CT scan of the neck and chest.
B. Arrange for bronchoscopy.
C. Review the individual spirometry efforts.
D. Increase the dose of the combination inhaled corticosteroid/long-acting β_2-agonist and add montelukast.

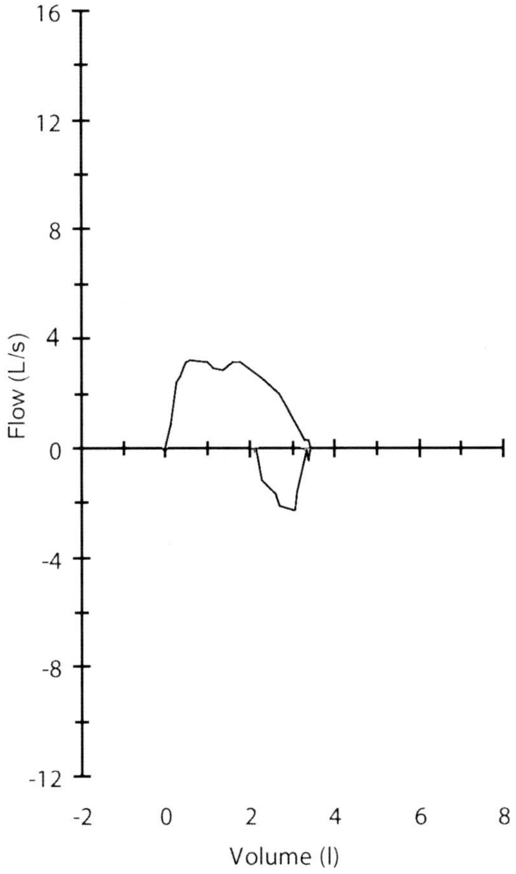

Figure 179-A

180. A 38-year-old woman was seen 2 years ago by a cardiologist for atypical chest pain, dyspnea on exertion, and palpitations. After an extensive evaluation, she received a diagnosis of probable idiopathic pulmonary arterial hypertension (IPAH), and a cardiac catheterization was recommended. The patient refused treatment and was lost to follow-up. She now comes to the pulmonary clinic for help because she can no longer perform her activities of daily living. She reports dyspnea at rest, with significant worsening with minimal exertion. She has also noted the onset of swelling in her legs. She is observed to be notably tachypneic after walking from the waiting room to the office. Her oxygen

saturation at rest is 89%, which decreases rapidly to 83% on ambulation. She has a right ventricular heave and edema of the lower extremities with 2+ pitting. She now consents to cardiac catheterization, which is remarkable for the following:

Right atrium pressure	15 mm Hg
Right ventricle pressure	70/15 mm Hg
PA pressure*	70/30 mm Hg
PA mean pressure	45 mm Hg
PA occlusion pressure	12 mm Hg
Cardiac index	1.7 L/min/m^2
Pulmonary vascular resistance	10 Wood U

* PA = pulmonary artery.

After vasodilator challenge, the mean PA pressure decreases to 38 mm Hg, and the cardiac index falls to 1.4 L/min/m^2.

In addition to oxygen, warfarin, and diuretics, her medical therapy should include:

A. Oral diltiazem.
B. Oral sildenafil.
C. Oral bosentan.
D. IV epoprostenol.

181. A 70-year-old man with advanced end-stage COPD complains of severe breathlessness that has been intractable despite aggressive conventional therapy.

Which of the following pharmacologic and nonpharmacologic interventions would you recommend as having the strongest evidence for effectiveness in reducing breathlessness?

A. Morphine sulfate taken orally.
B. Morphine sulfate administered by nebulization.
C. Acupuncture.
D. Air blown on the patient's face using a fan.

182. A 50-year-old man, who is a lifelong nonsmoker, has recently developed an enlarging right anterior chest lesion in the breast area. He is in the ICU after a prolonged hospitalization; he was initially admitted due to a right-sided pulmonary infiltrate that has continued to progress despite multiple antibiotics, including vancomycin, ceftazidime, piperacillin/tazobactam, and levofloxacin. Normal findings were obtained on a chest radiograph obtained 1 month prior to admission, as part of his routine follow-up for a history of successfully treated lymphoma 5 years ago. The patient underwent a bronchoscopy with BAL 2 weeks ago with negative results for routine cultures, including TB and fungi. BAL fluid cytologic findings were negative for malignancy. Multiple sputum samples are negative for TB by smear and culture.

Physical examination reveals a cachectic man with poor dentition and bilateral rhonchi more severe in the right chest than the left chest. The right anterior chest just below the nipple reveals a soft, slightly erythematous lesion measuring 10 × 8 cm in diameter that expands with each ventilator-delivered tidal volume. Exhaled and inhaled tidal volumes recorded on the ventilator are the same.

The patient's current chest radiograph (see Figure 182-A) and CT scans (see Figures 182-B and 182-C) are shown. Which of the following is the most likely diagnosis?

A. Squamous cell carcinoma.
B. Pneumococcal pneumonia and empyema.
C. Actinomycosis.
D. TB.

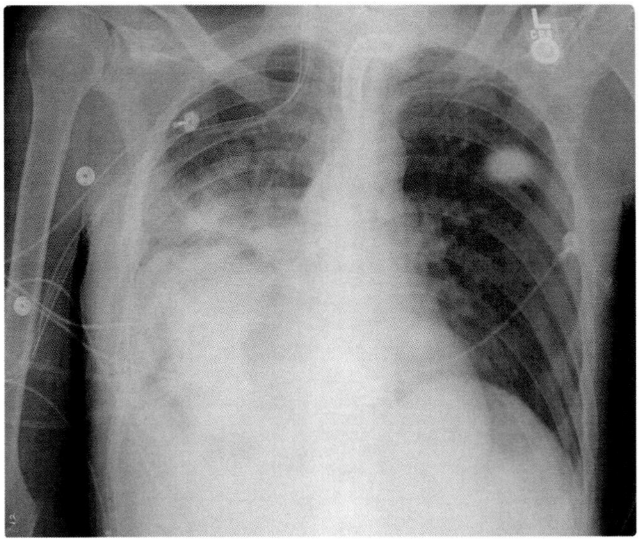

Figure 182-A

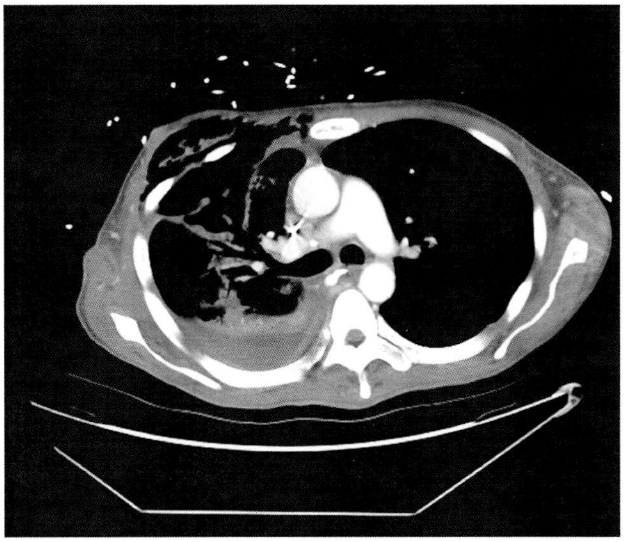

Figure 182-B

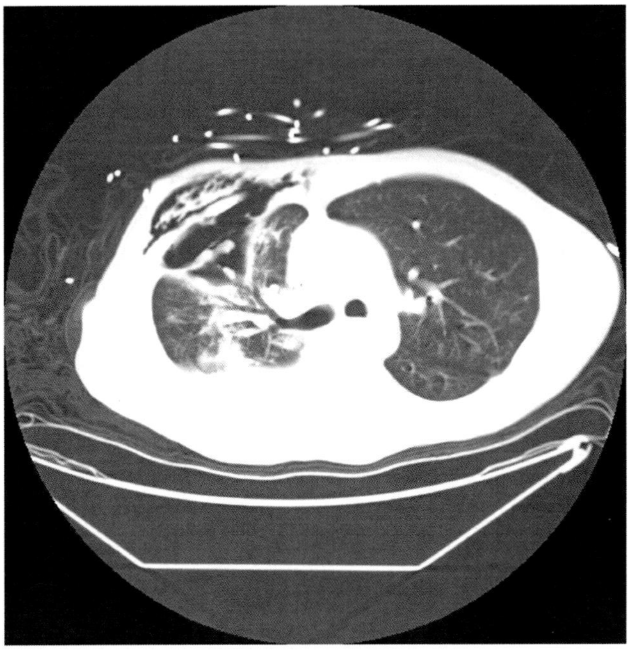

Figure 182-C

183. A 55-year-old postmenopausal woman with restless legs syndrome has been treated with carbidopa/levodopa, 25 to 100 mg, for the last 6 months and has been compliant with the prescribed treatment. Initially she had an excellent response, but on a return appointment, she complains that the symptoms occur earlier in the day, are more

intense, easier to provoke, and have spread to different sites. Laboratory testing reveals a ferritin level in the midrange of normal at 100 ng/mL (224 pmol/L). The best course of action is:

A. Start iron replacement therapy.
B. Continue the current dose of carbidopa/levodopa.
C. Switch to a benzodiazepine at nighttime.
D. Increase the dose of carbidopa/levodopa.

184. Which of the following laryngoscopic findings is most specific for vocal cord dysfunction syndrome?

A. Inspiratory and expiratory vocal cord adduction with a posterior glottic chink.
B. Expiratory vocal cord adduction.
C. Inspiratory abduction with posterior glottic chink.
D. Expiratory false vocal cord adduction.

185. Which of the following characteristics would portend improved clinical outcome in patients with emphysema undergoing lung-volume-reduction surgery?

A. Upper-lobe-predominant disease with low exercise capacity.
B. Non-upper-lobe-predominant disease with high exercise capacity.
C. Non-upper-lobe-predominant disease with low exercise capacity.
D. Upper-lobe-predominant disease with high exercise capacity.

186. Which of the following is true about endobronchial ultrasound-guided transbronchial needle aspiration (EBUS-TBNA)?

A. It is more accurate than mediastinoscopy in the diagnosis of lung cancer in subcarinal, posterior, and inferior mediastinal lymph nodes.
B. It can access all lymph nodes in the mediastinum.
C. It is not useful in the diagnosis of lymphoma.
D. It cannot obtain adequate samples for the diagnosis of sarcoidosis.

187. A 52-year-old man was well until 3 months prior to hospital admission when he developed increasing dyspnea and joint swelling. He first noticed painful swelling of his hands and, 2 weeks later, he developed painful swelling of his feet. An initial course of prednisone helped somewhat, but his dyspnea worsened, and he was admitted to the hospital for further management. He is a nonsmoker and has no HIV risk factors. On examination, his temperature was 38.6°C, BP was 105/66 mm Hg, pulse was 103/min, and respiratory rate was 24/min. There was painful swelling of both elbows, all the metacarpal-phalangeal joints of both hands, and all the proximal interphalangeal joints of both hands and both feet diffusely. Subungual telangiectasias and heliotrope discoloration periorbitally were noted. He had bibasal crepitations. Laboratory investigations indicated a normal hemoglobin level and WBC count. The following test results were negative or normal: renal function, liver function tests, urinalysis, anti-DNA, rheumatoid factor, antineutrophil antibody (ANA), cytoplasmic and perinuclear antineutrophil cytoplasmic antibody (C- and P-ANCA, respectively), anti-Jo-1 antibody, and complement. The C-reactive protein level was 76.7 mg/L (5,848.4 nmol/L), and the creatinine kinase level was 296 U/L (4.9 µkat/L). A chest radiograph and representative image of a chest CT scan are shown (see Figures 187-A and 187-B). A surgical lung biopsy was performed, and two representative sections are shown in Figures 187-C and 187-D.

The most likely diagnosis is:

A. Rheumatoid lung.
B. *Pneumocystis jirovecii* pneumonia.
C. Dermatomyositis-associated interstitial lung disease (ILD).
D. Idiopathic pulmonary fibrosis (IPF).

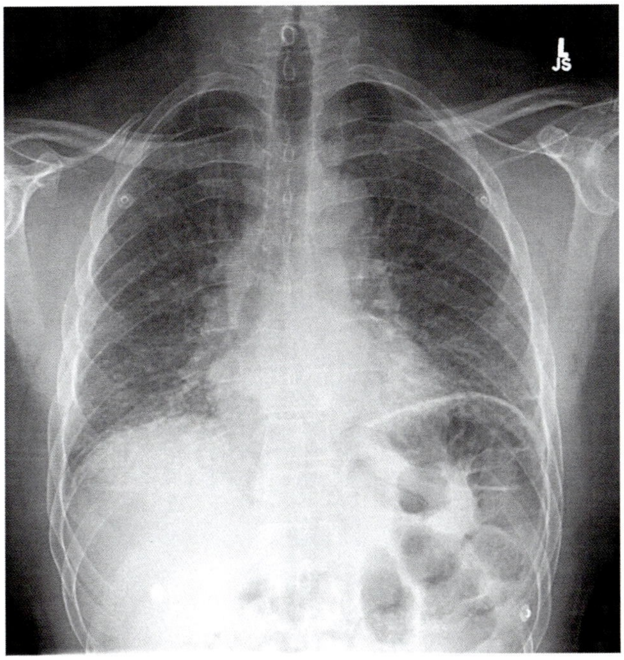

Figure 187-A

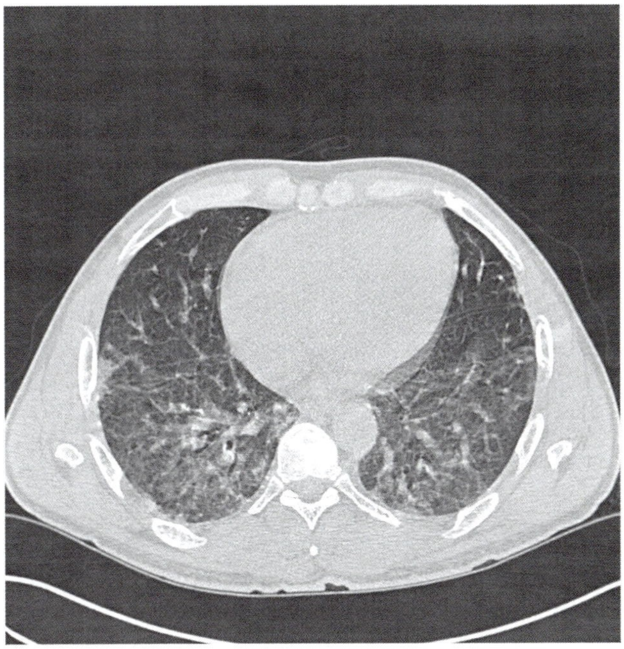

Figure 187-B

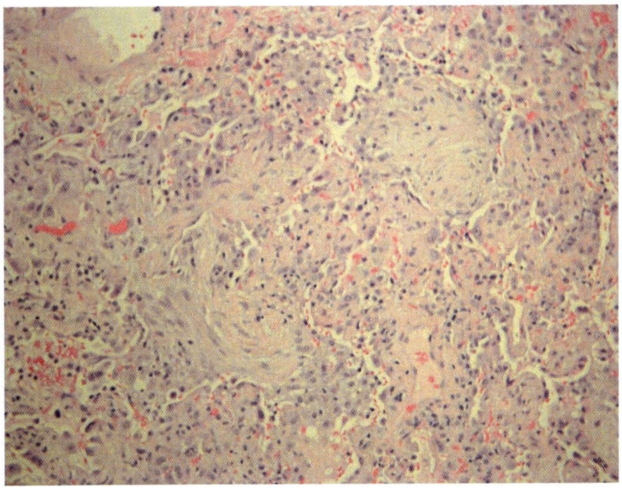

Figure 187-C
Hematoxylin-eosin

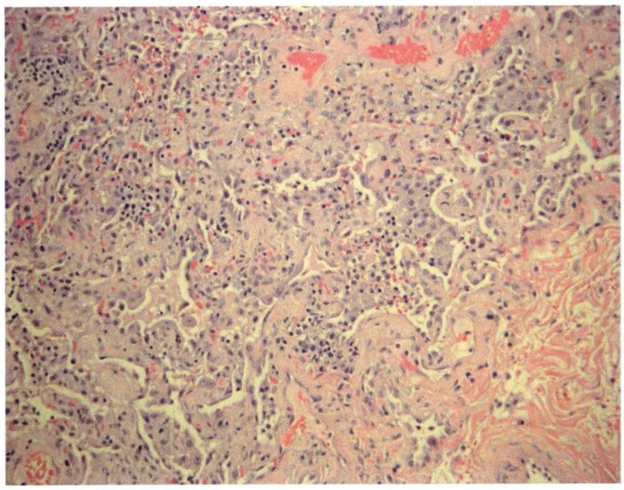

Figure 187-D
Hematoxylin-eosin

188. A 25-year-old man arrives at the clinic with a history of physician-diagnosed asthma since he was 5 years old. He had eczema in infancy and has had seasonal allergic rhinitis since the age of 12 years. His asthma worsened during childhood with upper respiratory infections and also with exposure to cats and dust. He required several emergency visits and hospitalizations in childhood for asthma, but symptoms became mild in his mid teens, and he had no need for regular asthma medications and no emergency visits until the age of 23 years. For the past 2 years, since changing to a new job, he has again noted worsening symptoms of cough, wheeze, chest tightness, and shortness of breath.

He works for a pulp and paper mill as a "debarker helper." Pine, spruce, and black spruce are processed by this mill. The job occasionally exposes him to high concentrations of wood, dust, and mold when the machines jam.

Within days of starting this work, he noted worsening of his asthma symptoms, occurring daily, with some improvement on weekends away from work and significant improvement when he was on vacation. He has had five ED visits for asthma in the past 2 years. He uses his short-acting bronchodilator two or three times a day on weekdays and usually once a day on weekends. He awakens with respiratory symptoms two or three times a week. His primary care physician had prescribed fluticasone, 220 μg twice daily, and he has been adherent to this regimen. He has never smoked. His physical examination results are normal, and spirometry shows mild airflow limitation in the Monday clinic after a weekend off work.

The best next step for this patient is:

A. Advise him to leave his workplace and add a long-acting β-agonist.
B. Advise him to stay in his current job and add a leukotriene receptor antagonist.
C. Advise him to be relocated to a cleaner area on a trial basis and add a long-acting β-agonist.
D. Suggest dust-control measures at home and add a leukotriene receptor antagonist.

189. A 70-year-old man undergoes a physical examination during which the physician orders a "routine" chest radiograph (see Figure 189-A). The physician then orders a CT of the chest (see Figures 189-B and 189-C) and sends the patient to you for consultation. The man notes no significant pulmonary symptoms, denies any significant past medical history, and is a lifelong nonsmoker. He has held many jobs throughout his life, including various jobs in construction in his 20s when he had exposure to asbestos, including the use of asbestos housing insulation.

Which of the following best describes the lesions seen on this patient's radiographs?

A. Not known to undergo malignant transformation.
B. Solely found with asbestos exposure.
C. An infrequent radiographic abnormality.
D. Calcification occurs within the first 10 years after asbestos exposure.

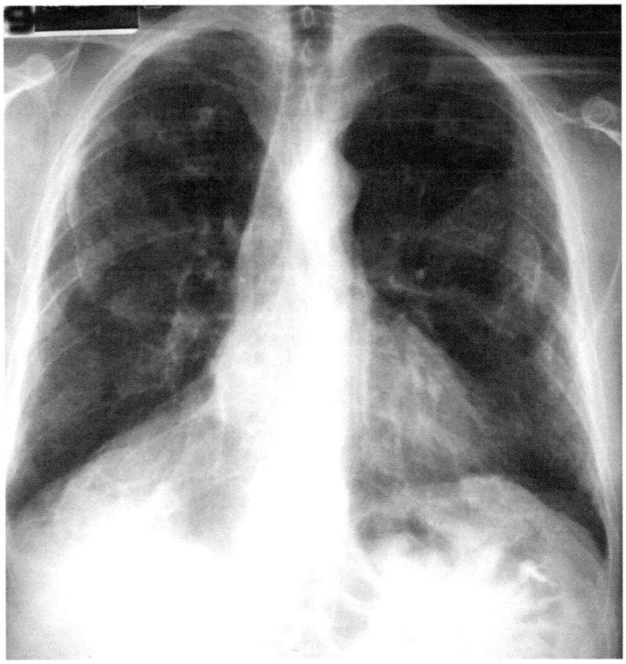

Figure 189-A

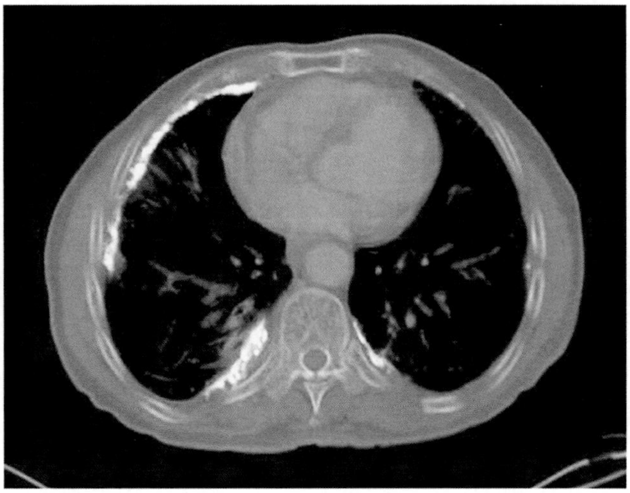

Figure 189-B

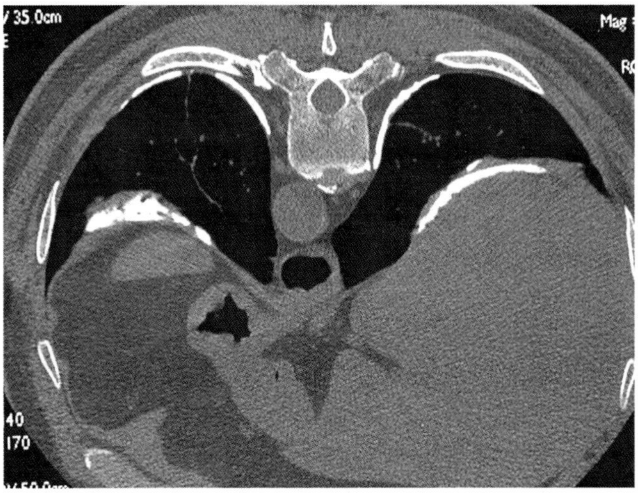

Figure 189-C

190. A 62-year-old former smoker (25 pack-year history) who quit 20 years ago arrives at your office and requests testing to determine whether she has lung cancer. She has no family history of lung cancer and has no other medical illnesses. She has no symptoms, and her examination is normal.

Which of the following should be recommended?

A. Perform serial chest radiographs.
B. Obtain serial sputum cytologies.
C. Order a low-dose chest CT scan.
D. Further testing is not necessary.

191. A 44-year-old woman comes to your office for evaluation with dyspnea on exertion and a nonproductive cough. She has been told she has "emphysema," and attempts at tobacco cessation have failed. On physical examination, crackles are detected. She undergoes a diagnostic evaluation. Her radiographic, pathologic, and lavage findings are shown in Figures 191-A, 191-B, 191-C, and 191-D.

Which of the following smoking-related lung diseases is most likely?

A. COPD.
B. Goodpasture syndrome with diffuse pulmonary hemorrhage.
C. Pulmonary Langerhans histiocytosis.
D. Desquamative interstitial pneumonia (DIP).

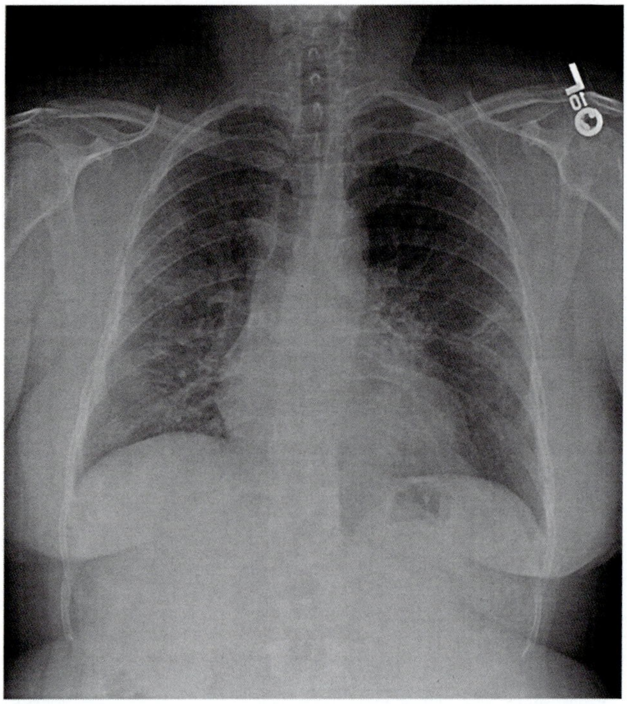

Figure 191-A

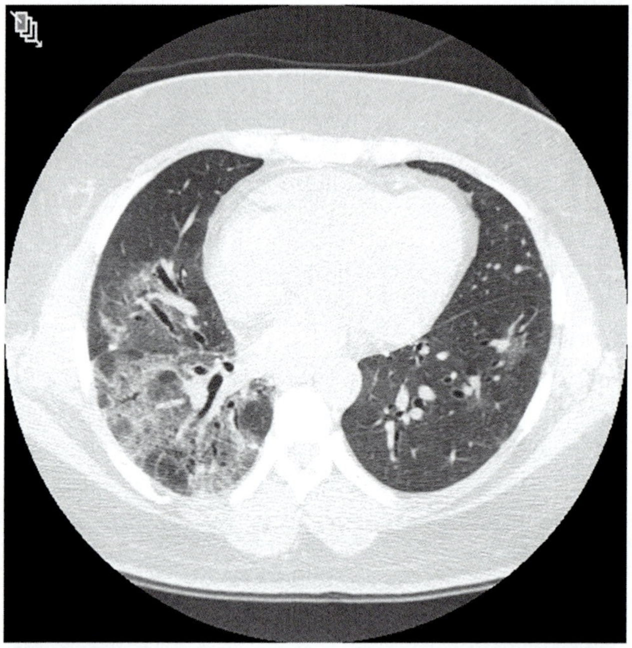

Figure 191-B

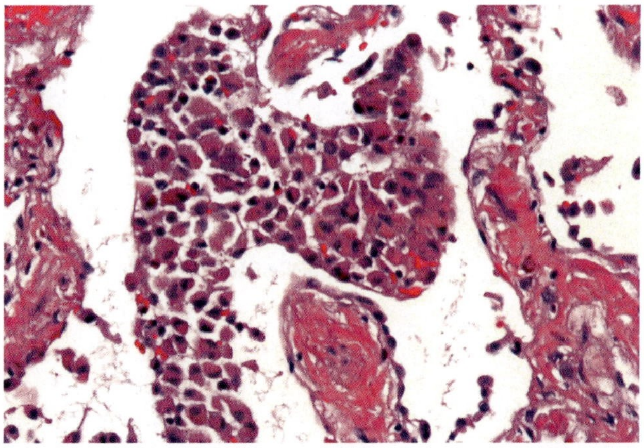

Figure 191-C
Hematoxylin-eosin

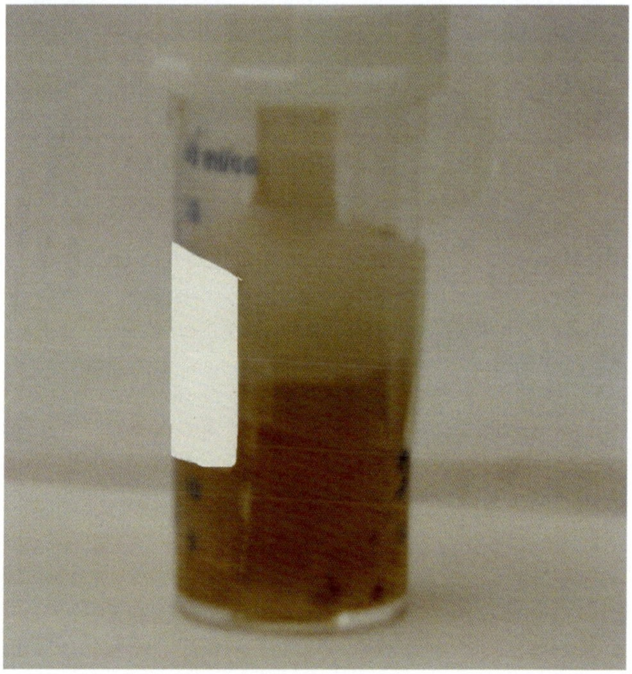

Figure 191-D

192. Well-established tests exist for measuring Histoplasma fungal antigens in urine, serum, and BAL fluid and antibody responses in serum. Which statement is true concerning assays of fungal antigens and antibody responses?

A. The incidence of antibody positivity in the general population is approximately 80% in areas endemic for asymptomatic histoplasmosis infection.
B. Detection of antigen in BAL fluid is at least as sensitive as urinary antigen for identifying active infection.
C. Antibody levels rise within 1 week of onset of acute infection and peak at 3 weeks.
D. In patients with AIDS with progressive disseminated histoplasmosis, the sensitivity of urinary antigen testing is $<25\%$.

193. Which of the following genetic mutations has been described in people with congenital central hypoventilation syndrome?

A. *PHOX2B.*
B. Casein kinase I ε (CKIε)-binding region of hPer2.
C. Type 2 hypocretin/orexin receptor gene.
D. Codon 178 of the prion protein gene.

194. A 45-year-old woman is referred for mild shortness of breath and the constellation of findings noted on the chest (see Figure 194-A) and abdominal (see Figure 194-B) CT scans. Which of the following statements is correct regarding this disease process?

A. Lung tissue will stain positive with S-100.
B. A cholesterol pleural effusion develops in one-third of patients.
C. The disease does not recur following lung transplantation.
D. Rapamycin (sirolimus) may be therapeutic.

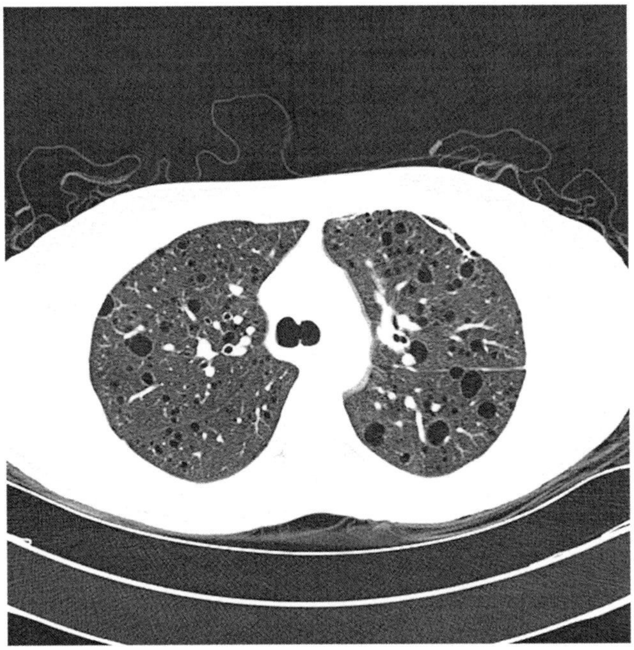
Figure 194-A

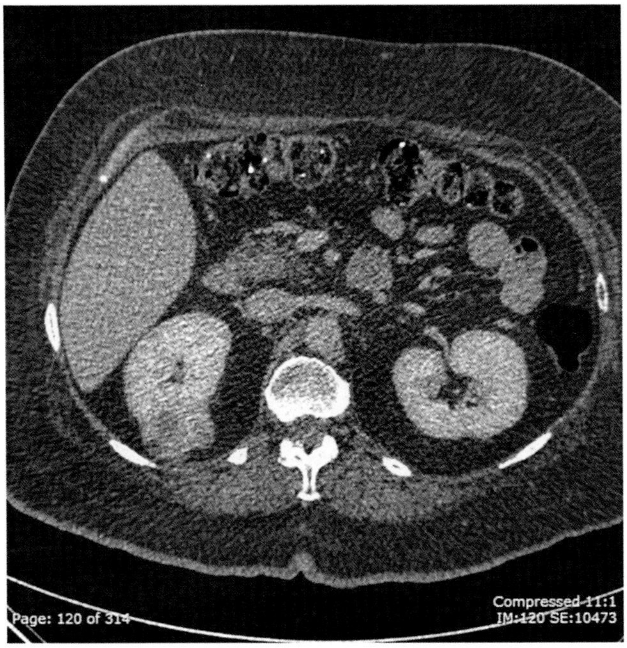

Figure 194-B

195. A 56-year-old man is intubated and placed on mechanical ventilation support for ARDS following a seizure and massive aspiration. His BP is 130/84 mm Hg, his pulse is 86/min, and his urine flow is 0.8 mL/kg/h. According to the large NIH ARDS Network fluid management trial, the best fluid management strategy (*ie,* liberal fluids prioritizing cardiac filling vs conservative fluids prioritizing "dry lungs") and the best method of monitoring (*ie,* central venous catheter [CVC] vs pulmonary artery catheter [PAC]) for this patient are:

A. Conservative fluids, monitoring devices equivalent.
B. Conservative fluids, monitoring with PAC.
C. Liberal fluids, monitoring devices equivalent.
D. Liberal fluids, monitoring with PAC.

196. A 27-year-old woman who is at 30 weeks' gestation with twins is admitted to the labor and delivery unit because of preterm labor. She is treated with bed rest and hydration. However, because regular, painful uterine contractions continue and some effacement of the cervix is noted, treatment with IV terbutaline is also started. Approximately 2 h later, the patient complains of shortness of breath. Physical examination is notable for a pulse of 96, BP of 126/82 mm Hg, and respiratory rate of 24/min. There is no jugular venous distension, and bibasilar inspiratory crackles are noted without bronchophony or egophony. Bilateral trace pedal edema is observed.

Her chest radiograph reveals a diffuse alveolar filling process but without cardiomegaly. Laboratory testing reveals that the prothrombin time, activated partial thromboplastin time, and platelet count are all within normal limits.

Which of the following is the most likely explanation for her dyspnea?

A. Amniotic fluid embolism.
B. Peripartum cardiomyopathy.
C. Pulmonary edema secondary to terbutaline.
D. Pulmonary embolism.

197. Regarding the interpretation of spirometry, individual spirograms are acceptable if:

A. They are free from artifacts, they have good starts, and they show satisfactory exhalation.
B. The two largest values of both FEV_1 and FVC are within 0.15 L of each other.
C. A maximum of eight tests have been performed.
D. The patient is tiring and cannot continue.

198. To answer the question of whether smoking increases the risk of lung cancer, the most appropriate study design would be a:

A. Randomized controlled trial (RCT).
B. Cohort study.
C. Case-control study.
D. Series of case reports.

199. A 25-year-old woman is admitted to the ED with respiratory failure and is rapidly intubated. She is a field researcher for the federal government, and in the past 6 months, has traveled throughout the United States to collect soil samples, with stops in Tennessee, Alabama, Iowa, Washington, Arizona, and California. She has no medical history of respiratory failure and does not smoke tobacco. One month ago, she developed a low-grade fever and a mild cough. Her primary physician obtained a sputum culture and prescribed levofloxacin. She noted no improvement but continued to work. One week prior to admission, she developed a mild wheeze and began treatment with a fluticasone proprionate inhaler, 110 μg twice daily, and an albuterol metered-dose inhaler, as well as resumed treatment with levofloxacin, 500 mg/d. Her symptoms did not improve after 2 days when she was switched to prednisone, 60 mg/d orally, and she had taken only four doses before admission.

On admission, she is profoundly short of breath. Her temperature is 38.2°C, pulse rate is 110/min, and BP is 145/90 mm Hg. Her WBC count is 11,500/μL (11.5×10^9/L) with 50% neutrophils, 20% lymphocytes, and 25% eosinophils. Her hematocrit concentration and platelet count are normal. Her chest radiograph is shown in Figure 199-A. Biopsy results of her lung are shown in Figure 199-B.

What is this patient's diagnosis?

A. Blastomycosis.
B. Histoplasmosis.
C. Sporotrichosis.
D. Coccidioidomycosis.

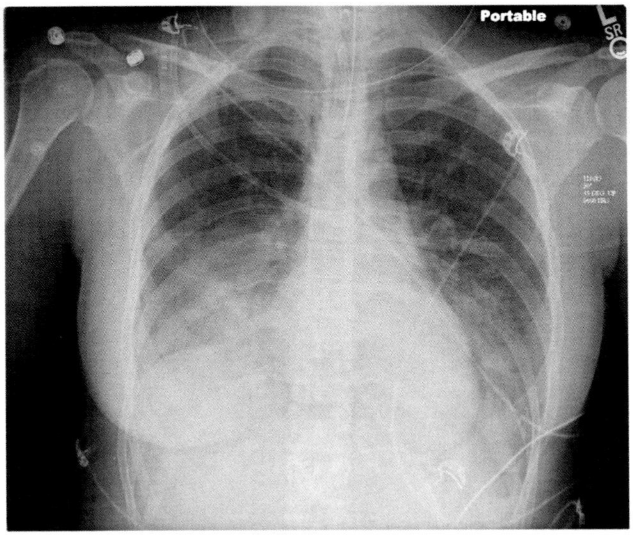

Figure 199-A

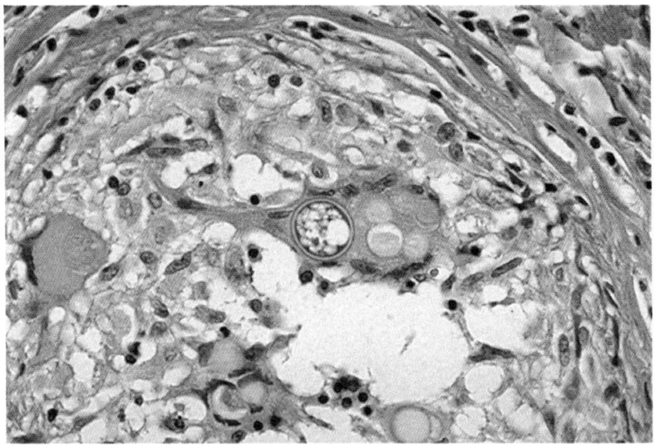

Figure 199-B
Hematoxylin-eosin

200. A 71-year-old man had a CT scan obtained following a motor vehicle accident (see Figure 200-A). A needle biopsy test of the mediastinal mass revealed a thymoma. Which of the following is true about this patient's disease?

A. Histologic absence of malignant features is the best indicator of survival.
B. Surgical resection should be attempted.
C. There is no indication for postoperative adjuvant radiation therapy if surgical resection is performed.
D. Myasthenia gravis portends a poor prognosis.

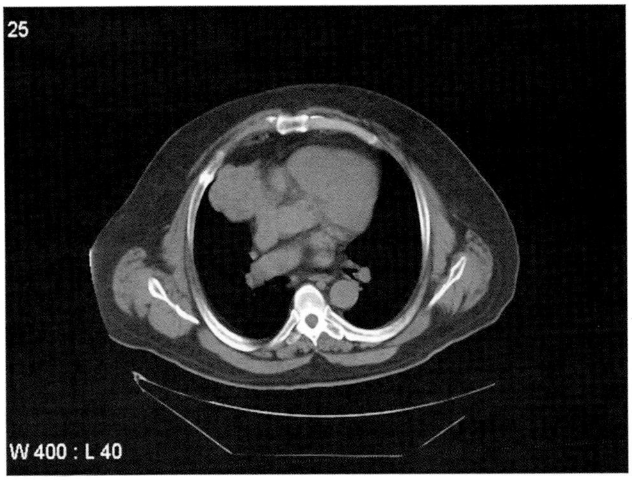

Figure 200-A

Part II

Response Key, Rationale, and References

1. D. High-intensity exercise.

Aerobic training is designed to improve the endurance of exercising muscles, and an essential component of all pulmonary rehabilitation programs is training of the muscles of ambulation. Clinical trials in patients with COPD show that high-intensity training of these muscles (at least 60 to 80% of that individual's maximal work rate) is generally well tolerated and is more effective than lower-intensity regimens in improving exercise performance, as measured by reduced minute ventilation and heart rate at comparable workloads, improved dyspnea, and increased timed walk distances (choice D is correct).

Pulmonary rehabilitation is a multidisciplinary and individualized intervention for symptomatic patients with chronic respiratory diseases designed to reduce breathlessness, anxiety, and depression; improve exercise tolerance; and increase participation in activities of daily living. Programs generally include exercise training, education, instruction in respiratory and chest physiotherapy techniques, and psychosocial support. The effectiveness of pulmonary rehabilitation is best validated in patients with COPD, but data are emerging to support its use in other chronic respiratory illnesses. The key component to all programs is endurance training of the lower extremities, although upper-extremity exercise training increases patients' work capacity while decreasing their oxygen consumption at comparable work levels. Strength training is intended to improve the ability of muscles to perform intense exercise over a short duration, as in running and lifting weights; in addition, patients who have weak muscles may benefit from strength training to perform simple tasks like rising from a chair. Although improving muscle strength and mass may improve peak exercise performance, it does not lead to major improvements in endurance, a more important component of ambulating and other activities of daily living (choice A is incorrect). When administered to patients with COPD, both growth hormone and anabolic steroids increase lean body mass and muscle mass but generally do not improve exercise performance or quality-of-life scores and carry the risk of serious side effects (choice B is incorrect). Many patients with COPD have weak inspiratory muscles, and a few randomized trials show that inspiratory muscle training may improve dyspnea and exercise capacity in select patients who have measurable respiratory muscle weakness (*eg,* PImax $\leq$ 60 cm H_2O) and breathlessness despite receiving optimal medical therapy. However, it is not effective in most patients with COPD and is not recommended as a routine intervention in pulmonary rehabilitation programs (choice C is incorrect).

Ries AL, Bauldoff GS, Carlin B, et al. Pulmonary rehabilitation: joint ACCP/AACVPR evidence-based clinical practice guidelines. Chest 2007; 131(suppl):4S–42S

American Thoracic Society, European Respiratory Society. ATS/ERS statement on pulmonary rehabilitation. Am J Respir Crit Care Med 2006; 173:1390–1413

Lotters F, van Tol B, Kwakkel G, et al. Effects of controlled inspiratory muscle training in patients with COPD: a meta-analysis. Eur Respir J 2002; 20:570–576

Lacasse Y, Goldstein R, Lasserson TJ, et al. Pulmonary rehabilitation for chronic obstructive pulmonary disease. Cochrane Database Syst Rev 2006; 4:CD003793

2. B. Placement of an esophageal stent.

The chest radiograph demonstrates hyperinflation and a vague left lower lobe infiltrate. The chest CT scan demonstrates left lower lobe airspace disease, confirming pneumonia and a very clearly defined esophageal-bronchial fistula. The diagnosis is aspiration pneumonia secondary to the fistula, and placing an esophageal stent is the correct answer (choice B is correct). Although antibiotic therapy is indicated for the treatment of aspiration pneumonia, the use of ceftriaxone and azithromycin (ordinarily good choices for community-acquired pneumonia) is inappropriate because these antibiotics do not have anaerobic coverage (choice A is incorrect). Squamous cell carcinoma of the esophagus responds poorly to cancer chemotherapy. Although a trial of chemotherapy at some point may be helpful, it is not an intervention that should be offered during infection (choice C is incorrect). The fistulous tract developed, in part, from the radiotherapy. There is no evidence that further radiotherapy would close the fistulous tract and may, in fact, aggravate the situation (choice D is incorrect).

The palliative treatment of esophageal cancer includes the placement of a self-expanding metallic stent into the esophagus. There are many different types of metallic stents on the market, covered and uncovered, some of which have antireflux valves. They are primarily used to palliate symptoms of dysphagia in patients with inoperable esophageal cancer and allow the patient to swallow food until the more advanced stages of the disease are reached. Inspection of the tracheobronchial tree to examine the impact of the esophageal stent on airway caliber is an important consideration. Treatment of the bronchoesophageal fistula in patients with advanced disease is dictated by the disease itself. The endoscopic placement of an expandable, coated stent may be the treatment of choice for closure of tracheoesophageal fistulas, and, later, another stent may be placed in the airway if necessary to maintain quality of life.

Adler DG, Baron TH. Endoscopic palliation of malignant dysphagia. Mayo Clin Proc 2001; 76:731–738

Miwa K, Mitsuoka M, Tayama K, et al. Successful airway stenting using silicone prosthesis for esophagobronchial fistula. Chest 2002; 122:1485–1487

3. C. Common variable immune deficiency (CVID).

The CT scan shows mediastinal lymphadenopathy (see Figure 3-A) and patchy areas of airspace disease (see Figure 3-B). The mediastinal lymph node biopsy (see Figure 3-C) reveals nonnecrotizing granulomatous inflammation, and the lung biopsy (see Figure 3-D) reveals organizing pneumonia and prominent lymphoid aggregates. This, combined with the history of recurrent episodes of infection dating back to childhood, is highly suggestive of CVID (choice C is correct). Subsequent testing in this patient confirmed markedly reduced IgG and IgA levels and an impaired ability to synthesize humoral antibodies.

The findings of pleural fibrovascular adhesions with prominent lymphoid aggregates, localized areas of organizing pneumonia, and nonnecrotizing granulomatous inflammation have been reported in patients with CVID. They are reaction patterns associated with the underlying immunopathology rather than representing sarcoidosis (choice A is incorrect) or COP (choice B is incorrect). Similarly, despite the fact that her CT scan shows mediastinal adenopathy suggestive of sarcoidosis (see Figure 3-A) and areas of confluent parenchymal disease, some showing air bronchograms (see Figure 3-B) consistent with COP, taken together, the diagnosis of CVID is unifying. There is no evidence of vasculitis in the biopsy specimens nor does the clinical picture fit with Wegener granulomatosis (choice D is incorrect).

CVID is the most common of the primary immune deficiency disorders, with a prevalence of 1:50,000 to 1:200,000. Although it is a congenital disease, it can be observed at any age, with the median age of both onset and diagnosis being higher in women. The disease is characterized by recurrent rhinosinusitis, respiratory tract infections, and bronchiectasis, and there is an increased incidence of autoimmune disease, lymphoid proliferation, and malignancy. Granulomatous lesions in both lymph nodes and solid organs have been reported in CVID, and the diagnosis of sarcoidosis is frequently mistakenly made prior to CVID being considered. Levels of angiotensin-converting enzyme may be elevated in CVID. COP has also been reported in CVID and has been reported to respond to oral corticosteroids. In addition, the pathologic findings in CVID may show follicular bronchiolitis. Treatment of CVID revolves around augmentation of antibody levels with IV immunoglobulin therapy and prompt treatment of infections. Mortality is most commonly due to acute-on-chronic respiratory infections, with a mean age of death of 55.4 years in women and 28.8 years in men. There is some evidence that the presence of granulomatous-lymphocytic disease shortens survival. Infliximab may have a role in treating these patients.

Thickett KM, Kumarratne DS, Banerjee AK, et al. Common variable immune deficiency: respiratory manifestations, pulmonary function, and high-resolution CT scan findings. Q J Med 2002; 95:655–662

Tanaka N, Kim JS, Bates CA, et al. Lung diseases in patients with common variable immunodeficiency: chest radiographic, and computed tomographic findings. J Comput Assisted Tomogr 2006; 30:828–838

Bates CA, Ellison MC, Lynch DA, et al. Granulomatous-lymphocytic lung disease shortens survival in common variable immune deficiency. J Allergy Clin Immunol 2004; 114:415–421

Thatayatikom A, Thatayatikom S, White AJ. Infliximab treatment for severe granulomatous disease in common variable immunodeficiency: a case report and review of the literature. Ann Allergy Asthma Immunol 2005; 95:293–300

4. B. 30-min delay to analysis.

The choice least likely to alter the pleural fluid pH and impact clinical decision making is the 30-min delay to analysis (choice B is correct). Pleural fluid pH remains stable at room temperature for 1 h; however, time delays of 4 and 24 h significantly alter pH to a level that has an impact on clinical decisions.

An accurate pleural fluid pH determination provides important diagnostic information for pleural effusions due to infection, rheumatoid arthritis, and esophageal rupture in which the pH can be quite low. Similarly, pleural fluid pH provides important prognostic information in malignant pleural effusions (lower pH portends poor prognosis and predicts pleurodesis failure) and pleural infections (pH < 7.20 indicates the need for drainage). However, the usefulness of pleural pH depends on accurate measurement. Clinicians must be aware of the factors that can adversely impact pH accuracy to ensure proper decisions are made based on the pH value reported.

A blood gas analyzer is considered the "gold standard" for pleural fluid pH determination. Significant inaccuracies occur with a pH meter (probe device placed in open container of pleural fluid being tested; choice C is incorrect), pH indicator paper, and a urine dipstick, all yielding significantly more alkalotic pH values. Sampling protocol errors can also significantly alter the pH obtained. One milliliter of retained air in the pH syringe significantly raises the pH (mean increase 0.08; choice D is incorrect); 0.2 mL and 0.4 mL of retained 2% lidocaine significantly decrease pH (mean decrease of 0.15 and 0.24, respectively; choice A is incorrect). Air in the syringe likely leads to rapid CO_2 diffusion through the fluid-air interface; similarly, this likely accounts for more alkaline pH values using a pH meter. Two-tenths of a milliliter of lidocaine, which is acidic, is compatible with the dead space of needles often used for thoracentesis and may contaminate the pleural fluid sampled. These value changes of pH due to air and lidocaine are of potential clinical significance. Heparin (0.4 mL, preloaded amount in syringe) significantly decreases the pH (mean decrease of 0.02), but this magnitude is of no clinical significance. Although pH alterations in pleural fluid glucose values are noted with air, lidocaine, heparin, and time, none is of clinical significance. Glucose and pH measurements of pleural fluid are strongly correlated, so glucose measures may provide a reasonable alternative to pH measurement.

In loculated parapneumonic pleural effusions, as is the likely diagnosis in this patient, the pH may vary considerably from one loculation to another. In three of seven patients in whom at least two different loculations were sampled, the variation in pH was of a magnitude to alter clinical practice (range, 0.40 to 0.94).

Rahman NM, Mishra EK, Davies HE, et al. Clinically important factors influencing the diagnostic measurement of pleural fluid pH and glucose. Am J Respir Crit Care Med 2008; 178:483–490

Sarodia BD, Goldstein LS, Laskowski DM, et al. Does pleural fluid pH change significantly at room temperature during the first hour following thoracentesis? Chest 2000; 117:1043–1048

Maskell NA, Gleeson FV, Darby M, et al. Diagnostically significant variations in pleural fluid pH in loculated parapneumonic effusions. Chest 2004; 126:2022–2024

Chandler TM, McCoskey EH, Byrd RP, et al. Comparison of the use and accuracy of methods of determining pleural fluid pH. South Med J 1999; 92:214–217

5. A. Strength training.

This patient has moderately severe COPD. He has had a recent exacerbation and has had a decline in his functional status. He should be offered pulmonary rehabilitation that includes lower and upper extremity training, education, and strength training (choice A is correct). Rehabilitation is indicated for patients with moderate to severe COPD and can be started soon after hospitalization. Pulmonary rehabilitation has been shown to reduce dyspnea, improve health-related quality of life, improve exercise tolerance, and reduce health-care utilization. The program consists of a variety of therapeutic interventions. Lower and upper extremity training is a key component of the program. Education is also a core component of the program. Various additional interventions also should be included. Strength training has been shown to be an effective addition to both upper and lower extremity training and should be included in all programs. This patient has developed significant muscular deconditioning and, thus, strength training should be included in his program.

This patient has lost a significant amount of weight and has a low BMI. The low BMI is associated with a higher mortality rate in patients with COPD. Nutritional counseling is an important component of a pulmonary rehabilitation program. However, there is little evidence that nutritional supplementation benefits patients when combined with pulmonary rehabilitation (choice B is incorrect). Anabolic steroids also have been used in association with exercise and strength training, but there is no conclusive evidence that these result in an improvement in exercise tolerance (choice C is incorrect). Depression is seen in up to 40% of patients with COPD. Screening for depression should be included in all rehabilitation programs by the rehabilitation staff, and referrals to health professionals should be offered by the rehabilitation staff when signs of depression are revealed. Although antidepressant therapy may be indicated, a more thorough evaluation should be performed prior to starting medications (choice D is incorrect). Pulmonary rehabilitation in and of itself has been shown to reduce symptoms of anxiety and depression.

Ries AL, Bauldoff GS, Carlin BW, et al. Pulmonary rehabilitation: joint ACCP/AACVPR evidence-based clinical practice guidelines. Chest 2007; 131:4S–42S

Maurer J, Reggapragada V, Borson S, et al. Anxiety and depression in COPD. Chest 2008; 134;43S–56S

Griffiths TL, Burr ML, Campbell IA, et al. Results at 1 year of outpatient multidisciplinary pulmonary rehabilitation: a randomized controlled trial. Lancet 2000; 355:362–368

6. D. Surgical consultation for resection of the lesion.

The patient has a bronchogenic cyst suggested on imaging with a well-defined homogeneous mass. Based on the location and symptoms, there was concern about pulmonary artery and left atrial compression (see Figures 6-C and 6-D) resulting in hemodynamic consequences during exertion. For this reason, he was referred for surgical resection (choice D is correct). A conservative approach with serial observation is appropriate in those patients who are asymptomatic, which is not the situation for our patient (choice A is incorrect). The location of the mass raises concern about an esophageal duplication cyst and foregut derivation, and further evaluation with either an esophagram or esophagogastroduodenoscopy would be indicated if anatomic structures could not be determined by imaging. The chronicity and absence of predisposing events and systemic features suggest that an esophageal perforation is less likely.

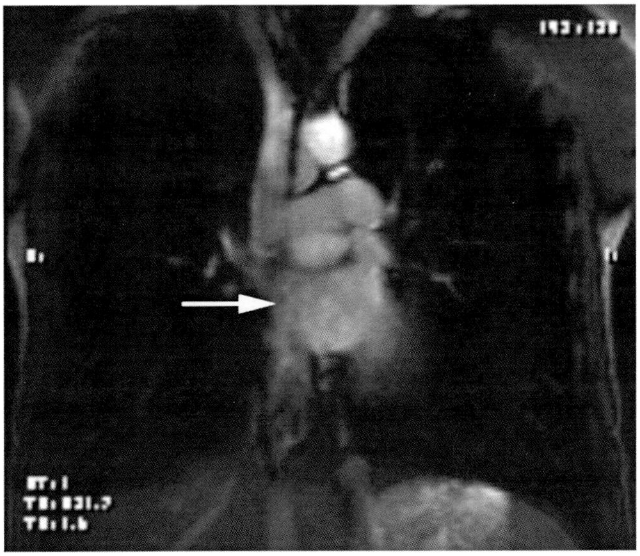

Figure 6-C

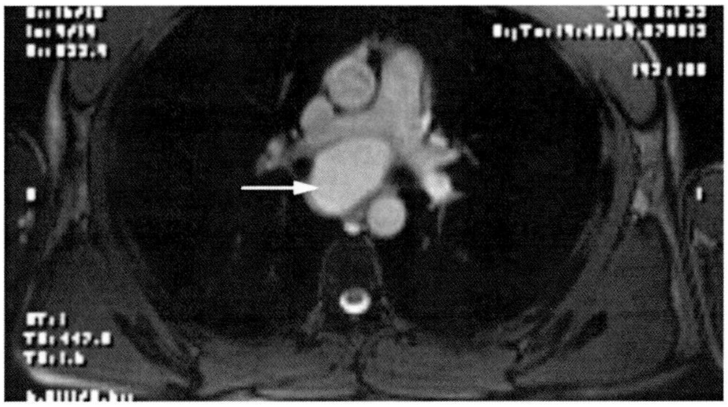

Figure 6-D

Endobronchial ultrasound-guided needle aspiration and/or drainage may be considered as a temporizing measure in acutely ill patients or in those who are poor surgical candidates. Recurrence, however, is common (choice C is incorrect). A definitive diagnosis can only be obtained with surgical resection, often via video-assisted thoracoscopic surgery (choice D is correct).

Foregut cysts, composed of either bronchogenic or esophageal duplication cysts, result from abnormal division of the primitive foregut. The cysts may occur in the anterior, middle, or posterior mediastinum but more commonly occur in the middle mediastinum and in the right paratracheal or hilar position. Up to one-third may be intraparenchymal and, in rare cases, have been reported in the presternal tissues, diaphragm, spine, pericardium, neck, and within the peritoneum. Patients may be seen who have an asymptomatic mediastinal mass on chest radiograph. Although most patients were previously thought to be asymptomatic, more recent reports suggest the majority (39 to 80%) of patients have symptoms. Common symptoms include retrosternal chest pain, cough, fever, and hoarseness. Acute rupture of the cyst and frank mediastinitis are uncommon. Chest radiography will identify bronchogenic cysts in the majority of patients, as was the case in our patient in whom a subcarinal mass was identified (see Figure 6-A). Chest CT is helpful to characterize bronchogenic cysts as round, well-circumscribed water-density lesions, which was seen in our patient on contrast-enhanced CT of the chest in the subcarinal position (see Figure 6-B). MRI, with T2-weighted imaging revealing cystic content, distinguishes solid and cystic masses. In Figures 6-C and 6-D, the complex, cystic subcarinal mass is identified by the arrows. Some physicians, because of the progressive symptomatic course and low operative morbidity and mortality, even in asymptomatic patients, have advocated surgical resection.

Funakoshi Y, Takeda S, Kadota Y, et al. Mediastinal bronchogenic cyst with respiratory distress from airway and vascular compression. Thorac Cardiovasc Surg 2007; 55:53–54

Takeda S, Miyoshi S, Minami M, et al. Clinical spectrum of mediastinal cysts. Chest 2003; 124:125–132

Aktogu S, Yuncu G, Halilcolar H, et al. Bronchogenic cysts: clinicopathological presentation and treatment. Eur Respir J 1996; 9:2017–2021

Patel SR, Meeker DP, Biscotti CV, et al. Presentation and management of bronchogenic cysts in the adult. Chest 1994; 106:79–85

7. C. Technetium-99m sulfur-colloid (SC) scan.

This patient's CT scan abnormalities are manifestations of intrathoracic and soft tissue splenosis, resulting from the ectopic growth of splenic tissue in the lung, pleural surface, and chest wall. Scintigraphy with indium 111–labeled platelets, technetium-99 SC, or technetium-99–labeled heat-damaged RBCs can demonstrate splenosis because these agents are sequestered by splenic tissue (choice C is correct). Tc-99 SC scanning was performed in this patient, and each of the masses identified by CT scan showed intense uptake consistent with splenosis (see Figure 7-D and the nuclear medicine scan oriented in the same plane as the CT scan, Figure 7-E).

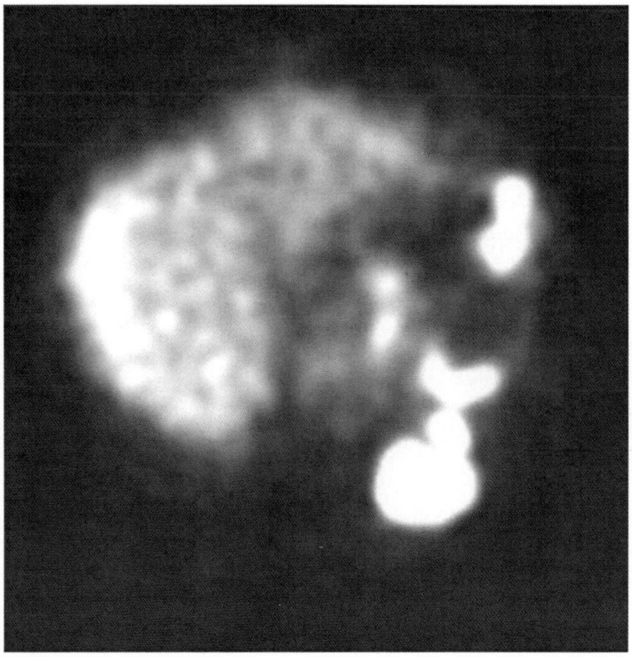

Figure 7-D

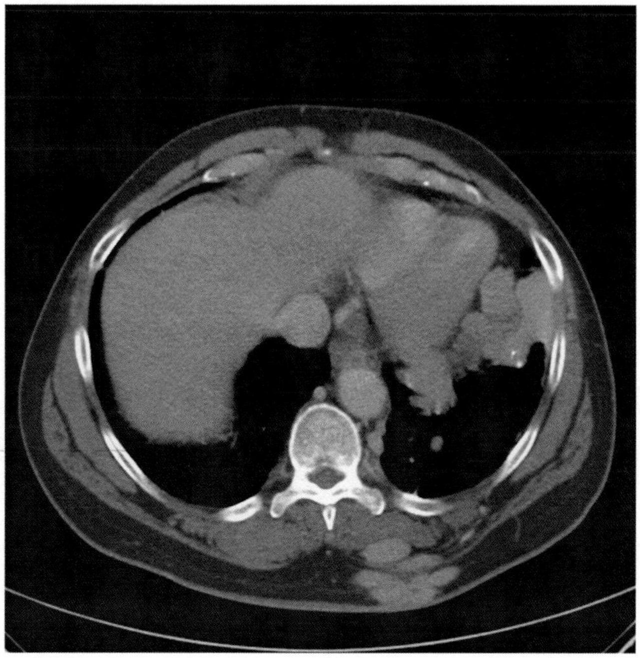

Figure 7-E

Splenosis can occur when splenic pulp cells spill to other sites following injury to the spleen and/or splenectomy. These cells may grow *in situ* and, in fact, can reconstitute splenic function after splenectomy. This patient had a peripheral blood smear performed that did not exhibit Howell-Jolly bodies, a marker of absent splenic function following splenectomy. Accordingly, despite the absence of the spleen itself, it is likely that he has normal splenic function and would not need management as an asplenic individual.

If traumatic splenic injury is accompanied by a diaphragmatic tear, implants can be present within the pleural or pericardial cavities. It is virtually certain that one aspect of this patient's original injury was diaphragm interruption and seeding of splenic cells along a track extending all the way to the posterior chest wall. The history given by the patient of a tissue mass arising in the months following the trauma is consistent with this process.

The findings of splenosis can be confused with those of a neoplasm or endometriosis. Ectopic splenic tissue is highly vascular, so biopsy is not recommended and would be unnecessarily invasive because imaging can often confirm the diagnosis (choice A is incorrect). In addition to being unnecessarily invasive, bronchoscopy would likely fail to obtain tissue, given the distal location of these masses (choice B is incorrect). This patient does not have symptoms suggesting granulomatous vasculitis, the masses are not consistent with such a diagnosis, and the history is very compelling for splenosis. Thus, serum tests for vasculitis are not appropriate (choice D is incorrect).

Hagnan TF, Winer-Muram HT, Meyer CA, et al. Intrathoracic splenosis. Chest 2001; 120:2097–2098
Naylor MF, Karstedt N, Finck SJ, et al. Noninvasive methods of diagnosing thoracic splenosis. Ann Thorac Surg 1999; 68:243–244

8. C. Bright light exposure during the morning.

This patient has delayed sleep phase syndrome (DSPS), a circadian rhythm sleep disorder characterized by a habitually delayed nocturnal sleep period. Individuals are usually unable to fall asleep until the early morning hours (1:00 AM to 6:00 AM) and have difficulty waking up until late morning or early afternoon (between 11:00 AM and 2:00 PM). Phototherapy using timed early morning light exposure *after* the core body temperature nadir (minimum core temperature [CTmin]) and avoidance of bright lights in the evening produce a phase advance and is an effective therapy for this condition (choice C is correct). His complaints are related to the shift in his major sleep period and not to a primary disorder of excessive sleepiness; therefore, a stimulant agent, although it may improve daytime alertness, does not correct the circadian rhythm sleep disturbance (choice A is incorrect). Furthermore, although hypnotic agents may shorten sleep latency, their benefits are often temporary, and these agents generally are not effective for long-term use (choice B is incorrect). Cognitive behavioral therapy for insomnia is an effective treatment for both primary insomnia and comorbid insomnia, but it is not primarily indicated for treating circadian rhythm sleep disorders (choice D is incorrect).

People with DSPS may present to the pulmonologist for evaluation of either insomnia and/or excessive sleepiness. Although people with DSPS are incapable of voluntarily advancing their sleep time, they have no difficulty remaining asleep, with a normal sleep quality and a normal (or prolonged) sleep duration, if sleep is allowed to continue *ad libitum* until spontaneous awakening. They often describe themselves as "night owls," having less difficulty staying up late at night than waking up early in the morning, as well as being most sleepy in the morning and most alert at night. Both sleep-onset insomnia and morning sleepiness develop if sleep is attempted closer to socially accepted bedtimes.

This disorder tends to affect adolescents and young adults with a prevalence of up to 16%. Both genders are affected equally. If untreated, the course tends to be persistent, but severity may lessen with increasing age. Diagnosis is based mainly on history and sleep diaries and may be aided by actigraphy. With actigraphy, accelerometers, typically worn over the wrist, produce a signal whenever movement is detected, thus discerning periods of rest-sleep or activity; when recorded over several days to weeks, a stable delay in the habitual sleep period is revealed.

Phototherapy is the principal therapy for DSPS. Light exposure can be timed prior to CTmin. CTmin is often 1 to 2 h after the habitual midsleep time. Both intensity and duration of light exposure should be individualized. Many clinicians start with a 10,000 lux exposure for 30 to 40 min each morning using commercially available medical light boxes. Phototherapy is contraindicated in patients with retinopathy or significant photosensitivity and can precipitate mania in those with bipolar disorder and possibly in those with migraines. An ophthalmologic exam is recommended for patients who have retinal and ocular disorders prior to initiating therapy.

Other therapies that have been described for DSPS are evening administration of melatonin and chronotherapy. Chronotherapeutic techniques include progressive phase delay (bedtime and wake times are delayed by about 2 to 3 h each day on successive days until the desired or conventional bedtime is reached), progressive phase advancement (gradually advancing bedtime by 30 to 60 min until the desired schedule is attained), and schedule shift technique (allowing six consecutive nights on the usual sleep schedule followed by a night of sleep deprivation and six subsequent days with a 90-min advance in sleep schedule; the protocol is then repeated until the desired bedtime is attained).

Morgenthaler TI, Lee-Chiong T, Alessi C, et al. Practice parameters for the clinical evaluation and treatment of circadian rhythm sleep disorders: an American Academy of Sleep Medicine report. Sleep 2007; 30:1445–1459

Sack R, Auckley D, Auger RR, et al. Circadian rhythm sleep disorders: Part 2. Advanced sleep phase disorder, delayed sleep phase disorder, free-running disorder, and irregular sleep-wake rhythm. Sleep 2007; 30:1484–1501

9. A. Trimethoprim-sulfamethoxazole.

This patient has developed an *S maltophilia* infection, formerly called *Xanthomonas maltophilia*, and trimethoprim-sulfamethoxazole is the initial antibiotic agent of choice (choice A is correct). The organism is a nonfermenting, Gram-negative bacillus and usually infects patients with chronic infection, such as those with cystic fibrosis, lung transplant recipients, and occasionally those with idiopathic bronchiectasis. Other susceptible hosts include patients who are immunosuppressed with hematologic malignancies or prolonged neutropenia, patients who are exposed to broad-spectrum antibiotics, and those requiring mechanical ventilation. The organism may cause catheter-related bacteremia, pneumonia, skin and soft tissue infection, meningitis, complicated biliary and urinary tract infection, prosthetic valve endocarditis, and ocular infections. Infection can be associated with high mortality, particularly in patients with hematologic malignancy, those in ICUs, and those with chronic illnesses, but it also causes chronic indolent infection. This patient's chest radiograph shows typical findings of advanced cystic fibrosis with areas of bronchiectasis and patchy infiltrates (see Figure 9-A).

S maltophilia is resistant to many antibiotics, and some microbiology laboratories do not routinely test sensitivities for this organism unless requested. Typically, resistance to expanded-spectrum penicillins, third-generation cephalosporins, aminoglycosides, and quinolones is found (choices B and D are incorrect). The organism is intrinsically resistant to carbapenems (choice C is incorrect), and exposure to these agents has been linked to selection of *S maltophilia.* Although trimethoprim-sulfamethoxazole is the agent most consistently used to treat *S maltophilia* infections, it is bacteriostatic, and increasing resistance is being reported. This is one of the few Gram-negative organisms that can be treated with single-agent therapy. Combination drug regimens and the inhaled route of administration (as may be used with aminoglycosides) might be necessary in difficult cases and may have *in vivo* synergy against this organism. Upon special request, *in vitro* susceptibilities to combination antibiotics can be assessed. Other possible drug combinations in the case of resistance, intolerance, or an allergy to sulfa drugs include ticarcillin/clavulanate with or without aztreonam; a combination including cephalosporins (ceftazidime or ceftriaxone), quinolones (ciprofloxacin), and/or doxycycline may be considered as alternative options beyond trimethoprim-sulfamethoxazole, but not as first-line therapy. Vancomycin, an antibiotic used to treat Gram-positive infections, would not treat this infection (choice D is incorrect).

Paez JI, Costa SF. Risk factors associated with mortality of infections caused by *Stenotrophomonas maltophilia*: a systematic review. J Hosp Infect 2008; 70:101–108

Falagas ME, Valkimadi PE, Huang YT, et al. Therapeutic options for *Stenotrophomonas maltophilia* infections beyond co-trimoxazole: a systematic review. J Antimicrob Chemother 2008; 62:889–894

Nicodemo AC, Paez JI. Antimicrobial therapy for *Stenotrophomonas maltophilia* infections. Eur J Clin Microbiol Infect Dis 2007; 26:229–237
Muder RR. Optimizing therapy for *Stenotrophomonas maltophilia*. Semin Respir Crit Care Med 2007; 28:672–677
Davies JC, Rubin BK. Emerging and unusual gram-negative infections in cystic fibrosis. Semin Respir Crit Care Med 2007; 28:312–321

10. B. Worsening lung compliance and oxygenation.

It is now widely accepted that lower tidal volumes and plateau pressures are lung protective in that excessive lung stretch is avoided. Reducing excessive stretch appears to reduce an acute lung injury termed ventilator-induced lung injury (VILI). These lower settings, however, may adversely affect lung physiology. For example, a reduced tidal volume without a concomitant increase in rate will reduce minute ventilation and thus reduce CO_2 clearance. The resulting "permissive hypercapnia," however, can be viewed as an acceptable trade-off if VILI can be reduced.

Less appreciated is the fact that a reduced tidal volume may also reduce the lung recruitment that can occur during positive-pressure lung inflation. This can result in more atelectasis, a worsening of lung compliance, and worsening of ventilation-perfusion matching, resulting in hypoxemia. However, in several recent clinical trials, the reduced VILI from the reduced end inspiratory stretch appears to be worth this physiologic deterioration (choice B is correct and the other options are incorrect). Indeed, in the seminal ARDS Network trial showing a mortality benefit from a 6 mL/kg IBW tidal volume strategy vs a 12 mL/kg IBW tidal volume strategy, respiratory system compliance and PaO_2/FIO_2 ratios were both significantly worse in the small tidal volume vs the large tidal volume group over the first 2 days of the trial. After the third day, however, these differences disappeared, and the small tidal volume group went on to a better survival. Like permissive hypercapnia described above, "permissive atelectasis/hypoxemia" may be a reasonable trade-off if overstretch-induced VILI can be reduced.

Dreyfuss D, Savmon G. Ventilator induced lung injury: lessons from experimental studies Am J Resp Crit Care Med 1998; 157:294–323
NIH ARDS Network. Ventilation with lower tidal volumes as compared with traditional tidal volumes for acute lung injury and the acute respiratory distress syndrome. New Engl J Med 2000; 342:1301–1308
Grasso S, Stripoli T, De Michele M, et al. ARDSnet ventilatory protocol and alveolar hyperinflation: role of positive end-expiratory pressure. Am J Resp Crit Care Med 2007; 176:761–767
Ferragni PP, Rosbosh G, Tealdi A, et al. Tidal hyperinflation during low tidal volume ventilation in acute respiratory distress syndrome. Am J Respir Crit Care Med 2007; 175:160–166

11. B. Hydroxocobalamin.

This patient was exposed to the products of combustion of plastics, which increases his risk of cyanide toxicity, so hydroxocobalamin should be administered promptly pending measurement of cyanide serum levels (choice B is correct). Cyanide is a potent toxin that acts by blocking oxidative phosphorylation. Exposures may be due to smoke inhalation (particularly during the combustion and pyrolysis of wool, silk, synthetic rubber, and plastics such as polyurethane, polyacrylonitriles, and melamine resins), industrial exposure (mining, pesticides, and electroplating), or its use as an agent of terrorism. Symptoms of acute exposure tend to be neurologic (headache, confusion, seizures, and coma), respiratory (tachypnea followed by bradypnea), and cardiac (bradycardia, hypotension, atrioventricular block, and ventricular dysrhythmias). Lactic acidosis and a narrowed arterial-venous oxygen difference may be observed because of interference with tissue oxygen utilization.

Because cyanide levels cannot be quickly obtained, treatment should begin when the diagnosis is suspected on clinical grounds. Until recently, treatment of cyanide poisoning in the United States centered on the use of nitrites to intentionally induce the formation of methemoglobin, which can complex with cyanide to form cyanomethemoglobin, a much less toxic moiety. However, methemoglobinemia is hazardous in the presence of significant carboxyhemoglobin concentrations because its oxygen-carrying capacity will be further compromised.

Therefore, nitrites should not be administered to this patient (choice A is incorrect), and a better choice would be hydroxocobalamin, a vitamin B_{12} precursor that directly binds cyanide. In addition to treatment with hydroxocobalamin or nitrites, all patients should be treated with sodium thiosulfate, a sulfur donor that can detoxify cyanide by converting it to thiocyanate.

Nitrates (as opposed to nitrites) have no established role in the treatment of cyanide poisoning (choice D is incorrect). Neither does pralidoxime, which is an important agent in treating poisonings by organophosphate nerve agents (choice C is incorrect).

Borron SW, Baud FJ, Barriot P, et al. Prospective study of hydroxocobalamin for acute cyanide poisoning in smoke inhalation. Ann Emerg Med 2007; 49:794–801

Morocco AP. Cyanides. Crit Care Clin 2005; 21:691–705

Sauer SW, Keim ME. Hydroxocobalamin: improved public health readiness for cyanide disasters. Ann Emerg Med 2001: 37:635–641

12. B. Prescribe participation in a pulmonary rehabilitation program.

This patient has stage 2 COPD (FEV_1 between 50 and 80% of predicted), has dyspnea classified as Medical Research Council Dyspnea grade 3 (has to stop for breath when walking at his own pace on a level surface), and has infrequent exacerbations (probably a single exacerbation about 2 years ago). He is currently being treated with combination long-acting bronchodilators and with a short-acting β_2-agonist as needed. To further improve his symptoms, and assuming his inhaler technique is good and he is adherent with the prescribed medication, participation in a pulmonary rehabilitation program would be the best recommendation (choice B is correct). Pulmonary rehabilitation would be expected to significantly improve exercise capacity, reduce breathlessness, reduce anxiety and depression associated with COPD, and reduce hospitalizations and days in the hospital.

This patient would not yet be a candidate for continuous oxygen because his room air oxygen saturation is 93% at rest, and he has no evidence of cor pulmonale (choice A is incorrect). Adding an inhaled corticosteroid would be appropriate only after pulmonary rehabilitation was instituted, as recommended by the Global Initiative for Chronic Obstructive Lung Disease and Canadian Thoracic Society Guideline Committees (choice C is incorrect). Initiating therapy with fluticasone/salmeterol or budesonide/formoterol could be considered in the setting of repeated exacerbations, but this patient has not had a prior exacerbation. There is no current evidence or agreement to suggest that one long-acting β_2-agonist is better or worse than any other in COPD; therefore, changing the long-acting β_2-agonist would not be expected to improve the patient's condition (choice D is incorrect).

O'Donnell DE, Aaron S, Bourbeau J, et al. Canadian Thoracic Society recommendations for management of chronic obstructive pulmonary disease: 2007 update. Can Resp J 2007; 14:5B–32B

Rabe KF, Hurd S, Anzueto A, et al. Global strategy for the diagnosis, management, and prevention of chronic obstructive pulmonary disease: GOLD executive summary. Am J Respir Crit Care Med 2007; 176:532–555

Ries AL, Bauldoff GS, Carlin BW, et al. Pulmonary rehabilitation: joint ACCP/AACVPR evidence-based clinical practice guidelines. Chest 2007; 131:4–42

13. C. An unprovoked initial event.

Up to 18% of patients who complete an initial adequate course of therapy with warfarin will experience a recurrent event in the 2 years following the completion of therapy. However, the rate varies based on the circumstances surrounding the initial event. In a prospective cohort of almost 600 patients followed after the completion of therapy, 17% of patients whose initial event was unprovoked (idiopathic) experienced a recurrent event, whereas in those whose initial event was in the setting of a surgical procedure, there were no recurrences (choice C is correct, and choice D is incorrect). Other studies have shown that the recurrence rate in those with either no risk factors or persistent risk factors is 10 to 20%, whereas in those with transient risk factors, the rate varies from 4 to 8%.

Several genetic and acquired hypercoagulable (or thrombophilic) states have been identified, with the factor V Leiden mutation being one of the most common (behind the antiphospholipid antibody syndrome). These factors increase the relative risk of an initial thrombotic event from 2 to 10 times the baseline risk. However, with the exception of the antiphospholipid antibody syndrome, newer evidence suggests that thrombophilia does not significantly increase the risk of recurrent thrombosis (choice A is incorrect). Two metaanalyses found an overall relative risk of recurrence of approximately 1.5 for hereditary thrombophilias, but this did not reach statistical significance in either analysis. Additionally, the relative risk of recurrence in those with the factor V Leiden mutation was also not significant, with a hazard ratio of 1.2 (95% CI, 0.7 to 1.9). On the basis of these data, authors of the eighth edition of the American College of Chest Physicians antithrombotic guidelines state that the presence of hereditary thrombophilia is not a major determinant of the risk of recurrence.

In an initial trial of > 800 patients who were prospectively followed for a median of 2 years after withdrawal of oral anticoagulants, the relative risk of recurrence in men vs women was 3.6. After 5 years, the likelihood of recurrence was 31% among men, compared with 8.5% among women (choice B is incorrect). A metaanalysis that included 15 trials with > 5,000 patients confirmed an increased risk of recurrence in men, with a relative risk of 1.6. The lower risk of recurrence in women in this and other studies could not be accounted for by a reduced rate of recurrence in those whose initial event was related to estrogen therapy.

Other factors that are associated with an increased risk of recurrence include age, malignancy, and an elevated d-dimer or thrombin level upon the completion of therapy.

Christiansen SC, Cannegieter SC, Koster T, et al. Thrombophilia, clinical factors, and recurrent venous thrombotic events. JAMA 2005; 293:2352–2361

Kearon C, Kahn SR, Agnelli G, et al. Antithrombotic therapy for venous thromboembolic disease. American College of Chest Physicians evidence-based clinical practice guidelines, 8th edition. Chest 2008; 133(suppl):454S–545S

Bauer KA. The thrombophilias: well-defined risk factors with uncertain therapeutic implications. Ann Intern Med 2001; 135:367–373

McRae S, Tran H, Schulman S, et al. Effect of patient's sex on risk of recurrent thromboembolism: a meta-analysis. Lancet 2006; 368:371–378

14. B. Improved self-perception of body image and perception of level of physical activity.

This patient's chest radiographs show pectus excavatum with mild scoliosis. Patients with this congenital chest wall disorder have a decreased self-perception of body image along with a lower perceived physical activity level, and surgical correction leads to improved body image and perceived level of physical activity (choice B is correct). Pulmonary function test results show restrictive dysfunction that is not associated with age, severity of the deformity, or the patient's body image and level of activity.

Pectus excavatum may be associated with a variety of congenital disorders, including scoliosis, congenital heart disease, and Marfan syndrome and appears be a phenotypic marker for those patients at risk of developing pulmonary nontuberculous mycobacterial disease (such as *Mycobacterium avium* complex). In two reports of patients with *M avium* complex infection, 11 to 27% had pectus excavatum, and 50 to 52% had scoliosis. However, surgical correction of skeletal deformities does not reduce the risk of developing infection (choice D is incorrect).

Surgical correction of pectus excavatum has traditionally involved resection of costal cartilage or sternal osteotomy and was done in early adolescence when the chest was relatively malleable. More recently, insertion of a retrosternal metal bar with subsequent anterior chest wall remodeling (Nuss procedure) is becoming more common because of its minimal invasiveness, lack of cartilage resection, short operating time, and quicker recovery time. The optimal age for surgical correction is between 5 and 20 years because of chest wall compliance and malleability. When performed in adults, the procedure has higher complication rates (pneumothorax), more postoperative pain, and less cosmetic improvement. Surgical intervention has *not* been shown to improve postoperative lung function, with some patients actually having lower TLC, FVC, and FEV_1 results despite improved physical activity perception (choices A and C are

incorrect). Correction of scoliosis, in severe cases, can reduce the likelihood of developing respiratory failure. However, the associated scoliosis in this case is mild and would not impact the patient's respiratory mechanics.

Iseman MD, Buschman DL, Ackerson LM. Pectus excavatum and scoliosis: thoracic anomalies associated with pulmonary disease caused by *Mycobacterium avium* complex. Am Rev Respir Dis 1991; 144:914–916

Kelly RE, Cash TF, Shamberger RC, et al. Surgical repair of pectus excavatum markedly improved body image and perceived ability for physical activity: a multicenter study. Pediatrics 2008; 122:1218–1222

Morshuis W, Folgering H, Barentsz J, et al. Pulmonary function surgery for pectus excavatum and at long term follow-up. Chest 1994; 105:1646–1652

Nuss D, Kelly RE. Minimally invasive surgical correction of chest wall deformities in children (Nuss procedure). Adv Pediatr 2008; 55:395–410

15. D. Methylprednisolone, 20 mg IV every 4 h for four doses.

This patient is at increased risk for postextubation stridor upon removal of the ET tube. Multiple doses of corticosteroids (*ie,* 20 to 40 mg of methylprednisolone or 5 mg dexamethasone for four doses every 4 to 6 h) administered prior to extubation have been demonstrated in placebo-controlled randomized clinical trials (RCTs) to reduce postextubation stridor (choice D is correct, and choice A is incorrect). In contrast, a single dose of dexamethasone or methylprednisolone administered shortly before extubation has been demonstrated in RCTs to be ineffective (choice B is incorrect). In the largest multicenter RCT of 698 adults who had been intubated > 36 h, administration of methylprednisolone, 20 mg IV every 4 h for four doses significantly reduced postextubation laryngeal edema to 3% compared with 22% for patients who received placebo. Reintubation was also significantly reduced from 8 to 4%. Metaanalyses confirm the different results for single-dose corticosteroid therapy and multiple-dose therapy. There is no evidence to support the higher doses, such as 250 mg of methylprednisolone every 6 h for a longer duration (choice C is incorrect).

Many patients develop postextubation stridor that requires intervention, often including reintubation. The following characteristics have been identified as risk factors for postextubation stridor: prolonged intubation (> 6 days), traumatic intubation or extubation, a large ET, and a reduced "cuff leak." A number of studies has demonstrated higher rates of postextubation stridor among patients who have absent or modest (*ie,* < 15 to 25% or < 150 mL) leak of exhaled tidal volume around the ET tube when a volume-targeted breath is administered and the ET tube cuff is deflated. The cuff leak test is less reliable as a predictor of postextubation stridor with shorter duration ET intubation, such as after cardiac surgery. This patient has multiple risk factors, including prolonged intubation, traumatic extubation, prior stridor, and poor cuff leak, so prophylactic corticosteroid administration to reduce the likelihood of postextubation stridor should be considered.

Francois B, Bellissant E, Gissot V, et al. 12-h pretreatment with methylprednisolone versus placebo for prevention of postextubation laryngeal oedema: a randomised double-blind trial. Lancet 2007; 369:1083–1089

Cheng KC, Hou CC, Huang HC, et al. Intravenous injection of methylprednisolone reduces the incidence of postextubation stridor in intensive care unit patients. Crit Care Med 2006; 34:1345–1350

Lee CH, Peng MJ, Wu CL. Dexamethasone to prevent postextubation airway obstruction in adults: a prospective, randomized, double-blind, placebo-controlled study [abstract]. Crit Care 2007; 11:72

Markovitz BP, Randolph AG, Khemani RG. Corticosteroids for the prevention and treatment of post-extubation stridor in neonates, children and adults. Cochrane Database Syst Rev 2008; CD001000

Roberts RJ, Welch SM, Devlin JW. Corticosteroids for prevention of postextubation laryngeal edema in adults. Ann Pharmacother 2008; 42:686–691

16. C. Initiation of colchicine therapy.

The mutation in the *MEFV* gene is diagnostic of familial Mediterranean fever (FMF). The recurrent episodes of inflammation may lead to amyloidosis with subsequent proteinuria, nephrotic syndrome, and premature death from renal failure. Once the diagnosis is established, the prompt initiation of colchicine, 0.6 mg bid, is recommended

(choice C is correct). This is not only helpful in greatly reducing the frequency of attacks, but it also prevents, or greatly delays, the development of amyloidosis. The benefits of colchicine have been established in two controlled clinical trials.

There is no good evidence for recurrent thromboembolic events in this case. Therefore, there is no indication for initiation of warfarin therapy (choice A is incorrect). Even in patients with a slightly increased risk of thromboembolic events because of the presence of factor V Leiden, there is no indication to start anticoagulation therapy in the absence of a family or personal history of thrombotic events. The risk of a thrombotic event in patients with factor V Leiden who are taking high-dose estrogen is about 50 to 70 times the risk in women not taking estrogen and who do not have factor V Leiden. However, the absolute risk remains very low, and there are no data linking a 20-μg oral contraceptive with thromboembolic events. This, combined with the fact that the current patient developed severe pelvic pain off of her oral contraceptive, means that the latter should be continued (choice B is incorrect). Finally, there is no role for low-dose aspirin therapy in preventing pulmonary thromboembolic events or attacks of FMF (choice D is incorrect).

FMF is an autosomal recessive disorder found mostly in individuals of non-Ashkenazi Jewish, Armenian, Arab, or Turkish background. It is characterized by brief, recurrent episodes of peritonitis, pleuritis, and arthritis that are usually accompanied by fever. Occasionally, small amounts of pericardial fluid, presumably related to pericarditis, can be seen, as in the current case. FMF should be suspected in patients with an appropriate genetic background or positive family history who have a history of at least four episodes of abdominal or chest pain, or both, lasting 24 to 72 h; who are asymptomatic between attacks; who do not have another condition that could explain the symptoms; and who respond to colchicine. Genetic testing now offers a confirmatory test. More then 80 MEFV mutations causing FMF have been identified, and the finding of this mutation is 100% specific for the disease. The *MEFV* gene is necessary for making a protein, called *pyrin*, that is found mostly in WBCs. Whereas the exact function of pyrin is unknown, it is felt to keep the inflammatory response under control—perhaps by directing the migration of WBCs to sites of inflammation and turning the process off when it is no longer required. Recurrent episodes of inflammation can lead to the development of amyloidosis, which greatly worsens prognosis. For patients who do not respond to colchicine, the drugs thalidomide, etanercept, and infliximab have been shown to be useful.

Blickstein I. Thrombophilia and women's health: an overview. Obstet Gynecol Clin North Am 2006; 33:347–356

Onen F. Familial Mediterranean fever. Rheumatol Int 2006; 26:489–496

Samuels J, Aksentijevich I, Torosyan Y, et al. Familial Mediterranean fever at the millennium: clinical spectrum, ancient mutations, and a survey of 100 American referrals to the National Institutes of Health. Medicine (Baltimore) 1998; 77:268–297

17. A. Lower extremity involvement is common.

The pathology image (see Figure 17-C in the stem) shows well-formed noncaseating granulomas with adjacent skeletal muscle compatible with the diagnosis of nodular tumorous sarcoidosis involving muscle. The diagnosis of sarcoidosis is supported by the bilateral hilar lymphadenopathy seen on the chest radiograph and the mediastinal views of the chest CT scan (see Figures 17-A and 17-B in the stem). Lower extremity involvement occurs in 90% of cases of nodular tumorous sarcoidosis skeletal muscle involvement (choice A is correct), with upper extremities involved in 43% of cases. However, palpable nodules or mass lesions involving the muscles of patients with sarcoidosis are uncommon, with only 60 published cases from 1908 to 1999. Multiple nodules are present in 80%; only 20% exhibit a single mass lesion, as in this case. The most common complaint is weakness (70%) followed by pain or tenderness (60%), neither of which are found in this patient. In 12 of the 60 reported cases, functional limitations are exhibited, but these are poorly described. Accompanying evidence of extramuscular sarcoidosis is frequent with the most common manifestations, including peripheral lymphadenopathy, cutaneous and subcutaneous involvement, and uveitis. Results of chest radiographs are abnormal in 73% of patients at presentation (23 of 31 patients where available), with stage I or II disease in 19 of 31 patients (61%) (choice C is incorrect). Laboratory abnormalities are nonspecific, with normal serum calcium and creatine phosphokinase levels (choice D is incorrect). ^{67}Ga scintigraphy may be used to distinguish muscular sarcoidosis from soft tissue malignancies. The optimal treatment of sarcoidosis nodules and masses involving

skeletal muscle is undefined, as the response to corticosteroids is variable and difficult to assess given different reported dosages, routes of administration, and duration (choice B is incorrect). Spontaneous tumor regression and success with surgical excision have been reported.

Asymptomatic involvement of muscles is reported in 25 to 75% of patients with sarcoidosis. Symptomatic involvement is rare in retrospective series, suggesting an occurrence of $< 0.5\%$. Patterns of sarcoidosis symptomatic muscle involvement include chronic progressive myopathy, an acute polymyositis-like syndrome, and nodular or tumorous sarcoidosis affecting the muscle. Chronic myopathy is the most common form of symptomatic skeletal muscle involvement, with acute and subacute myositis being the rarest form.

This patient's lesion is quite unlike the most common cutaneous manifestation of sarcoidosis, erythema nodosum. Erythema nodosum is usually found on the shins as indurated, painful, and symmetrical red lesions.

Lynch JP, Sharma OP, Baughman RP. Extrapulmonary sarcoidosis. Semin Respir Infect 1998; 13:229–254

Zisman DA, Biermann JS, Martinez FJ, et al. Sarcoidosis presenting as a tumorlike muscular lesion: case report and review of the literature Medicine 1999; 78:112–122

Zisman DA, Shorr AF, Lynch JP. Sarcoidosis involving the musculoskeletal system. Semin Respir Crit Care Med 2002, 23:555–570

18. C. Dexbrompheniramine with pseudoephedrine.

While the potential differential diagnostic possibilities (see Figure 18-A) to explain the patient's acute cough include the common cold (upper respiratory tract infection), acute bronchitis (lower respiratory tract infection), asthma, and pneumonia, this patient has the classic presentation of an uncomplicated common cold. Of the medications listed, only dexbrompheniramine with pseudoephedrine has been shown to be effective for this cough (choice C is correct). While the older antihistamine dexbrompheniramine is efficacious probably because of its anticholinergic activity, the newer antihistamine loratadine has not been shown to favorably affect cough due to the common cold in randomized, double-blind, placebo-controlled trials (choice D is incorrect). The only other medication that has been shown to improve cough due to the common cold is the nonsteroidal antiinflammatory agent naproxen, which is not listed as a choice. Therefore, choices A and B are incorrect.

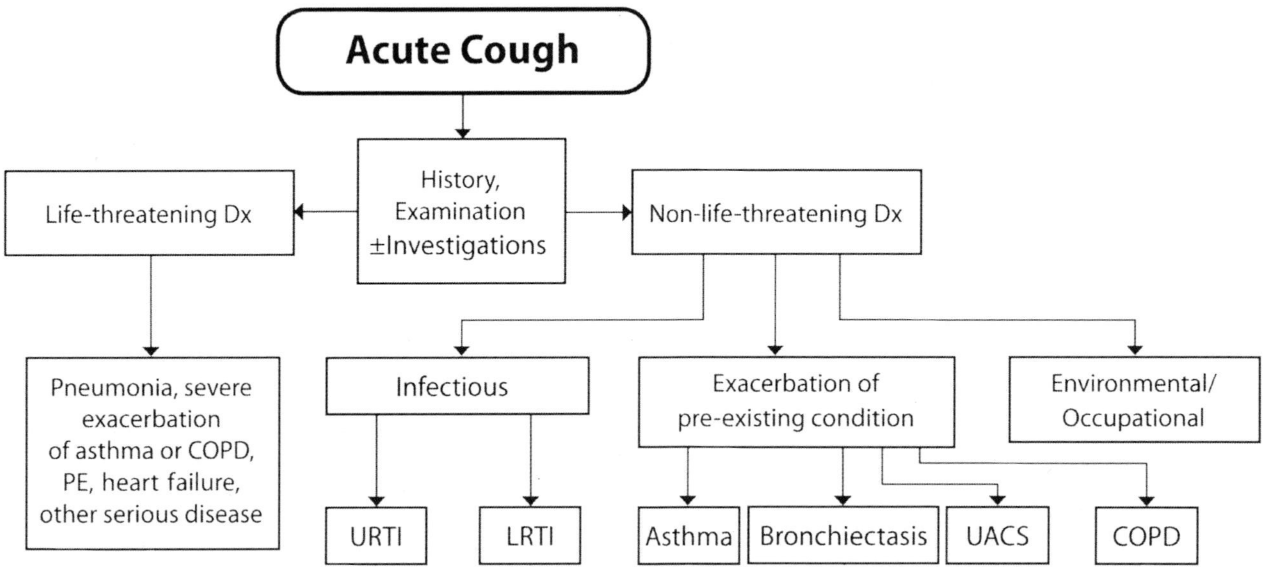

Figure 18-A

LRTI = lower respiratory tract infection; PE = pulmonary embolism; UACS = upper airway cough syndrome; URTI = upper respiratory tract infection.

It is becoming more difficult for patients to purchase antihistamines with decongestants over the counter, so physicians may need to prescribe trade name combination products.

The common cold and acute bronchitis are defined in similar terms and it is not often appreciated that cough due to the common cold can be productive of discolored phlegm, so acute cough due to the common cold is often misdiagnosed as being due to acute bronchitis, a term that implies a lower airway infection. Misdiagnosing cough due to the common cold as acute bronchitis can lead to inappropriate overprescribing of antibiotics. For example, even though antibiotics have been shown to be without benefit in acute bronchitis, physicians often prescribe them (65 to 80% of the time) when the diagnosis of acute bronchitis is made. Furthermore, patients expect them to be prescribed when the diagnosis of acute bronchitis, rather than a cold, is made (44% vs 11%).

While antibiotics have not been shown to be of benefit in randomized, controlled, clinical trials in patients with acute bronchitis, they should be prescribed for other conditions that present as an acute cough (*eg*, upper airway cough syndrome due to bacterial sinusitis, a severe acute exacerbation of chronic bronchitis or bronchiectasis, or *Bordetella pertussis* infection [whooping cough]). These conditions can complicate the common cold and should be suspected when acute cough either worsens (*ie*, biphasic course) or does not get better after a week following the common cold.

When the diagnosis of acute bronchitis is made, inhaled albuterol has only been shown to be of benefit in a subgroup of subjects with wheezing. Because wheezing was not part of this patient's acute cough syndrome, choice B is incorrect. There are data to suggest that this subgroup of subjects that has benefited from inhaled albuterol actually had another condition, such as an acute exacerbation of chronic bronchitis or asthma, for which inhaled albuterol would be expected to provide benefit. For example, up to 30% of patients misdiagnosed with acute bronchitis or 65% with recurrent acute bronchitis actually have had an acute exacerbation of chronic bronchitis from cigarette smoking or asthma. Therefore, clinicians should not diagnose acute bronchitis unless acute exacerbation of chronic bronchitis or asthma, as well as the common cold, has been ruled out.

Braman SS. Cough due to acute bronchitis: ACCP evidence-based clinical practice guidelines. Chest 2006; 129:95S–103S
Pratter MR. Cough and the common cold: ACCP evidence-based clinical practice guidelines. Chest 2006; 129:72S–74S

19. C. Langerhans cell histiocytosis.

This patient exhibits most of the recognized features of pulmonary Langerhans cell histiocytosis (LCH), previously known as eosinophilic granuloma and histiocytosis X: pulmonary changes involving the middle and upper parts of the lungs with irregularly shaped cystic and nodular lesions of varying size; involvement of a flat bone (the rib) (see Figure 19-C, arrow); and diabetes insipidus in a young person who smokes (choice C is correct). The only frequently encountered complication that is not present in this patient is a history of spontaneous pneumothorax. The radiographic findings, especially when a high-resolution CT scan shows cystic and nodular lesions (see Figure 19-D), are highly suggestive of LCH; in fact, most authorities accept this constellation of findings as proof of LCH. Cystic, nodular, and fibrotic lesions seen on high-resolution CT scans are the most frequent findings, followed by the presence of bone lesions in up to 20% of patients and diabetes insipidus in up to 15% of patients. Spontaneous pneumothorax occurs in 15 to 25% of patients (although not seen in this patient). Other manifestations contributing to morbidity and mortality include pulmonary hypertension and the development of a pulmonary neoplasm. The most important treatment for pulmonary LCH is cessation of smoking. Glucocorticoids and immunosuppressive agents have been tried but have not been proven to be effective. Smoking cessation alone will not alleviate pain in the symptomatic rib lesions.

Radiation therapy has been useful in controlling progression and reducing pain. Similarly, smoking cessation alone will not control diabetes insipidus, and therefore, replacement therapy should continue.

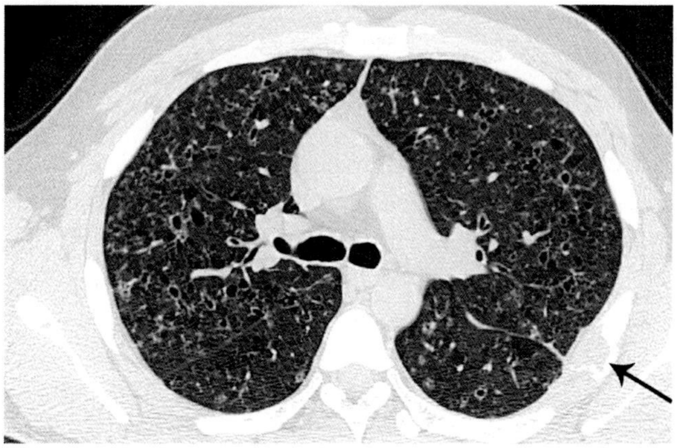

Figure 19-C

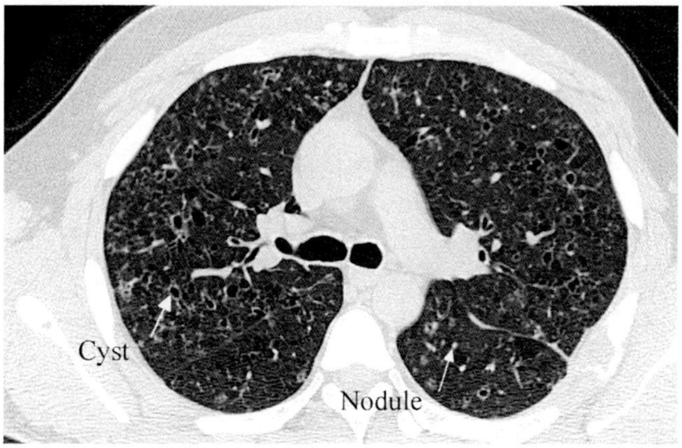

Figure 19-D

The bone lesion could be due to a metastatic cancer, but the chest radiograph does not show distinct nodules and is not consistent with metastatic cancer (choice A is incorrect). Patients with sarcoidosis may present with diabetes insipidus and may have extensive fibrosis late in the disease, but bone lesions are rare (choice B is incorrect). While the fibrotic lesions may be similar to those found in patients with idiopathic pulmonary fibrosis (IPF), bone lesions are not found in IPF and diabetes insipidus is not associated with IPF (choice D is incorrect).

Vassallo R, Jesen EA, Colby TV, et al. The overlap between respiratory bronchiolitis and desquamative interstitial pneumonia in pulmonary Langerhans cell histiocytosis: high-resolution CT, histologic, and functional correlations. Chest 2003; 124:1199–1205.

Vassallo R, Ryu JH, Colby TV, et al. Pulmonary Langerhans cell histiocytosis. N Engl J Med 2000; 342:1969–1978.

Vassallo R, Ryu JH, Schroeder DR, et al. Clinical outcomes of pulmonary Langerhans cell histiocytosis in adults. N Engl J Med 2002; 346:484–490.

20. C. Reduced hospitalization rates for acute myocardial infarction.

Exposure to environmental tobacco smoke (secondhand smoke) is known to increase health risks in nonsmoking adults and children, prompting major public health efforts around the world to ban smoking in workplaces and public spaces, with the expectation that the risk of developing tobacco-related illnesses in nonsmokers will decline correspondingly. Indeed, several studies confirm that hospitalization rates for acute myocardial infarction decline within a year after enactment of regulations banning smoking in public spaces and workplaces and that this effect is sustained over at least a few years (choice A is correct.)

Environmental tobacco smoke contains potentially toxic particulates, hydrocarbons, and carbon monoxide, and exposure to secondhand smoke is associated with numerous health-care risks to all age groups. The 2006 US Surgeon General's Report presents evidence "sufficient to infer a causal relationship of secondhand smoke exposure to sudden infant death syndrome, lower respiratory illnesses in infants and children, middle ear disease and asthma in children, as well as lung cancer and coronary artery disease in adults." Other illness may also be linked to secondhand smoke exposure, but the evidence for a causal link is less robust. Local, regional, and national laws that regulate smoking in the workplace and indoor public spaces were enacted to reduce these risks in exposed individuals and have been largely successful. Population studies confirm that levels of the nicotine metabolite, cotinine, have declined among US nonsmokers following implementation of nonsmoking regulations. In addition, these laws motivate many smokers to reduce their tobacco intake or stop smoking completely, amplifying the public health benefits.

Studies assessing the impact of smoke-free air laws consistently found that after implementation, there are marked improvements in both secondhand smoke exposure and air quality. Some short-term health outcomes have also been shown to improve in addition to a reduced rate of hospitalization due to myocardial infarction. In a study of bartenders, 74% reported respiratory symptoms such as cough and wheeze before a smoke-free workplace law took effect, compared with 41% 8 weeks after; this was accompanied by significant improvement in their mean FVC and FEV_1.

The US Environmental Protection Agency classifies secondhand smoke as a group A carcinogen, defined as a substance known to cause cancer in humans, and an estimated 3,000 lung cancer deaths in the United States per year in nonsmokers are attributed to secondhand smoke. Although limiting or eliminating secondhand smoke exposure is expected to eventually lead to a reduced incidence of tobacco-related lung, nasopharyngeal, and other cancers in nonsmokers, antismoking regulations have been adopted too recently to be able to measure an effect on these outcomes; it would probably take two or more decades after wide implementation to achieve a measureable reduction in cancers in nonsmokers (choices A and B are incorrect). Despite claims that antismoking regulations inevitably lead to an adverse economic impact on bars and restaurants, objective studies of retail sales generally find either no significant change or an increase in revenues and employment (choice D is incorrect).

Centers for Disease Control and Prevention. Reduced hospitalizations for acute myocardial infarction after implementation of a smoke-free ordinance: City of Pueblo, Colorado, 2002–2006. MMWR 2009; 57:1373–1377

Eisner MD, Smith AK, Blanc PD. Bartenders' respiratory health after establishment of smoke-free bars and taverns. JAMA 1998; 280:1909–1914

U.S. Department of Health and Human Services. The health consequences of involuntary exposure to tobacco smoke: a report of the Surgeon General. Atlanta, GA: U.S. Department of Health and Human Services, Centers for Disease Control and Prevention, Coordinating Center for Health Promotion, Office on Smoking and Health, 2006

U.S. Environmental Protection Agency. Respiratory health effects of passive smoking: lung cancer and other disorders. Washington, DC: U.S. Environmental Protection Agency, Office of Research and Development, Office of Air Radiation, 1992. Report No. EPA/600/6-90/0006F

21. C. Lymphocytic interstitial pneumonia (LIP).

This patient has had a long-standing productive cough unresponsive to many interventions. Investigations initially indicated mild bronchiectasis, but subsequently airspace disease developed, as seen best in the right lower lobe on CT scanning. Results of the lung biopsy demonstrate increased cellularity in the lung interstitium with lymphocytes, characteristic of LIP (choice C is correct). She subsequently was treated with a prolonged course of oral corticosteroids, with complete resolution of the lung infiltrates and symptoms. Although the patient had evidence of mild bronchiectasis, the normal sweat chloride test result makes the diagnosis of cystic fibrosis very unlikely in this context (choice A is incorrect). The patient did not have a rheumatologic disorder, and the negative rheumatoid factor also makes the diagnosis of rheumatoid lung with bronchiolitis unlikely (choice B is incorrect). The lung biopsy result is not in keeping with IPF (choice D is incorrect). Although LIP is usually a diffuse disease, occasionally focal disease has been described.

LIP has been described as a hyperplastic disorder of the mucosa-associated lymphoid tissues (MALT), which lies on a spectrum of pathologic abnormalities that extends from follicular bronchiolitis to pseudolymphoma to LIP. Although some have considered it a preneoplastic condition with a high likelihood of progression to lymphoma, immunohistochemical and molecular analyses indicate that malignant transformation is unusual. The pathologic finding has been associated with a variety of clinical conditions, such as connective tissue disorders, especially Sjögren syndrome, and other immune system abnormalities, such as dysproteinemia, AIDS, and bone marrow transplantation. In the absence of any comorbid illness predisposing a patient to LIP, the diagnosis of idiopathic LIP can be made (as in this case). Most patients respond to or stabilize with corticosteroid therapy. The prognosis is variable and often unpredictable from clinical, morphologic, and radiographic parameters. In general, death occurs in approximately 33 to 50% of patients within 5 years of diagnosis. Most patients die from infectious complications related to immunosuppression, progressive pulmonary fibrosis, or transformation to malignant lymphoma. In the past, LIP had been reported to progress to malignant lymphoma in up to 30% of cases. In retrospect, many of these cases were reclassified by immunohistochemical or molecular techniques as malignant lymphoma from the outset and were not LIP. The risk of transformation to malignant lymphoma is not known but is likely infrequent. A more recent and realistic estimate is that closer to 5% of patients with LIP acquire malignant, low-grade, B-cell lymphoma.

Cha SI, Fessler MB, Cool CD, et al. Lymphoid interstitial pneumonia: clinical features, associations and prognosis. Eur Respir J 2006; 28:364–369

Swigris JJ, Berry GJ, Raffin TA, et al. Lymphoid interstitial pneumonia: a narrative review. Chest 2002; 122:2150–2164

22. A. Initiate therapy with low-molecular-weight heparin.

The current CT angiogram clearly shows a large filling defect (see Figure 22-E, arrow) diagnostic of a pulmonary embolus so that immediate anticoagulation is the treatment of choice (choice A is correct). One might contemplate discontinuation of methotrexate and treatment with corticosteroids if there was evidence of methotrexate toxicity or progressive disease with therapy, but neither is present in this patient. The parenchymal changes have not worsened with therapy (see Figures 22-B and 22-D), and the pulmonary function has actually improved slightly with therapy (choice B is incorrect). Although *Pneumocystis jirovecii* has been reported to complicate low-dose methotrexate therapy, this complication is rare, and the absence of new pulmonary infiltrates argues strongly against this (choice C is incorrect). The elevated JVP and mild pedal edema suggest that there might be some right ventricular dysfunction related to the pulmonary emboli, but this is secondary to the acute problem and immediate anticoagulation is a much more important first step (choice D is incorrect).

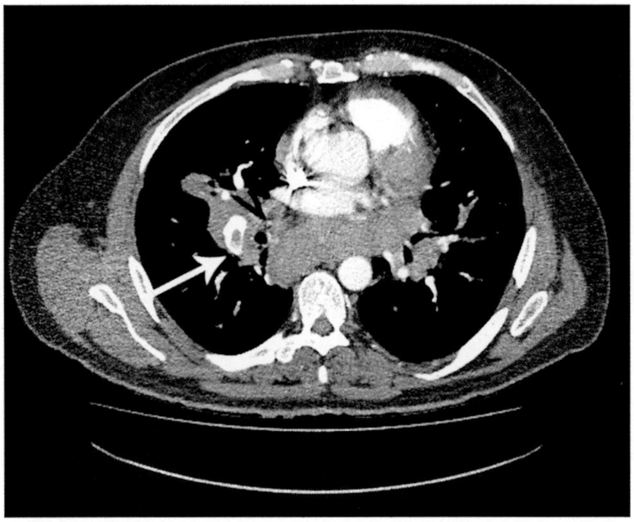

Figure 22-E

Pulmonary hypertension is an increasingly recognized complication of pulmonary sarcoidosis. This is most commonly seen in patients with extensive parenchymal involvement, but other potential causes such as granulomatous involvement of the pulmonary arteries, pulmonary venoocclusive disease, or extrinsic compression of the pulmonary arteries by enlarged mediastinal nodes have also been described. The latter may mimic a pulmonary embolism particularly on ventilation-perfusion scanning, but a CT angiogram, can clearly differentiate intraluminal clot vs external compression. Multiple venous thromboses secondary to regional lymph node involvement have been reported in sarcoidosis, but reports of pulmonary emboli in the disease have been extremely rare. Sarcoidosis very rarely has been associated with the presence of antiphospholipid antibodies, thereby increasing the risk of pulmonary emboli. The current patient had a negative test result for antiphospholipid antibodies.

Vahid B, Wildemore B, Marik PE. Multiple venous thromboses in a young man with sarcoidosis: is there a relation between sarcoidosis and venous thrombosis? South Med J 2006; 99:998–999

Morello FA, Ali S, Cesani F. Sarcoid: an unusual mimicker of classic pulmonary embolus. Clin Nucl Med 1998; 23:654–656

Esen BA, Kiyan E, Kucukkaya RD, et al. Antiphospholipid syndrome presenting as massive pulmonary embolism in a patient with sarcoidosis. Eur J Gen Med 2006; 2:173–176

Shigemitsu H, Nagai S, Sharma OP. Pulmonary hypertension and granulomatous vasculitis in sarcoidosis. Curr Opin Pulm Med 2007; 13:434–438

Kaneko Y, Suwa A, Ikeda Y, et al. *Pneumocystis jirovecii* pneumonia associated with low-dose methotrexate treatment for rheumatoid arthritis: report of two cases and review of the literature. Mod Rheumatol 2006; 16:36–38

23. D. Usually does not require biopsy for diagnostic confirmation.

This patient's chest radiograph (see Figure 23-F, arrows) and CT (see Figures 23-B, 23-C, and 23-D) demonstrate calcification in the anterior and lateral walls of the submucosa of the airways coinciding with airway cartilaginous structures. This, in combination with the bronchoscopic findings (see Figure 23-E), is diagnostic for tracheobronchopathia osteochondroplastica (TO; also known as tracheopathia osteoplastica or osteochondroplastica), a rare, benign disease. Biopsy of the airway lesions is usually not required to make the diagnosis, given the typical radiographic and bronchoscopic findings as described (choice D is correct). Bronchoscopic biopsy of these lesions can be difficult with the use of the usually small biopsy forceps and the inability to obtain adequate specimens. Successful biopsy using larger forceps during rigid bronchoscopy of these lesions shows heterotopic bone formation with abnormal cartilage proliferation and calcium deposits. Importantly, if involvement of the posterior wall of the airway is seen by CT imaging or on bronchoscopy, other entities need consideration, including amyloidosis, relapsing polychondritis, endobronchial sarcoidosis, papillomatosis, tracheobronchomalacia, and Wegener granulomatosis; all of these produce submucosal soft tissue abnormalities, and bronchoscopic biopsy may be necessary to confirm a diagnosis.

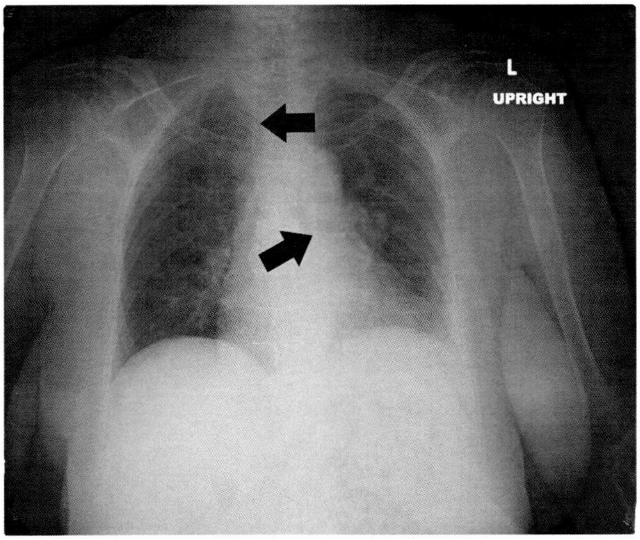

Figure 23-F

The diagnosis of TO usually occurs in patients in their fourth through sixth decade of life (choice A is incorrect), with a mean age of 51 years for women and 42 years for men. The majority of reported cases are asymptomatic, as in this patient (choice B is incorrect), but if patients are symptomatic, common symptoms include progressive dyspnea, cough, wheezing, and recurrent respiratory tract infections. Symptoms are due to progression of the airway lesions and are related to narrowing and thickening of the airway walls. There is no clear relationship between smoking or systemic disorders (choice C is incorrect). Despite past speculation, a relationship with amyloidosis has not been proven. No clear pathogenesis has been defined.

Most reports note tracheal involvement, but bronchial involvement, as in this patient, is described. Conversely, the trachea may be spared, and only the lobar and more distal (bronchial) airways may be involved. As noted, the radiographic, especially CT, and bronchoscopic appearance alone may make the diagnosis. However, foci of calcium may not be apparent on chest radiographs or CT. The CT may only show nodular and irregular narrowing of the airway lumen.

Prognosis is usually good and depends on the severity of airway compromise. Treatment is supportive, although interventional bronchoscopic techniques may play a role in relieving symptoms in more advanced cases.

Chroneou A, Zias N, Gonzalez AV, et al. Tracheobronchopathia osteochondroplastica: an unrecognized entity? Monaldi Arch Chest Dis 2008; 69:65–69

Restrepo S, Pandit M, Villamil MA, et al. Tracheobronchopathia osteochondroplastica: helical CT findings in 4 cases. J Thorac Imaging 2004; 19:112–116
White BD, Kong A, Khoo E, et al. Computed tomography diagnosis of tracheobronchopathia osteochondroplastica. Australas Radiol 2005; 49:319–321
Prakash UB. Tracheobronchopathia osteochondroplastica. Semin Respir Crit Care Med 2002; 23:167–175

24. C. Pulmonary hypertension.

This man has severe COPD associated with daytime hypoventilation and relative hypoxemia. He also has moderate obstructive sleep apnea (OSA). Pulmonary hypertension is often associated with the "overlap syndrome" (choice C is correct). It is estimated that ≤ 15% of patients with COPD have concomitant OSA. When seen together, the term overlap syndrome is used. This combination is not more common than would be expected on the basis of the prevalence of each of these conditions alone in the population. One does not predispose a person to the other. From a clinical standpoint, hypoxemia is exaggerated in patients with overlap syndrome compared with those with OSA alone. The presence of pulmonary hypertension is often mild and does not correlate directly with the severity of the nocturnal oxyhemoglobin desaturation. Survival is decreased in patients with both conditions compared with those with OSA alone.

There are several factors that worsen oxygenation and ventilation during sleep in healthy people. Physiologically, sleep induces muscle hypotonia (*eg*, accessory muscles). The ventilatory responses to hypercapnia and hypoxemia are blunted during sleep. The recumbent position is associated with a decrease in ventilation and respiratory rate (choice D is incorrect). These all contribute to the hypoventilation and hypoxemia during sleep. For patients with COPD, these responses can lead to exaggerated hypoxemia. Specific causes of sleep-associated hypoxemia in patients with COPD include a heightened airway resistance (choice B is incorrect) and the loss of chest hyperexpansion (due to the skeletal muscle hypotonia occurring during REM sleep). Diaphragmatic hypotonia has not been noted to occur during sleep (choice A is incorrect).

Gay P. Chronic obstructive pulmonary disease and sleep. Respir Care 2004; 49:39–51
Sander MH, Newman AB, Haggerty CL, et al. Sleep and sleep-disordered breathing in adults with predominantly mild obstructive airway disease. Am J Respir Crit Care Med 2003; 167:7–14

25. C. Pulmonary angiogram.

The patient has an arteriovenous malformation (AVM) secondary to trauma from his prior motor vehicle accident, identified on his CT scan (see Figure 25-C, arrows) as an enhancing lesion in the right lower lobe (thick white arrow) with a feeding vessel (thin white arrow). Conservative management of his AVM, in the setting of progressive dyspnea and hypoxia, would not be appropriate (choice A is incorrect). Bronchoscopy with transbronchial biopsy has no role in the evaluation of an AVM and may result in significant morbidity due to hemorrhage. An echocardiogram, which was not listed as an additional diagnostic measure, may be helpful in further characterizing pulmonary AVMs. Late transit of contrast within the left atrium, after five to eight cardiac cycles, is suggestive of an AVM, whereas early transit of contrast within one cardiac cycle is consistent with an intracardiac shunt. The chest radiograph is abnormal in almost all patients with symptomatic pulmonary AVMs (98%). Lesions appear as oval masses with a uniform density, ranging in size from 1 to 5 cm in diameter. Feeding vessels may be present (see Figure 25-C, thin white arrow), which are highly suggestive of a pulmonary AVM. CT with angiography is the most sensitive imaging technique, identifying 98% of lesions in one series. Contrast angiography remains the gold standard for a diagnosis, given the ability to therapeutically intervene and perform endovascular embolization (see Figures 25-D, 25-E, and 25-F) once the diagnosis is confirmed (choice C is correct). Treatment is recommended for those with symptoms, enlarging lesions or lesions > 2 cm, and afferent arteries > 3 mm. Surgery with vascular ligation, local excision, lobectomy, or pneumonectomy was the preferred treatment; embolization has since replaced surgical intervention for the vast majority of cases (choice D is incorrect).

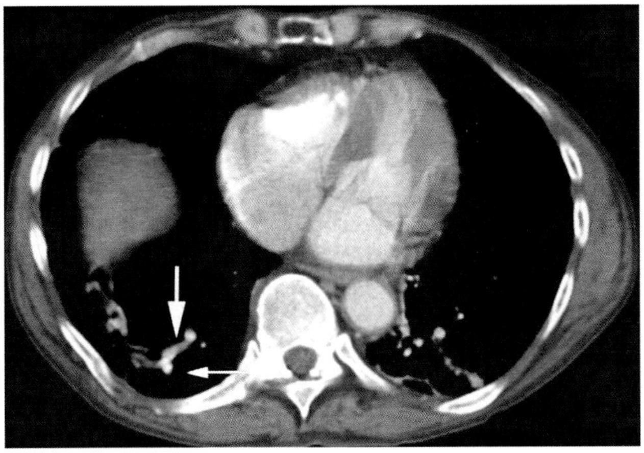

Figure 25-C

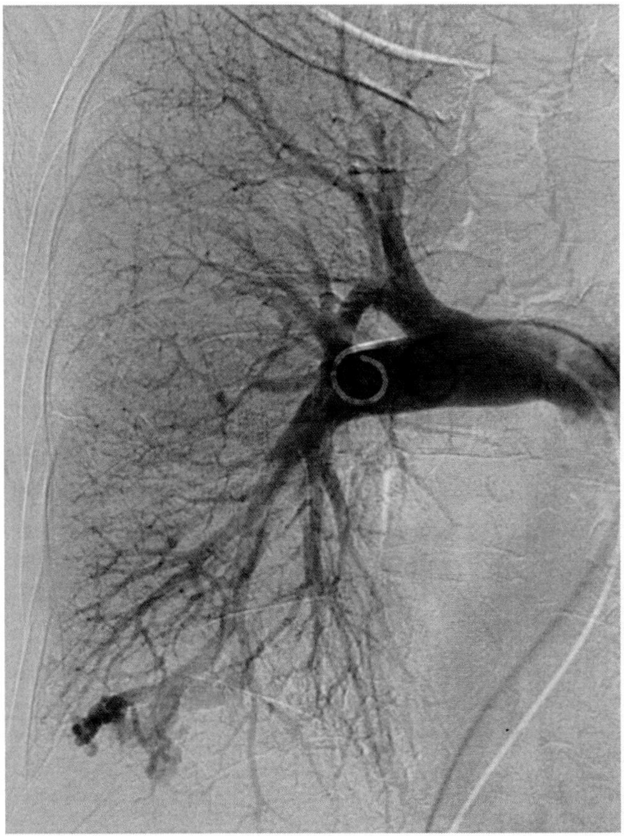

Figure 25-D

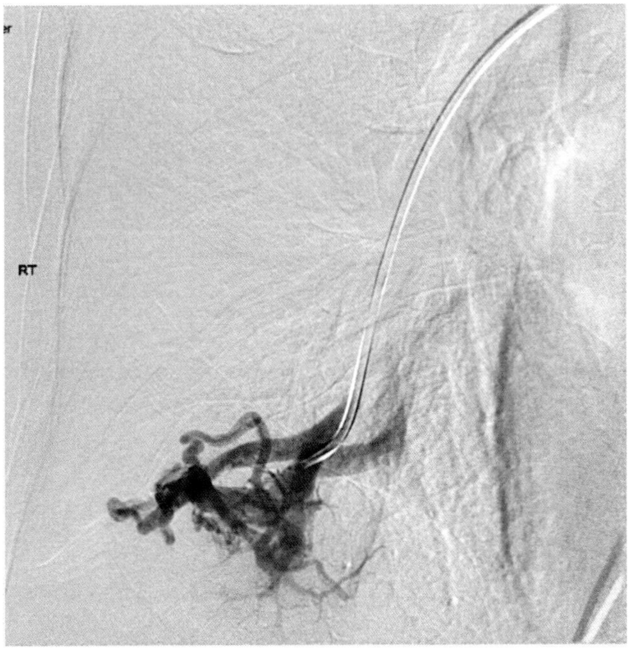

Figure 25-E

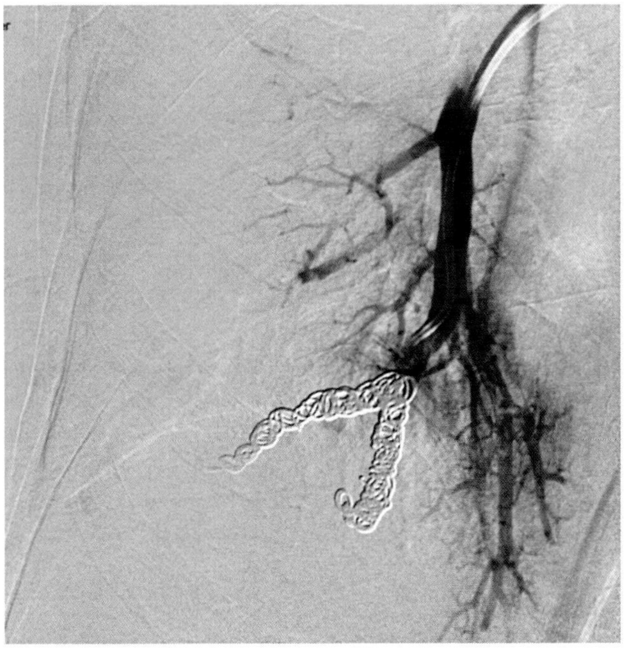

Figure 25-F

Pulmonary AVMs are abnormal communications between pulmonary arteries and veins. Most pulmonary AVMs are congenital in nature and, in >70% of cases, associated with hereditary hemorrhagic telangiectasia (HHT). Additional causes of pulmonary AVMs include trauma, mitral stenosis, hepatopulmonary syndrome, complications of prior thoracic surgery, Fanconi syndrome, metastatic thyroid carcinoma, pulmonary vein atresia, and suppurative bronchiectasis. Most AVMs, 53 to 70%, are found in the lower lobes, with 75% being unilateral. Up to one-third of patients may have multiple AVMs, which may be bilateral in distribution. In 80 to 90% of cases, the AVMs have one

afferent and efferent vessel and are supplied by the pulmonary vasculature. In suppurative bronchiectasis, the vascular communications may be between the pulmonary and bronchial (systemic) circulations.

In HHT-related AVMs, epistaxis is a common presenting symptom due to mucosal AVMs. Dyspnea is another common complaint, which is often progressive. Hemoptysis is the third most common presenting symptom, which may be massive. Platypnea and orthodeoxia, manifestations of dynamic pulmonary circulation in response to changes in position, also may be present.

Bosher LH Jr, Blake DA, Byrd BR. An analysis of the pathologic anatomy of pulmonary arteriovenous aneurysms with particular reference to the applicability of local excision. Surgery 1959; 45:91–104

Ekstrom D, Weiner M, Baier B. Pulmonary arteriovenous fistula as a complication of trauma. Am J Roentgenol 1978; 130:1178–1180

Remy J, Remy-Jardin M, Wattinne L, et al. Pulmonary arteriovenous malformations: evaluation with CT of the chest before and after treatment. Radiology 1992; 182:809–816

McAllister KA, Grogg KM, Johnson DW, et al. Endoglin, a TGF-beta binding protein of endothelial cells, is the gene for hereditary haemorrhagic telangiectasia type 1. Nat Genet 1994; 8:345–351

Gossage JR, Kanj G. Pulmonary arteriovenous malformations: a state of the art review. Am J Respir Crit Care Med 1998; 158:643–661

26. C. Discontinue both vancomycin and piperacillin/tazobactam. Initiate meropenem.

This patient has an infection due to a multidrug-resistant (MDR) organism, with resistance conferred by production of an extended-spectrum β-lactamase, which inactivates many antibiotics. In this case, the organism isolated is an AmpC β-lactamase–producing *E cloacae.* In all cases of MDR infections, appropriate infection control measures should be implemented in an attempt to prevent horizontal transmission. Additionally, efforts should be made to remove any intravascular catheters that may be associated with the nosocomial infection. Antibiotics targeted to this organism should be started and unnecessary antibiotics stopped (choice C is correct).

Risk factors for MDR nosocomial infection include indwelling catheters, frequent admissions, and previous antimicrobial therapy with a third-generation cephalosporin, which are all present in this patient. The previous use of cephalosporin therapy is associated with the subsequent selection and emergence of AmpC β-lactamase–producing organisms (Serratia spp, indole-positive Proteus spp, Citrobacter spp, and Enterobacter spp). Production of AmpC β-lactamase can be either constitutive (all the time) or by induction (in the presence of an antibiotic). The most potent inducers are the cephalosporins and imipenem. However, imipenem is chemically stable to the hydrolyzing enzymes and maintains its potency in the presence of AmpC β-lactamase–producing organisms. Additionally, many AmpC β-lactamase–producing organisms acquire other antibiotic-resistant genes, conferring resistance to other drug classes including fluoroquinolones and some aminoglycosides. AmpC β-lactamase–producing organisms are not inhibited by β-lactamase inhibitors, such as clavulanate and tazobactam (choice A is incorrect). Traditional microbiology testing methods would be unable to identify resistance to piperacillin/tazobactam in this case. Identification of common patterns of phenotypic expression of resistance is also key in selecting appropriate antimicrobial therapy.

Carbapenems remain stable against these hydrolyzing enzymes and are considered the drug class of choice for the therapy of AmpC β-lactamase–secreting organisms. Aminoglycoside monotherapy would be inappropriate because this class of drugs penetrates lung tissue poorly and is inactivated by low pH, as is often present in the local microenvironment of lung infections (choice B is incorrect). In this case, meropenem is the correct choice. Using pharmacokinetic parameters by maximizing dosing regimens should be implemented for effective therapy and prevention of emergence of hyperresistant organisms. Another point is to narrow therapy as appropriate. Thus, in this case, vancomycin can be discontinued because *E cloacae* was the only organism isolated (choice D is incorrect).

Jacoby GA, Munoz-Price LS. The new beta-lactamases. N Engl J Med 2005; 354:380–391

Endimiani A, Luzzaro F, Perilli M, et al. Bacteremia due to *Klebsiella pneumoniae* isolates producing TEM-52 extended-spectrum beta-lactamase: treatment outcome of patients receiving imipenem or ciprofloxacin. Clin Infect Dis 2004; 38:243–251

Yang K, Guglielmo J. Diagnosis and treatment of extended-spectrum and AmpC beta-lactamase-producing organisms. Ann Pharmacother 2007; 41:1427–1435

27. A. Expose to bright lights in the workplace.

Work during nonconventional daytime hours may be associated with significant sleepiness during night work as well as daytime sleep disturbance because of a recurrent or persistent mismatch between the habitual sleep-wake schedules and endogenous circadian rhythms. Excessive sleepiness occurs during night work because of a circadian trough in alertness and an increase in the homeostatic sleep drive and can increase the risk of work-related accidents and impair work performance. Conversely, sleep attempted during the day is often of poor quality and shortened duration because of circadian rhythm–related alerting influences. Exposure to bright lights in the workplace has been shown to decrease sleepiness during night shift work (choice A is correct). Neither increasing physical activity nor taking frequent rest periods during night shift work are consistently effective countermeasures for sleepiness during shift work (choices B and C are incorrect). Although the use of melatonin or hypnotic agents during morning sleep after shift work can enhance sleep quality, these agents do not improve nocturnal alertness (choice D is incorrect).

Shift work includes permanent night or early morning hour shifts, rotating schedules, or random work assignments. An estimated 10% of the night and rotating shift work population describe insomnia, excessive sleepiness, or both, and thus qualify for a diagnosis of shift work sleep disorder.

Provision of bright ambient lights during night work can enhance performance efficiency, decrease sleepiness, augment alertness, and improve mood. Timing, intensity, and duration of light treatment have not been standardized, and published studies have used different treatment schedules as well as various light intensities.

Administration of wake-promoting agents (*eg,* caffeine or modafinil) during night shift work can counter sleepiness and enhance performance. Nevertheless, these agents should not be used chronically to replace obtaining a sufficient amount of sleep. Scheduled napping before, or during, night work also has beneficial effects on alertness and vigilance. It appears that combined caffeine ingestion and napping is superior in improving alertness compared with caffeine use alone.

Hypnotic medications, including melatonin and benzodiazepine receptor agonists, can improve daytime sleep quality and duration and enhance quality of life among night shift workers. Their effects on nighttime alertness and psychomotor performance are inconsistent. Finally, nonphotic external stimulation (*eg,* loud noises) and behavioral modification (*eg,* frequent changes in posture or increasing levels of physical activity) are of limited efficacy.

Yoon IY, Jeong DU, Kwon KB, et al. Bright light exposure at night and light attenuation in the morning improve adaptation of night shift workers. Sleep 2002; 25:351–356

Moon CA, Hindmarch I, Holland RL. The effect of zopiclone 7.5 mg on the sleep, mood and performance of shift workers. Int Clin Psychopharmacol 1990; 5(suppl):79–83

Czeisler CA, Walsh JK, Roth T, et al. U.S. Modafinil in Shift Work Sleep Disorder Study Group: modafinil for excessive sleepiness associated with shift-work sleep disorder. N Engl J Med 2005; 353:476–486

28. A. Chemotherapy and radiation.

This patient has small cell lung cancer as noted in the histopathologic results (see Figure 28-A). The pathology is characterized by small blue cells with prominent nucleoli, sparse cytoplasm, a high nuclear/cytoplasmic ratio, and indistinct nucleoli. Nuclear molding and crush artifact are often noted. Mitotic rates are high, and necrosis is common. Small cell cancer is found nearly exclusively in smokers and comprises 13 to 20% of all lung cancers. It is one of the centrally located bronchogenic carcinomas, typically has a short doubling time, and frequently has widely spread metastases at presentation. It originates from a neuroendocrine cell line.

Small cell lung cancer, in contrast to non-small cell lung cancer, is most often staged on the basis of limited vs extensive disease. Limited disease is defined as disease confined to the ipsilateral hemithorax that can be contained in a single radiation port. Extensive disease is defined as disease outside the ipsilateral hemithorax. The majority of patients with small cell lung cancer have extensive stage disease (60 to 70%) vs limited disease (30 to 40%) at presentation. Combination platinum-based chemotherapy and concurrent thoracic radiation significantly prolong survival in small cell lung cancer and are the treatment of choice for limited-stage disease. This patient should receive combination therapy for limited disease with combination platinum-based chemotherapy and concurrent radiation (choice A is correct). Response rates of 80 to 90% are reported, with 50 to 60% complete response. Although the tumor is highly responsive to chemotherapy and radiation, relapse is common. Extensive disease is treated with platinum-based chemotherapy alone (choice C is incorrect). Extensive disease is associated with a 60 to 80% response rate but only a 15 to 20% complete response. Five-year survival rates are <3 to 8%. Radiation therapy alone is not part of standard treatment for small cell lung cancer (choice B is incorrect).

Surgery is rarely an option for small cell cancer except for extremely early-stage disease (which applies to $<10\%$ of patients; choice D is incorrect). In this small subset, invasive mediastinal staging and extrathoracic imaging should be performed, and adjuvant chemotherapy given. Surgical evaluation would be appropriate for stage IIB or lower non-small cell cancer but not in this patient who has small cell cancer. If this was non-small cell cancer, this would be clinical stage IIB (T2 N1), and surgical evaluation would be indicated.

Other components of staging for small cell cancer in addition to chest and abdominal scans include a bone scan and head CT scan. Bone marrow biopsies are no longer a routine part of staging in patients with apparent limited-stage disease. The role of routine PET scanning in small cell cancer staging is not routinely recommended but appears promising. If complete remission is achieved in limited disease, prophylactic cranial irradiation should be offered.

Gaspar LE, Gay EG, Crawford J, et al. Limited-stage small cell lung cancer (stages I-III): observations from the National Cancer Data Base. Clin Lung Cancer 2005; 6:355–360

Samson DJ, Seidenfeld J, Simon GR, et al. Evidence for management of small cell lung cancer: ACCP evidence-based clinical practice guidelines, 2nd edition. Chest 2007; 132(suppl):314S–323S

Simon GR, Turrisi AT. Management of small cell lung cancer: ACCP evidence-based clinical practice guidelines (2nd edition). Chest 2007: 132(suppl):324S–339S

Jänne PA, Freidlin B, Saxman S, et al. Twenty-five years of clinical research for patients with limited-stage small cell lung carcinoma in North America. Cancer 2002; 95:1528–1538

Alberts WM. Diagnosis and management of lung cancer executive summary: ACCP evidence-based clinical practice guidelines, 2nd edition. Chest 2007; 132(suppl):1S–19S

29. C. Worsen air trapping, which will further impair cardiac function and possibly raise $Paco_2$ through increased dead space.

In patients with obstructive lung disease who are requiring mechanical ventilation, the combination of a high minute ventilation, a short expiratory time, and a long expiratory time constant (resistance × compliance) will often lead to air trapping and intrinsic PEEP. This can be determined during controlled mechanical ventilation by the use of an expiratory pause maneuver that equilibrates circuit and alveolar pressure at the end of the normal expiratory period. In this patient, the expiratory pause shows that there is 18 cm H_2O pressure remaining in the alveolus when the next breath is given. This pressure is added to the inspiratory pressure to produce an elevated mean and end inspiratory plateau pressure. This pressure buildup is likely contributing to impaired cardiac filling and the hypotension in the patient.

The only way to reduce or eliminate intrinsic PEEP in this patient is to reduce the minute ventilation, lengthen the expiratory time, or improve lung mechanics such that resistance is better. Increasing the minute ventilation and not affecting expiratory time (*ie,* a constant I:E ratio) will worsen the air trapping, increase the mean intrathoracic pressure, and further impair cardiac filling. Moreover, the higher intrathoracic pressures from the worsening air

trapping could also increase dead space, further worsening the respiratory acidosis (choice C is correct, and choices A, B, and D are incorrect).

In addition to overdistending the lung, intrinsic PEEP can also serve as an inspiratory pressure triggering load if the patient was spontaneously triggering mechanical breaths. Under these conditions, equilibrating circuit PEEP and the intrinsic PEEP can help reduce this inspiratory triggering threshold and, thus, make it easier for the patient to trigger the machine. However, in this patient, only controlled breaths are being given, so triggering is not an issue.

Pepe PE, Marini JJ. Occult postive end-expiratory pressure in mechanically ventilated patients with airflow obstruction. Am Rev Respir Dis 1982; 126:166–170

Marini JJ, Crooke PS. A general mathematical model for respiratory dynamics relevant to the clinical setting. Am Rev Resp Dis 1993; 147:14–24

Truwit JD, Marini JJ. Evaluation of thoracic mechanics in the ventilated patient: Part 1. Primary measurements. J Crit Care 1988; 3:133–150

Truwit JD, Marini JJ. Evaluation of thoracic mechanics in the ventilated patient: Part 2. Applied mechanics. J Crit Care 1988; 3:192–213

30. C. Epoprostenol.

The patient has idiopathic pulmonary arterial hypertension (IPAH) and requires treatment with continuous IV epoprostenol because of the high mortality associated with pregnancy in this condition (choice C is correct). IPAH is a diagnosis of exclusion when cardiac catheterization documents a mean pulmonary arterial pressure >25 mm Hg at rest or >30 mm Hg with exercise, when pulmonary artery occlusion pressure is <15 mmHg, and when appropriate studies have excluded conditions known to be associated with pulmonary hypertension such as collagen vascular diseases, systemic-to-pulmonary shunts, portal hypertension, HIV infection, and exposure to drugs such as cocaine, amphetamines, and certain diet drugs. Additional conditions that must be excluded include significant pulmonary disease, alveolar hypoventilation, left-sided cardiac disease, chronic thromboembolic disease, chronic hemolysis, and schistosomiasis.

IPAH affects both sexes and all ages but is more common among women and in the fourth decade of life. Pregnancy may accelerate the presentation of the condition because of its associated physiologic requirements, such as increased blood volume and increased cardiac output.

Mortality associated with pulmonary hypertension of any cause is high during pregnancy and requires management by a coordinated team of obstetricians, perinatologists, anesthesiologists, and specialists in pulmonary hypertension if the pregnancy is not terminated due to maternal health. IPAH is treated in this setting with diuretics, oxygen, and, in some centers, anticoagulation with heparin. Warfarin would be contraindicated in this pregnant patient because it would cross the placenta (choice B is incorrect). Specific treatment of IPAH during pregnancy has traditionally involved continuous IV epoprostenol because it has the longest record of efficacy and safety in this setting. IV or subcutaneous treprostinil or inhaled iloprost may be acceptable alternatives, and oral sildenafil has been used in cases of mild disease.

Endothelin receptor antagonists, such as bosentan and ambrisentan, are US Food and Drug Administration (FDA) pregnancy risk category X (contraindicated) and should never be used when pregnancy is established or if highly effective contraception practices are not in place (choice A is incorrect). In addition, angiotensin-converting enzyme inhibitors are FDA pregnancy risk category D (positive evidence of risk), if administered during the second or third trimesters.

Calcium channel antagonists, such as nifedipine, amlodipine, and diltiazem, have a role in the treatment of IPAH only when a patient exhibits significant pulmonary vasoreactivity in response to a short-acting pulmonary vasodilator, such as inhaled nitric oxide, IV epoprostenol, or IV adenosine. A significant response is defined as a decrease in mean pulmonary artery pressure by ≥ 10 mm Hg and decrease to a value of <40 mm Hg with no decrease in

cardiac output and a minimally reduced or unchanged systemic BP. This patient does not meet these criteria, so calcium channel antagonists will not be helpful (and may be harmful) and, therefore, should not be used (choice D is incorrect).

Bendayan D, Hod M, Oron G, et al. Pregnancy outcome in patients with pulmonary arterial hypertension receiving prostacyclin therapy. Obstet Gynecol 2005; 106:1206–1210
Chin KM, Rubin LJ. Pulmonary arterial hypertension. J Am Coll Cardiol 2008; 51:1527–1538
Huang S, DeSantis ER. Treatment of pulmonary arterial hypertension in pregnancy. Am J Health Syst Pharm 2007; 64:1922–1926

31. **A.** 3 months.

The eighth edition of the American College of Chest Physicians' (ACCP) evidence-based guidelines for antithrombotic and thrombolytic therapy, published in 2008, recommends treatment with a vitamin K antagonist for 3 months in patients with PE secondary to a transient risk factor. The prolonged air travel (or estrogen therapy) would be considered a transient risk factor for a thrombotic event (choice A is correct). This recommendation is based on the only trial to focus exclusively on patients who had PE only, as well as the many studies that included patients with deep vein thrombosis with or without PE. These studies are consistent with the observation that vitamin K antagonists are effective in preventing recurrences while they are taken. However, extending the duration beyond 3 months does not affect the rate of recurrence once the anticoagulant is stopped (choices B and C are incorrect).

For patients who experience an unprovoked PE or have a continuing or permanent risk factor, the recommendation is to consider indefinite treatment with a vitamin K antagonist. This patient's event would certainly not be considered unprovoked, but some might consider the underlying factor V Leiden mutation as a permanent risk factor that would predict a higher likelihood of recurrence and thus necessitate long-term treatment. The factor V Leiden mutation and other genetic and acquired thrombophilias clearly increase the relative risk of an initial thrombotic event (from 2 to 10 times the baseline risk). Two metaanalyses found an overall relative risk of recurrence of approximately 1.5 for hereditary thrombophilias, but this did not reach statistical significance in either analysis. Additionally, the relative risk of recurrence in those with the factor V Leiden mutation was also not significant, with a hazard ratio of 1.2 (95% CI, 0.7 to 1.9). Based on these data, the ACCP antithrombotic guidelines state that the presence of hereditary thrombophilia is not a major determinant of the risk of recurrence (choice D is incorrect).

Given that this patient's thrombosis was likely related to prolonged air travel (in addition, perhaps, to the estrogen therapy), she should be counseled about using preventive measures for future travel. The guidelines recommend general measures such as avoidance of constrictive clothing around the lower extremities or waist, maintenance of adequate hydration, and frequent calf muscle contraction for all travelers taking flights longer than 8 h. For travelers with additional risk factors for venous thromboembolism, such as this patient, more active thromboprophylaxis can be considered (properly fitted, below-knee grated compression stocking or a single prophylactic dose of low-molecular-weight heparin [LMWH] injected prior to departure).

Most patients with a thrombotic event should receive a vitamin K antagonist for the period of secondary prophylaxis. Small studies in patients with acute PE suggest that LMWH is equally efficacious in preventing recurrences. In the subgroup of patients who experience a PE in the setting of malignancy, LMWH appears to be superior to vitamin K antagonists. The guidelines thus recommend treatment with LMWH for the first 3 to 6 months of therapy and then continuing treatment with either LMWH or a vitamin K antagonist indefinitely (or for as long as the cancer is active). Patients who experience a second unprovoked PE should always receive indefinite therapy with a vitamin K antagonist unless they develop a true contraindication.

Kearon C, Kahn SR, Agnelli G, et al. Antithrombotic therapy for venous thromboembolic disease: American College of Chest Physicians evidence-based clinical practice guidelines, 8th edition. Chest 2008; 133(suppl):454S-545S
Dalen JE. Should patients with venous thromboembolism be screened for thromophilia? Am J Med 2008; 121:458–463

Geerts WH, Bergqvist D, Pineo GF, et al. Prevention of venous thromboembolism: American College of Chest Physicians evidence-based clinical practice guidelines, 8th edition. Chest 2008; 133(suppl):381S-453S
Lee AY, Levin MN, Baker RI, et al. Low-molecular-weight heparin versus a coumarin for the prevention of recurrent venous thromboembolism in patients with cancer. N Engl J Med 2003; 349:146–153

32. C. Methacholine challenge testing should move to the next level of dosing (2 mg/mL).

At least three forced expiratory maneuvers are recommended to ensure consistency and reproducibility at baseline and at each level of testing throughout the challenge, with the best attempt of the three being recorded. The best attempt for this patient, corresponding to the highest FEV_1 at 1.0 mg/mL, was a 12.1% decline. This did not meet the 20% threshold decline for a positive bronchoprovocation challenge test, so testing should be continued at 2 mg/mL methacholine (choice C is correct). Full FVC efforts lasting ≥ 6 s should be performed at baseline (and after diluent, if applicable). However, if the FEV_1 is the only outcome being measured, the expiratory maneuver can be shortened to about 2 s, with caution. If a shortened expiratory time is used, care should be taken that the inspiration is complete because incomplete inhalations will result in a false reduction in FEV_1, and abbreviated flow-volume tracings may not show an inadequate inhalation. If other spirometric outcome variables are used or if vocal cord dysfunction is suspected, full FVC maneuvers should be performed throughout the test. The highest FEV_1 value from acceptable tests is selected for the outcome variable after each dose.

The stepwise approach to bronchoprovocation challenge testing begins with baseline spirometry maneuvers. If the baseline FEV_1 is > 70% of predicted for age, height, and sex, then challenge testing is continued, and if it is below 60 to 70% of predicted, challenge testing may not be considered safe and is performed on the basis of the clinical need. A variety of bronchoprovocation challenge testing methods and protocols exist, with multiple dosing regimens for methacholine administration. Regardless of the method used, three forced expiratory maneuvers should be performed, with the best result recorded after each dosing level to ensure consistency and reproducibility (choice D is incorrect). Most methacholine dosing regimens consist of a "test" dose followed by an increase of the methacholine to a maximum dose of 16 to 32 mg/mL. In this case, the 2-min tidal breathing dosing protocol was used (a five-breath dosimeter protocol is used at some testing centers). Administration of the methacholine dose by nebulization should occur during a 2-min period, with an appropriate flow rate and pressure with tidal volume breathing. Flow rates of > 1 L/s can affect the deposition of the methacholine, which affects results. Additional tilting of the nebulizer or lack of nasal occlusion can dilute the dose and diminish the effect. In this case, the flow rate was appropriate, with administration of the dose lasting 2 min, so inappropriate administration was not likely to affect the results (choice A is incorrect). Forced expiratory maneuvers should be performed starting at 30 s after the methacholine dosing has stopped, with all maneuvers performed within 180 s (3 min) after administration of the dose (choice B is incorrect).

Crapo RO, Casaburi R, Coates AL, et al. Guidelines for methacholine and exercise challenge testing: 1999. Am J Respir Crit Care Med 2000; 161:309–329
Miller MR, Hankinson J, Bursasco V, et al. Standardisation of spirometry. Eur Respir J 2005; 26:319–338
Miller MR, Crapo RO, Hankinson J, et al. General considerations for lung function testing. Eur Respir J 2005; 26:153–161

33. A. Administer alteplase via a peripheral vein over 2 h.

This patient has a massive acute pulmonary embolism, as indicated by imaging evidence of pulmonary embolism, and hypotension or shock that has persisted despite administration of a fluid challenge. Treatment that rapidly dissolves or mechanically removes thromboembolic material within the pulmonary artery sufficient to relieve shock is indicated. The most appropriate intervention under the circumstances presented is the IV administration of a thrombolytic agent, such as alteplase, via a peripheral vein for a short duration, such as 2 h (choice A is correct). The other options presented are inferior choices primarily because of higher risks for adverse events and lack of evidence for superior

outcomes. Prolonged infusion ($\geq$ 12 h) of thrombolytic agents has been demonstrated in RCTs to have higher rates of bleeding, as well as slower clot lysis compared with short-duration thrombolysis (choice B is incorrect). Although the infusion of a thrombolytic agent directly into the pulmonary artery in close proximity to the clot seems likely to produce more rapid clot dissolution or less of a systemic lytic state, the evidence for superiority to peripheral vein infusion is lacking. Bleeding from the catheter venipuncture site is significantly more frequent (choice C is incorrect).

Extraction or fragmentation of the clot within the pulmonary artery can be accomplished using a number of catheter devices. This technique is not available at many hospitals but, if available, can result in relief of life-threatening pulmonary artery obstruction. However, thus far, evidence of safety and efficacy is limited to case series without prospective controlled trial results. Experts recommend that this technique be considered if thrombolysis is absolutely contraindicated or has failed or if the patient's clinical status is so critical (such as cardiac arrest or profound shock) that systemic thrombolysis will not be achieved rapidly enough. In this case, there are no absolute or relative contraindications to thrombolysis (choice D is incorrect), as follows:

Absolute
- History of hemorrhagic stroke or stroke of unknown origin
- Ischemic stroke in the previous 6 months
- CNS neoplasm
- Major trauma, surgery, or head injury in the past 3 weeks

Relative
- Transient ischemic attack in previous 6 months
- Oral anticoagulation
- Pregnancy or first postpartum week
- Noncompressible puncture sites
- Traumatic resuscitation
- Refractory hypertension
- Advanced liver disease
- Infective endocarditis
- Active peptic ulcer

Recent interventional approaches combine local administration of a thrombolytic agent with mechanical clot disruption and removal. Finally, surgical embolectomy can be lifesaving in select cases but carries a higher risk.

Kearon C, Kahn SR, Agnelli G, et al. Antithrombotic therapy for venous thromboembolic disease: American College of Chest Physicians evidence-based clinical practice guidelines, 8th edition. Chest 2008; 133(suppl):454S–545S

Konstantinides S. Clinical practice: acute pulmonary embolism. N Engl J Med 2008; 359:2804–2813

Verstraete M, Miller GA, Bounameaux H, et al. Intravenous and intrapulmonary recombinant tissue-type plasminogen activator in the treatment of acute massive pulmonary embolism. Circulation 1988; 77:353–360

34. A. Transjugular intrahepatic portosystemic shunt (TIPS).

As shown in the radiograph (see Figure 34-A), this patient has a massive right pleural effusion with contralateral shift of the mediastinum and has developed a hepatic hydrothorax. Hepatic hydrothoraces are seen in up to 4 to 10% of patients with end-stage liver disease (ESLD) and ascites and have been described in patients with ESLD in the absence of ascites, as well. The pathophysiology is thought to be due to movement of ascitic fluid into the pleural space through diaphragmatic defects, likely due to pressure differences across the diaphragm. Hepatic hydrothoraces

are most commonly seen unilaterally on the right in >70% of normal anatomic patients but can occur bilaterally or unilaterally on the left. Thoracentesis chemistry results are consistent with a transudate as in this case. The diagnosis can be made presumptively in the appropriate clinical setting and can be made definitively by a radionucleotide study of the ascites, observing tracer entering the pleural space.

This patient is refractory to standard diuretic therapy, so the most definitive treatment for the hepatic hydrothorax is the placement of a transjugular intrahepatic portosystemic shunt (TIPS) to reduce portal pressures and decrease ascitic pressure in the abdomen (choice A is correct). TIPS can be partially or completely effective in approximately 75% of patients with refractory hepatic hydrothorax. Encephalopathy can develop following TIPS, and this procedure should not be performed in patients with preexisting encephalopathy. Because of the large amount of pleural fluid and fluid shifts, it is often difficult to achieve pleural symphysis, making chemical pleurodesis difficult and usually unsuccessful, and this can actually result in the further development of ascites (choice C is incorrect). Large-volume paracentesis may be a transient approach but would not permanently correct this problem (choice D is incorrect). A pleural peritoneal shunt would not work in this patient because it would actually worsen the problem (choice B is incorrect). Video-assisted thoracoscopic surgery with talc poudrage and repair of the anatomic diaphragmatic defects can also be successful but may be associated with significant morbidity and mortality. Liver transplantation is also a possible permanent solution to this problem but is not offered as a choice and would not be appropriate in a patient who is still actively consuming alcohol. TIPS can be used as a "bridge" to liver transplantation in some cases of hepatic hydrothorax.

Gordon FD, Anastopoulos HT, Crenshaw W, et al. The successful treatment of symptomatic, refractory hepatic hydrothorax with transjugular intrahepatic portosystemic shunt. Hepatology 1997; 25:1366–1369

Spencer EB, Cohen DT, Darcy MD. Safety and efficacy of transjugular intrahepatic portosystemic shunt creation for the treatment of hepatic hydrothorax. J Vasc Interv Radiol 2002; 13:385–390

Siegerstetter V, Deibert P, Ochs A, et al. Treatment of refractory hepatic hydrothorax with transjugular intrahepatic portosystemic shunt: long-term results in 40 patients. Eur J Gastroenterol Hepatol 2001; 13:529–534

de Campos M Jr, Filho LO, de Campos Werebe E, et al. Thoracoscopy and talc poudrage in the management of hepatic hydrothorax. Chest 2000; 111:13–17

Lazaridis KN, Frank JW, Krowka MJ, et al. Hepatic hydrothorax: pathogenesis, diagnosis, and management. Am J Med 1999; 107:262–267

35. D. Repeat the physical examination.

This patient presents with a sudden onset of cough, chest pain, and hemoptysis, and his chest radiograph and CT scan indicate multiple nodules of varying size and shape. There is nothing in his history to suggest infection, and he has no risk factors for HIV infection. The most likely diagnosis of multiple nodules in this young man is metastatic disease, and the likely source is testicular cancer. The correct choice is to repeat the physical examination with a careful examination of the testes (choice D is correct). In fact, this patient had a small but palpable right testicular mass, which was confirmed on testicular ultrasound. Occasionally, the physical examination will not identify an abnormal testis despite the presence of a mass, and testicular ultrasound would be appropriate in those cases. Careful physical examination is also appropriate to identify possible thyroid or soft tissue (sarcoma) tumors that can be associated with multiple pulmonary nodules. In this case, the chorionic gonadotropin level was >200,000 U/L, and choriocarcinoma was eventually documented. Bronchoscopy with BAL, aspiration needle biopsy of the lung, and thoracoscopic lung biopsy are all unnecessary to establish the diagnosis at this time (choices A and C are incorrect), and HIV infection is unlikely in this young man with essentially no risk factors (choice B is incorrect). The finding of an elevated LDH level is common in metastatic germ cell tumors, and in some cases, pulmonary nodules may be calcified.

More than 8,000 new cases of testicular cancer are diagnosed annually in the United States. Germ cell tumors are relatively uncommon, comprising only 2% of all human tumors, but they are the most common solid tumors in men between the ages of 15 and 34 years. A prior history of a germ cell tumor, positive family history, cryptorchism,

testicular dysgenesis, and Klinefelter syndrome have been identified as risk factors. Germ cell tumors are classified as seminoma or nonseminoma. Nonseminomatous tumors include embryonal cell carcinoma, choriocarcinoma (as in our patient), yolk sac tumor, and teratoma. Nonseminoma is the more aggressive tumor. A painless, solid testicular mass is a common presentation, but, often, patients will present with testicular discomfort or swelling. Choriocarcinoma is diagnosed in younger men. Unlike other cancers, choriocarcinoma metastasizes by hematogenous routes, the testicular primary is often small or even "burned-out," and the mortality rate is high. Rarely, the disease may originate in the lung and be associated with a syndrome resembling diffuse alveolar hemorrhage. This tumor usually responds poorly to radiation and chemotherapy. Surgery is usually limited to radical orchiectomy for tissue diagnosis. β-Human chorionic gonadotropin has a 24-h half-life and is secreted by syncytiotrophoblast cells within the tumor. β-Human chorionic gonadotropin is usually markedly elevated in pure choriocarcinoma. Pure choriocarcinoma is not as sensitive to chemotherapy as mixed nonseminomatous germ cell tumors. The standard chemotherapy for this disease is bleomycin, etoposide, and cisplatin for four cycles.

Prow DM. Germ cell tumors: staging, prognosis, and outcome. Semin Urol Oncol 1998; 16:82–93

Shintaku M, Hwang MH, Amitani R. Primary choriocarcinoma of the lung manifesting as diffuse alveolar hemorrhage. Arch Pathol Lab Med 2006; 130:540–543

36. A. Administration of positive airway pressure therapy is the treatment of choice for this patient.

The polysomnographic tracing indicates episodes of obstructive apneas (*ie*, absence of airflow in the nasal pressure [NPRES] and airflow [FLOW] channels) (see Figure 36-B) associated with continued respiratory efforts seen in the thoracic (THO) and abdominal (ABD) belts and snoring on the microphone (MICRO). Administration of positive airway pressure (PAP) therapy is the treatment of choice for most patients with obstructive sleep apnea (OSA) (choice A is correct). PAP is believed to act like a pneumatic splint maintaining the patency of the vulnerable portions of the upper airway, and it is generally recommended for all patients with an apnea-hypopnea index (AHI) greater than 15/h, or for symptomatic patients (*eg*, excessive daytime sleepiness) with an AHI of 5 to 30/h (choice B is incorrect).

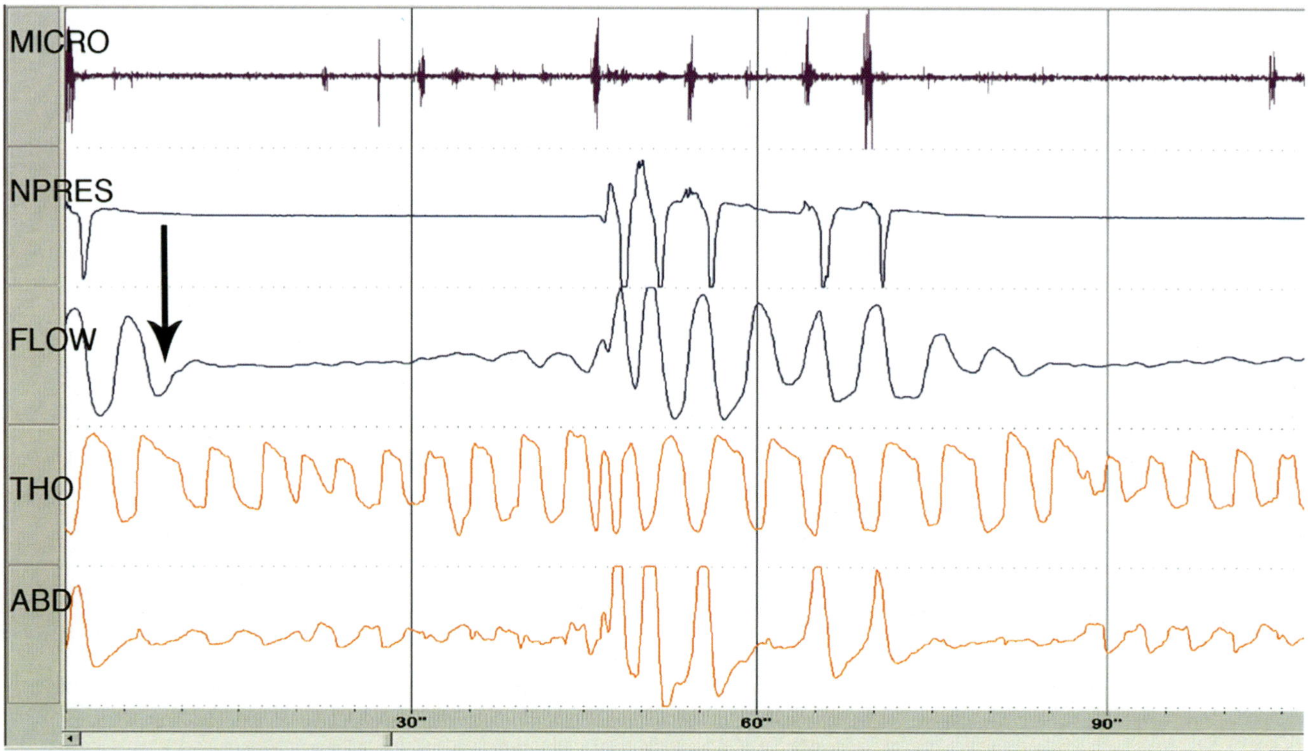

Figure 36-B

MICRO = microphone; NPRES = nasal pressure; FLOW = airflow; THO = thoracic belt; ABD = abdominal belt.

The current standard of practice for determining optimal CPAP pressures involves an attended pressure titration using laboratory polysomnography to identify a single, fixed pressure that eliminates apneas, hypopneas, snoring, and respiratory effort-related arousals; maintains adequate oxygen saturation; and improves sleep in all body positions and all sleep stages. A split-night study, in which an initial diagnostic portion is followed by CPAP titration on the same night, is a common alternative.

PAP therapy has salutary effects on sleep quality and sleepiness, as well as on mortality, hypertension, neurocognitive function, mood, and health-care utilization. However, less-than-optimal CPAP utilization is a significant problem in clinical practice, and patients often overestimate their actual CPAP use. Among the reasons for nonadherence to CPAP therapy include perception of lack of benefit, inconvenience, discomfort from the mask or pressure, air leaks, nasal problems (*eg*, congestion or epistaxis), claustrophobia, and difficulty with exhaling against high expiratory pressures. Patterns of use can often be discerned within the first few days or weeks of initiating treatment. The addition of heated humidification and systematic educational programs can enhance adherence to CPAP use, as may proper selection of the CPAP interface, desensitization procedures for CPAP, adjustment of the pressure ramp, correction of nasal problems, early follow-up, and prompt management of adverse effects related to CPAP use.

Autotitrating positive airway pressure (APAP) may be used to identify a fixed pressure for subsequent treatment with conventional CPAP (APAP titration) or utilized in a self-adjusting mode for nightly therapy of OSA (APAP treatment), but its usefulness for these purposes needs further validation. Required PAP pressure can differ considerably depending on sleep posture and sleep stages, and optimal PAP may vary significantly during one night or on different nights. Mean delivered pressure is generally lower during APAP compared with CPAP, but peak airway pressures may be higher. Not all APAP systems are comparable in efficacy, and different devices may utilize different algorithms for monitoring respiratory events and adjusting delivered pressures. APAP is not recommended for patients with concurrent congestive heart failure, significant COPD, daytime hypoxemia and respiratory failure, and nocturnal arterial oxygen desaturation due to disorders other than OSA (choice D is incorrect).

Patients with OSA who have persistent oxygen desaturation due to hypoventilation despite CPAP therapy, complain of being unable to exhale against high CPAP expiratory pressures, have mouth leaks or aerophagia, or have hypoventilation or concurrent COPD may benefit from bilevel positive airway pressure (BPAP). Studies in those with isolated OSA have not shown consistent advantages of BPAP over CPAP in patient preference and device utilization (choice C is incorrect). Nocturnal nasal positive pressure ventilation may be necessary in patients with sleep-related hypoventilation and CO_2 retention.

Berry RB, Parish JM, Hartse KM. The use of auto-titrating continuous positive airway pressure for treatment of adult obstructive sleep apnea: an American Academy of Sleep Medicine review. Sleep 2002; 25:148–173

Hack M, Davies RJ, Mullins R, et al. Randomised prospective parallel trial of therapeutic versus subtherapeutic nasal continuous positive airway pressure on simulated steering performance in patients with obstructive sleep apnoea. Thorax 2000; 55:224–231

Hirshkowitz M, Lee-Chiong T. Positive airway pressure therapy for obstructive sleep apnea. In: Lee-Chiong TL, ed. Sleep: a comprehensive handbook. Hoboken, NJ: John Wiley & Sons, 2006; 355–365

Kushida CA, Littner MR, Hirshkowitz M, et al. Practice parameters for the use of continuous and bilevel positive airway pressure devices to treat adult patients with sleep-related breathing disorders. Sleep 2006; 29:375–380

Littner M, Hirshkowitz M, Davila D, et al. Practice parameters for the use of auto-titrating continuous positive airway pressure devices for titrating pressures and treating adult patients with obstructive sleep apnea syndrome: an American Academy of Sleep Medicine report. Sleep 2002; 25:143–147

37. C. Anion gap metabolic acidosis with appropriate respiratory compensation.

In this problem, the patient has an anion gap metabolic acidosis and has appropriate ventilatory compensation that increases the pH (choice C is correct). Metabolic acidosis is confirmed by a reduced pH and $Paco_2$. Normal respiratory compensation for metabolic acidosis is calculated as $Paco_2 = 1.5 \times [HCO_3^-] + 8 \pm 2$, which, in this case, is 32 ± 2. This patient's $Paco_2$ was 32 mm Hg, indicating appropriate respiratory compensation for the primary metabolic

acidosis. Note that this patient's respiratory rate was 32/min; a modestly reduced $Paco_2$ at this rapid respiratory rate suggests that either tidal volumes were low, the dead space fraction was high, or both.

Solving acid-base problems requires a stepwise approach to determine whether the measurements are internally consistent and whether there are one or more physiologic abnormalities. The first step is to assess the internal consistency of the data using the Henderson-Hasselbach or Henderson equation. The latter states $[H^+] = 24 \times Paco_2/[HCO_3^-]$. At pH 7.32, $[H^+]$ is 48 mEq/L. In this problem, $48 = 24 \times 32/16$, so the data are consistent, and the primary abnormality is metabolic acidosis (choice A is incorrect).

The next step is to calculate the anion gap: $[Na^+] - ([Cl^-] + [HCO_3^-])$. In this case, the anion gap is $140-(100 + 16)$, or 24. Because the normal anion gap is 12 ± 4 mEq/L, this patient has an anion gap acidosis. As acids are buffered by bicarbonate, each milliequivalent per liter increase in the anion gap leads to a 1 mEq/L decrease in the serum bicarbonate. If this is not the case in an acid-base problem, then there is a mixed disorder. Departures from the principle that an increased anion gap would correspond to a reduction in serum bicarbonate are expressed as the "delta gap," or [(anion gap − 12) − (24 − bicarbonate)]. In pure anion gap metabolic acidosis, the delta gap should be zero, but measurement errors result in a normal delta gap in practice of 0 ± 6. If the delta gap is positive, a simultaneous metabolic alkalosis or respiratory acidosis exists, whereas if it is a negative number, there is a concomitant hyperchloremic (nonanion gap) acidosis or chronic respiratory alkalosis. In this problem, the delta gap is (24 − 12) − (24 − 16), or 4, which rules out significant hyperchloremic acidosis and metabolic alkalosis (choices B and D are incorrect).

Narins RG, Emmet M. Simple and mixed acid-base disorders: a practical approach. Medicine (Baltimore) 1980; 59:161–187
Adrogué HJ, Madias NE. Management of life-threatening acid-base disorders: Part 1. N Engl J Med 1998; 338:26–34
Adrogué HJ, Madias NE. Management of life-threatening acid-base disorders: Part 2. N Engl J Med 1998; 338:107–111

38. A. Exchange transfusion.

The chest radiograph demonstrates bilateral lung infiltrates, and this patient is deteriorating despite appropriate therapy for the acute chest syndrome (ACS). The principles of management include oxygen supplementation to correct hypoxia, respiratory therapy including use of incentive spirometry, antibiotic therapy (include coverage for community-acquired and atypical pathogens), monitoring intake and output, maintaining euvolemia, pain management to minimize chest splinting, avoiding oversedation, and bronchodilator therapy if reactive airway disease is present (consider an empiric trial in all patients). RBC transfusion is recommended if respiratory compromise or clinical deterioration occurs.

Transfusion therapy is often used in the treatment of ACS (choice A is correct). Reports of dramatic improvement in clinical condition after initiation of transfusion are well documented in the literature. In addition, both the Pao_2 and oxygen saturation have been shown to significantly improve with transfusion. The mechanism by which this therapy works is not entirely known, but it is likely related to improved oxygenation and lowering of the hemoglobin S concentration. The latter mechanism may promote blood flow through the pulmonary vasculature. The options for transfusion include simple or exchange technique. No randomized controlled trials comparing simple vs exchange transfusion for ACS have been done. The degree of improvement of oxygenation does not differ depending on the transfusion technique. Simple transfusion is often recommended in patients with mild events associated with severe anemia and is usually tried first. Exchange transfusion is then reserved for those who deteriorate, as in our patient. Hypotonic fluid resuscitation and avoidance of hemoglobin concentrations > 10 g/dL (100 g/L) are also advocated to avoid hyperviscosity. The end point of exchange transfusion is, ideally, a hemoglobin S concentration $< 30\%$.

All patients with ACS should receive antibiotics at presentation, which should include a third-generation cephalosporin to cover *Streptococcus pneumoniae*, *Haemophilus influenzae*, and *Klebsiella pneumoniae*, and a macrolide to cover *Mycoplasma pneumoniae* and *Chlamydophila pneumoniae*. Further changes should depend on culture results.

There is no reason to switch to moxifloxacin because the antimicrobial coverage is virtually identical to that obtained with the macrolide/cephalosporin combination (choice D is incorrect).

IV dexamethasone was found to be beneficial in one randomized controlled trial of 43 episodes of ACS in children, reducing the length of hospital stay and need for transfusion. Steroid therapy in adults has not been evaluated in clinical trials, and there are no data to support its use (choice C is incorrect). A prospective multicenter study analyzed 671 episodes of ACS in 538 patients to determine the cause, clinical course, and outcomes. For those patients ≥ 20 years with an etiology identified, infection was most common and included a substantial incidence of atypical organisms; however, 26% sustained a pulmonary fat embolism. Thromboembolism is not thought to be an important part of this syndrome, and routine anticoagulation is not recommended (choice B is incorrect).

Lottenberg R, Hassell KL. An evidence-based approach to the treatment of adults with sickle cell disease. Hematology 2005; 2005:58–65
Bernini JC, Rogers ZR, Sandler ES, et al. Beneficial effect of intravenous dexamethasone in children with mild to moderately severe acute chest syndrome complicating sickle cell disease. Blood 1998; 92:3082–3089
Vichinsky EP, Neumayr LD, Earles AN, et al. Causes and outcomes of the acute chest syndrome in sickle cell disease. N Engl J Med 2000; 342:1855–1865
Gladwin MT, Vichinsky E. Pulmonary complications of sickle cell disease. N Engl J Med 2008; 359:2254–2265

39. B. Histoplasmosis.

The CT scan shows abnormal soft tissue in the mediastinum with some calcification encasing the right bronchial tree, as well as thrombus within the superior vena cava (see Figures 39-A and 39-B) and calcifications within the liver and spleen (see Figures 39-B and 39-C). The perfusion scan (see Figure 39-D) reveals poor perfusion to the entire right lung, and the ventilation scan (see Figure 39-E) shows poor ventilation to the right lung, where perfusion is not as extensively diminished as that shown in the perfusion scan. These findings are most in line with fibrosing mediastinitis. Although many cases are idiopathic, of the known causes, histoplasmosis is the most common and consistent with the liver and splenic calcifications in this patient (choice B is correct), in addition to being a consequence of his exposure to chicken coops in childhood. The soft tissue structure seen on the right in Figure 39-B is a diaphragmatic eventration unrelated to the current problem.

Silicosis can certainly cause hilar and mediastinal calcifications but does not cause fibrosing mediastinitis, and splenic calcifications are unheard of (choice A is incorrect). Sarcoidosis can cause mediastinal calcifications, has very rarely been associated with fibrosing mediastinitis, and even more rarely has splenic calcifications, but there is nothing else to suggest the disease in this patient (choice C is incorrect). Lymphoma, particularly Hodgkin disease, has rarely been reported to cause fibrosing mediastinitis, but mediastinal calcifications have been reported in < 1% of mediastinal lymphomas, and none of the choices has had all three: hepatic, splenic, and mediastinal calcifications (choice D is incorrect).

Fibrosing mediastinitis is a rare benign disorder caused by proliferation of dense fibrous tissue within the mediastinum. Affected patients tend to be younger and have symptoms attributable to obstruction of mediastinal structures such as arteries, veins, the esophagus, or the airways. Although granulomatous reactions caused by *Histoplasma capsulatum* infection are most commonly associated with this condition, the relationship remains speculative in most cases because definitive demonstration of organisms is usually absent. Other infections such as TB, aspergillosis, blastomycosis, mucormycosis, and cryptococcosis have been reported to cause fibrosing mediastinitis, as have Behçet disease, radiation therapy, trauma, and Hodgkin disease. It may also be present as part of a spectrum with other idiopathic fibrosing diseases, such as sclerosing cholangitis, Riedel thyroiditis, and retroperitoneal fibrosis.

The disease has an unpredictable course. Death may be attributable to pulmonary hypertension, hemoptysis, or recurrent chest infections. There is no clearly effective therapy. Case reports have suggested that ketoconazole may stabilize the disease when caused by histoplasmosis, but this has never been documented with randomized, controlled trials. Similarly, there is little or no evidence that corticosteroids are helpful. Surgery may be helpful in resecting very

limited mediastinal disease but generally has been associated with very high morbidity and mortality. There have been case reports of successful endovascular stent placements to treat pulmonary artery compression due to the disease.

Rossi SE, McAdams HP, Rosada-de-Christenson ML, et al. Fibrosing mediastinitis. Radiographics 2001; 21:737–757

Devaraj A, Griffin N, Nicholson AG, et al. Computed tomography findings in fibrosing mediastinitis. Clin Radiol 2007; 62:781–786

Apter S, Avigdor A, Gayer G, et al. Calcification in lymphoma occurring before therapy: CT features and clinical correlation. Am J Roentgenol 2002; 178:935–938

Guerrero A, Hoffer EK, Hudson L, et al. Treatment of pulmonary artery compression due to fibrous mediastinitis with endovascular stent placement. Chest 2001; 119:966–968

Hamper UM, Fishman EK, Khouri NF, et al. Typical and atypical CT manifestations of pulmonary sarcoidosis. J Comput Assist Tomogr 1986; 10:928–936

40. C. Endotracheal intubation.

This patient was likely bitten by a crotalid, given the area and the characteristic "two-bite mark" nature of the bite. A more severe envenomation was likely present, considering the relative hypotension, borderline tachycardia, and progression of the local signs of inflammation over a period of < 1 h. Given the location of the bite itself (in this case, on the neck), securing the airway should be the first and foremost concern in the management regimen. Elective endotracheal intubation should be performed because subsequent edema can make attempts at intubation difficult or even impossible (choice C is correct).

In the United States, there are approximately 20 species of venomous snakes inflicting about 1,500 snakebites annually. Most of the snakebites are caused by pit vipers (Croatalidae), which include rattlesnakes, cottonmouths, and copperheads. A minority of bites are inflicted by coral snakes (Elapidae). The croatilid venom are complex mixtures of enzymes and toxic proteins and cause local tissue injury, coagulopathy (depletion of fibrinogen and disseminated intravascular coagulation), and other systemic manifestations (*eg,* vasodilation, hypotension, shock, myocardial ischemia, myoglobinuria, and renal failure).

The symptoms associated with snakebite depend on the degree of envenomation. In the case of the croatalid bites, this degree can be estimated by the presence and progression of signs and symptoms. Minimal envenomation is characterized by the presence of local findings with slow progression and absence of systemic signs and symptoms. In cases of severe envenomation, local findings progress more rapidly, and systemic complications appear early. Laboratory data, including monitoring of the coagulation system (*eg,* prothrombin time, partial thromboplastin time, platelet count, fibrinogen levels, fibrinogen degradation products), and hemoglobin and myoglobin concentrations should be obtained on admission and every 4 h thereafter.

Antivenom should be administered as soon as it is available, although the acute administration is not as vital as endotracheal intubation (choice A is incorrect). Antivenoms bind to and neutralize the venom, halting further damage, but do not reverse damage already done. Thus, they should be administered as soon as possible after the venom has been injected, but they are of some benefit as long as venom is present in the body. Diphenhydramine should be administered only to those patients who exhibit (approximately 20%) a reaction to the anitvenom infusion itself (choice B is incorrect). Immediate excision of the bite down to the fascia (and damaged muscle) has been advocated but can be effective only in cases of recent envenomation and in the absence of local diffusion of venom or systemic symptoms (choice D is incorrect). In this patient, endotracheal intubation should be performed at this point to ensure maintenance of an adequate airway, followed by management of the hypotension.

Moss ST, Bogdan G, Dart RC, et al. Association of rattlesnake bite location with severity of clinical manifestations. Ann Emerg Med 1997; 30:58–61

Gold BS, Barish RA, Dart RC. North American snake envenomation: diagnosis, treatment, and management. Emerg Med Clin North Am 2004; 22:423–433

41. A. Perform flexible bronchoscopy and BAL.

The patient underwent bronchoscopy and BAL (choice A is correct) that identified *Mycobacterium avium* complex, for which he was successfully treated with three-drug therapy with significant symptomatic and radiographic improvement of the peripheral, right lower lobe infiltrate. The incidence of community-acquired infection may be increased in patients receiving chronic immunosuppressive therapy, and therefore, consideration for empiric therapy may be warranted. Patients with RA maintained on chronic immunosuppressive therapy, particularly corticosteroids and cyclophosphamide, are at increased risk for infection with atypical or opportunistic organisms. Empiric treatment for community-acquired pathogens should not be pursued in light of the subacute-chronic nature of his symptoms (choice B is incorrect), and a definitive assessment should be considered with bronchoscopy and BAL. Organizing pneumonia is a common manifestation of RA-related lung injury and may be seen in association with medication-related toxicity. Although corticosteroids would be the treatment of choice for this condition, infectious complications from chronic tumor necrosis factor-α (TNF-α) antagonist therapy should be excluded prior to escalating immunosuppressive therapy for RA-related lung injury (choice C is incorrect). The peripheral location of the infiltrate makes it amenable to video-assisted thoracoscopic surgical lung biopsy. The radiographic characteristics do not suggest a mass, and therefore, bronchoscopy with BAL would be the most appropriate initial study to assess for infectious pathogens, with less morbidity than a surgical lung biopsy (choice D is incorrect). If lymphoma were of concern, a better diagnostic intervention would be to proceed with video-assisted thoracoscopic lung biopsy.

RA may manifest within the lungs in up to 15% of patients. Asymptomatic radiographic abnormalities have been identified in up to 70 to 80% of patients by thin-cut, high-resolution CT imaging. A multitude of case reports document the association of chronic immunosuppressive therapy with an increased risk of infection and pneumonia, in contrast to those data from randomized clinical trials that validated the efficacy of agents used for the treatment of RA. Atypical pathogens, such as *M avium* complex, *Mycobacterium xenopi*, *Mycobacterium tuberculosis*, adenovirus, Nocardia sp, Aspergillus sp, *Histoplasma capsulatum*, and *Pneumocystis jirovecii* have all been associated with TNF-α inhibitors. In those patients with a productive cough, sputum studies may be diagnostic and would be the initial diagnostic study. If *H capsulatum* is considered to be a relevant pathogen, serologic studies and urinary histoplasmosis antigen testing may be diagnostic in the appropriate context. Noninfectious, medication-related lung injury has also been reported in patients using leflunomide, infliximab, etanercept, and methotrexate for the treatment of RA and should be considered in all RA patients while on disease-modifying antirheumatic drugs or biological therapy. The differential diagnosis for new pulmonary infiltrates in patients with RA must be considered carefully because it includes infectious, rheumatologic, and medication-related complications of the disease.

Doraiswamy VA. Nocardia infection with adalimumab in rheumatoid arthritis. J Rheumatol 2008; 35:542–543

Bernatsky S, Hudson M, Suissa S. Anti-rheumatic drug use and risk of serious infections in rheumatoid arthritis. Rheumatology (Oxford) 2007; 46:1157–1160

Weisman MH, Paulus HE, Burch FX, et al. A placebo-controlled, randomized, double-blinded study evaluating the safety of etanercept in patients with rheumatoid arthritis and concomitant comorbid diseases. Rheumatology (Oxford) 2007; 46:1122–1125

Ostor AJ, Chilvers ER, Somerville MF, et al. Pulmonary complications of infliximab therapy in patients with rheumatoid arthritis. J Rheumatol 2006; 33:622–628

Wolfe F, Caplan L, Michaud K. Treatment for rheumatoid arthritis and the risk of hospitalization for pneumonia: associations with prednisone, disease-modifying antirheumatic drugs, and anti-tumor necrosis factor therapy. Arthritis Rheum 2006; 54:628–634

Zimmer C, Beiderlinden M, Peters J. Lethal acute respiratory distress syndrome during anti-TNF-alpha therapy for rheumatoid arthritis. Clin Rheumatol 2006; 25:430–432

42. A. Macrolide antibiotics should be used in management regardless of culture results.

The clinical course and radiologic findings in this patient are consistent with the biopsy, which is diagnostic for diffuse panbronchiolitis (DPB). DPB is a syndrome characterized by upper and lower airway abnormalities, which manifests as progressive airway obstruction with nodular lung densities and often a "tree-and-bud" appearance on CT, reflecting mucous impaction in respiratory bronchioles (see this patient's CT scan in Figure 42-D). The most effective treatment

identified to date is long-term administration of macrolides, which likely result in benefit apart from their antibacterial effects because improvement occurs independent of culture results (choice A is correct).

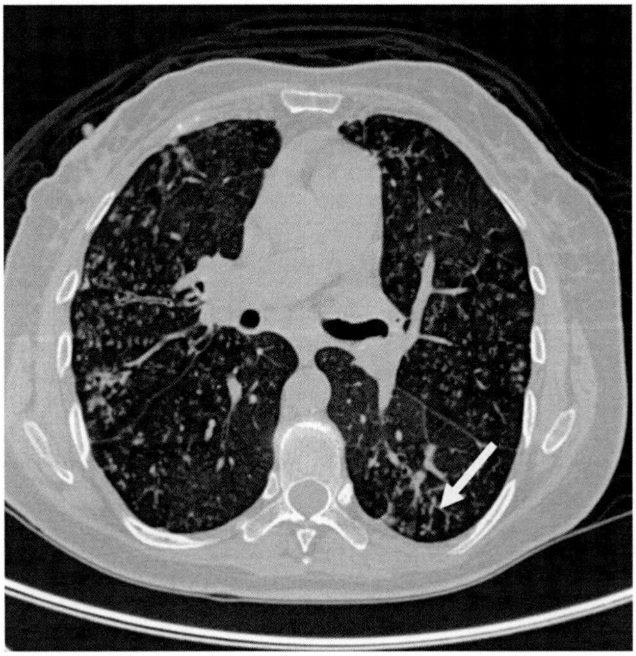

Figure 42-D

DPB was originally described in Japan, and the majority of series involve Japanese patients, although cases have been identified in North and South America and Europe, raising the possibility of underdiagnosis in these locales. Genetic factors are likely important in disease pathogenesis because familial cases have been identified, and there is an association with specific human leukocyte antigen haplotypes.

Typical clinical features include a history of chronic sinusitis in a majority of patients, often having a cough with purulent sputum, breathlessness with activity, wheezing, and weight loss. Nodular densities on chest CT are typical but in no way specific, and other causes of bronchiolitis and bronchiectasis should be sought and excluded. Pathologic findings include neutrophilic infiltrates obstructing respiratory bronchioles (BAL fluid often demonstrates this marked neutrophilia), with macrophage and lymphocyte infiltration of the airway walls. Disease progression often leads to bronchiectasis and fibrosis.

General management should include bronchodilators and physical measures such as flutter valves, chest wall percussive devices, or physical therapy to enhance mucous clearance. Nonsteroidal antiinflammatory drugs have been used, resulting in reduced mucous production. Corticosteroids have been used in treatment, with no clear evidence of benefit, and aggressive immunosuppression is not warranted (choice C is incorrect). Like patients with other causes of bronchiectasis, superinfection with mycobacterial species and resistant bacteria such as Pseudomonas spp can occur, but antimicrobial treatment should be reserved for those patients whose culture results are positive (choice B is incorrect). Immunoglobulin deficiency is a cause of bronchiectasis but is not a pathogenic mechanism for DPB, and treatment with IV immunoglobulin is not warranted (choice D is incorrect).

Many patients with DPB have been reported to progress to end-stage lung disease and respiratory failure. Several reports have shown a benefit from chronic (at least 6 to 12 months) treatment with macrolides for this disorder, with subjects in an uncontrolled series showing an improvement in survival and small randomized trials showing a significant improvement in lung function for many patients.

Poletti V, Casoni G, Chilosi M, et al. Diffuse panbronchiolitis. Eur Resp J 2006; 28:862–864
Kudoh S, Azuma A, Yamamoto M, et al. Improvement in survival in patients with diffuse panbronchiolitis treated with low dose erythromycin. Am J Resp Crit Care Med 1998; 157:1829–1834

43. D. Sleep disturbances persist for several years following cessation of alcohol use.

Sleep disturbance and insomnia can persist for many years during abstinence from alcohol, with reductions in total sleep time (TST) and nonrapid eye movement (NREM) stage N3 sleep (choice D is correct) as shown in Table 43-1.

Table 43-1. Polysomnographic Features of Alcohol Use, Withdrawal, and Abstinence

	Alcohol Use	Alcohol Withdrawal	Alcohol Abstinence
Sleep onset latency	↓	↑	
TST	↓ (↑ in some)	↓	↓
Awakenings	↓	↑	↑
NREM stage N3 sleep	↑ (during first half of sleep period)	↓	↓
REM sleep	↓ (during first half of sleep period)	↑	
REM sleep latency	↑	↓	

Acute ingestion of alcohol is associated with a biphasic effect on arousal. It is stimulatory at low doses and during the rising phase of alcohol levels and is sedating at high doses and during the falling phase of alcohol levels (choice A is incorrect).

Its sedative action is additive to that of benzodiazepines, and coingestion of the two agents can result in considerable sleepiness and increased risk for accidents. Acute ingestion of alcohol at bedtime decreases sleep onset latency. It also increases NREM stage N3 sleep and reduces REM sleep during the first half of the sleep period. Latency to stage REM from sleep onset is prolonged (choice B is incorrect). Some individuals may use alcohol only for its sedative effects and do not exhibit other patterns of behavior compatible with overt alcoholism, a condition referred to as alcohol-dependent sleep disorder. Alcohol use can exacerbate snoring, obstructive sleep apnea, and restless legs syndrome, and may precipitate nightmares and disorders of arousal, such as confusional arousals, sleepwalking, and sleep terrors. As alcohol is metabolized, its concentration in the blood rapidly decreases during the sleep period. This, in turn, causes an increase in the frequency of arousals and awakenings, as well as a REM sleep rebound during the second part of the night. Individuals can awaken with headaches and diaphoresis at this time.

Alcohol withdrawal is generally characterized by significant sleep disturbance, with an increase in sleep onset latency, decrease in total sleep time, and increase in frequency of awakenings. NREM stage N3 sleep is reduced, as is REM sleep latency. REM sleep duration increases (choice C is incorrect). Delirium tremens is often accompanied by markedly decreased total sleep time.

Stein MD, Friedmann PD. Disturbed sleep and its relationship to alcohol use. Subst Abus 2005; 26:1–13
Qureshi A, Lee-Chiong T Jr. Medications and their effects on sleep. Med Clin North Am 2004; 88:751–766

44. B. Begin isoniazid, rifampin, and ethambutol.

With a few caveats, treatment of active TB in a pregnant woman is similar to that of treatment in the nonpregnant individual. In the 2003 TB treatment guidelines by the American Thoracic Society, Centers for Disease Control and

Prevention, and the Infections Diseases Society of America, standard treatment for active TB during pregnancy is isoniazid (INH), rifampin, and ethambutol for ≥ 9 months, depending on results of susceptibility testing (choice B is correct). INH, rifampin, and ethambutol cross the placenta but have not been shown to have teratogenic effects. These drugs are all category C drugs and can be continued during lactation without compromise to the infant. Patients who are INH-resistant can be treated with rifampin and ethambutol. Multidrug-resistant patients may have to consider therapeutic abortion. It is recommended that pyridoxine always be administered with INH during pregnancy to decrease the incidence of INH neurotoxicity (optic and peripheral neuropathy). Four-drug therapy that includes moxifloxacin, a category C drug, is not an approved treatment for active TB during pregnancy (choice A is incorrect). Isoniazid and rifampin for 9 months was the previously recommended treatment regimen during pregnancy in a patient without suspected INH resistance but is no longer the accepted initial therapy (choice D is incorrect).

In general, pyrazinamide (PZA; category C) containing regimens (choice A), streptomycin (category D), and ethionamide (category C) should be avoided during pregnancy. There are situations in which treatment with these drugs may outweigh the potential risks of using them. The teratogenicity of streptomycin is primarily fetal ototoxicity due to nerve damage, congenital auditory malformations, and/or congenital deafness. PZA has been avoided traditionally in the United States because there is a lack of data for use during pregnancy, compared with the data available for other category C agents, and PZA is not recommended for initial therapy of TB during pregnancy by the 2003 TB treatment guidelines. However, PZA has been recommended routinely by the World Health Organization and the International Union Against Tuberculosis and Lung Disease. Non-PZA–containing regimens require 9 months of treatment compared with 6 months of treatment with PZA-containing regimens. PZA should be included when treating HIV-positive patients or if drug resistance is suspected.

The prognosis for recovery from TB in pregnant women has been debated. At one time, it was thought that TB had an increased incidence of dissemination in the pregnant woman. Most recent data show that there is no difference in the susceptibility to infection, course of disease, obstetrical outcome, prognosis, and incidence of TB in nonpregnant or pregnant individuals, unless immunosuppression coexists. Nevertheless, untreated active TB is associated with significant morbidity and mortality, and therefore, treatment should not be deferred (choice C is incorrect).

The following table shows the US Food and Drug Administration's classification of pharmaceutical agents in pregnancy:

Category	Definition
A	Controlled studies show no fetal risk
B	No evidence of fetal risk in humans
C	Fetal risk cannot be ruled out
D	Positive evidence of fetal risk
X	Contraindicated in pregnancy

Blumberg HM, Burman WJ, Chaisson RE, et al. American Thoracic Society/Centers for Disease Control and Prevention/Infectious Diseases Society of America: treatment of tuberculosis. Am J Respir Crit Care Med 2003; 167:603–662
Davidson PT. Managing tuberculosis during pregnancy. Lancet 1995; 346:199–200
Ormerod P. Tuberculosis in pregnancy and the puerperium. Thorax 2001; 56:494–499
Laibl VR, Sheffield JS. Tuberculosis in pregnancy. Clin Perinatol 2005; 32:739–747

45. B. Increased plateau but unchanged esophageal pressures.

During a controlled mechanical breath (*ie,* one in which patient activity is not present), the change in airway pressure reflects both lung and chest wall mechanical properties, whereas the change in esophageal pressure reflects only the chest wall mechanical properties. Thus the difference between the airway plateau pressure (*ie,* the end-inspiratory pressure under no-flow conditions) and the esophageal pressure at end inspiration reflects only lung distending forces.

In this patient, a massive aspiration has caused an acute lung injury that is expected to worsen lung compliance. It, however, should have no effect on chest wall mechanics. Accordingly, the plateau pressure will be substantially elevated, but because this will be entirely due to lung abnormalities, the pleural pressure (*ie,* esophageal pressure) will be unchanged (choice B is correct). Choices A and C are incorrect because they both describe changes in esophageal pressure that are not present in this patient. Choice D is incorrect because the plateau pressure will rise in the patient.

Knowing the chest wall mechanical properties can be helpful in selecting lung-protective mechanical ventilator settings. This is particularly true in patients with severely reduced chest wall compliance (*eg,* obesity and ascites), where the effect of the stiff chest wall on measurements of airway plateau pressure may be underappreciated and ventilator settings are unnecessarily reduced.

Truwit JD, Marini JJ. Evaluation of thoracic mechanics in the ventilated patient: Part 1. Primary measurements. J Crit Care 1988; 3:133–150
Truwit JD, Marini JJ. Evaluation of thoracic mechanics in the ventilated patient: Part 2. Applied mechanics. J Crit Care 1988; 3:192–213
Ranieri VM, Brienza N, Santostasi S, et al. Impairment of lung and chest wall mechanics in patients with acute respiratory distress syndrome: role of abdominal distension. Am J Respir Crit Care Med 1997; 156:1082–1091
Talmor D, Sarge T, Malhotra A. Mechanical ventilation guided by esophageal pressure measurements in acute lung injury. New Engl J Med 2008; 359:2095–2104
Sarge T, Talmor D. Transpulmonary pressure: its role in preventing ventilator-induced lung injury. Minerva Anestesiologica 2008; 74:335–339

46. A. Chylothorax.

The pleural fluid triglyceride concentration of > 110 mg/dL (1.24 mmol/L) is diagnostic of chylothorax (choice A is correct). Chylothorax develops when lipids from chyle collect in the pleural space, usually as a result of injury to the thoracic duct or other regional lymphatic tributaries. Such disruption can either be traumatic or nontraumatic. Traumatic chylothorax can follow thoracic surgery, penetrating chest trauma, pacemaker placement, or central line placement. Because of the location of the terminus of the thoracic duct, procedures involving the left subclavian vein are higher-risk than right-sided central vascular procedures. In this case, during pacemaker insertion, the thoracic duct was injured at its junction with the left subclavian vein.

Empyema is unlikely in this patient given the high pH. Empyema, heart failure, and pulmonary embolism would not yield an elevated pleural triglyceride concentration (choices B, C, and D are incorrect).

Nontraumatic causes of chylothorax are usually related to malignant involvement of the mediastinum leading to lymphatic disruption (most commonly with lymphoma or metastatic lung cancer) but can also be seen in association with other metastatic malignancies, such as sarcoidosis, histoplasmosis, TB, lymphangioleiomyomatosis, multiple myeloma, chronic lymphocytic leukemia, amyloidosis, thoracic irradiation, superior vena cava syndrome, or subclavian vein thrombosis.

Patients with chylothorax typically have dyspnea and fatigue, and pleuritic chest pain is less common than in the presence of inflammatory effusions. Diagnosis is by pleural fluid analysis. The effusion may appear grossly white or milky, although the absence of such an appearance does not exclude the diagnosis. The pleural fluid pH is generally > 7.40, and a triglyceride concentration of > 110 mg/dL (1.24 mmol/L) or detection of chylomicrons in the pleural fluid is considered diagnostic. Most chylous effusions are exudative in nature.

Treatment of chylothorax generally involves dietary modification, including a low-fat diet and limited oral intake with or without medium-chain triglyceride supplementation. In some cases, parenteral nutrition with full bowel rest is required, and octreotide or somatostatin may be useful as adjunctive therapy. Should these conservative measures fail, surgical repair may be attempted in certain situations. Talc pleurodesis, an indwelling pleural catheter, or percutaneous catheterization and embolization of the thoracic duct have been employed in some cases. In any event, prolonged chest tube drainage should be avoided because of the risk of nutritional compromise and immunosuppression due to lymphocyte depletion.

Agrawal V, Sahn SA. Lipid pleural effusions. Am J Med Sci 2008; 335:16–20

Boffa DJ, Sands MJ, Rice TW, et al. A critical evaluation of a percutaneous diagnostic and treatment strategy for chylothorax after thoracic surgery. Eur J Cardiothorac Surg 2008; 33:435–439

Doerr CH, Miller DL, Ryu JH. Chylothorax. Semin Respir Crit Care Med. 2001; 22:617–626

Maldonado F, Hawkins FJ, Daniels CE, at al. Pleural fluid characteristics of chylothorax. Mayo Clin Proc 2009; 84:129–133

47. A. Referral for genetic testing.

The patient has had recurrent pneumothoraces over a 30-year period in the setting of no known lung disease, normal lung function, previously excised skin lesions, and multiple bilateral thin-walled cysts in both subpleural and central locations. A similar history of recurrent pneumothoraces in an otherwise healthy sibling is an important highlight and suggestive of an underlying inherited condition, specifically Birt-Hogg-Dube syndrome. Genetic testing will confirm the diagnosis in this setting (choice A is correct) and reveal a deletion of the single base (delT) at nucleotide 59 of the *FLCN* (familial cancer syndrome) gene on chromosome 17p11.2. Mutations of this gene have been associated with bullous lung disease. Test results confirm the diagnosis of the autosomal dominant Birt-Hogg-Dube syndrome, which also predisposes patients to benign skin tumors (fibrofolliculomas) and renal tumors, although full expression of the phenotype may not always be present. In the absence of a family history, cigarette smoking, or a specific underlying lung disease, spontaneous pneumothorax also occurs with increased frequency in patients with Marfan syndrome and homocystinuria.

Patients with an established diagnosis of Birt-Hogg-Dube syndrome should be offered appropriate genetic counseling and family testing (children have a 50% chance of inheriting the tendency toward spontaneous pneumothorax). In addition, initial and ongoing screening for renal tumors would be indicated, including urinalysis and imaging.

A CT scan of the head would be appropriate for assessment of patients with lymphangioleiomyomatosis (LAM) because of the increased incidence of meningiomas and its association with tuberous sclerosis. However, although genetic abnormalities have been documented in LAM, a genetic predisposition is not present and, therefore, genetic testing would not confirm the diagnosis. Although approximately one-third of patients with LAM have normal pulmonary function tests at diagnosis, abnormalities typically develop over time. This patient, at age 58 years, has normal lung function 30 years after her initial pneumothorax and did not have a history of pleural effusions or ascites, hemoptysis, signs of pulmonary hypertension, or neurologic complaints (choice B is incorrect). The CT scan findings are not characteristic of emphysema (choice C is incorrect), and there is no indication to proceed to lung biopsy at this time (choice D is incorrect).

Painter JN, Tapanainen H, Somer M, et al. A 4-bp deletion in the Birt-Hogg-Dube gene (FLCN) causes dominantly inherited spontaneous pneumothorax. Am J Hum Genet 2005; 76:522–527

Schmidt LS, Nickerson ML, Warren MB. Germline BHD-mutation spectrum and phenotype analysis of a large cohort of families with Birt-Hogg-Dube syndrome. Am J Hum Genet 2005; 76:1023–1033

Toro JR, Pautler SE, Stewart L, et al. Lung cysts, spontaneous pneumothorax, and genetic associations in 89 families with Birt-Hogg-Dube syndrome. Am J Respir Crit Care Med 2007; 175:1044–1053

48. D. Refer for embolotherapy.

The tortuous collection of vessels and feeding artery seen on the CT scan (see Figure 48-C, arrows) is suggestive of an isolated pulmonary arteriovenous malformation (PAVM). The mild hypoxemia seen with an arterial blood gas test suggests an elevated shunt fraction, which is confirmed by arterial blood gas testing done after breathing 100% oxygen (showing a shunt fraction of 9.49%, which also is consistent with a PAVM). Although the equation for a shunt fraction is somewhat complicated,

$$Q_S/Q_T = \frac{100 \times [0.0031 \times D_{A\text{-}a}O_2]}{[0.0031 \times D_{A\text{-}a}O_2]}$$

where the A-a gradient is the alveolar-to-arterial oxygen gradient calculated for the appropriate barometric pressure and inspired oxygen, it does not have to be calculated in this case because a $Pao_2 < 575$ mm Hg after breathing 100% oxygen is consistent with an abnormal shunt fraction of > 5%. Because of considerable morbidity and mortality of untreated PAVMs, patients who are symptomatic or have a PAVM > 2 cm or a PAVM with a feeding vessel > 3 mm should be treated with embolotherapy or surgery. Embolotherapy is preferable in most cases because it avoids the risks of major surgery and anesthesia and minimizes the loss of lung parenchyma (choice D is correct). Embolotherapy generally starts with conventional pulmonary angiography to characterize the PAVM, followed by placement of embolic material, such as steel or wood coils, detachable balloons, or polyvinyl alcohol, into the feeding artery of the PAVM. The most common complication is pleuritic chest pain. More serious complications are infrequent and have included transient air embolization, pulmonary infarct, migration of the balloon or coil, and transient ischemic attack or stroke. Postembolotherapy management includes lifelong periprocedural antibiotics and follow-up chest CT scanning every 2 to 3 years to monitor for progression or new PAVMs. Figures 48-D and 48-E are from this patient's successful embolotherapy procedure. Follow-up arterial blood gas measurement on 100% oxygen for 20 min revealed that the shunt fraction had decreased to 2.8%. Surgery can be considered for those patients with an untreatable allergy to contrast dye or with PAVMs not amenable to embolotherapy (choice C is incorrect).

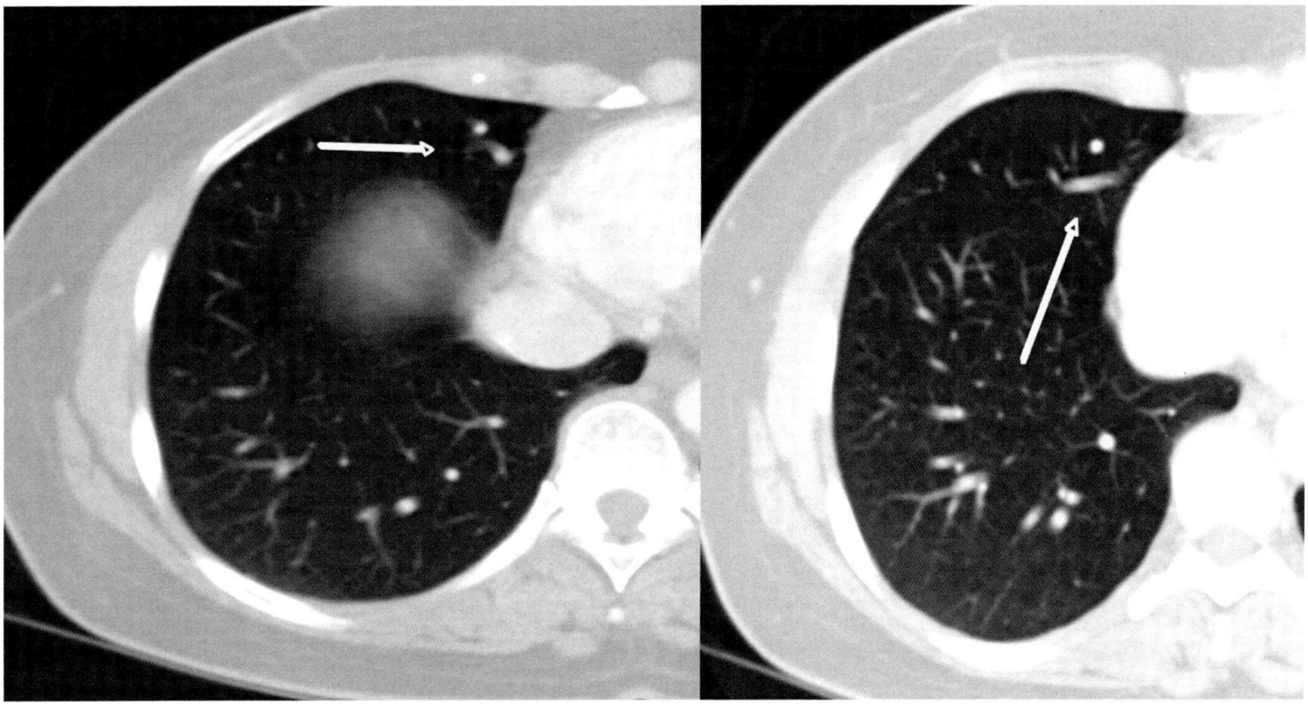

Figure 48-C

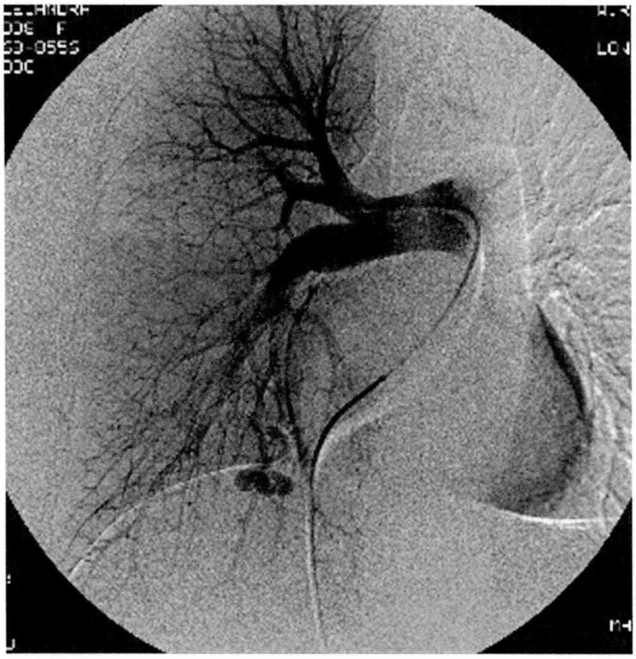

Figure 48-D

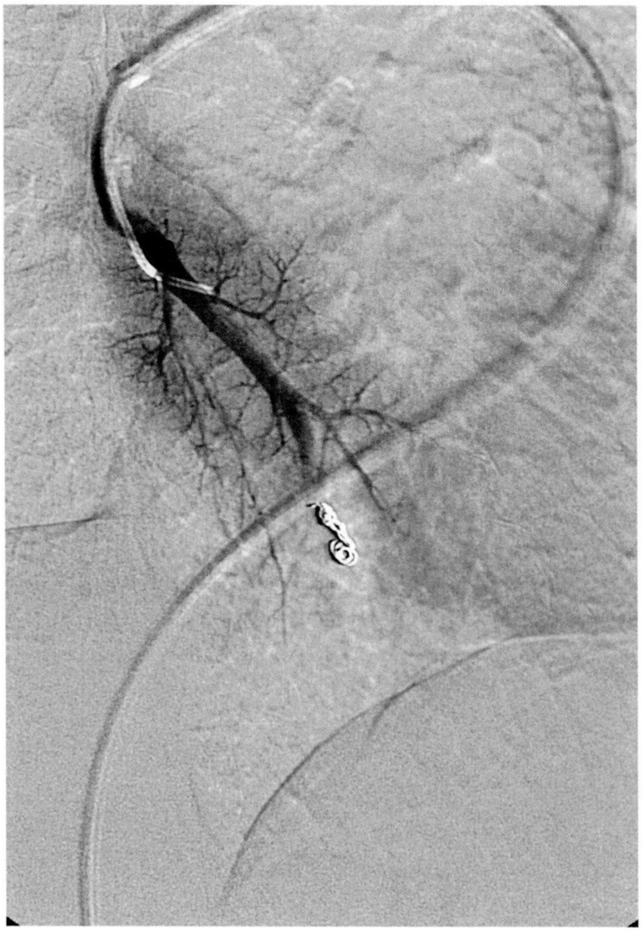

Figure 48-E

Patients who have PAVMs in the setting of hereditary hemorrhagic telangiectasia (HHT) also may be candidates for pharmacologic therapy. In small studies, a variety of hormonal treatments (estrogen preparations, tamoxifen, danazol, and octreotide) have shown promise in the management of epistaxis and GI bleeding. In addition, isolated case reports have noted an association between immunosuppressive agents and resolution of telangiectasias of the skin, buccal mucosa, and upper GI tract of patients with HHT. This patient does not manifest signs of HHT, at least in the upper airway or GI tract. In addition, pharmacologic agents have not been used to treat PAVMs (choices A and B are incorrect).

Khalil A, Farres MT, Mangiapan G, et al. Pulmonary arteriovenous malformations. Chest 2000; 117:1399–1403

Gossage JR, Kanj G. Pulmonary arteriovenous malformations: a state of the art review. Am J Respir Crit Care Med 1998; 158:643–661

White RI Jr, Lunch-Nyhan A, Terry P, et al. Pulmonary arteriovenous malformations: techniques and long-term outcome of embolotherapy. Radiology 1988; 169:663–669

Jameson JJ, Cave DR. Hormonal and antihormonal therapy for epistaxis in hereditary hemorrhagic telangiectasia. Laryngoscope 2004; 114:705–709

49. D. Phosgene.

This patient has acute respiratory failure roughly 24 h after exposure to an unknown chemical agent, and that exposure has led to signs of acute lung injury and pulmonary edema after a slight delay of 12 to 24 h. A number of chemical agents can cause pulmonary irritation, but the most common are chlorine gas, ammonia, and phosgene. Chlorine and ammonia, due to their water solubility, cause acute-onset lung injury. Phosgene, which is more lipid-soluble, has a delay of 12 to 24 h before the onset of acute lung injury (choice D is correct).

These agents are common in industrial use and recently have gained additional attention as agents used by terrorists. Early symptoms of exposure include nose, throat, and eye irritation and cough, chest pain, and bronchospasm.

In high-dose exposure, severe airway irritation, edema, and bronchospasm can occur rapidly and lead to death. Airway hyperreactivity and obstructive airflow associated with inhalation of a pulmonary irritant is called reactive airways dysfunction syndrome. With less exposure, a latent period of 12 to 36 h before the onset of acute lung injury and pulmonary edema can occur. Onset of acute lung injury within 4 h of exposure carries a poor prognosis. Because of the potential delay in symptoms, these patients must be observed for ≥ 48 h after exposure. Detection based on odor (phosgene can smell like freshly mowed hay) has been reported but is not a reliable indicator. At room temperature, chlorine and phosgene exist as a gas that is heavier than air.

Supportive care is the main form of treatment for these patients, and, although secondary transmission to health-care professionals is limited, all patients should be thoroughly decontaminated. Intervention at the site of exposure includes removal from the site and increased ventilation. Organophosphates are common in agricultural locations, and symptoms consist of bronchorrhea, bronchospasm, and in rare cases, acute lung injury. Additional symptoms of bradycardia, hypotension, diarrhea, and urinary incontinence also occur (choice A is incorrect). Isocyanate, a component of paint and paint products, is often seen in individuals with occupational asthma and is not associated with acute lung injury with a latency period (choice B is incorrect). Pyrethrin is a common insecticide that is used frequently and has gained attention due to use in mosquito vector control in urban areas. Wheezing, but not acute lung injury, has been reported after exposure (choice C is incorrect).

Parrish JS, Bradshaw DA. Toxic inhalational injury: gas, vapor, and vesicant exposure. Respir Care Clin N Am 2004; 10:43–59

Greenfield RA, Brown BR, Hutchins JB, et al. Microbiological, biological, and chemical weapons of warfare and terrorism. Am J Med Sci 2002; 323:326–340

Mapp CE, Boschetto P, Mastrelli P, et al. Occupational asthma. Am J Respir Crit Care Med 2005; 172:280–305

50. C. Briefly disconnect the ET from ventilator tubing and then reduce the set rate to 12/min.

This patient with severe asthma has evidence of progressive hyperinflation that is now producing cardiopulmonary compromise with systemic hypotension and hypoxemia. Among the options presented, the best combination of an intervention and a ventilator adjustment to relieve hyperinflation is to briefly disconnect the ET from ventilator tubing and then reduce the set rate to 12/min (choice C is correct). Immediate relief of the patient's hyperinflated state can be achieved by disconnecting the ventilator circuit from the ET, allowing exhalation to functional residual capacity and prevention of the delivery of additional breaths until full exhalation has occurred. Often, BP and Spo_2 will return to baseline within seconds of completing this maneuver. Although deep tracheal suction with saline lavage may be appropriate if mucus plugging is present, there is no clinical evidence of overt plugging in this case, and prolonged suctioning during positive pressure ventilation may worsen hyperinflation (choices A and B are incorrect).

Adjustments in the ventilator settings must be made in order to prevent recurrence of hyperinflation. A major determinant of progressive hyperinflation is the delivery of a breath before the last breath is entirely exhaled. In the setting of significant airflow obstruction, an expiratory time of only 2 s, as in this case (*ie,* with a respiratory rate of 20/min and a 1-s inspiratory time), would be likely to lead to progressive hyperinflation. Accordingly, reducing the set rate from 20/min to 12/min would double the expiratory time from 2 to 4 s in a patient who is deeply sedated and/or therapeutically paralyzed and not breathing above the set rate (choice C is correct). This benefit would not be realized, however, if the patient's spontaneous respirations increase. Reducing the set rate will reduce minute ventilation; however, in a pressure-targeted mode, some of the reduction will be offset by relief of dynamic hyperinflation and subsequent increases in tidal volume. Although the reduction in minute ventilation may worsen hypercapnia, relief of hyperinflation will likely reduce dead space, thus partially offsetting the drop in alveolar ventilation and rise in $Paco_2$. The observation that tidal volume has decreased significantly in the setting of pressure-targeted ventilation is an important clue that air trapping and auto-PEEP or intrinsic-PEEP are developing. Increasing the inspiratory pressure would tend to increase tidal volume but worsen hyperinflation (choices A and D are incorrect).

Levy BD, Kitch B, Fanta CH. Medical and ventilatory management of status asthmaticus. Intensive Care Med 1998; 24:105–117
Papiris S, Kotanidou A, Malagari K, et al. Clinical review: severe asthma. Crit Care 2002; 6:30–44
Smyth RJ. Ventilatory care in status asthmaticus. Can Respir J 1998; 5:485–490

51. B. Left lower lobe atelectasis.

The findings of sharply marginated retrocardiac opacity without air bronchograms, elevation of the left hemidiaphragm, displacement of the mediastinum to the left, and approximation of the left ribs are most consistent with left lower lobe atelectasis (choice B is correct). The retrocardiac opacity is demarcated laterally by caudal and medial displacement of the left major fissure, illustrated in Figures 51-A (see the stem) and 51-B. Compensatory hyperinflation may be apparent in the remaining aerated lobes, but this finding is often subtle. This patient had a carcinoma completely obstructing the left lower lobe bronchus.

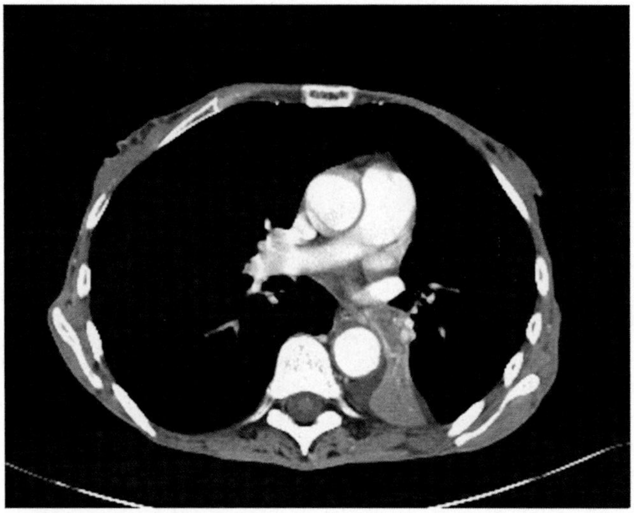

Figure 51-B

A left pleural effusion would cause an increased retrocardiac density without air bronchograms, but the left hemidiaphragm would be in a normal or depressed position; the mediastinum would be at midline or displaced to the right; and the cardiac silhouette would probably not be visualized below the level of fluid (choice A is incorrect). The chest radiograph after left lower lobe resection could resemble atelectasis. Although there are surgical clips present, they are below the diaphragm and, therefore, not the result of a pneumonectomy (choice C is incorrect). Left lower lobe pneumonia is unlikely because there are no air bronchograms in the retrocardiac opacity (choice D is incorrect). However, some patients with pneumonia also have significant atelectasis complicating the respiratory infection.

Atelectasis. In: Fraser RS, Müller NL, Colman N, et al, eds. Fraser and Paré's diagnosis of diseases of the chest. 4th ed. Philadelphia, PA: WB Saunders Co, 1999; 513–562
Woodring JH, Reed JC. Types and mechanisms of pulmonary atelectasis. J Thorac Imag 1996; 11:92–108

52. B. Organizing pneumonia.

The CT scan reveals patchy airspace disease bilaterally, with areas of ground-glass opacities. The biopsy specimen shows granulation tissue plugs within the airspaces, with no evidence of granulomatous inflammation, viral inclusions,

eosinophilic infiltration, or vasculitis. These findings, taken together, are suggestive of cryptogenic organizing pneumonia, also called *bronchiolitis obliterans with organizing pneumonia*. Because this patient has an associated connective tissue disease, it is not truly cryptogenic, so many prefer the term *organizing pneumonia* (OP) (choice B is correct).

Rheumatoid arthritis is an autoimmune disorder with predominantly articular features, but pleuropulmonary complications can be present. Two less common complications include bronchiolitis obliterans (BO) and OP. BO is a particularly severe and often fatal complication of rheumatoid arthritis that is more common in women. Histologically, peribronchiolar fibrosis ultimately results in complete cicatrization of the bronchiolar lumen, so some pathologists prefer the term *constrictive bronchiolitis*. The chest radiograph is usually normal or reveals hyperinflation. The characteristic patchy airspace consolidation with ground-glass components favoring the lower lung zones peripherally (as in the current case) that is seen in OP are not present. In addition, patients with OP commonly present with cough associated with constitutional symptoms, as opposed to patients with BO, who normally have little malaise, weight loss, or fever. Physical examination can reveal crackles in both entities, but OP has a restrictive pattern with a reduced DLCO on pulmonary function tests, whereas BO shows severe obstruction and normal or elevated lung volumes, and diffusing capacity is often normal (choice A is incorrect).

Methotrexate pulmonary toxicity most commonly occurs within the first year of treatment and may present with dyspnea, cough, and fever. CT scanning frequently shows patchy airspace disease with thickened interlobular septa and scattered ground-glass changes, the so-called "crazy paving" picture. BAL fluid may show an increased CD4/CD8 cell ratio. Occasionally, hypersensitivity reactions to methotrexate can result in a high BAL fluid eosinophil count. Pathologic specimens reveal poorly formed granulomas with eosinophilic infiltration. Delayed reactions years after discontinuing the drug have not been reported with methotrexate (choice C is incorrect). Sarcoidosis has protean presentations and may mimic the radiographic picture seen in the current case. The BAL fluid of patients with sarcoidosis normally has a high CD4/CD8 cell ratio, and noncaseating granulomas are seen on transbronchial biopsies (choice D is incorrect).

Findings in BAL fluid in patients with OP are similar to those seen in hypersensitivity pneumonitis, with lymphocytosis and a decreased CD4/CD8 cell ratio, although this is not consistently found or diagnostic. Foamy macrophages are also seen. Histologic findings (see Figure 52-B in the stem) consist of a uniform temporal appearance of intraluminal organizing fibrosis in distal airspaces with a patchy distribution. There is, however, preservation of lung architecture differentiating it from other idiopathic interstitial lung diseases. While diagnosis may be suggested through transbronchial biopsies interpreted within proper clinical context, surgical lung biopsy may be required. Figure 52-C shows a good example of OP from a video-assisted thoracic surgery biopsy specimen.

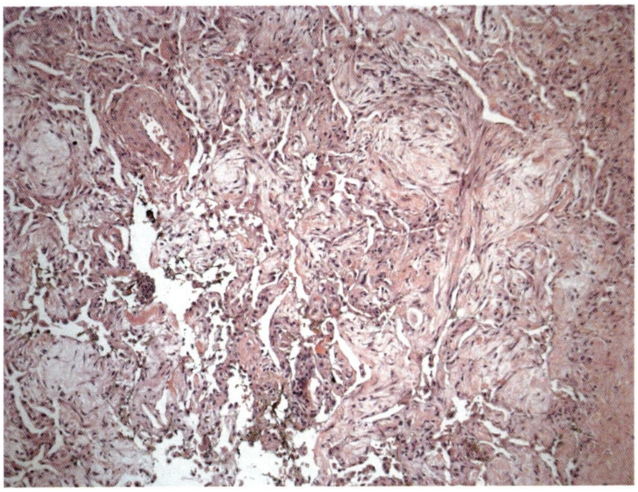

Figure 52-C
Hematoxylin-eosin

The mainstay of treatment for OP is corticosteroids, starting with 0.75 to 1.5 mg/kg, with a slow taper over 3 to 12 months, depending on clinical response. Prognosis is generally good, but rate of relapse can be high if corticosteroids are tapered too quickly. Nonetheless, it appears that a relapse responds as well as to initial treatment with corticosteroids; therefore, attempts at faster tapering are reasonable to avoid potential side effects in patients with a good initial response.

Cannon GW. Methotrexate pulmonary toxicity. Rheum Dis Clin North Am 1997; 23:917–937

Cordier JF. Cryptogenic organising pneumonia. Eur Respir J 2006; 28:422–446

Kaushik P, Cooper ES, Banda VR, et al. Bronchiolitis obliterans with organizing pneumonia in rheumatoid arthritis: a fatal case and short review of literature. Rheumatol Int 2005; 25:391–393

Oymak FS, Demirbas HM, Mavili E, et al. Bronchiolitis obliterans organizing pneumonia: clinical and roentgenological features in 26 cases. Respiration 2005; 72:254–262

Tanaka N, Kim JS, Newell JD, et al. Rheumatoid arthritis-related lung diseases: CT findings. Radiology 2004; 232:81–91

53. B. Immediate IV diphenhydramine and corticosteroids; hold aspirin overnight; restart the provocative aspirin dose.

This patient has aspirin-exacerbated respiratory disease (AERD). Continuing desensitization after treatment of his urticaria and respiratory symptoms with IV corticosteroids and diphenhydramine and an overnight hiatus in aspirin dosing is the appropriate treatment choice. The titration dose of aspirin creating the reactions described is called the *provocative dose* and should be restarted the next day (choice B is correct). Aspirin desensitization in patients with AERD followed by daily aspirin administration is generally recommended because it produces significant reductions in sinus infections and in the number of short courses of prednisone. Additionally, there are improvements in the sense of smell and general nasal-sinus and asthma symptoms. Up to 87% of patients completing a year or more of aspirin treatment following desensitization experience improvements. Exacerbations of sinusitis, as suffered by this patient despite surgical intervention, may increase asthma severity, potentially requiring systemic corticosteroids and hospitalization. Hence, despite prior significant aspirin-induced symptoms, including anaphylaxis, this patient can substantially benefit from completion of aspirin desensitization. Aspirin dosing is continued until a final dose of 325 to 650 mg of aspirin is reached. The aspirin dose timing and addition of ranitidine described in this case are an accepted desensitization approach. Importantly, prior to the desensitization effort, the patient's asthma management was optimized as much as possible. Aspirin desensitization followed by daily aspirin is efficacious for at least 6 months after treatment and continues to be effective for up to 5 years of follow-up.

After desensitization, oral aspirin must be continued indefinitely, as sensitivity will recur within 7 days of discontinuation. The dose of aspirin to treat AERD can be up to 650 mg bid. However, some recommend decreasing this dose after a year of aspirin treatment in responders or earlier if gastric side effects occur.

Abandoning desensitization is unwarranted, especially given this patient's current relatively limited symptoms, nonthreatening vital signs, and monitoring in the hospital (choice A is incorrect). Choice A is also incorrect because it provides no additional treatment of his acute aspirin reaction. Choice C is incorrect because, similarly, the treatment does not address the need for completion of aspirin desensitization. Immediate intubation without an initial medical intervention is unwarranted given his current stability, regardless of a prior history of an anaphylactoid reaction requiring intubation (choice D is incorrect).

Berges-Gimeno MP, Simon RA, Stevenson DD. Long-term treatment with aspirin desensitization in asthmatic patients with aspirin-exacerbated respiratory disease. J Allergy Clin Immunol 2003; 111:180–186

Stevenson DD. Aspirin and NSAID sensitivity. Immunol Allergy Clin N Am 2004; 24:491–505

54. C. Segmental resection with mediastinal lymph node sampling.

In this case, the fine needle aspirate shows uniform, round-to-polygonal cells with small oval nuclei containing finely granular chromatin, scant-to-moderate eosinophilic cytoplasm, and no mitotic activity. These findings are most consistent with a typical carcinoid, a diagnosis also consistent with the clinical course. Typical carcinoids are most effectively treated by surgical resection. For peripheral tumors <2 cm in diameter, segmental resection is

recommended, provided that systematic sampling of hilar and mediastinal nodes is also performed (choice C is correct, and choice B is incorrect). Lymph node involvement provides important prognostic information, with 5-year survival rates reported as >90% with no lymph node involvement and around 67% with lymph node involvement. Complete excision of involved lymph nodes might improve prognosis.

An important clue to the diagnosis of this slowly growing nodule comes from the history of Cushing syndrome. A pituitary source of adrenocorticotropic hormone (ACTH) production had not been identified to explain the adrenal hyperplasia; ACTH production from a nonpituitary (ectopic) source causes Cushing syndrome in about 10% of cases. The most common source of ectopic ACTH production is a pulmonary carcinoid. Typical carcinoids can cause Cushing syndrome years before they are detected radiographically. In this case, special stains showing that the tumor contained ACTH confirmed that it was the cause of this patient's Cushing syndrome. Rarely, atypical carcinoid and small-cell carcinoma will secrete ACTH and cause Cushing syndrome, but cytologic findings would have shown greater pleomorphism and mitotic activity, and regional and systemic spread would have been expected.

Pulmonary carcinoids represent about 25% of all carcinoids (most carcinoids originate in the GI tract) and about 1% of all lung tumors. Although immunohistochemical studies show that carcinoids contain cytokeratin and desmoplakin, suggesting derivation from bronchial epithelium, carcinoids are probably derived from Kulchitsky or enterochromaffin cells, which are part of the diffuse neuroendocrine cells of the gut. Pulmonary carcinoids are categorized as neuroendocrine tumors because they have neurosecretory granules. These may be immunoreactive for a variety of peptides, such as ACTH, serotonin, melanocyte-stimulating hormone, and growth hormone, explaining the association of carcinoids with various paraneoplastic syndromes. The current World Health Organization classification of neuroendocrine tumors includes three categories: typical carcinoid, atypical carcinoid, and large-cell and small-cell carcinomas. Distinguishing among the various types of neuroendocrine tumors can be difficult, especially with cytologic material. Pulmonary carcinoids occur more often in women than men and present in patients in their 50s more often than lung cancer. Typical carcinoids are usually located in the proximal bronchial tree, but about 20% present as peripheral nodules. They grow slowly, with a low likelihood for regional lymph node involvement or systemic metastases.

Combined chemoradiotherapy is the accepted approach to limited-stage, small-cell carcinoma, but the clinical course and cytologic findings are not consistent with this diagnosis (choice A is incorrect). Pulmonary carcinoids are not particularly radiosensitive, although radiation therapy may be useful for palliation (choice D is incorrect).

Ilias I, Torpy DJ, Pacak K, et al. Cushing's syndrome due to ectopic corticotropin secretion. J Clin Endocrinol Metab 2005; 90:4955–4962

Kulke MH, Mayer RJ. Carcinoid tumors. N Engl J Med 1999; 340:858–867

Martini N, Zaman MB, Bains MS, et al. Treatment and prognosis in bronchial carcinoids involving regional lymph nodes. J Thorac Cardiovasc Surg 1995; 107:1–7

Mineo T, Guggino G, Mineo D, et al. Relevance of lymph node micrometastases in radically resected endobronchial carcinoid tumors. Ann Thorac Surg 2005; 80:428–433

Modlin IM, Lye KD, Kidd M. A 5-decade analysis of 13,715 carcinoid tumors. Cancer 2003; 97:934–959

55. C. 37 patients.

In this study, approximately 37 patients who met inclusion and exclusion criteria would need to receive the silver-coated tube (*ie*, the number needed to treat [NNT]) to prevent one case of VAP (choice C is correct, and other choices are incorrect). The NNT is calculated as the inverse of the absolute risk reduction (ARR) and can be derived from the data presented in this problem using the following calculations:

CER, % = Number of events/Number of control subjects × 100
EER, % = Number of events/Number of experimental subjects × 100
ARR = CER − EER
RRR = (CER − EER)/CER
NNT = 1/ARR

CER = control event rate; EER = experimental event rate; ARR = absolute risk reduction; RRR = relative risk reduction.

To determine whether an intervention is beneficial, there should be a strong association between receiving that intervention and either an increased likelihood of benefit or, in this case, a reduced risk of a bad outcome. The strength of this association is estimated by comparing the odds (or risk) of the adverse outcome with or without exposure to the intervention. In this study, the risk of developing pneumonia in 766 patients who received the silver-coated endotracheal tube was 37/766 or 4.8%, and the risk of developing pneumonia in patients who received an uncoated tube was 56/743 (7.5%). The relative risk of developing pneumonia in patients who received the silver-coated tube was 4.8/7.5 or 0.64. Alternatively, this can be expressed as a relative risk reduction of 36%: patients who received the silver-coated tube were about 36% less likely to develop VAP than patients who received the standard tube. Evaluating the potential clinical impact of that intervention should be refined by calculating the "absolute" risk reduction or the difference in rates of the adverse outcome between experimental and control patients. In this study, the ARR is 7.5% − 4.8% = 2.7%. In other words, the risk of developing VAP was reduced by 2.7% with the silver-coated tube. This concept may also be expressed as the NNT, or number of patients who must receive the intervention to prevent one bad outcome. This is calculated as 1/ARR; in this case, the NNT is 1/0.027 or 37 (choice C is correct). Thus, 37 patients would need to receive the silver-coated tube to prevent one case of VAP.

The NNT can only be expressed for binary outcomes and not for continuous variables. In this example, the outcomes are "pneumonia" and "no pneumonia." NNT calculations also express the frequency of the outcome and not its utility, such as cost, side effects, and ease of use. Finally, NNT calculations apply only to the population that was studied and may not hold for patients who are at especially high or low risk of developing an adverse outcome. For example, in a study of approximately 3,000 patients with diabetes receiving either a statin or a placebo, the NNT to prevent a first cardiovascular event over a 5-year period was 20. However, in patients who had occlusive arterial disease on enrollment, the NNT was 12, and in those without arterial disease, the NNT was 33. In the case of VAP, the use of silver-coated endotracheal tubes would also be likely to be most beneficial in patients at especially high risk of developing the disease.

In addition, although prevention of VAP is itself a desirable outcome, decisions on whether to use the silver-coated tube must also be made in the context of the incremental cost and whether other important outcomes are achieved. In this study, although the incidence of VAP was reduced, there were no statistically significant differences in the two groups in duration of intubation, length of ICU stay and hospital stay, and mortality.

Kollef MH, Afessa B, Anzueto A, et al. Silver-coated endotracheal tubes and the incidence of ventilator-associated pneumonia. JAMA 2008; 300:805–813

Levine M, Walter SD, Lee H, et al. Users' guides to the medical literature, IV: how to use an article about harm. JAMA 1994; 271:1615–1619

McAlister FA. The "number needed to treat" turns 20 and continues to be used and misused. Can Med Assoc J 2008; 179:549–553

Sackett DL, Richardson WS, Rosenberg W, et al. Evidence-based medicine: how to practice and teach EBM. Edinburgh: Churchill Livingstone, 2000

Collins R, Armitage J, Parish S, et al. MRC/BHF heart protection study of cholesterol-lowering with simvastatin in 5,693 people with diabetes: a randomized placebo-controlled trial. Lancet 2003; 14:361:2005–2016

56. C. It has led to a decrease in the number of penicillin-resistant pneumococcal strains among adults ≥ 65 years.

In 2000, a seven-serotype pneumococcal conjugate vaccine was introduced for routine use in infants even though there are more than 90 pneumococcal serotypes. Only 23 serotypes produce the majority of cases. The strains selected included five of the seven serotypes usually associated with resistance (6B, 9V, 14, 19F, and 23F; the other two are serotypes 4 and 18C). The vaccine is recommended for all children < 2 years and for children ages 2 to 4 years with chronic illnesses or high-risk conditions. One of the pleasant surprises associated with the introduction of this vaccine was a 49% decline in the rate of penicillin-nonsusceptible disease from 16.4/100,000 in 1999 to 8.4/100,000 among adults ≥ 65 years in 2004 (choice C is correct). Similar observations have been made among HIV-infected adults. There has been an overall decrease in invasive pneumococcal disease among HIV-infected adults, despite increased disease caused by nonvaccine serotypes (choice A is incorrect). The effectiveness of the vaccine in healthy children

has been measured as 96% and as 81% in those with coexisting disorders (choice B is incorrect). In a Spanish study, virulent clones of non-PCV7 serotypes have emerged, comprising 72% of infecting serotypes (choice D is incorrect).

Conjugate pneumococcal vaccines reduce the risk of carriage and transmission of vaccine-type strains among recipients of the vaccine and their household members. The vaccine interrupts the transmission of resistant pneumococci from children to adults. This property has been termed "herd immunity," whereby reduction in disease in part of the population offers some degree of protection to the entire population. Although use of the polyvalent pneumococcal vaccine has increased throughout North America, experts agree that the decrease in invasive pneumococcal disease, particularly of resistant strains, is largely related to the seven-serotype pneumococcal conjugate vaccine. This is mainly because there has been no reduction in the incidence of resistant disease caused by serotypes included in the 23-valent polysaccharide vaccine but not in the seven-valent conjugate vaccine. There has been an increase in resistant disease caused by nonvaccine serotypes (replacement disease) but, so far, the magnitude of this is small.

Kyaw MH, Lynfield R, Schaffner W, et al. Effect of introduction of the pneumococcal conjugate vaccine on drug-resistant *Streptococcus pneumoniae.* N Engl J Med 2006; 354:1455–1463

Flannery B, Heffernan RT, Harrison LH, et al. Changes in invasive pneumococcal disease among HIV-infected adults living in the era of childhood pneumococcal immunization. Ann Intern Med 2006; 144:1–9

Whitney CG, Pilishvili T, Farley MM, et al. Effectiveness of seven-valent pneumococcal conjugate vaccine against invasive pneumococcal disease: a matched case-control study. Lancet 2006; 368:1495–1502

57. D. Bronchiolitis obliterans attributable to her rheumatoid arthritis.

The presence of fixed airflow obstruction with a normal diffusing capacity and evidence of air trapping on her expiratory (see Figure 57-B) compared with her inspiratory (see Figure 57-A) CT scan is highly suggestive of bronchiolitis obliterans (BO). This was proven with an open lung biopsy (see Figure 57-C) showing a bronchiole with complete luminal obliteration by fibrous tissue (choice D is correct). The bronchiole is demarcated by the discontinuous bundles of smooth muscle around what would have been the lumen.

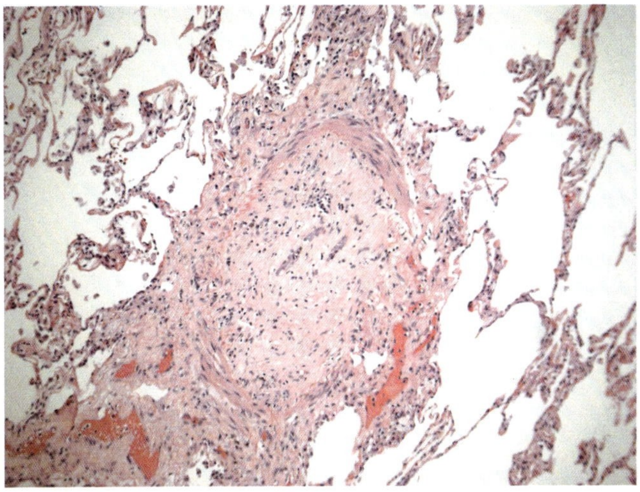

Figure 57-C
Hematoxylin-eosin

Reports of methotrexate lung toxicity complicating therapy of RA vary widely, with quotes between 0.86% and 6.9%. Most clinicians think that the true incidence is toward the lower range because the drug only has to be stopped in approximately 1 of 108 patient-treatment years because of pulmonary toxicity. In this patient, the slowly progressive nature of the symptoms combined with the lack of evidence for interstitial disease, both on physiologic testing and CT scan, rules out this condition (choice A is incorrect). Interstitial lung disease complicating RA is found in 20 to 40% of patients at autopsy, but clinically apparent disease is much less common, affecting 3 to 14% of patients with RA.

The normal diffusing capacity and lung volumes combined with the absence of interstitial changes on CT scan rules this out (choice B is incorrect). Emphysema is certainly a cause of fixed airflow obstruction, and the incidence of the disease is higher in patients with RA; however, the normal diffusing capacity combined with the absence of destructive changes on CT scan is not consistent with this disorder (choice C is incorrect).

BO is a rare but severe complication of RA and can also, less commonly, complicate other connective tissue diseases. It is much more common in women and rarely is reported in men with RA. Dyspnea is the most common symptom and might be severe. Physical examination may be normal or reveal some inspiratory crackles or a midinspiratory squeak. The chest radiograph usually shows hyperinflation but may show normal findings. Pulmonary function tests usually show severe, fixed airflow obstruction with gas trapping. There are two predominant pathologic patterns seen: constrictive bronchiolitis or intraluminal granulation tissue plugs, with the latter having a much better prognosis. Treatment with oral steroids is often tried, but there is little evidence of benefit. There is at least one report of a favorable response to prolonged erythromycin therapy in a group of seven patients with RA and constrictive bronchiolitis, but overall prognosis is poor.

Geddes DM, Corrin B, Brewerton DA, et al. Progressive airway obliteration in adults and its association with rheumatoid arthritis. Q J Med 1977; 184:427–444

Gauhar UA, Gaffo AL, Alarcón GS. Pulmonary manifestations of rheumatoid arthritis. Semin Respir Crit Care Med 2007; 28:430–440

Hayakawa H, Sato A, Toyoshima M, et al. Bronchiolar disease in rheumatoid arthritis. Am J Respir Crit Care Med 1996; 154:1531–1536

Sarvanan V, Kelly CA. Reducing the risk of methotrexate pneumonitis in rheumatoid arthritis. Rheumatology 2004; 43:143–147

Kim DS. Interstitial lung disease in rheumatoid arthritis: recent advances. Curr Opin Pulm Med 2006; 12:346–353

58. A. Curve A.

Curve A represents a normal pressure/volume curve (pleural elastance) and is the most likely of the three curves to be compatible with a subsequent successful pleurodesis (choice A is correct; therefore, choice D is incorrect). This curve indicates that the lung is reexpanding with removal of pleural fluid, with a minimal drop in pleural pressure. Provided enough fluid is removed to ensure reapproximation of the parietal and visceral pleural surfaces, as revealed by a follow-up chest radiograph, subsequent pleurodesis has the highest chance of success compared with curves B and C.

Curve B represents an "entrapped lung" or "lung entrapment." Patients with this curve have an active process, either inflammatory or malignant pleural disease, creating visceral pleural restriction and preventing normal lung reexpansion. The curve has an initial normal portion followed by a steep drop indicating limited lung reexpansion. Specific therapy is directed toward the active process. In the case of a malignant pleural effusion, limited lung reexpansion will limit the success of pleurodesis (choice B is incorrect).

Curve C represents a relatively uncommon diagnosis, a trapped lung. Trapped lung is related to a remote pleural inflammatory process creating a fibrous visceral pleural peel and preventing lung reexpansion. Cardiac surgery is one of the most common causes. Other causes include pleural infection, uremia, hemothorax, and rheumatoid arthritis. Trapped lung represents a chronic condition wherein the initiating process, often inflammatory, has resolved, and pleural analysis usually reveals a transudative effusion. Patients often have a chronic asymptomatic pleural effusion. The initial pleural pressure, as in this patient, is negative and continues to fall steeply with fluid removal. Pleurodesis is not indicated in these patients, and given that the lung cannot reexpand and reapproximate the visceral and parietal pleural surfaces, pleurodesis would not be successful (choice C is incorrect). Surgical intervention may be indicated but only if the patient has dyspnea proven to be due to the effusion.

Given the perception that manometry is difficult to perform, its use is limited. (For more information on manometry, see the Web-based Interactive Physiology Grand Rounds series in the online January 2009 issue of *CHEST,* which demonstrates how to perform manometry, along with the accompanying editorial that describes how the diagrams work.) Alternatively, a chest radiograph after thoracentesis (see Figure 58-B) or CT of the chest (see Figure 58-C), showing incomplete reexpansion of the lung and a thickened visceral pleural surface suggests either a trapped or entrapped lung.

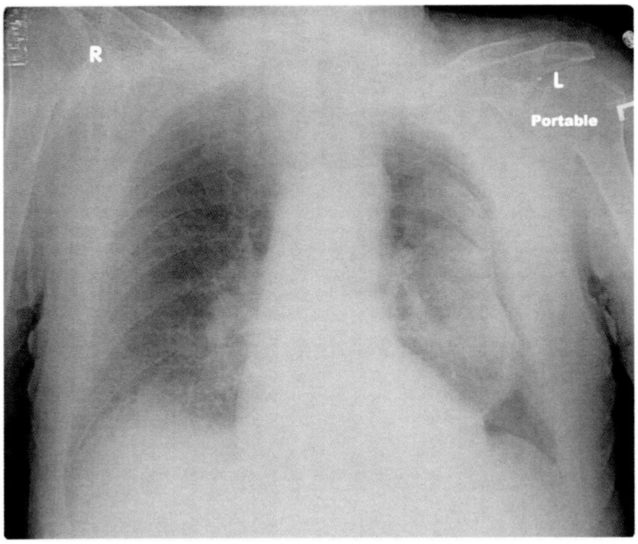

Figure 58-B

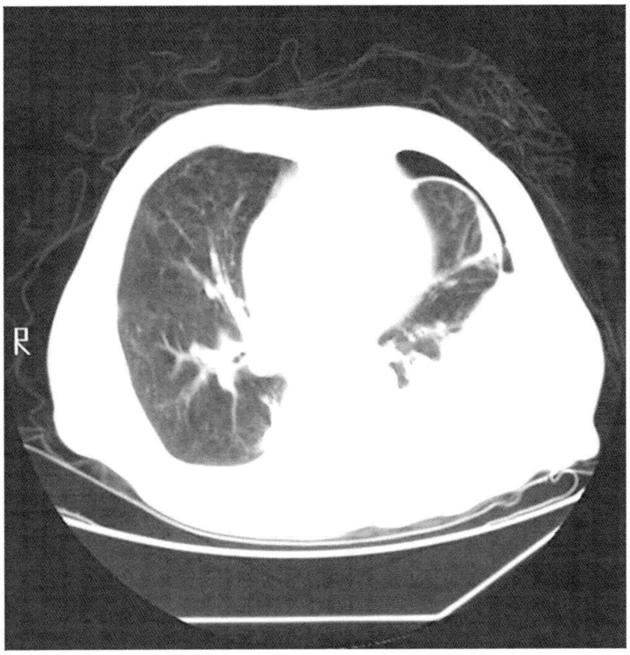

Figure 58-C

Doelken P, Huggins JT, Pastis NJ, et al. Pleural manometry: technique and clinical implications. Chest 2004;126:1764–1769
Huggins JT, Sahn SA, Heidecker J, et al. Characteristics of trapped lung: pleural fluid analysis, manometry, and air-contrast chest CT. Chest 2007; 131:206–213
Lan RS, Lo SK, Chuang ML, et al. Elastance of the pleural space: a predictor for the outcome of pleurodesis in patients with malignant pleural effusion. Ann Intern Med 1997; 126:768–774
Feller-Kopman D, Parker MJ, Schwartzstein RM. Assessment of pleural pressure in the evaluation of pleural effusions [interactive diagram 3]. Chest 2009; 135:201–209. Available at www.chestjournal.org/content/135/1/201.full. Accessed February 10, 2009
Schwartzstein RM, Parker MJ. Interactive physiology grand rounds: introduction to the series. Chest 2009; 135:6–8. Available at www.chestjournal.org/content/135/1/6.full. Accessed February 10, 2009

59. C. Obtain CT scan of the abdomen.

This woman has preeclampsia associated with hemolysis, elevated liver enzymes, and low platelets (HELLP). Patients with HELLP syndrome are usually older and more frequently multiparous than other women with preeclampsia. Hepatocellular injury (the cause for the elevated liver function test results) is often due to vasospasm and may also be associated with hepatic infarction, intrahepatic hemorrhage, and subcapsular hematoma. In this instance, a subcapsular hematoma with rupture should be suspected, given the development of hemodynamic instability. Prompt diagnosis by a CT scan of the abdomen should help to determine the presence of the subcapsular hematoma (choice C is correct).

The overall treatment is generally supportive. Treatment of the hemolytic anemia seldom requires specific treatment, other than fetal delivery. Treatment with magnesium sulfate is used for preeclampsia, but this patient does not have typical features of that illness (choice A is incorrect). Treatment with platelet transfusion is usually necessary only for Cesarean delivery or other major surgery (choice B is incorrect). Emergency Cesarean section could be considered after the cause for the hemodynamic instability has been determined but should not be performed at this point (choice D is incorrect).

Sibai BM. Diagnosis, controversies, and management of the syndrome of hemolysis, elevated liver enzymes, and low platelet count. Obstet Gynecol 2004; 103:981–991
Wicke C, Pereira PL, Neeser E, et al. Subcapsular liver hematoma in HELLP syndrome: evaluation of diagnostic and therapeutic options: a unicenter study. Am J Obstet Gynecol 2004: 190:106–112

60. A. Institution of noninvasive mechanical ventilation.

The patient has a myasthenia gravis crisis (MGC) with marked hypercapnic and hypoxemic respiratory failure. Supportive therapy with mechanical ventilation may be necessary (choice A is correct), but the use of succinylcholine should be avoided in patients with myasthenia gravis (MG) because of increased sensitivity, particularly with depolarizing agents (choice D is incorrect), that may result in acute, severe hyperkalemia and cardiac dysrhythmias. Patients with severe hypothyroidism may develop a myopathy and should be considered in the differential diagnosis of MG. Thyroid hormone replacement would be appropriate if hypothyroidism is suspected. In the absence of bradycardia and altered temperature regulation, hypoventilation secondary to severe hypothyroidism is less likely (choice B is incorrect).

An electromyogram is helpful in accurately diagnosing MG when the diagnosis is in question. In the acute setting with hypercapnic ventilatory failure, the study would be of limited value until the patient is stabilized. To objectively determine respiratory muscle function, bedside spirometry should be performed. In normal individuals, an FVC >65 mL/kg is noted. Indications for mechanical ventilation support occur with an FVC <15 mL/kg. At the time of evaluation, this patient's FVC was 0.99 L, or 16 mL/kg. She was supported by noninvasive ventilation and recovered following the institution of plasmapheresis.

MG is an antibody-mediated autoimmune disease affecting 3 to 4 million individuals each year in the United States. Women are affected twice as often as men. Respiratory involvement, with ventilatory failure requiring ventilatory support, called an MGC, occurs in up to 20% of patients, most commonly within the first 2 years of diagnosis. An MGC may be the initial presentation of the disease in some patients. A precipitating event or trigger often precedes an MGC, most commonly an antecedent infection (40%). Additional triggers include new medication or changes in medications, aspiration, surgery, trauma, or botulinum injections. Aminoglycosides, fluoroquinolone antibiotics, and antihypertensive medications, such as β-blockers and calcium channel blockers, have been reported to trigger MGCs. Acetylcholine receptor antibodies are detected in 90% of patients with generalized MG but in only 70% who manifest predominantly ocular symptoms. In patients who are ACR-negative antibodies to other proteins can be detected, such as muscle-specific kinase (MuSK), calcium and potassium channels in the motor nerve terminal, and titin and ryanodine receptor intracellularly in the muscle cells. MG may be paraneoplastic in 10 to 15% of patients, as a coexisting thymoma may be present. In those with MuSK antibodies, bulbar and respiratory weakness occurs out of proportion to limb weakness. Therapy for MGC is to restore appropriate synaptic transmission across the neuromuscular junction. Plasma exchange or IV immunoglobulin (IVIG) therapy is typically used in the setting of MGC but may be complicated with excessive secretions, predisposing patients to atelectasis. The efficacy for plasma exchange approaches 75%, with immediate improvement after two to three sessions. Improvement is delayed with IVIG and typically occurs after 4 to 5 days of therapy. Controlled trials have failed to demonstrate a clear advantage of one therapy over another. Maintenance therapy with prednisone, azathioprine, cyclosporine, mycophenolate mofetil, or pyridostigmine should be considered depending on disease activity, side effects profile, and response. Corticosteroids are the mainstay of chronic therapy but should be titrated up carefully because a transient exacerbation of weakness may occur (choice C is incorrect). In those patients with a thymoma, resection is recommended.

Bershad EM, Feen ES, Suarez JI. Myasthenia gravis crisis. South Med J 2008; 101:63–69

Diaz-Manera J, Rojas-Garcia R, Gallardo E, et al. Antibodies to AChR, MuSK and VGKC in a patient with myasthenia gravis and Morvan's syndrome. Nat Clin Pract Neurol 2007; 3:405–410

Gold R, Schneider-Gold C. Current and future standards in treatment of myasthenia gravis. Neurotherapeutics 2008; 5:535–541

Cosi V, Lombardi M, Erbetta A, et al. Azathioprine as a single immunosuppressive drug in the treatment of myasthenia gravis. Acta Neurol (Napoli) 1993; 15:123–131

61. D. Lorazepam.

Renal failure is a common complication of sepsis and respiratory failure, and it is important to identify reversible causes to enhance the likelihood of early recovery. Medications are a common cause of renal dysfunction, and only one

of the medications listed is a likely cause of renal dysfunction—lorazepam—particularly when infused intravenously at infusion rates > 8 mg/h over an extended period of time (choice D is correct). Under these conditions of administration, it is the stabilizing agent propylene glycol rather than the lorazepam that is the cause of injury.

Lorazepam is mixed in propylene glycol for IV administration. Each 1 mL lorazepam contains 830 mg propylene glycol. Serum concentrations of propylene glycol in excess of 0.18 mg/mL are associated with an osmolar gap, renal dysfunction that may progress to renal failure, and lactic acidosis manifesting as a metabolic acidosis with an anion gap. In this patient, the bicarbonate level is low, indicating a metabolic acidosis, and the anion gap is increased at 21. Confirmation of an increased lactate concentration would be appropriate. The calculated osmolarity is two times the sodium concentration + the glucose concentration/18 + the BUN concentration/2.8 = 296 mOsm. The measured osmolarity is 348, so the osmole gap is increased at 52 mOsm/kg, or approximately 42 mOsm/kg above the expected. In the absence of other common causes of unmeasured osmoles (mannitol, ethanol, ethylene glycol, and methanol), the difference here is almost certainly due to a significant serum concentration of propylene glycol. The appropriate therapy would be to discontinue the lorazepam infusion immediately and use an alternative sedative regimen. Identified risk factors for the development of renal toxicity due to lorazepam infusions are high doses (> 8 mg/h) and/or a prolonged period of infusion (> 7 days).

Famotidine, moxifloxacin, and ceftriaxone are extremely unlikely causes of renal dysfunction and would not explain the increased anion gap metabolic acidosis and osmolar gap present in this case (choices A, B, and C are incorrect).

Yaucher NE, Fish JT, Smith HW, et al. Propylene glycol toxicity associated renal toxicity from lorazepam infusion. Pharmacotherapy 2003; 23:1094–1099

Arthur RB. Propylene glycol toxicity related to high-dose lorazepam infusions: case report and discussion. Am J Crit Care 1999; 8:499–506

Bejerus L, Baker C, Fenton J, et al. Propylene glycol as a cause of elevated serum osmolality. Am Soc Clin Pathol 1979; 72:633–636

Hayman M, Seidl EC, Ali M, et al. Acute tubular necrosis associated with propylene glycol from concomitant administration of intravenous lorazepam and trimethoprim-sulfamethoxazole. Pharmacotherapy 2003; 23:1190–1194

62. D. Discontinue zolpidem.

The differential diagnoses of complex sleep-related behavior are extensive and include disorders of arousal (sleepwalking, sleep terrors, and confusional arousals), rapid eye movement (REM) sleep behavior disorder, nightmares, nocturnal seizures, arousals related to sleep-related breathing disorders, nocturnal psychogenic dissociative disorders, panic attacks, posttraumatic stress syndrome, sundowning, malingering, and alcohol, substance, or medication use. Administration of hypnotic agents, such as zolpidem, has resulted in complex behaviors, and it is reasonable to discontinue these medications before proceeding with more extensive evaluation (choice D is correct).

Clonazepam is an effective therapy for REM sleep behavior disorder, which is characterized by dream-enacting behavior, rapid awakening with full alertness, and good recall of the preceding dream, none of which are present in this patient. Also, REM sleep behavior disorder is predominantly seen in men and in elderly adults ≥ 50 years. Thus, it is less likely that this patient has this disorder (choice A is incorrect).

Although a history of recent-onset bedwetting should prompt a consideration of nocturnal seizures, the former also has been described with other sleep disorders, including hypnotic-induced complex sleep behaviors. Thus, electroencephalography may be indicated if enuresis persists following discontinuation of all possibly offending medications or if other clinical features suggestive of a seizure disorder are present; it is, however, not the first step in this patient's diagnostic evaluation (choice B is incorrect). A trial of sleep extension may be considered in people who are sleep deprived, but this would be difficult to accomplish in those who are chronically suffering from sleep-initiation and sleep-maintenance insomnia (choice C is incorrect).

In addition to sleepwalking, other complex behaviors related to the use of hypnotic agents have included eating, cooking, driving, shopping, sexual activity, and painting the front door while seemingly asleep. These behaviors have been induced by nonbenzodiazepine benzodiazepine receptor agonists (NBBRAs), including zolpidem. Risk factors are not well characterized.

Aside from discontinuing medications that can potentially precipitate complex sleep-related behaviors and possibly avoidance of sleep deprivation, there is no consensus regarding management and prevention of NBBRA-related sleep behaviors. A trial of sleep extension may be beneficial and should be considered.

Sleep-related eating disorders must be distinguished from nighttime feeding behavior triggered by hypoglycemia or to relieve gastroesophageal reflux or gastric dyspepsia, compulsive eating following arousals from sleep, and Kleine-Levin syndrome (recurrent periods of hypersomnia, hypersexuality, and hyperphagia).

Dolder CR, Nelson MH. Hypnosedative-induced complex behaviours: incidence, mechanisms and management. CNS Drugs 2008; 22:1021–1036
Howell MJ, Schenck CH, Crow SJ. A review of nighttime eating disorders. Sleep Med Rev 2009; 13:23–34

63. C. Measure maximal expiratory and inspiratory pressures.

This patient has developed "shrinking or vanishing lung syndrome," which is a rare pulmonary manifestation of SLE. The diagnosis can be further supported by obtaining maximal inspiratory and expiratory pressures (choice C is correct) to assess for respiratory muscular weakness that is found in the large majority of patients with this diagnosis. The etiology of this syndrome is unclear, and the postulated pathophysiology has included myositis or myopathy and phrenic nerve dysfunction, which have been disputed in some diaphragmatic studies. The muscle weakness does not appear to correlate with corticosteroid use. Pleural inflammation causing pain, resulting in a reflex inhibition of diaphragmatic activity, has also been postulated.

In small series, patients with this diagnosis are a mean age of 36 years, and the ratio for the diagnosis is 6:1 in women and men. This syndrome often develops in the latter stages of SLE. The usual findings in shrinking lung syndrome include unexplained dyspnea progressing over weeks or months and pleuritic chest pain in 40 to 65% of cases. Less than 20% of patients have clinical evidence of myositis. The chest radiograph usually reveals elevated hemidiaphragms and small lung volumes, and there is an absence of interstitial lung disease (ILD) and/or pleural disease even when examined by high-resolution CT. Results of pulmonary function tests show restriction, with reduced absolute diffusion, but normal diffusing capacity when adjusted for alveolar volume, as in this case. Interpretation of the latter parameter can be controversial, but, in general, restriction with a diffusing capacity that is reduced but normal when adjusted for lung volume implies an extraparenchymal cause of restriction but does not always exclude ILD. Decreased transdiphragmatic pressures may be found. Laboratory results are usually normal, and the process does not correlate with antinuclear and anti-DNA antibody levels or complement levels. Treatment for shrinking lung syndrome has included theophylline, corticosteroids, β-agonists, nonsteroidal inflammatory agents, and an increase in immunosuppression, with variable results.

A bronchoscopy with transbronchial biopsy (choice A is incorrect) would not be indicated in this patient because the high-resolution CT does not show evidence of ILD. Although this patient has a lupus anticoagulant and is thus at high risk for a pulmonary embolism (PE), a PE would not explain the marked restriction or the chest radiograph findings. In addition, with PE, one might expect the diffusion to be reduced even when adjusted for alveolar volume (choice B is incorrect). An echocardiogram might assist with the evaluation of pulmonary hypertension but, again, would not explain the marked restriction, chest radiograph findings, normal cardiac examination, and normal diffusing capacity when adjusted for lung volume (choice D is incorrect).

Other pulmonary complications of SLE include pleural effusions, pleuritis, acute lupus pneumonitis, bronchiolitis obliterans, ILD, diffuse alveolar hemorrhage, pulmonary hypertension, pulmonary embolism, and infection.

Warrington KJ, Moder KG, Brutinel WM. The shrinking lungs syndrome in systemic lupus erythematosus. Mayo Clin Proc 2000; 75:467–472
Karim MY, Miranda LC, Tench CM, et al. Presentation and prognosis of the shrinking lung syndrome in systemic lupus erythematosus. Semin Arthritis Rheum 2002; 31:289–298
Orens JB, Martinez FJ, Lynch JP III. Pleuropulmonary manifestations of systemic lupus erythematosus. Rheum Dis Clin North Am 1994; 20:59–193
Singh R, Huang W, Menon Y, et al. Shrinking lung syndrome in systemic lupus erythematosus and Sjogren's syndrome. J Clin Rheumatol 2002; 8:340–345
Toya SP, Tzelepis GE. Association of the shrinking lung syndrome in systemic lupus erythematosus with pleurisy: a systematic review. Semin Arthritis Rheum 2008; Jun 26, Epub ahead of print

64. D. Excellent exercise rehabilitation candidate.

One of the major components of pulmonary rehabilitation is aerobic exercise. This can have profound effects on cardiovascular fitness along with skeletal muscle conditioning. For aerobic exercise to have significant conditioning effects, however, the cardiovascular system needs to be stressed and pushed to near maximal heart rates. In the patient with lung disease, the ability to achieve a significant heart rate increase may be limited by lung function. Thus, the beneficial effects of exercise therapy may be limited.

In our patient, an exercise test shows severe disability (a $\dot{V}O_2$ of only 42% of predicted). Importantly, it does not appear that his lung function is the rate-limiting step to exercise in that his SpO_2 at peak exercise is still adequate (93%) and his exercise ventilation is only 60% of his known maximum voluntary ventilation. Instead, his heart rate has exceeded 100% of predicted, indicating that he has reached cardiovascular maximum. Although this may represent undiagnosed heart disease, in our patient with no cardiac history and a normal exercise ECG, it is more likely that this represents cardiovascular and skeletal muscle deconditioning, a situation ideal for aerobic exercise training.

This patient is thus an excellent candidate for exercise rehabilitation (choice D is correct). Choice A is incorrect because the high heart rate indicates that his lung function did not prevent him from reaching cardiovascular maximum. Choice B is incorrect because the low exercise ventilation with respect to his maximum voluntary ventilation indicates the ventilatory reserve exists and is therefore available for use during aerobic exercise training. Choice C is incorrect because the low $\dot{V}O_2$ is reflecting poor function, and the low $\dot{V}O_2$/heart rate is consistent with cardiovascular (deconditioning) limitations to exercise. Again, this is a pattern that is amenable to aerobic exercise during pulmonary rehabilitation.

Plankeel J, McMullen B, MacIntyre NR. Exercise outcomes after pulmonary rehabilitation depend upon initial mechanisms of limitation in non-oxygen dependent COPD patients. Chest 2005; 127:110–116
Gallagher CG. Exercise limitation and clinical exercise testing in chronic obstructive pulmonary disease. Clin Chest Med 1994; 15:305–326
Casaburi R, Porszasz J, Burns MR, et al. Physiologic benefits of exercise training in rehabilitation of patients with severe chronic obstructive pulmonary disease. Am J Respir Crit Care Med 1997; 155:1541–1551
Maltais F, LeBlanc P, Jobin J, et al. Intensity of training and physiologic adaptation in patients with chronic obstructive pulmonary disease. Am J Respir Crit Care Med 1997; 155:555–561
Casaburi R, Patessio A, Ioli F, et al. Reductions in exercise lactic acidosis and ventilation as a result of exercise training in patients with obstructive lung disease. Am Rev Respir Dis 1991; 143:9–18

65. A. Begin treatment with isoniazid.

Because of her recent contact with an individual with active TB, this patient's tuberculin skin test is considered positive because it exceeds the threshold of 5 mm of induration, and treatment of latent TB infection with isoniazid is appropriate (choice A is correct). Tuberculin skin test reactivity is unaffected by pregnancy, and if the patient's initial test after learning of her exposure was negative, then repeating a surveillance 5-TU tuberculin skin test every 12 weeks

for 1 to 2 years would be appropriate. However, because the patient's initial postexposure PPD test result is positive, it is not useful to repeat a 5-TU tuberculin skin test (choice D is incorrect). The 250-TU ("second strength") PPD test was widely used in the past but currently has no role in the diagnosis of latent TB infection (choice C is incorrect). There is no evidence of active TB in this patient, so starting her on a four-drug regimen is not appropriate (choice B is incorrect).

The effect of pregnancy on the risk of developing active TB is somewhat controversial but is not thought to be great. Thus, in the absence of treatment, this patient would be expected to have the standard risk of an immunocompetent new skin test converter: an approximately 2 to 5% risk of developing active TB within 2 years and a 10 to 20% lifetime risk of developing active disease. These risks can be reduced by up to 90% if isoniazid therapy is administered.

Isoniazid, usually administered to adults at a 300-mg/day dose for a period of 9 months, is the first-line agent for the treatment of latent TB infection, regardless of HIV status, age, and chest radiograph results showing the presence or absence of fibrotic lesions. Isoniazid is classified as US Food and Drug Administration pregnancy category C but is widely used and generally considered safe during pregnancy. Guidelines of the American Thoracic Society, the Infectious Diseases Society of America, and the Centers for Disease Control and Prevention state that initiation of isoniazid therapy should not be delayed on the basis of pregnancy alone, even during the first trimester, in patients with a high risk of reactivation such as recent converters (such as this patient) or in patients infected with HIV. In lower risk patients, some experts recommend postponing therapy until after delivery. Routine pyridoxine supplementation and monitoring of liver function tests are recommended when isoniazid is used during pregnancy.

Horsburgh CR Jr. Priorities for the treatment of latent tuberculosis infection in the United States. N Engl J Med 2004; 350:2060–2067
Lee E, Holzman RS. Evolution and current use of the tuberculin test. Clin Infect Dis 2002; 34:365–370
Centers for Disease Control and Prevention, American Thoracic Society. Targeted tuberculin testing and treatment of latent tuberculosis infection: a Joint Statement of the American Thoracic Society (ATS) and the Centers for Disease Control and Prevention (CDC). Am J Respir Crit Care Med 2000; 161:S221–S247

66. D. Arrange follow-up assessment and pulmonary function testing in 6 months.

Family genetic screening for A1AT deficiency in this patient detected the homozygote PI*ZZ phenotype, with a markedly reduced A1AT level of 0.38 g/L (normal values are 1.5 to 3.5 g/L), confirming the diagnosis of A1AT deficiency. However, he is asymptomatic and has normal pulmonary function, normal chest radiograph results, and the absence of emphysema on CT scanning, with no extrapulmonary manifestations of disease. Therefore, management should include close clinical follow-up and pulmonary function testing on a regular basis, appropriate vaccinations, genetic counseling, and prompt treatment for any infections (choice D is correct).

The PI*ZZ phenotype is characterized by markedly reduced A1AT plasma levels and an 80 to 100% risk of developing COPD. In appropriate patients with the PI*ZZ phenotype, reduced plasma levels of A1AT, and airflow obstruction, particularly in those with an FEV_1 between 30 and 65% of predicted, both IV (weekly or monthly) and aerosolized administrations have been shown to be of benefit. In the absence of airflow obstruction, there is no evidence of benefit in preventing COPD with A1AT replacement therapy, and current guideline recommendations do not support its administration in this clinical setting. Choices A, B, and C involve the administration of replacement therapy and would therefore not be correct. Other phenotypes carry a lower risk of developing COPD (MM, normal phenotype and average risk; MZ and SS, possible mild increased risk; and SZ, moderate increased risk of 20 to 50%). The null phenotype in a subject is associated with absent measurable A1AT levels and carries a 100% risk of developing COPD at a young age.

American Thoracic Society/European Respiratory Society. American Thoracic Society/European Respiratory Society statement: standards for the diagnosis and management of individuals with alpha-1 antitrypsin deficiency. Am J Respir Crit Care Med 2003; 168:818–900
Demeo DL, Sandhaus RA, Barker AF, et al. Determinants of airflow obstruction in severe alpha-1-antitrypsin deficiency. Thorax 2007; 62:806–813
Sandhaus RA, Turino G, Stocks J, et al. Alpha1-antitrypsin augmentation therapy for PI*MZ heterozygotes. Chest 2008; 134:831–834
Tanash, Nilsson PM, Nillson J-A, et al. Clinical course and prognosis of never-smokers with severe alpha-1-antitrypsin deficiency (PiZZ). Thorax 2008; 63:1091–1095

67. A. Repeat thoracentesis with pleural manometry.

Patients commonly develop pleural effusions related to CABG. The time course of the effusion helps narrow the cause and define the management. Post-CABG effusions are typically categorized as (1) perioperative (within the first week); (2) early (within the first month); (3) late (2 to 12 months); and (4) persistent (after 6 months). There are four distinct causes of late effusions: postcardiac injury syndrome (PCIS), lymphocytic effusions of uncertain cause, constrictive pericarditis, and lung entrapment. All of these can often be exudative, lymphocyte-predominate effusions.

It is relatively easy and important to recognize a trapped lung because pleural fluid drainage will not alleviate the patient's symptoms or treat the underlying pathophysiology. The diagnosis of a trapped lung can be confirmed physiologically with pleural manometry demonstrating an initial negative intrapleural pressure and a change in intrapleural pressure of > 14.5 cm H_2O after removal of 1 L of fluid (choice A is correct). The diagnosis can also be made by CT scanning after thoracentesis demonstrating a thickened visceral pleura and failure of the lung to reexpand. Figure 67-C shows the patient's chest radiograph after thoracentesis, demonstrating that the lung has failed to reexpand (see arrows). Trapped lung represents dysfunctional healing of the pleura as a result of an inflammatory process. The lung is unable to expand completely, and the chest wall cannot conform, resulting in a persistently negative pressure in the pleural space. In an attempt to normalize the intrapleural pressure, the space fills with fluid. Although this more commonly occurs on the left side, it can also be seen on the right side, as in this patient. As mentioned earlier, a chest tube placed into the pleural space will not result in complete lung expansion (choice B is incorrect). Pleural decortication should be considered in patients with significant symptoms related to the lung restriction.

Constrictive pericarditis is an uncommon cause of late pleural effusions following CABG. Symptoms include dyspnea on exertion, peripheral edema, and weight gain. Physical examination reveals jugular venous distension, hepatomegaly, and edema. Thoracentesis will often reveal a transudate, although a bloody exudate may be seen with constriction from PCIS. The pleural effusions from constrictive pericarditis resolve following pericardiectomy. This patient has no clinical symptoms or signs of constriction, so pericardiectomy would not be the initial step (choice C is incorrect).

PCIS is thought to be an exaggerated immune response to myocardial injury. Patients typically have pleuritic chest pain, fever, pericardial rub, and dyspnea that occur in a period from weeks to months after CABG. The pleural fluid is typically a hemorrhagic exudate. Patients with PCIS may require antiinflammatory therapy, including prednisone, for relief of symptoms. Because of the potential deleterious effect of prednisone on wound healing, antiinflammatory therapy with either aspirin or nonsteroidal antiinflammatory agents is often used as the first-line treatment. The timing, lack of fever, and nonbloody exudates make PCIS less likely in this scenario, and antiinflammatory agents would not be indicated until other causes of a late effusion have been excluded (choice D is incorrect). Table 67-1 reviews the typical presentation and management of early post-CABG plural effusions related to PCIS. The typical features of late post-CABG pleural effusions are shown in Table 67-2.

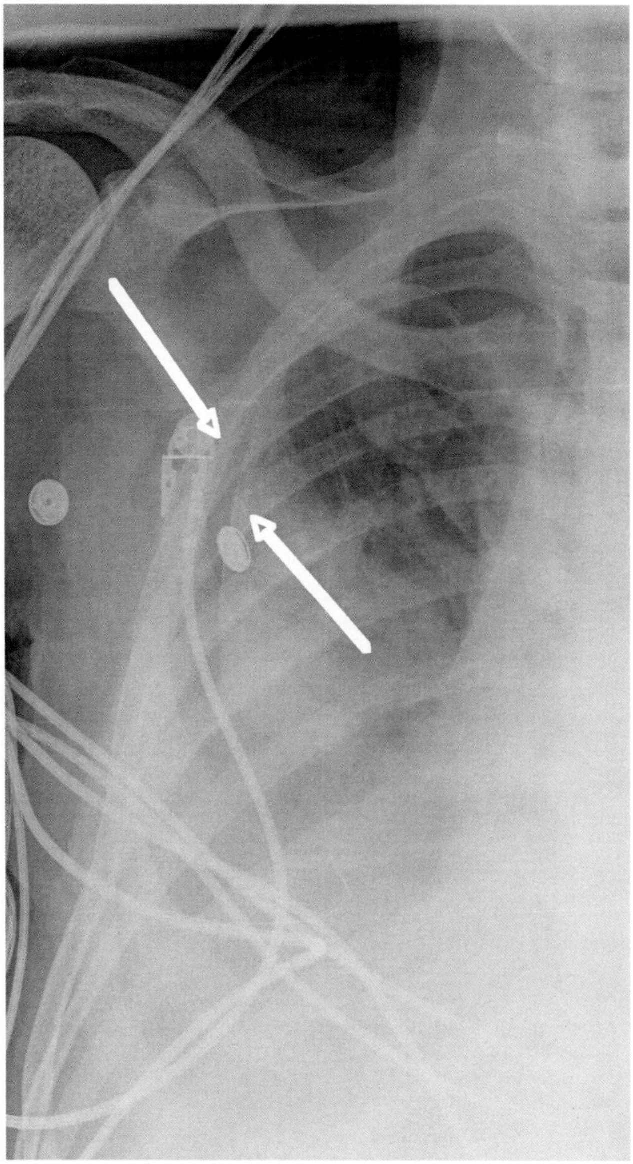

Figure 67-C

Table 67-1. Early Post-CABG Pleural Effusions Related to PCIS*

Clinical characteristics	Occurs weeks after CABG; chest pain, fever, rub, leukocytosis, elevated ESR
Radiograph findings	Moderate-to-large left pleural effusion; often left pulmonary infiltrates
Pleural fluid analysis	Exudate; neutrophilic initially, then lymphocytic; bloody; antimyocardial antibodies present
Proposed mechanism	Immune response to myocardium antigens
Management	Spontaneous resolution; NSAIDs and prednisone; often recurs
Sequelae	Can lead to constrictive pericarditis or trapped lung

*Within 1 month following surgery. ESR = erythrocyte sedimentation rate; NSAIDs = nonsteroidal antiinflammatory drugs. Adapted from Heidecker.

Table 67-2. Typical Features of Late Post-CABG Pleural Effusions*

	Clinical Characteristics	Radiograph Findings	Pleural Fluid Analysis	Proposed Mechanism	Management	Sequelae
Lymphocytic effusion of uncertain etiology	Small-to-large effusion; usually apparent within days of CABG	Usually left-sided, small-to-large effusion	Exudative; nonhemorrhagic; lymphocyte predominant	May represent a chronic form of PCIS or persistent pleural injury from CABG	Usually resolves with conservative management	Can progress to trapped lung requiring decortication
Constrictive pericarditis	Occurs months after CABG; dyspnea, edema, jugular venous distention, Kussmaul sign	Bilateral effusions; may have calcified pericardium	Lymphocyte-predominant transudate	Persistent PCIS results in pericardial thickening with cardiac restriction and venous hypertension	Careful diuretic use if mild; if severe, pericardiectomy	
Lung entrapment	Small-to-large effusion; possible dyspnea	Usually left-sided, small-to-large effusion; may have ipsilateral volume loss	Exudative; nonbloody; lymphocyte predominant; pleural manometry shows biphasic elastance curve	Persistent inflammation results in exudative effusion with pleural restriction	May resolve with conservative management	Can progress to trapped lung requiring decortication

*Occurring 2 to 12 months following CABG. Adapted from Heidecker.

Doelken P, Huggins JT, Pastis NJ, et al. Pleural manometry: technique and clinical implications. Chest 2004; 126:1764–1769
Huggins JT, Sahn SA, Heidecker J, et al. Characteristics of trapped lung: pleural fluid analysis, manometry, and air-contrast chest CT. Chest 2007; 131:206–213
Heidecker JT. A new classification for pleural effusions after CABG surgery. Pulmonary and Critical Care Update (PCCU) 2007; 21(Lesson 15). www.chestnet.org/education/online/pccu/vol21/lessons15_16/index.php

68. D. Patient A is generating flow rates of 80 L/min vs 40 L/min by patient B.

ATC is an option found on many newer-generation mechanical ventilators that is designed to support spontaneous breaths with an amount of airway pressure calculated to overcome the resistance that accompanies airflow through the tracheal tube. Resistance, and therefore pressure required to overcome resistance, are related to flow through the tracheal tube in a curvilinear fashion: the higher the flow rate, the higher the pressure (choice D is correct). Resistance is also directly correlated to the length of the tube and inversely related to the fourth power of the radius (which is proportional to the internal diameter) of the tube. Accordingly, greater resistance is present, and therefore, higher airway pressure is required for endotracheal tubes (ETs), which are longer than tracheostomy tubes (choice B is incorrect). Similarly, airflow through smaller diameter tubes generates higher resistance and requires higher airway pressure (choice C is incorrect). The operator enters data regarding tube type (ET vs tracheostomy) and internal diameter of the tube into the ventilator processor for that individual patient. The percent compensation is typically set at 100%; however, the pressure will be proportionally lower if the percent compensation is set to a lower value, such as 40% (choice A is incorrect). This is rarely done.

Automatic tube compensation is designed to deliver pressure to compensate for the calculated resistance associated with airflow through the tube and, therefore, be a suitable form of ventilation to accurately compensate for the tube-imposed work of breathing during a spontaneous breathing trial (SBT). Flow and, by extension, resistance, change rapidly, so the required pressure is recalculated by the ventilator processor every 5 ms. Research suggests that automatic tube compensation preserves a natural breathing pattern, reduces work of breathing, and improves patient comfort and patient-ventilator synchrony. In two single-center randomized controlled trials, automatic tube compensation was shown to have trends for higher success rates for SBTs than pressure support ventilation (PSV), T-piece, or continuous positive airway pressure (CPAP). In one study, patients randomized to automatic tube compensation had significantly better overall success (defined as passing the SBT and remaining extubated for > 48 h) than CPAP.

Cohen JD, Shapiro M, Grozovski E, et al. Extubation outcome following a spontaneous breathing trial with automatic tube compensation versus continuous positive airway pressure. Crit Care Med 2006; 34:682–686

Mols G, Rohr E, Benzing A, et al. Breathing pattern associated with respiratory comfort during automatic tube compensation and pressure support ventilation in normal subjects. Acta Anaesthesiol Scand 2000; 44:223–230

Haberthur C, Mols G, Elsasser S, et al. Extubation after breathing trials with automatic tube compensation, T-tube, or pressure support ventilation. Acta Anaesthesiol Scand 2002; 46:973–979

Guttmann J, Haberthur C, Mols G. Automatic tube compensation. Respir Care Clin N Am 2001; 7:475–501

69. C. Thoracic endometriosis.

The most likely diagnosis for this patient is thoracic endometriosis (choice C is correct). This syndrome includes four well-recognized clinical entities, namely catamenial pneumothorax, catamenial hemothorax, catamenial hemoptysis (as was the case with this patient), and lung nodules. Endometriosis refers to the presence of endometrial tissue outside the uterine cavity and myometrium. It has been identified in virtually all tissues and organs in the female body with the exception of the spleen, which seems to resist implantation of endometrial tissue. Endometriosis is rare before menarche and after menopause, when women are deficient in estrogen. In contrast, endometriosis is present in 5% of women of reproductive age. Most patients present with pelvic or back pain that is exacerbated by menses (dysmenorrhea), sexual intercourse (dyspareunia), and/or bowel movements (dyschezia). Diagnosis is usually made by laparoscopy or laparotomy.

Pulmonary endometriosis can be categorized as pleural or parenchymal. Pleural lesions are more likely to cause pneumothorax and hemothorax with associated chest pain and/or dyspnea in most cases. Parenchymal lesions most commonly result in isolated catamenial hemoptysis, but chest pain and dyspnea have been reported. Symptoms are generally cyclical, occurring within 24 to 48 h after menses. Pneumothoraces are believed to occur either by air from the genital tract entering the pleural space through diaphragmatic defects or by rupture of pleural endometrial implants.

Chest radiograph results are often normal in cases of pulmonary endometriosis or they may reveal transient infiltrates caused by bleeding. Chest CT scanning is more sensitive for demonstrating abnormalities. CT scans should be performed during menses because lesions enlarge at this time. Bronchoscopy rarely produces a tissue diagnosis, although it may be helpful in the assessment and treatment of hemoptysis or excluding other pulmonary pathology. Pleural fluid cytologic studies are rarely useful for diagnosis, although it has been reported.

The optimal management of endometriosis is controversial, as current evidence is derived from case reports and small clinical series. Surgery, hormonal treatments, and combined approaches have all been proposed, with variable results in terms of short- and long-term outcome. Endometrial tissue is completely dependent on estrogen for continued growth, so effective therapy for endometriosis requires hormonal suppression of estrogen production by the ovaries or surgical ablation of endometrial lesions. Hormonal suppressive therapy can be accomplished surgically or medically

using oral contraceptives, danazol, or gonadotropin-releasing hormone analogues. Birth control pills have been used most commonly, but there is a high recurrence rate (50%). Gonadotropin-releasing hormone agonists suppress gonadotropin secretion and desensitize the ovarian response to gonadotropin to achieve hypoestrogenemia. This is accomplished without androgenic side effects.

TB is unlikely in this patient with no other systemic signs or symptoms consistent with the disease (choice A is incorrect). Wegener granulomatosis would be unusual in a young woman with no other symptoms and an isolated nodule (choice B is incorrect). Choriocarcinoma is not a consideration in a patient with a negative pregnancy test (choice D is incorrect).

Alifano M, Roth T, Broet SC, et al. Catamenial pneumothorax: a prospective study. Chest 2003; 124:1004–1008
Alifano M, Trisolini R, Cancellieri A, et al. Thoracic endometriosis: current knowledge. Ann Thorac Surg 2006; 81:761–769
Johnson MM. Catamenial pneumothorax and other thoracic manifestations of endometriosis. Clin Chest Med 2004; 25:311–319

70. A. Positional therapy with avoidance of a supine sleep position.

Positional therapy might benefit those whose obstructive sleep apnea (OSA) occurs exclusively or predominantly during a supine sleep position, with polysomnography (PSG) demonstrating a normal apnea-hypopnea index (AHI) in the lateral posture. Patients with positional OSA are more likely to be less overweight and have lower AHIs compared with patients whose apnea is present in all sleep positions. Positional therapy involves the avoidance of a supine sleep position and promotion of a lateral or upright sleep position (choice A is correct). Patients can be instructed to place three to four tennis balls in a pocket sewn on the back of a well-fitted pajama top; pin a sock filled with tennis balls to the back of a sleep garment; sleep with a Styrofoam-filled backpack; or use a posture alarm that is triggered whenever the person remains in a supine position.

The goals of therapy for OSA include improving sleep quality, relieving daytime symptoms such as excessive sleepiness, preventing long-term neurocognitive and cardiovascular consequences associated with OSA, and enhancing quality of life.

Many medications, such as acetazolamide, methylxanthines, medroxyprogesterone, estrogen, and serotonin-active agents, have been investigated for the therapy of OSA. However, these pharmacologic agents are not currently recommended for the therapy of patients with OSA because of lack of proven efficacy (choice B is incorrect).

Supplemental oxygen is not indicated as a primary therapy for OSA. Although oxygen supplementation can decrease central and mixed apneas, it generally fails to reverse OSA. In patients with OSA, it may improve nocturnal oxygen saturation but at the risk of increasing apnea duration (choice D is incorrect).

Oral devices worn during sleep, including mandibular advancers and tongue retainers, may be considered for persons who snore, who have mild-to-moderate OSA and do not tolerate positive airway pressure therapy, or whose OSA persists following upper airway surgery. These devices are designed to reposition the mandible and tongue in an anterior or forward position to enlarge the dimensions of the upper airways during sleep. Oral devices should be avoided in patients who are unable to breathe nasally, have high resistance to nasal airflow, or whose sleep apnea is primarily central in nature. Mandibular advancers cannot be used for patients without teeth (choice C is incorrect).

Upper airway surgery may be considered in patients who are either unwilling or unable to use positive airway pressure therapy or who have significant craniofacial or upper airway abnormalities. Surgical procedures for OSA are designed to increase the dimensions of the retropalatal airspace (uvulopalatopharyngoplasty), retrolingual airway (genioglossal advancement, hyoid myotomy, and suspension or mandibular advancement), or both (uvulopalatopharyngoglossoplasty and maxillomandibular advancement). In select patients with severe OSA, a tracheostomy to bypass the upper airway might be necessary. Surgery is commonly sequentially staged. Polysomnography is recommended following upper airway surgery to determine its therapeutic efficacy.

Uvulopalatopharyngoplasty may negatively impact the subsequent use of CPAP therapy. Data on long-term surgical effectiveness are limited.

Weight reduction for patients who are overweight is essential. Methods include restriction of dietary caloric consumption, increase in physical activity, and even bariatric surgery in select individuals with morbid obesity. The magnitude of weight reduction needed to improve OSA varies across patients, and weight loss alone is often insufficient to reverse OSA related to morbid obesity or an abnormal upper airway anatomy. Finally, optimal weight can be difficult to maintain, and OSA may recur in some individuals despite maintenance of weight loss.

Bailey DR. Dental therapy for obstructive sleep apnea. Semin Respir Crit Care Med 2005; 26:89–95

Jokic R, Klimaszewski A, Crossley M, et al. Positional treatment vs continuous positive airway pressure in patients with positional obstructive sleep apnea syndrome. Chest 1999; 115:771–781

Kushida CA, Morgenthaler TI, Littner MR, et al. Practice parameters for the treatment of snoring and obstructive sleep apnea with oral appliances: an update for 2005. Sleep 2006; 29:240–243

Morgenthaler TI, Kapen S, Lee-Chiong T, et al. Practice parameters for the medical therapy of obstructive sleep apnea. Sleep 2006; 29: 1031–1035

Sher AE. Upper airway surgery for obstructive sleep apnea. Sleep Med Rev 2002; 6:195–212

71. B. Start antibiotic therapy in the ED and send the patient home with appropriate follow-up.

This patient has community-acquired pneumonia, and two tools developed to assess severity of illness would suggest that he is of very low risk for a poor outcome and likely could be managed with appropriate antibiotic therapy as an outpatient (choice B is correct). The pneumonia PORT prediction rule used a derivation cohort of 14,199 inpatients and was independently validated in 38,039 inpatients and in 2,287 inpatients and outpatients prospectively enrolled in a cohort study. Patients were stratified into five severity classes using a two-step process that evaluated a number of demographic factors, especially age, comorbid illnesses, physical findings, laboratory results, and radiographic data. The final score was based on the numerical age supplemented by additional points assigned for the risk factors identified. In the derivation and validation groups, mortality ranged from 0.1 to 0.4% in class I ($<$ 50 points), 0.6 to 0.7% in class II ($\leq$ 70 points), and 0.9 to 2.8% in class III (71 to 90 points). Mortality was intermediate for class IV (8.2 to 9.3%) (91 to 130 points) and high for class V (27.0 to 31.1%) ($>$ 130 points). This patient has a PORT score $<$ 50, because he is $<$ 50 years of age and has no identified risk factors for a poor outcome. This indicates a low risk of mortality and the possibility of home management. It should be recognized that the PORT score was derived as a mortality prediction rule and not as a tool for admission/discharge decisions. The PORT score is used infrequently in practice because of its complex calculations.

The British Thoracic Society prediction rule was derived using 453 inpatients and independently validated in 246 inpatients. The rule defines a patient as at high risk for mortality if at least two of three features are present: respiratory rate $\geq$ 30/min, diastolic BP $<$ 60 mm Hg, and BUN concentration $>$ 7.0 mmol/L ($>$ 19.1 mg/dL). Patients with two or more of these prognostic factors had a relative risk of death of 21.1 (19.4% vs 0.9%) and 9.1 (28.6% vs 3.1%) in the derivation and validation cohorts, respectively. Recently, confusion and age were added to the model to strengthen the mortality prediction. Data from three prospective studies of community-acquired pneumonia conducted in the United Kingdom, New Zealand, and the Netherlands were combined. A derivation cohort, comprising 80% of the data, was used to develop the model. A five-point score, one point for each of Confusion, Urea $>$ 7 mmol/L, Respiratory rate $\geq$ 30/min, low systolic ($<$ 90 mm Hg) or diastolic ($\leq$ 60 mm Hg) BP and age $\geq$ 65 years (CURB-65 score), is based on information available at initial hospital assessment and enables patients to be stratified according to increasing risk of mortality: score 0, mortality of 0.7%; score 1, mortality of 3.2%; score 2, mortality of 3%; score 3, mortality of 17%; score 4, mortality of 41.5%; and score 5, mortality of 57%. This patient has a CURB-65 score of 0, again suggesting a very minimal risk of death, and consideration should be given for management of the patient in an ambulatory setting.

There appears to be no medical or social reason to recommend hospitalization (choice A is incorrect). The patient appears to have uncomplicated community-acquired pneumonia, so there is no rationale to obtain a chest CT scan (choice C is incorrect). Studies have demonstrated that delaying antibiotic therapy while awaiting the results of laboratory investigations is associated with worse outcomes (higher mortality, prolonged length of hospital stay), at least among patients requiring hospital admission (choice D is incorrect).

Fine MJ, Auble TE, Yealy DM, et al. A prediction rule to identify low-risk patients with community-acquired pneumonia. N Engl J Med 1997; 336:243–250

Houck PM, Bratzler DW, Nsa W, et al. Timing of antibiotic administration and outcomes for medicare patients hospitalized with community-acquired pneumonia. Arch Intern Med 2004; 164:637–644

Lim WS, van der Eerden MM, Laing R, et al. Defining community-acquired pneumonia severity on presentation to hospital: an international derivation and validation study. Thorax 2003; 58:377–382

72. C. Pleural effusion with ascites.

The image shows echo-free spaces indicating the presence of pleural fluid (PF), surrounded by normal chest wall, diaphragm, and visceral pleura, as well as an echo-free space below the diaphragm, indicating ascites (see Figure 72-B, label A; choice C is correct, and choice B is incorrect).

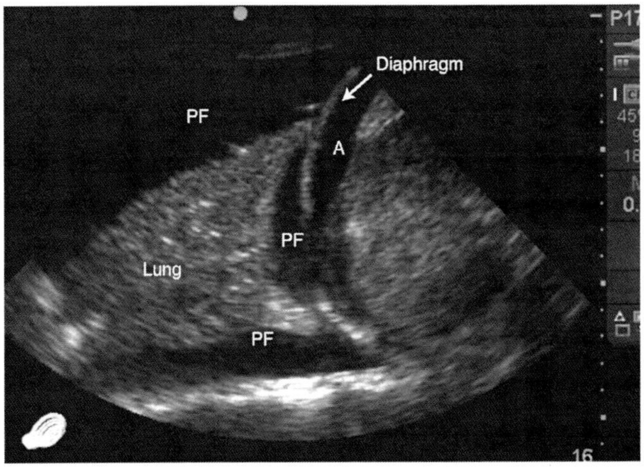

Figure 72-B

Ultrasonography is very useful in both the diagnosis and treatment of pleural disorders. Compared with chest radiography and CT scans, ultrasonography has the advantages of portability, lack of radiation, ease of performing immediate and serial evaluations, and increased sensitivity compared with chest radiographs in detecting PF and pneumothorax. In addition, it increases the safety of thoracentesis by identifying the appropriate locations, angle, and depth of needle placement. Although not yet in wide use by pulmonary and critical care specialists, ultrasonographic evaluation of the pleura is not difficult to learn.

Ultrasonography is often useful in distinguishing transudates from exudates because transudates are almost always anechoic. Exudates may also be anechoic, but pleural thickening in association with parenchymal abnormality, echogenic effusions, and septation generally indicates inflammatory diseases or hemorrhage. Figure 72-B shows anechoic pleural spaces, and empyema is very unlikely (choice D is incorrect). Although the lung is compressed by pleural fluid, it appears normal otherwise, with no visible mass (choice A is incorrect).

In addition to evaluating pleural effusions, thoracic ultrasonography is useful at the bedside to rule out pneumothorax and detect pleural thickening and masses. The use of ultrasonography is expanding in the ICU to include training and routine use by intensivists, including vascular imaging to increase safety of intravascular access and diagnose DVT and pulmonary embolism, abdominal imaging in the evaluation of acute renal failure, and echocardiography in the evaluation of hypotension and shock.

Feller-Kopman D. Ultrasound-guided thoracentesis. Chest 2006; 129:1709–1714
Mayo P, Doelken P. Pleural ultrasonography. Clin Chest Med 2006; 27:215–227
Mayo PH, Goltz HR, Tafreshi M, et al. Safety of ultrasound-guided thoracentesis in patients receiving mechanical ventilation. Chest 2004; 125:1059–1062

73. B. Thoracic surgery consultation.

The chest radiograph results demonstrate several right-sided healed rib fractures. The lung projects beyond the confines of the rib cage in the anteroposterior (AP) view. Review of a CT scan indicates that a segment of the right lower lobe is partially herniated through an intercostal defect (see Figure 73-B, circle). The defect measures 14 cm in the AP dimension and 8 cm in a craniocaudal orientation. The findings are in line with a posttraumatic right intercostal muscle rupture with partial herniation of the right lower lobe through the above described defect. The appropriate action at this time is referral to a thoracic surgeon for an opinion regarding the role of surgery in correcting the trauma-induced hernia (choice B is correct). Although a pulmonary exercise study might determine the contribution of the underlying lung disease and deconditioning to the patient's complaint of dyspnea, it would not deal with the major underlying problem: the mechanical effect of the lung herniation (choice A is incorrect). A CT angiogram is not indicated because there is no clinical suspicion of pulmonary embolic disease and the diffusing capacity is normal (choice C is incorrect). With an FEV_1 in the 50% range, a methacholine challenge study is relatively contraindicated (choice D is incorrect).

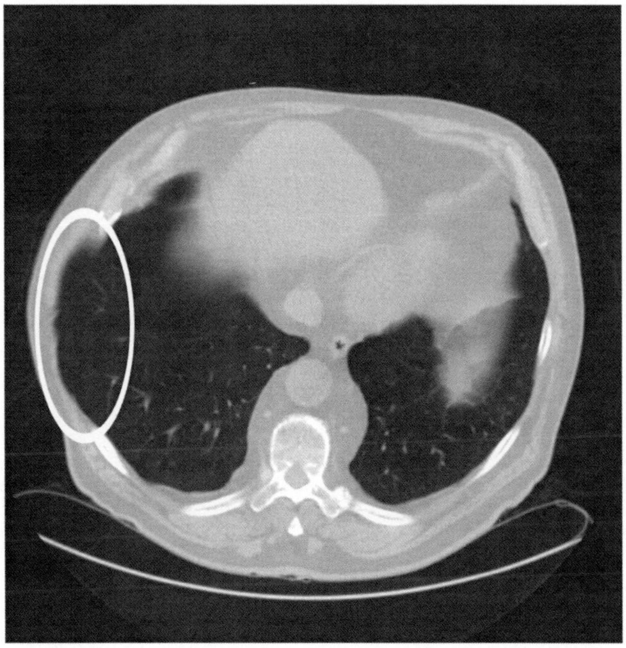

Figure 73-B

Extrathoracic lung herniation is defined as the protrusion of lung tissue through an abnormal opening in the chest wall. It can be congenital or acquired, and the latter can be related to trauma, a pathologic process, or spontaneous occurrence. Spontaneous lung hernias have been linked to strenuous coughing and presumably are related to increased intrathoracic pressure. Posttraumatic lung hernia can be recognized immediately after chest wall trauma has occurred or be delayed for months or years, as in this patient. It is more common after penetrating rather than blunt trauma and may be associated with multiple costal fractures (as in this patient), direct sternal injury, and clavicle-sternal or costal-sternal dislocation. With the advent of three-point restraint systems in automobiles, an unusual form of blunt chest trauma may develop. In this case, the shoulder harness may compress the lung on one side, increasing intrathoracic pressure. This increase may result in herniation of the lung through a defect in the costal cartilages. Usually it is a parasternal hernia because external intercostal muscles are absent in this area and the chest wall is at its thinnest. It may present as a chest wall mass that increases in size with coughing and a Valsalva maneuver. Incarceration and strangulation of the hernia have been reported. Large hernias are treated surgically, whereas smaller, asymptomatic ones may be treated conservatively.

Lykissas MG, Zikos N, Kazakos N, et al. Post-traumatic intercostal lung hernia. Injury Extra 2006; 37:258–260
Beran E, Dimitri WR, Marzouk JFK. Posttraumatic anterior lung herniation in a restrained front seat passenger. Injury Extra 2007; 38:433–435

74. C. Referral for counseling.

Figure 74-A shows crystalloid or fiber-like substances within capillaries and small vessels. Figure 74-B is the exact same field, imaged with polarized light. The material is strongly birefringent with polarized light, suggesting the abuse of IV substances. Appropriate next steps would include questioning regarding drug abuse and referral to a drug counselor (choice C is correct). In retrospect, similar findings were seen in the explanted native lungs (see Figure 74-C). This shows abundant crystalline material in and around a small pulmonary artery, associated with a foreign body granulomatous reaction (characterized by numerous multinucleated giant cells that have engulfed the material).

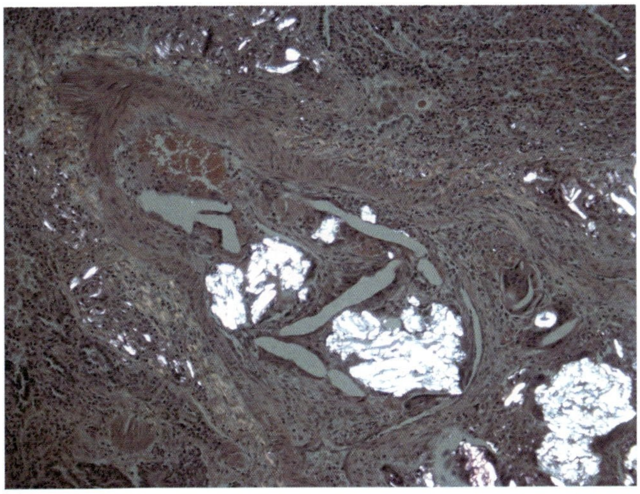

Figure 74-C
Hematoxylin-eosin

Rejection is one of the most feared complications of lung transplantation. The initial manifestation of acute rejection is a cellular, lymphocyte-predominant inflammatory response centered around blood vessels and/or airways, whereas chronic rejection is characterized by bronchiolitis obliterans (BO). There is nothing to suggest either of these from this patient's biopsy or spirometry results, respectively, so there is no indication to increase immunosuppression (choice A is incorrect). Aspiration is characterized by peribronchiolar acute and/or chronic inflammation, with or without surrounding pneumonia. In cases of chronic aspiration, there may be associated constrictive or obliterative bronchiolitis, characterized by narrowing or obliteration of bronchiolar lumens by fibrosis. Patients who undergo lung transplant probably are at increased risk for reflux or aspiration, given the denervation of the airways and loss of protective reflexes, and this is postulated as a risk factor for the development of BO in this population. However, the current biopsy results show no evidence for inflammation, and spirometry does not suggest BO (choice B is incorrect). There is nothing from the history, physical, or roentgenographic examination that is suggestive of infection (choice D is incorrect).

The nonmedical use of prescription pain killers is well recognized and a problem particularly among adolescents and young adults. Pharmaceutical agents intended for oral consumption contain a variety of inactive filler substances (excipients) that are used as a vehicle for the drug or play a role in binding or absorption of the medications. These may include microcrystalline cellulose, talc, cornstarch, or povidone. These excipients are harmless if ingested, but if crushed and injected as part of an aqueous solution, they are filtered by the pulmonary circulation and can cause occlusion, thrombosis, and inflammation of the pulmonary arterial microvasculature. The current patient had been crushing his pain medications for some time and injecting them into his peripherally inserted central catheter line, which was removed after the biopsy, and he was referred to a drug counselor. The material in the biopsy stained

positive with Congo Red, periodic acid-Schiff, and Gomori methenamine silver stains, which is characteristic for microcrystalline cellulose and helps differentiate it from talc.

Fields TA, McCall SJ, Reams BD, et al. Pulmonary embolization of microcrystalline cellulose in a lung transplant recipient. J Heart Lung Transplant 2005; 24:624–627

Ott MC, Khoor A, Scolapio JS, et al. Pulmonary microcrystalline cellulose deposition from intravenous injection of oral medication in a patient receiving parenteral nutrition. J Parenter Enteral Nutr 2003; 21:1–2

Smith KJ, Elidemir O, Dishop MK, et al. Intravenous injection of pharmaceutical tablets presenting as multiple pulmonary nodules and declining pulmonary function in an adolescent with cystic fibrosis. Pediatrics 2006; 118:924–928

Boehler A, Estenne M. Post-transplant bronchiolitis obliterans. Eur Respir J 2003; 22:1007–1018

Blondeau K, Mertens V, Vanaudenaerde BA, et al. Gastro-oesophageal reflux and gastric aspiration in lung transplant patients with or without chronic rejection. Eur Respir J 2008; 31:707–713

75. C. Transbronchial biopsies aid diagnosis in > 50% of cases.

This patient's most recent chest radiograph (see Figure 75-A) showing a miliary pattern and the acid-fast positive bacilli seen in the bone marrow biopsy (see Figure 75-B) are diagnostic of miliary TB. A diagnosis of miliary TB, whether in an HIV-positive or -negative patient, often presents a challenge. No large series on miliary TB in the HIV-positive population has been published. Sputum staining results for AFB are is negative in one-third of patients with miliary TB, but can be culture positive in up to 60%. Similarly, AFB staining for bronchial brushings/lavage in miliary TB has a yield of slightly less than one-third. Transbronchial lung biopsy yields granulomas in > 60% of cases (choice C is correct); the impact of HIV status is not well studied, but granulomas are often less well formed in the HIV population. Bone marrow biopsy results reveal granulomas, on average, in > 60% (range 33 to 100%, case series reports), reflecting the hematogenous dissemination of the TB bacillus. In general, given the greater bacillus load in the HIV-positive population with miliary TB, staining and culture yields of these tests are greater than in the non-HIV population. Repeat sputum testing with staining and culture, in nonmiliary pulmonary TB patients with or without HIV, remains the initial diagnostic approach.

The CD4 count in HIV-positive patients correlates well with clinical manifestations of HIV-related TB. The presence of extrapulmonary TB (as in this patient with pancytopenia and bone marrow involvement) is found in 70% of patients with a CD4 count of 0 to 100 cells/μL (0 to 0.10×10^9/L) (as opposed to 28% of patients with a CD4 count of > 300 cells/μL [0.30×10^9/L]) (choice A is incorrect). This patient's CD4 count 2 weeks before admission was 22 cells/μL (0.022×10^9/L). Blood culture results, particularly in patients with low CD4 counts (< 100 cells/μL [< 0.10×10^9/L], are positive in upto 50% (choice B is incorrect), and patients may appear septic. A positive tuberculin skin test result (≥ 5 mm) may be found in ≤ 91% of HIV-positive patients with TB and a CD4 count > 300 cells/μL (> 0.30×10^9/L) vs 0% of patients with a CD4 count of 0 to 100 cells/μL (0 to 0.10×10^9/L) (choice D is incorrect).

Miliary TB results from massive lymphohematogenous dissemination of *Mycobacterium tuberculosis* bacilli to the vascular bed of various organs, particularly those with high blood flow (spleen, liver, lungs, bone marrow, and kidneys). This dissemination results in the gross pathologic findings in various organs, particularly the lung, of lesions resembling the size and shape of millet seeds (average diameter < 2 mm). The resulting chest radiographic findings may not be evident in ≤ 50% of patients. Miliary TB is more common in the immunocompromised patient. Clinical presentation is nonspecific and includes fever for several weeks, anorexia, weight loss, and cough. Treatment in the absence of meningeal involvement is for 6 months (2 months initial treatment with isoniazid, rifampicin, pyrazinamide, and ethambutol followed by 4 months of isoniazid and rifampicin). Mortality for miliary TB in adults ranges from 25 to 30%, with delayed diagnosis being a primary driver for high mortality.

Sharma SK, Mohan A, Sharma A, et al. Miliary tuberculosis: new insights into an old disease. Lancet Infect Dis 2005; 5:415–430

Burman WJ, Jones BE. Clinical and radiographic features of HIV-related tuberculosis. Semin Respir Infect 2003; 18:263–271

Kinoshita M, Ichikawa Y, Koga H, et al. Re-evaluation of bone marrow aspiration in the diagnosis of miliary tuberculosis. Chest 1994; 106:690–692

Maartens G, Willcox PA, Benatar SR. Miliary tuberculosis: rapid diagnosis, hematologic abnormalities, and outcome in 109 treated adults. Am J Med 1990; 89:291–296

76. A. Prescribe modafinil.

This patient has obstructive sleep apnea. She has persistent daytime sleepiness despite adequate compliance with CPAP therapy. Modafinil is approved for use in such circumstances (choice A is correct). Several studies have shown objectively improved wakefulness and improved functional status over a 12-week period with the use of modafinil. It is well tolerated and has no adverse effects on CPAP use. Other stimulants have not been tested and are not recommended for this purpose.

This woman is compliant with CPAP monitoring, based on her history and objective documentation, but her daytime sleepiness is persistent. The MSLT showed a reduced mean sleep latency without REM sleep present in any of the nap periods. A mean sleep latency of > 8 min is interpreted as normal, < 5 min is indicative of pathologic daytime sleepiness, and between 5 and 8 min is in the "gray zone." Narcolepsy would be suggested by the presence of REM sleep in at least two of the five nap periods.

Narcolepsy treatment would include methylphenidate; however, the MSLT results are not consistent with that diagnosis (choice B is incorrect). The effectiveness of CPAP therapy was demonstrated by the sleep study, and thus, performing another study with the use of bilevel ventilation is not necessary (choice C is incorrect). Oral appliance therapy results in similar improvements to CPAP with regard to daytime hypersomnolence; however, because the patient did have adequate titration in the sleep laboratory and is compliant with the CPAP therapy, this option would not be recommended at this time (choice D is incorrect).

Black JE, Hirshkowitz M. Modafinil for treatment of residual excessive sleepiness in nasal continuous positive airway pressure-treated obstructive sleep apnea/hypopnea syndrome. Sleep 2005; 28:464–471

Roth T, Schwartz JR, Hirschkowitz M, et al. Evaluation of the safety of modafinil for treatment of excessive sleepiness. J Clin Sleep Med 2007; 3:595–602

77. D. Pulmonary artery balloon catheter occlusion and aspiration for cytologic examination.

The patient had tumor emboli syndrome (TES), which may occur with many different malignancies but is most commonly reported to occur in mucin-secreting adenocarcinomas (breast, colon, gastric, prostate, pancreas, and lung adenocarcinomas). Urothelial carcinomas, as occurred in this case, may also be complicated by this devastating complication. The clinical presentation of TES is highly suggestive of an acute thromboembolic event, which must be excluded because most patients are at increased risk for thromboembolic disease with their underlying malignancy. Acute pulmonary hypertension and right heart strain occur because of tumor emboli, resulting in pulmonary microvascular occlusion and *in situ* microthrombi. Tumor emboli are not metastatic foci because *in situ* proliferation and local spread do not occur. A definitive antemortem diagnosis is rare, and in most patients, a presumptive diagnosis is made and confirmed at autopsy by documenting malignant cells within the pulmonary vasculature. Lung sections obtained at the time of necropsy (see Figure 77-C) confirmed the diagnosis in this patient because malignant cells were identified within the pulmonary artery (arrow). Malignant cells may be identified by cytologic findings from pulmonary artery balloon catheter placement and aspiration of blood from the pulmonary vasculature (choice D is correct). The diagnostic yield, however, is low.

New-onset, subacute pulmonary hypertension may occur in patients with newly diagnosed HIV. Although the patient underwent transfusion during her radical cystectomy, the risk of acquiring HIV from a transfusion is less likely with current screening protocols (choice A is incorrect). A subacute-acute right-sided myocardial infarction was seen in this patient. The absence of myocardial injury in the setting of progressive deterioration makes this less likely (choice B is incorrect). A ventilation-perfusion scan may be suggestive of TES, with a "mottled" appearance and small peripheral perfusion defects with intact ventilation. In the appropriate clinical setting, these subtle findings support a diagnosis of TES but are not definitive (choice C is incorrect).

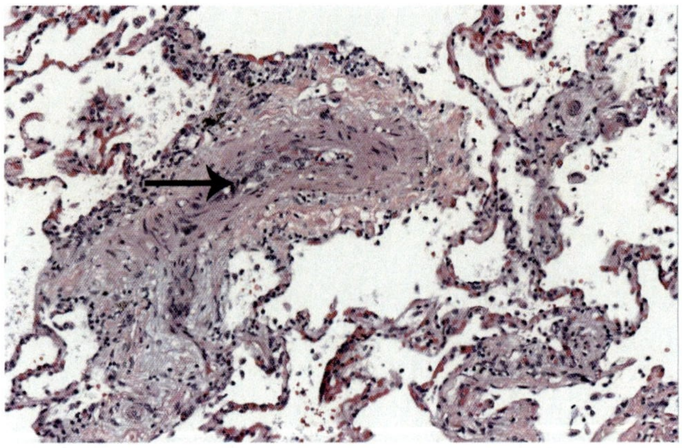

Figure 77-C
Hematoxylin-eosin

Yutani C, Imakita M, Ishibashi-Ueda H, et al. Pulmonary hypertension due to tumor emboli: a report of three autopsy cases with morphological correlations to radiological findings. Acta Pathol Jpn 1993; 43:135–141
Chakeres DW, Spiegel PK. Fatal pulmonary hypertension secondary to intravascular metastatic tumor emboli. Am J Roentgenol 1982; 139:997–1000
Abati A, Landucci D, Danner RL, et al. Diagnosis of pulmonary microvascular metastases by cytologic evaluation of pulmonary artery catheter-derived blood specimens. Hum Pathol 1994; 25:257–262
Miyano S, Izumi S, Takeda Y, et al. Pulmonary tumor thrombotic microangiopathy. J Clin Oncol 2007; 25:597–599

78. B. Refer for surgical resection.

This patient has experienced massive hemoptysis as a result of a broncholith and bronchiectasis of an airway segment of the left lung. On the basis of her history and pulmonary function tests, she is a good surgical candidate: her pattern of hemoptysis appears to be accelerating and will likely continue to be life-threatening, and surgery will definitively resolve this problem (choice B is correct). When underlying lung disease is advanced and the patient is not a good surgical candidate, angiography with embolization of the bleeding site may be a useful intervention.

Broncholithiasis (from the Greek, "spitting of stones") occurs when a calcified mass erodes into a central airway. The most typical causes are calcified lymph nodes that follow a Histoplasma or mycobacterial infection and are thought to migrate into the airway as a result of the effects of respiratory and cardiac motion on these structures. Silicosis is a recognized cause of broncholithiasis as well. In this patient, the multiple calcified granulomata and calcified central hilar nodes suggest prior histoplasmosis as a cause of this process.

Broncholithiasis may cause a number of symptoms and complications, including expectoration of calcified tissue, cough, airway obstruction, recurrent pneumonia, hemoptysis, and bronchoesophageal fistula. When these calcified masses are present in central airways and are causing obstruction, flexible or rigid bronchoscopy is an attractive alternative to surgery for removal, although success rates reported in the literature are not extremely high. When massive hemoptysis is present, the broncholith is located more distally, and coexisting bronchiectasis may contribute to bleeding—as in this patient. Rigid bronchoscopy is not an attractive option and should not impede surgical resection (choice D is incorrect). Even though histoplasmosis is a likely prior infectious cause of broncholithiasis in this patient, there is no evidence or likelihood of active disease at this point, and there is no role for treatment with a systemic antifungal agent such as itraconazole (choice C is incorrect). Another manifestation of fungal disease that is a cause of massive hemoptysis—mycetoma formation in cystic lung disease—has been treated by some with intracavitary amphotericin when other measures are contraindicated or exhausted, but there is no evidence of mycetoma in this patient (choice A is incorrect).

Menivale F, Deslee G, Vallerand H, et al. Therapeutic management of broncholithiasis. Ann Thorac Surg 2005; 79:1774–1776
Wahidi MM, Herth FJ, Ernst A. State of the art: interventional pulmonology. Chest 2007; 131:261–274

79. C. Decreased febrile response to endotoxin and antibody titers to influenza vaccination.

SD is associated with considerable adverse effects on several physiologic processes, including decreased febrile response to endotoxin and antibody titers to influenza vaccination (choice C is correct), decrease in leptin levels and increase in ghrelin (choice A is incorrect), hyperactive gag and deep tendon reflexes (choice B is incorrect), and decreased secretion of growth hormone and prolactin (choice D is incorrect).

SD can be acute and total (one to several nights of complete lack of sleep), acute and partial (one to several nights of insufficient sleep), chronic and partial (at least a week of inadequate sleep), or consist of fragmented sleep (diminished sleep time as a result of repeated awakenings). Adverse consequences of acute total SD differ from those generally observed with chronic partial SD. In addition, there are considerable differences in vulnerability to SD, with some individuals demonstrating more adverse physiologic, neurocognitive, and behavioral effects from sleep loss than others.

The most important consequence of SD is sleepiness due to an increase in homeostatic sleep drive. A sleep-deprived person has a greater propensity to fall asleep and may experience frequent napping, sleep attacks, or episodes of microsleep. This increase in sleep pressure is reflected in shortened sleep latencies during polysomnography, multiple sleep latency test, and maintenance of wakefulness test. Other polysomnographic features include enhanced sleep efficiency, decreased wake time after sleep onset, increase in nonrapid eye movement stage N3 sleep, and, in some instances, greater total sleep time.

It appears that SD may be associated with excess mortality and cardiovascular morbidity, although the mechanisms responsible for these associations are unknown. It also has a negative impact on mood, cognition, and executive function. The likelihood of errors of both omission and commission is increased. Ptosis and nystagmus can develop during total SD. Pain sensitivity increases.

Changes in endocrine function and metabolism include increase in evening levels of cortisol and levels of ghrelin, blunting of sleep-dependent secretion of growth hormone and prolactin, and decreases in glucose tolerance and serum levels of thyroxine and leptin. The combination of high ghrelin and low leptin concentrations may lead to weight gain despite an increase in metabolic rate. Hypothermia may occur with prolonged SD.

Decreased febrile response to endotoxin and decreased antibody titers to influenza vaccination can accompany SD, as can altered levels of interleukin-6, tumor necrosis factor-α, and leukocytes, as well as activity of natural killer cells.

Malik SW, Kaplan J. Sleep deprivation. Prim Care 2005; 32:475–490

Carskadon MA. Sleep deprivation: health consequences and societal impact. Med Clin North Am 2004; 88:767–776

Dorkova Z, Petrasova D, Molcanyiova A, et al. Effects of continuous positive airway pressure on cardiovascular risk profile in patients with severe obstructive sleep apnea and metabolic syndrome. Chest 2008; 134:686–692

80. D. Bronchiolitis obliterans (BO).

This patient has developed constrictive BO (choice D is correct), which is shown by the transbronchial biopsy findings. The chest radiograph shows the right transplanted lung without infiltrate and a hyperinflated native left lung. BO syndrome is the leading cause of morbidity and mortality after the first posttransplant year and is considered the *sine qua non* of chronic rejection in the lung transplant (LT) recipient. Chronic rejection has been equated with the histologic finding of BO. The current incidence of BO ranges from 35 to 50% among different centers. More than 50% of recipients will develop some degree of BO by 5 years after the transplant. The mean time for a diagnosis of BO is 16 to 20 months after the LT procedure but has been reported as early as 3 months after transplantation. The etiology and risk factors for BO remain unclear. The most consistently identified risk factor is acute rejection (as occurred in this patient), in particular, recurrent, high-grade episodes of acute rejection. It is probable that lymphocytic bronchitis or bronchiolitis, CMV pneumonitis, and primary graft dysfunction are also important risk factors for BO. Clinically, BO can manifest as an upper respiratory tract infection and can be mistakenly treated as such. Other

patients have no clinical symptoms, but PFT reveals gradual obstructive dysfunction. Typically, chest radiographs are not helpful in the diagnosis of BO because most patients have radiograph findings that are unchanged from their baseline posttransplant radiographs, as in this case. High-resolution CT may reveal peripheral bronchiectasis, patchy consolidation, decreased peripheral vascular markings, air trapping, mosaicism (on inspiratory/expiratory films), and bronchial dilation, which may aid in the diagnosis of BO.

Transbronchial biopsy is used to diagnose BO but primarily is used to exclude other diagnoses, such as acute rejection, infection, or anastomotic complications. The classic pathologic finding is constrictive bronchiolitis (see Figure 80-B). Unfortunately, the sensitivity for the diagnosis of BO by transbronchial biopsy is low (a range of 15 to 87%), and the diagnosis of BO is often made by exclusion and graded physiologically based on the degree of change in pulmonary function (FEV_1) from baseline. Because of the variability in obtaining bronchioles by transbronchial biopsy, the International Society for Heart and Lung Transplantation has established a bronchiolitis obliterans syndrome (BOS) staging system, revised in 2002. This staging is based on a reduction in midflows and/or FEV_1 in comparison to a posttransplant baseline FEV_1 with or without the pathologic documentation of BO (see Table 80-1). Treatment includes augmentation of immunosuppression, often with minimal improvement. Recently, it has become apparent that gastroesophageal reflux has been associated with chronic rejection, and aggressive treatment for gastroesophageal reflux is indicated. Newer data also suggest that the macrolide, azithromycin, may play a therapeutic role in BOS, likely through an antiinflammatory mechanism.

Table 80-1. Clinical Staging System for BOS*

Stage†	**FEV_1**	
BOS 0	No OB	FEV_1 > 90% of baseline and $FEF_{25\text{-}75\%}$ > 75% of baseline
BOS 0-p	Potential OB	FEV_1 81 to 90% of baseline and/or $FEF_{25\text{-}75\%}$ ≤ 75% of baseline
BOS 1	Mild OB	FEV_1 66 to 80% of baseline
BOS 2	Moderate OB	FEV_1 51% to 65% of baseline
BOS 3	Severe OB	FEV_1 ≤ 50% of baseline

*Adapted from Estenne et al. $FEF_{25\text{-}75\%}$ = forced expiratory flow, midexpiratory phase.

†Each stage is subdivided into a and b, where a is without histologic documentation of OB and b is with histologic documentation of OB.

Acute rejection usually occurs early after transplant and is characterized by a drop in PFT results with a clear or only mildly abnormal chest radiograph and with lymphocytic vasculitis on transbronchial biopsy (choice A is incorrect). CMV pneumonia can develop in the LT recipient but usually earlier following the LT and in those with a mismatched CMV status (*ie,* donor-positive, recipient-negative) and an interstitial infiltrate. A diagnosis of CMV can be determined pathologically by the presence of intranuclear inclusion bodies. Polymerase chain reaction testing is also helpful in this diagnosis. With gancyclovir prophylaxis, the incidence of this complication has decreased significantly (choice B is incorrect). Pulmonary drug toxicity is rarely described in the posttransplant recipient, and none of this patient's drugs have been reported to cause BO (choice C is incorrect). There have been rare case reports of BO with organizing pneumonia from tacrolimus.

Estenne M, Maurer JR, Boehler A, et al. Bronchiolitis obliterans syndrome 2001: an update of the diagnostic criteria. J Heart Lung Transplant 2002; 21:297–310

Stewart S, Fishbein MC, Snell GI, et al. Revision of the 1996 working formulation for the standardization of nomenclature in the diagnosis of lung rejection. J Heart Lung Transplant 2007; 26:1229–1242

Sharples LD, McNeil K, Stewart S, et al. Risk factors for bronchiolitis obliterans: a systematic review of recent publications. J Heart Lung Transplant 2002; 21:271–281

Boehler A, Kesten S, Weder W, et al. Bronchiolitis obliterans after lung transplantation. Chest 1998; 114:1411–1426

Belperio JA, Weigt SS, Fishbein MC, et al. Chronic lung allograft rejection: mechanisms and therapy. Proc Am Thorac Soc 2009; 6:108–121

Yates B, Murphy DM, Forrest IA, et al. Azithromycin reverses airflow obstruction in established bronchiolitis obliterans syndrome. Am J Respir Crit Care Med 2005; 172:772–775

Blondeau K, Mertens V, Vanaudenaerde BA, et al. Gastro-oesophageal reflux and gastric aspiration in lung transplant patients with or without chronic rejection. Eur Respir J 2008; 31:707–713

81. D. Increase plateau pressures and not affect mortality.

In patients with acute lung injury and ARDS, alveolar collapse is a prominent feature. This contributes to worsening lung compliance and poor ventilation/perfusion ($\dot{V}/\dot{Q}$) matching, leading to hypoxemia. A common strategy to improve these physiologic abnormalities is to add PEEP, which serves to prevent derecruitment of alveoli opened during the delivery of positive-pressure breaths. By improving $\dot{V}/\dot{Q}$ matching, FIO_2 exposure and, thus, the risk for oxygen toxicity are presumably decreased.

In recent years, the notion has developed that avoiding cyclical lung collapse-reopening may also reduce ventilator-induced lung injury and improve mortality and outcomes. This has led to the concept of the "open lung" approach to mechanical ventilation: the approach of putting as much expiratory pressure as is needed to keep the lung as maximally recruited as possible. It is important to realize, however, that additions of expiratory pressure will often increase the end-inspiratory pressure (plateau pressure) because the tidal breath is now being added to a higher baseline. Although improvements in respiratory system compliance with the addition of PEEP may mitigate this increase, there is almost always some increase in plateau pressure.

Recently, three large clinical trials have addressed this issue. In all three of these trials, an aggressive PEEP strategy was compared with a more conservative PEEP strategy for its effect on mortality in patients with ARDS. These strategies were all based on balancing gas exchange and FIO_2 exposure. An example of one of these strategies is shown in Table 81-1. In all three trials, the higher PEEP strategy was associated with better lung recruitment, in that PaO_2/FIO_2 was considerably higher and FIO_2 exposure was considerably lower. Moreover, in one trial (with the lowest PEEP settings of any of the trials), there was an increase in ventilator-free days with the high PEEP strategy. More importantly, in all three trials, the mortality was no different with either strategy. Thus choice D is correct, and the others are incorrect.

Table 81-1. NIH ARDS Network Comparison of PEEP Strategies*

Conservative PEEP Approach																	
FIO_2	0.300	0.40	0.400	0.500	0.50	0.600	0.700	0.70	0.700	0.800	0.90	0.90	0.90	1.0	1.0	1.0	1.0
PEEP	5	5	8	8	10	10	10	12	14	14	14	16	18	18	20	22	24

Liberal PEEP Approach														
FIO_2	0.30	0.30	0.40	0.40	0.50	0.50	0.6	0.6	0.70	0.8	0.8	0.9	1.0	1.0
PEEP	12	14	14	16	16	18	18	20	20	20	22	22	22	24

*Target: PO_2, 55–80 mm Hg; SpO_2, 88–95%.
Move up one step if below target and down one step if above target.

It is unclear why the improved lung recruitment with aggressive PEEP strategies did not translate into a mortality benefit. One possible explanation is that in all three trials, there was an increase in the end-inspiratory plateau pressure with the aggressive PEEP approach. Although this increase did not produce serious barotraumas, it is possible that any benefit of reduced atelectasis was counteracted by an increase in the end inspiratory lung stretch, an important cause of ventilator-induced lung injury. Another explanation is that, in the setting of small tidal volume ventilation, which has become so common in the management of patients with acute lung injury, the added benefit of some reduced atelectasis is not clinically important. Similarly, the reduction in FIO_2 from only moderately high levels, such as in this patient, may also not be particularly clinically relevant.

Meade MO, Cook, DJ, Guyatt GH, et al. Ventilation strategy using low tidal volumes, recruitment maneuvers, and high positive end-expiratory pressure for acute lung injury and acute respiratory distress syndrome: a randomized controlled trial. JAMA 2008; 299:637–645

Mercat A, Richard JC, Vielle B, et al. Positive end-expiratory pressure setting in adults with acute lung injury and acute respiratory distress syndrome: a randomized controlled trial. JAMA 2008; 299:646–655

NIH ARDS Network. Higher versus lower positive end-expiratory pressures in patients with the acute respiratory distress syndrome. N Engl J Med 2004; 351:327–336

Grasso S, Stripoli T, De Michele M, et al. ARDSnet ventilatory protocol and alveolar hyperinflation: role of positive end-expiratory pressure. Am J Resp Crit Care Med 2007; 176:761–767
Talmor D, Sarge T, Malhotra A. Mechanical ventilation guided by esophageal pressure measurements in acute lung injury. New Engl J Med 2008; 359:2095–2104

82. C. Switch to an oral antibiotic and discharge now.

Because the patient is clinically improving and meets criteria for clinical stability, it is most appropriate to switch her to an oral antibiotic and discharge her to complete her course of therapy as an outpatient (choice C is correct). In general, patients with community-acquired pneumonia should be switched from IV to oral therapy when they are hemodynamically stable and improving clinically, are able to ingest medications, and have a normally functioning GI tract. Observation for stability on oral antibiotics is not required, and patients generally should be discharged (assuming there are no other active medical problems and there is a safe outpatient environment for care) when they meet criteria for clinical stability, including temperature ≤ 37.8°C, heart rate ≤ 100/min, respiratory rate ≤ 24/min, systolic BP ≥ 90 mm Hg, Sao_2 ≥ 90% or Pao_2 ≥ 60 mm Hg on room air, and the presence of a normal mental status and a normal ability to maintain oral intake. Of note, in cases of pneumococcal pneumonia, the presence of bacteremia does not require a longer duration of IV antibiotics once the above criteria are met.

There is no benefit to completing a fixed period of IV antibiotics (choice A is incorrect) or overlapping IV and oral antibiotics (choice B is incorrect). As previously noted, maintaining inpatient status for observation on oral antibiotics in an otherwise stable patient is not indicated (choice D is incorrect).

Mandell LA, Wunderink RG, Anzueto A, et al. Infectious Diseases Society of America/American Thoracic Society consensus guidelines on the management of community-acquired pneumonia in adults. Clin Infect Dis 2007; 44(suppl):S27–S72
Nathan RV, Rhew DC, Murray C, et al. In-hospital observation after antibiotic switch in pneumonia: a national evaluation. Am J Med 2006; 119:512.e1–e7
Oosterheert JJ, Bonten MJ, Schneider MM, et al. Effectiveness of early switch from intravenous to oral antibiotics in severe community acquired pneumonia: multicentre randomised trial. Br Med J 2006; 333:1193
Ramirez JA, Srinath L, Ahkee S, et al. Early switch from intravenous to oral cephalosporins in the treatment of hospitalized patients with community-acquired pneumonia. Arch Intern Med 1995; 155:1273–1276
Ramirez JA, Vargas S, Ritter GW, et al. Early switch from intravenous to oral antibiotics and early hospital discharge: a prospective observational study of 200 consecutive patients with community-acquired pneumonia. Arch Intern Med 1999; 159:2449–2454

83. A. Begin therapy with clarithromycin for 1 week, discharge from the ED, and arrange a follow-up visit in 1 week.

This patient has community-acquired pneumonia, so initiating therapy with a macrolide antibiotic and arranging appropriate follow-up would, therefore, be the most appropriate option in this patient (choice A is correct). Although she is a health-care worker, her illness is of very short duration and was likely acquired outside the hospital setting when she was on vacation for 2 weeks. The patient's chest radiograph confirms a right upper lobe, posterior segment infiltrate with no volume loss or cavitation. Thus, her chest radiograph and physical examination results are consistent with her clinical presentation. Antibiotic therapy for community-acquired pneumonia is typically begun on an empiric basis, and more intensive investigations are usually reserved for patients requiring hospitalization. Indications for hospitalization often include severe illness or comorbid conditions, confusion, impaired renal function, significant respiratory distress, hypoxemia, hypotension, or advanced age. She has no known risk factors for drug resistance such as advanced age, recent antibiotic therapy (including macrolides), alcohol abuse, serious comorbidities, immunosuppressive therapy, or exposure to children in a day care setting.

Although the chest radiograph reveals an upper lobe, posterior segment infiltrate, this finding in itself does not suggest a diagnosis of TB. Although symptoms of pulmonary TB are varied and can be absent, there is no history of indolent fever, chills, weight loss, chest pain, hemoptysis, or shortness of breath, and she has had no recent known contacts with patients with TB. She is known to have had a tuberculin skin test result of 0 mm during an employment screening

1 year ago, so given the concerns of the referring physician, it would be prudent to repeat the tuberculin skin test (the patient's repeat tuberculin skin test result was 0 mm). However, the clinical usefulness of tuberculin skin testing in diagnosing current TB disease is limited. In the absence of a lack of response to initial empiric antibiotic therapy or the development of new signs or symptoms, respiratory isolation, bronchoscopy, and/or anti-TB therapy would not be appropriate (choices B, C, and D are incorrect). In this instance, a prompt clinical response (see Figure 83-C, 1 week following initiation of antibiotics; and Figure 83-D, 2 months following initiation of antibiotics) to therapy would serve to reassure both the patient and the referring ED physician.

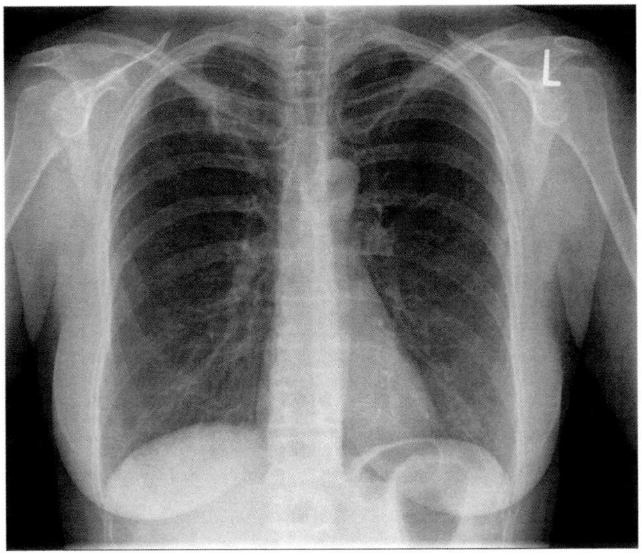

Figure 83-C

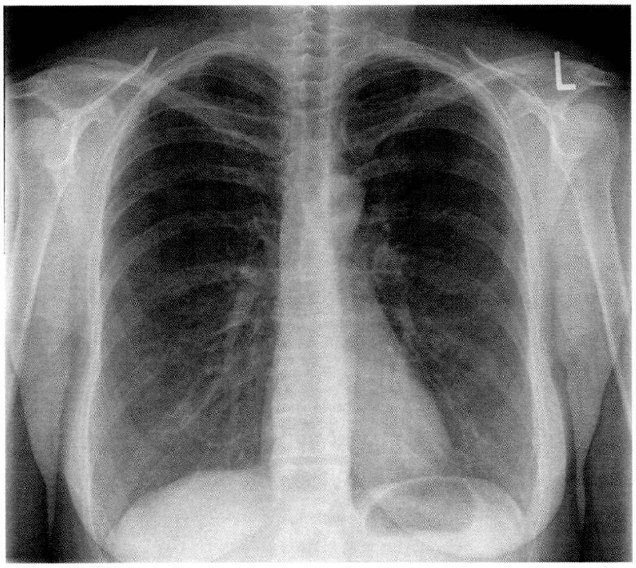

Figure 83-D

File TM, Garau J, Blasi F, et al. Guidelines for empiric antimicrobial prescribing in community-acquired pneumonia. Chest 2004; 125:1888–1901
Mandell LA, Wunderink RG, Anzueto A, et al. Infectious Diseases Society of America/American Thoracic Society consensus guidelines on the management of community-acquired pneumonia in adults. Clin Infect Dis 2007; 44(suppl):S27–S72
Woodring JH, Vandiviere HM, Fried AM, et al. Update: the radiographic features of pulmonary tuberculosis. Am J Roentgenol 1986; 146:497–506

84. C. Trimethoprim-sulfamethoxazole.

The lung tissue smear reveals the characteristic branching, filamentous, weakly acid-fast organisms typical of the Nocardia species (see Figure 84-B, arrow). Sulfonamides remain the treatment of choice for nocardiosis (choice C is correct). Minocycline is an alternative choice for an oral medication for patients who have sulfa allergies. IV regimens include amikacin, ceftriaxone, cefotaxime, ceftizoxime, and imipenem. Because of the risk of relapse, patients who have intact host defenses are generally treated from 6 to 12 months, whereas immune-deficient patients and those with CNS involvement are treated for 12 months.

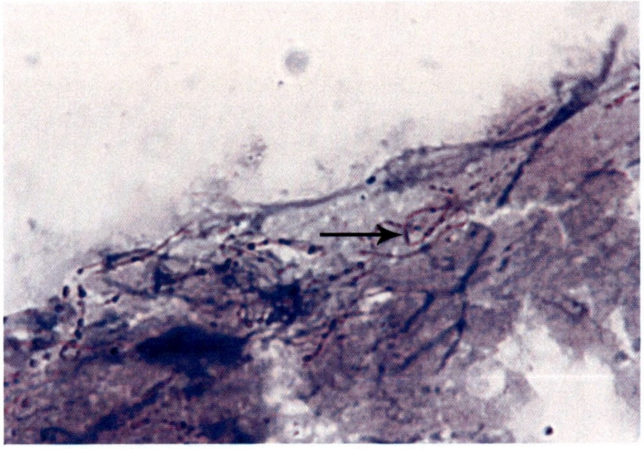

Figure 84-B
Modified Kinyoun acid-fast

Nocardia asteroides is the most common species associated with invasive disease. Pulmonary infection is increasingly being seen in immunosuppressed patients, with pneumonia being the most common respiratory tract syndrome. The presentation is often subacute, with several weeks of cough, purulent sputum, occasional blood-streaked sputum, night sweats, and pleuritic pain. Pleural involvement with an empyema occurs in approximately one-third of cases. Often, the initial respiratory tract involvement does not elicit symptoms. In approximately 50% of pulmonary cases, extrapulmonary dissemination occurs, most commonly to the brain.

As mentioned, nocardiosis is frequently recognized as an opportunistic disease, especially among patients with cell-mediated immune deficiencies, which include patients who undergo transplantation and those who have lymphoma and AIDS. Nocardiosis also has been reported to be associated with pulmonary alveolar proteinosis, mycobacterial diseases, and chronic granulomatous disease. The most frequent chest radiographic manifestation is an air space consolidation, usually with cavitation. In most cases of pneumonia, sputum smear results are negative. Bronchoscopy may be necessary to obtain an adequate specimen.

Although this immunosuppressed patient could certainly be at risk for disseminated infection with toxoplasmosis involving the lung and brain, the smear is not suggestive of the rounded tachyzoites of *Toxplasma gondii* (choice D is incorrect). Infection with actinomycetes is often confused with that of Nocardia because the two organisms appear similar on Gram stain. However, Actinomyces species will not stain positive on acid-fast staining. In addition, infection with Actinomyces usually occurs in immunocompetent hosts, more commonly involves chest wall invasion, and does not typically involve metastatic spread, particularly to the brain (choice B is incorrect). Finally, the weakly positive acid-fast stain could certainly suggest a mycobacterial infection. In addition, the cerebrospinal fluid features of tuberculous meningitis are similar to those seen in nocardial infection, and tuberculomas are radiographically similar to nocardial abscesses. However, the branching, filamentous forms on this stain are not characteristic of mycobacterium, which appear as shorter, more strongly acid-fast rods, which are only weakly gram-positive (choice A is incorrect).

Yildiz O, Doganay M. Actinomycoses and Nocardia pulmonary infections. Curr Opin Pulm Med 2006; 12:228–234
Husain S, McCurry K, Dauber J, et al. Nocardia infection in lung transplant recipients. J Heart Lung Transplant 2002; 21:354–359

85. A. A majority are benign and do not impact mortality.

Pleural effusions are common in patients in the medical ICU, with a prevalence of more than 60%. Studies evaluating pleural effusions in patients in the ICU supported by mechanical ventilation for more than 24 h found that most are small (92% in one study) and that they rarely cause significant complications (choice A is correct). A minority of these effusions (41%) are present on admission, with the remainder occurring during the ICU stay (choice B is incorrect). The most common cause was heart failure (35%), followed by atelectasis (23%) and parapneumonic

effusion (11%). Heart failure is the most common cause of bilateral effusions as well. Patients with pleural effusions were more likely to be older, have a lower albumin concentration, and have a higher severity of illness on admission (higher Acute Physiology and Chronic Health Evaluation [APACHE] II score). Patients with pleural effusions in the ICU tend to have longer mechanical ventilation support times when compared with those without a pleural effusion, but there is no evidence that tidal volume size (mL/kg) has an impact on development of an effusion (choice D is incorrect). Thoracentesis on a nonmassive effusion has been shown to decrease work performed by the ventilator and pleural liquid pressure in patients who are intubated and supported by mechanical ventilation. Despite these changes, compliance and resistance of the respiratory system, gas exchange, and ability to liberate from the mechanical ventilator were not changed (choice C is incorrect).

Evaluation of a pleural effusion in an ICU patient should carry a clinical suspicion, such as fever or a postprocedure complication. In febrile medical ICU patients, 62% had infectious-related exudates (27% empyema) and 30% had transudates. With ultrasound guidance for thoracentesis, complication rates are low (2%), with complications of hemothorax and pneumothorax being the most common.

Mattison LE, Coppage L, Alderman DF, et al. Pleural effusions in the medical ICU: prevalence, causes, and clinical implications. Chest 1997; 111:1018–1023

Doelken P, Abreu R, Sahn SA, et al. Effects of thoracentesis on respiratory mechanics and gas exchange in the patient receiving mechanical ventilation. Chest 2006; 130:154–161

Tu, CY, Hsu WH, Hsia TC, et al. Pleural effusions in febrile medical ICU patients: chest ultrasound study. Chest 2004; 126:1274–1280

Mayo PH, Goltz HR, Tafreshi M et al. Safety of ultrasound-guided thoracentesis in patients receiving mechanical ventilation. Chest 2004; 125:1059–1062

Light RW. Diseases of the pleura. Curr Opin Pulm Med 1995; 1:313–317

86. D. Arrange laser therapy of the lesions.

The lesions shown in the bronchoscopy image are classic for vocal cord papillomatosis. These are caused by the human papilloma virus, the same virus responsible for cutaneous or genital warts. Similar to warts, vocal cord papillomas tend to recur and often require recurrent therapy. Because of their propensity to recur, they are often referred to as recurrent respiratory papillomatosis (RRP). Lesions visualized on biopsy should be sampled and resected. The use of a carbon dioxide laser is preferred to surgical debridement, as the risk of local airway complications is less (choice D is correct). Appropriate respiratory precautions are required during laser therapy to avoid risk of transmission of aerosolized virus.

Although a history of gastroesophageal reflux is occasionally obtained from patients with RRP, reflux is not felt to contribute to the development of these lesions, and treatment of reflux is not effective therapy for RRP (choice A is incorrect). Inhaled corticosteroids can cause dysphonia by causing a vocal cord myopathy; however, their use has not been associated with the development of RRP, and discontinuing the medication will merely lead to worsening of this patient's asthma (choice B is incorrect).

RRP is the most common benign neoplasm affecting the vocal cord and upper respiratory tract. Laryngeal involvement occurs in more then 95% of infected individuals, although, rarely, the trachea alone is involved. The diagnosis is made with direct laryngoscopy or bronchoscopy. The lesions can very rarely undergo malignant transformation to squamous cell carcinomas; therefore, biopsy and resection of lesions is recommended. Chest radiograph results are usually normal, although, occasionally, an intratracheal density is visible. Distal bronchial obstruction has rarely been reported, and this may lead to a postobstructive pneumonia. RRP is much more common in children and can lead to upper airway obstruction. The course in adults is often not as severe, and single excision may sometimes be all that is required for cure. However, recurrence is common, even in adults. As a result, a number of adjunctive therapies to surgery have been examined. Interferon alfa-2a therapy for 6 months following surgical or laser excision has been reported to lead to lower recurrence rates but is not effective as monotherapy. Similarly, methotrexate may be useful, but very limited experience is available with this drug. Cruciferous vegetables, such as broccoli and cabbage, contain indole-3-carbinol, which slows the growth pattern of RRP and may be a useful adjunctive therapy in patients with frequent recurrences.

Cidofovir is an antiviral medication that may add to the benefits of therapy if injected into the lesions at the time of resection. Acyclovir may have a mild adjunctive effect postoperatively but has no role as primary therapy (choice C is incorrect).

Andrus JG, Shapshay SM. Contemporary management of laryngeal papilloma in adults and children. Otolaryngol Clin North Am 2006; 39:135–158
Armbruster C, Kreuzer A, Vorbach H, et al. Successful treatment of severe respiratory papillomatosis with intravenous cidofovir and interferon alpha-2b. Eur Respir J 2001; 17:830–831
Auborn KJ. Therapy for recurrent respiratory papillomatosis. Antivir Ther 2002; 7:1–9

87. A. Surgical resection with lung volume reduction surgery.

The best treatment outcomes for lung cancer come with surgical resection of the primary tumor, provided that there is no evidence of mediastinal or systemic metastases and that the patient can tolerate the planned removal of lung tissue. This patient's bronchoscopy confirmed that the nodule was lung cancer. The nodule size of 2.2 cm suggests a favorable long-term prognosis if surgical resection is possible. The clinical and radiographic screening evaluations showed no evidence of either mediastinal or systemic metastases. Potentially precluding surgical resection, however, is the patient's very poor lung function. The patient's postbronchodilator FEV_1 of <30% (29% in this patient) and the product of her FEV_1 % predicted and DLCO % predicted totaling <1,650% (29% × 26% = 754% in this patient) suggest that there is a very high risk for both perioperative death and cardiopulmonary complications and long-term pulmonary disability with lung cancer resection. Of note, extensive upper lobe emphysema with relative sparing of the lower lobes is indicated on the CT scan. Treatment of emphysema has been advanced through the National Emphysema Treatment Trial, which compared outcomes between lung volume reduction surgery (LVRS) and medical therapy. Overall survival was not improved by LVRS, but subgroup analysis showed marked differences in outcomes based on physiology and distribution of emphysema. Patients with an FEV_1 <20% of predicted and either a DLCO <20% of predicted or homogeneous emphysema indicated with CT scan had worse survival after surgery than with medical therapy. Patients with predominantly upper lobe emphysema (as in this patient) and a low baseline exercise capacity (<25 W, as with in this woman) had a survival benefit with LVRS. Thus, combining lung cancer resection with LVRS provides an attractive option for this patient (choice A is correct). Preliminary studies of patients who have undergone both lung cancer resection and LVRS suggest that both FEV_1 and quality of life improve postoperatively.

Advances in radiation therapy have improved outcomes for medically inoperable patients with non-small cell lung cancer. Three-dimensional conformal radiation therapy may allow the radiation dose to be escalated above 60 Gy without a significant increase in treatment-related toxicity and may be associated with more effective local tumor control and improved long-term survival. Radiation therapy might be considered but would not be able to provide the dual advantages of surgical resection of the lung cancer and LVRS (choice B is incorrect). Deferring radiation therapy until symptoms develop (choice C is incorrect) because it would eliminate the possibility of improving survival. CT scan–guided percutaneous radiofrequency ablation is a minimally invasive and generally well-tolerated approach to treating non-small cell lung cancer in marginal surgical patients, although long-term outcomes with this technique are not known. However, relative contraindications to the percutaneous placement of the needle electrode are extensive emphysema surrounding the cancer, as is the case with this patient, making choice D incorrect.

Beckles MA, Spiro SG, Colice GL, et al. The physiologic evaluation of patients with lung cancer being considered for resectional surgery. Chest 2003; 123:105S–114S
Fernando HC, De Hoyos A, Landreneau RJ, et al. Radiofrequency ablation for the treatment of non-small cell lung cancer in marginal surgical candidates. J Thorac Cardiovasc Surg 2005; 129:639–644
Kong FM, Zhao L, Hayman JA. The role of radiation therapy in thoracic tumors. Hematol Oncol Clin North Am 2006; 20:363–400
National Emphysema Treatment Trial Research Group. A randomized trial comparing lung-volume-reduction surgery with medical therapy for severe emphysema. N Engl J Med 2003; 348:2059–2073
Pompeo E, Dominicis E, Ambrogi V, et al. Quality of life after tailored combined surgery for stage I non-small cell lung cancer and severe emphysema. Ann Thorac Surg 2003; 76:1821–1827

88. C. Assume this clinical presentation is consistent with "shrinking lung syndrome," and continue to treat with immunosuppressives, with a consideration for escalating treatment.

Assuming this clinical presentation is consistent with shrinking lung syndrome, the best management would be to continue treatment with immunosuppressives, with a consideration for escalating treatment (choice C is correct).

This patient's main findings are a well-established and long-standing diagnosis of systemic lupus erythematosus (SLE), with long-standing symptoms of pleurisy and months of dyspnea associated with moderate-to-severe lung restriction by pulmonary function testing. By high-resolution CT scan, there is no evidence of severe pleural disease or evidence of lung fibrosis or ground-glass densities consistent with chronic lupus pneumonitis. All of these findings are consistent with shrinking lung syndrome, a well-described but poorly understood disorder seen in adult patients with SLE. Conflicting data exist to explain the source of restriction in this disorder, but there is agreement in the literature that lung fibrosis, hemorrhage, and inflammation must be excluded to entertain this diagnosis, typically by CT scan. Typical chest radiograph findings are consistent with those seen in this patient—low lung volumes with variable degrees of atelectasis. Some small series have suggested that myositis or isolated diaphragm dysfunction cause some cases of shrinking lung syndrome on the basis of weakness, but many patients have been described with normal muscle strength, as seen in this patient. Corticosteroids, other immunosuppressive therapies, and theophylline have been used to treat this disorder with variable success.

Dyspnea is a common complaint in patients with SLE and has a multitude of potential explanations that must be evaluated methodically. Anemia is common in SLE and occurs via a number of different mechanisms, but in this patient, the hemoglobin level is neither extremely low nor changed sufficiently to explain her progressive dyspnea over recent months. Pericardial effusions, cardiomyopathy, and coronary artery disease are common in patients with SLE, and this patient has had a long-standing pericardial effusion. However, this patient's pericardial effusion has been stable over time, and no cardiac compromise was noted with echocardiogram. While coronary artery disease may present relatively early in patients with SLE, particularly during treatment with corticosteroids or when antiphospholipid antibodies and hypercoagulopathies are present, noninvasive exercise testing is an adequate screening tool for this possibility (choice D is incorrect). Similarly, cardiomyopathy may occur in patients with SLE, and pulmonary hypertension may arise secondary to heart disease or as a primary pulmonary vascular phenomenon. Echocardiography is a reasonable screening tool for these possibilities, and specific findings on an endocardial biopsy that will guide therapy are not likely to be present (choice B is incorrect).

Some involvement of the respiratory system occurs in most adult patients with SLE and includes lung parenchymal, pulmonary vascular, pleural, and diaphragmatic abnormalities. Pleuritic chest pain occurs in as many as 50% of patients with SLE and was a long-standing complaint in this patient. Acute lupus pneumonitis is a much less common manifestation of lupus and presents as fever, cough, and pleurisy, with pulmonary infiltrates on chest radiograph and crackles on lung examination. This presentation has obvious overlap with acute infectious processes, and often both possibilities require treatment. Chronic lupus pneumonitis can also be seen, with a more protracted course and high-resolution CT scan findings of ground-glass opacities and/or reticular patterns consistent with fibrosis. Pulmonary hypertension, with or without parenchymal lung disease, and pulmonary hypertension arising secondary to pulmonary embolization are well described. This patient's high-resolution CT scan does not reveal parenchymal abnormalities, and ventilation-perfusion scanning is a reasonably sensitive test to exclude chronic pulmonary embolization. Pulmonary hemorrhage is a relatively rare complication of SLE and may present acutely with dyspnea, hemoptysis, and cough. Chest radiographs and high-resolution CT scans invariably show prominent bilateral infiltrates. This disorder has a high mortality and is typically treated with aggressive immunosuppression, including high-dose corticosteroids and cyclophosphamide. A variety of disorders of the respiratory muscles may be seen in patients with SLE, including diaphragm dysfunction or weakness related to myopathy associated with treatment with corticosteroids. This patient has findings inconsistent with severe muscle weakness producing her lung restriction. Her negative inspiratory force is normal, and her peak expiratory flow is only modestly diminished, the latter explicable by its measurement at low lung volumes. In addition, the patient's residual volume is not elevated, as would typically be seen in a patient with pure muscle weakness as an explanation for restrictive lung physiology. Tapering and stopping corticosteroids would not be an appropriate recommendation for this patient (choice A is incorrect).

Karim MY, Miranda LC, Tench CM, et al. Presentation and prognosis of the shrinking lung syndrome in systemic lupus erythematosus. Semin Arthritis Rheum 2002; 31:289–298
Keane MP, Lynch JP. Pleuropulmonary manifestations of systemic lupus erythematosus. Thorax; 2000; 55:159–166
Warrington KJ, Moder KG, Brutinel WM. The shrinking lungs syndrome in systemic lupus erythematosus. Mayo Clin Proc 2000; 75:467–472

89. B. Nasal polypectomy followed by aspirin desensitization and treatment.

The patient under discussion meets the criteria for aspirin-exacerbated respiratory disease (AERD) because she has underlying respiratory conditions, such as chronic rhinosinus disease, nasal polyps (see Figure 58-A in the stem), and asthma, that are exacerbated by aspirin or nonsteroidal antiinflammatory drugs (NSAIDs). A characteristic of AERD is the existence of cross-reactions with a variety of cyclooxygenase (COX-1) inhibitors. There does not appear to be cross-reactivity to any of the COX-2 inhibitors. While acetaminophen and salsalate are poor inhibitors of COX-1 enzyme, these drugs do cross-react when given in high concentrations, such as $\geq$ 1,000 mg. The therapy that has the best chance of providing the patient with long-term relief (*ie*, preventing recurrence of nasal polyposis for up to 5 years) is nasal polypectomy followed by aspirin desensitization and treatment (choice B is correct). With the possible exception of regular maintenance therapy with systemic corticosteroids (not a choice offered in this question), no other form of therapy has been shown to prevent the need for recurrent nasal polypectomies. Therefore, choices A and D are incorrect. Once AERD starts, it continues, even in the absence of aspirin and NSAIDs. Therefore, decreasing the dose of acetaminophen in this patient will not prevent the progression of the disease (choice C is incorrect).

Aspirin desensitization is the process through which a state of tolerance to aspirin is induced. If standardized protocols are followed, desensitization can be done safely. Once tolerance is induced and aspirin is ingested on a continuous basis (a usual starting dose is 650 mg bid), the aspirin-desensitized state can be maintained indefinitely. The dose can be gradually decreased over time. The desensitized state will persist for no more than 2 to 5 days, with return of full sensitivity after 7 days of stopping aspirin, so it is advisable to reperform the desensitization protocol once aspirin has been stopped for more than 1 to 2 days before reinstituting aspirin therapy. In patients who have complete 1 year of daily aspirin therapy, approximately 87% respond favorably (reductions in sinus infections, improvement in smell, reduction in doses of systemic and topical corticosteroids). For patients who do not complete 1 year of therapy, aspirin has to be discontinued in approximately 13% because of side effects such as gastritis and, occasionally, hives. To minimize gastric complications, acid suppression therapy should be given.

Berges-Gimeno MP, Simon RA, Stevenson DD. The natural history and clinical characteristics of aspirin-exacerbated respiratory disease. Ann Allergy Immunol 2002; 89:474–478
Berges-Gimeno MP, Stevenson DD. Nonsteroidal anti-inflammatory drug-induced reactions and desensitization. J Asthma 2004; 41:375–384

90. B. Figure 90-B.

Figure 90-B shows the internal jugular vein, the anechoic structure to the right of the internal carotid artery. Of the images shown, insertion of a catheter in this vein is likely to be successful and the safest approach because it is lateral to the artery (choice B is correct). An estimated 5 million central venous catheters are placed each year in the United States, but these procedures carry the risks of lack of success and require multiple passes, each associated with complications that include bleeding, arterial puncture, and pneumothorax. Ultrasound visualization to guide the choice of the vessel and approach to catheter placement is shown to decrease the rate of complications compared with the traditional anatomic landmark approach, especially in patients at high risk of complications due to coagulation disorders and obesity. Although several professional societies and regulatory agencies consider ultrasound-guided central venous access to be a "best practice," acceptance by clinicians has been suboptimal, in part because of resistance to adopt new methods, along with lack of proper equipment and training. Nevertheless, the 2008 American Board of Internal Medicine Training and Procedural Requirements states that "proficiency in use of ultrasound to guide central line placement and thoracentesis is strongly recommended."

B-mode ultrasound is usually employed to facilitate placement of central venous catheters. Ultrasound is most useful for imaging the internal jugular and femoral veins. The subclavian vein is more difficult to visualize because of its deeper location and the presence of the overlying clavicle, but experienced operators describe considerable success. Fluid (including blood) is hypoanechoic or anechoic and appears dark on images, whereas tissue appears gray. Distinguishing arteries from veins depends on dynamic images: arteries tend to be noncompressible and pulsatile, whereas veins are usually not. There is considerable anatomic variation in the positions of corresponding arteries and veins, accounting for the frequency of unsuccessful arterial punctures when landmark approaches are used. In each of the images in this question, the probe is placed on the skin corresponding to the top of the image. Figure 90-A shows a large vein that overlies the artery, and an attempted placement of a catheter would risk arterial puncture if the vein is compressed and traversed by the needle (choice A is incorrect). Inadvertent carotid arterial puncture is particularly problematic. Figure 90-C shows a femoral vein with an intramural thrombus; this vessel should not be used because the catheter could dislodge the clot (see Figure 90-E, arrow) or the catheter's presence would increase the risk of clot propagation (choice C is incorrect). Figure 90-D shows a subcutaneous echogenic structure that may be mistaken for a vein, but it is unsuitable for attempted cannulation because it is echogenic and would not be compressible on dynamic imaging. In fact, this is a lymph node (choice D is incorrect).

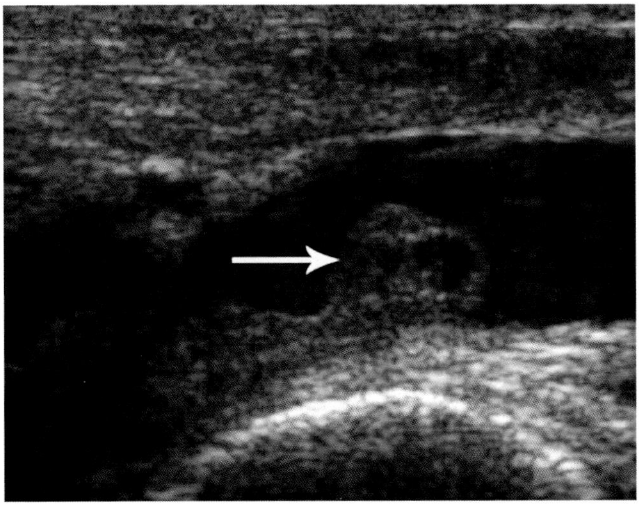

Figure 90-E

Feller-Kopman D. Ultrasound-guided internal jugular access: a proposed standardized approach for training and practice. Chest 2007; 132: 302–309

Mey U, Glasmacher A, Hahn C, et al. Evaluation of an ultrasound-guided technique for central venous access via the internal jugular vein in 493 patients. Support Care Cancer 2003; 11:135–136

Beaulieu Y, Marik PE. Bedside ultrasonography in the ICU: Part 1. Chest 2005; 128:881–895

Beaulieu Y, Marik PE. Bedside ultrasonography in the ICU: Part 2. Chest 2005; 128:1766–1781

91. C. Improved oxygenation.

A high-quality metaanalysis of 13 randomized controlled trials with appropriate grading of the methodology of these studies concluded that mechanical ventilation in the prone position improved oxygenation. The overall improvement was in the range of 34% in the PaO_2/FIO_2 ratio, and this improvement occurred on the first day (choice C is correct). This improvement continued into the second and third days after initiation of prone positioning. The ratio was still 6% higher the morning after the patients had returned to the supine position, compared with patients assigned to the supine position from the beginning. Unfortunately, 10 of 13 trials that reported mortality indicated that prone positioning did not reduce mortality among patients with hypoxemic respiratory failure (risk ratio 0.96, 95% CI, 0.84 to 1.09, p = 0.52; choice A is incorrect). This lack of effect was demonstrated even among studies that examined prolonged prone positioning. In the five trials that examined the effect of prone positioning on the risk of acquiring

ventilator-associated pneumonia (VAP), there was a 19% decreased risk of acquiring VAP (relative risk 0.81, 95% CI, 0.66 to 0.99, p = 0.04) but no change in the duration of ventilation (choice B is incorrect). Prone positioning was associated with an increased risk of pressure ulcers (risk ratio 1.36, 95% CI, 1.07 to 1.71, p = 0.01; choice D is incorrect). Although, in general, prone positioning is safe, the procedure is labor intensive, requiring four to six people to turn a patient. The only other major complication reported was a slight increased risk of tube blockage. A survey of more than 700 ICUs in Germany reported many more complications than those seen in the randomized controlled trials, suggesting that specialized centers with local experience and interest may be required to implement this ventilatory strategy.

Sud S, Sud M, Friedrich JO, et al. Effect of mechanical ventilation in the prone position on clinical outcomes in patients with acute hypoxemic respiratory failure: a systematic review and meta-analysis. Can Med Assoc J 2008; 178:1153–1161

Gattinoni L, Vagginelli F, Carlesso E, et al. Decrease in $Paco_2$ with prone position is predictive of improved outcome in acute respiratory distress syndrome. Crit Care Med 2003; 31:2727–2733

Gattinoni L, Tognoni G, Presenti A, et al. Effect of prone positioning on the survival of patients with acute respiratory failure. N Engl J Med 2001; 345:568–573

Bein T, Ritzka M, Schmidt F, et al. Positioning therapy in intensive care medicine in Germany: results of a national survey [German]. Anesthetist 2007; 56:226–231

92. A. Recurrent aspiration.

The CT scan (see Figures 92-A and 92-B) reveals patchy ground-glass densities mostly centered around airways, with some nodules in the lower lobes. The mixed inflammatory and obstructive bronchiolitis picture shown on biopsy combined with the CT and clinical picture is most consistent with recurrent aspiration (choice A is correct). Histologically, aspiration is characterized by peribronchiolar acute and/or chronic inflammation, with or without surrounding pneumonia. Food particles or other exogenous materials, such as barium or exogenous lipids, may be present. Another section of the biopsy in this patient is shown in Figure 92-E and demonstrates a bronchiole with adjacent food particles. In cases of chronic aspiration, there may be associated constrictive or obliterative bronchiolitis, characterized by the narrowing or obliteration of bronchiolar lumens by fibrosis as seen in this patient.

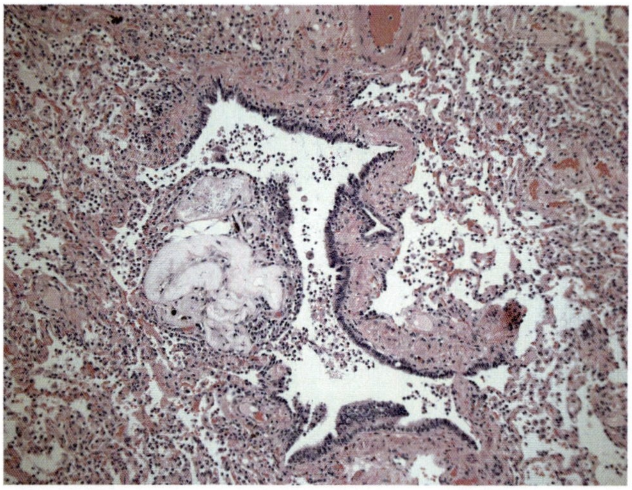

Figure 92-E
Hematoxylin-eosin

Sarcoidosis can cause systemic symptoms, although the waxing and waning pattern seen in this patient would be very unusual. In addition, ground-glass changes on CT scan can be consistent with sarcoidosis. However, no evidence of granulomatous inflammation is seen on the biopsy in the current patient, and the flow cytometry failed to reveal a high CD4/CD8 ratio characteristic of this disease (choice B is incorrect). The clinical picture is consistent with

vasculitis, and the ground-glass changes seen on CT might represent alveolar hemorrhage, but the biopsy results show no evidence for vasculitis or capillaritis (choice C is incorrect). Cryptogenic organizing pneumonia can show evidence of obliterative bronchiolitis on biopsy, but this should involve the airspaces (not seen on the current biopsy), and inflammation of the airways is not characteristic (choice D is incorrect).

Aspiration may lead to a number of different pulmonary syndromes depending on the amount and type of material aspirated (*eg*, oropharyngeal contents, stomach contents, and exogenous material), the frequency of the aspiration, and the host's response to the aspirated material. Aspiration pneumonitis is an acute lung injury caused by inhalation of gastric contents. It was first described by Mendelson in patients who aspirated while undergoing general anesthetics and, occasionally, is referred to as Mendelson syndrome. It is more commonly seen acutely in individuals after drug overdoses but can occur on a chronic basis in individuals with esophageal disorders, such as in this patient. The patient had frequent solid food dysphagia and underwent several esophageal dilatation procedures before finally undergoing a fundoplication that alleviated his recurrent symptoms.

In a review of cases of recurrent aspiration of particulate matter undergoing pathologic examination, organizing pneumonia was the most common pathologic finding seen, usually in combination with multinucleated giant cells, acute bronchopneumonia/bronchiolitis, and/or suppurative granulomas. Foreign material, including food remnants, was identified in all cases, as seen in the current patient. The average age of patients in the review of cases was 57 years, with a 2:1 male to female ratio. Bilateral infiltrates were found in half of the cases. Aspiration was suspected in only 9% of cases prior to biopsy. Predisposing factors for aspiration included esophageal or gastric causes in 59% of the cases and drug use or neurologic cause in most of the remainder. The most common symptoms included dyspnea, fever, and cough, similar to those reported by the current patient.

Mukhopadhyay S, Katzenstein AL. Pulmonary disease due to aspiration of food and other particulate matter: a clinicopathologic study of 59 cases diagnosed on biopsy or resection specimens. Am J Surg Pathol 2007; 31:752–759

Barnes TW, Vassallo R, Tazelaar HD, et al. Diffuse bronchiolar disease due to chronic occult aspiration. Mayo Clin Proc 2006; 81:172–176

Marik PE. Aspiration pneumonitis and aspiration pneumonia. N Engl J Med 2001; 344:665–671

Mendelson CL. The aspiration of stomach contents into the lungs during obstetric anesthesia. Am J Obstet Gynecol 1946; 52:191–205

93. A. Patient's age.

This patient developed bilateral reexpansion pulmonary edema (RPE; right much greater than left) 2 h after chest tube placement (see Figure 93-C). The patient's age is the most likely factor listed that is associated with development of RPE (choice A is correct).

Multiple factors potentially associated with RPE have been reported. The volume of pleural fluid frequently has been cited. The American Thoracic Society statement on the management of malignant pleural effusions suggests removing only 1.0 to 1.5 L of pleural fluid at one time as long as the patient does not develop dyspnea, chest pain, or severe cough. More recently, a study of the largest series of patients (185 patients) prospectively enrolled while undergoing large-volume thoracentesis (≥ 1.0 L of fluid) found that clinically apparent RPE (as in this patient) is rare and not statistically associated with the volume of fluid removed (choice B is incorrect). The clinical diagnosis of only one case of RPE (0.5%) and the radiograph diagnosis of four cases (2.2%) occurred in this series. All four of the radiographically diagnosed cases of RPE improved symptomatically after thoracentesis and required no therapy. Only if the clinical case and the radiographic cases are aggregated is any significance found with the volume of fluid removed and RPE development. No statistically significant association between the absolute change in pleural pressure, pleural elastance, or symptoms (cough, chest discomfort, worsening dyspnea, hypoxia, tachypnea, and hemodynamic instability) and the development of RPE has been found (choices C and D are incorrect).

Interestingly, a separate study notes that the development of vague chest discomfort (vs sharp chest pain [likely related to catheter irritation of the diaphragm] or cough) is associated with potentially dangerously low absolute pleural

pressures (< −20 cm H_2O). Although no clear link has been established between low absolute pleural pressures (or pleural elastance) and RPE, it has been suggested that therapeutic thoracentesis be discontinued if the patient develops vague chest discomfort.

RPE may occur with removal of either pleural fluid or air. A study of spontaneous pneumothorax associated RPE found a statistically significant association between RPE and age (higher rate in patients aged 20 to 39 years compared with patients older than 40 years) and greater extent of lung collapse. The mechanism of this age association is unknown and may include protective changes within the lung itself that evolve with age, such as changes in lung mechanics or the permeability properties of the alveolar-capillary interface. Also, greater chest wall compliance in the younger population may permit greater pleural pressure changes. Other incompletely established associations with RPE have been suggested and include duration of lung collapse (>72 h, experimentally), intrapleural suction by chest tube, and rapid removal of fluid or air.

Antony VB, Loddenkemper R, Astoul P, et al. Management of malignant pleural effusions. Am J Respir Crit Care Med 2000; 162:1987–2001

Feller-Kopman D, Berkowitz D, Boiselle P, et al. Large-volume thoracentesis and the risk of reexpansion pulmonary edema. Ann Thorac Surg 2007; 84:1656–1662

Matsurra Y, Nomimura T, Murakami H, et al. Clinical analysis of reexapansion pulmonary edema. Chest 1991; 100:1562–1566

Feller-Kopman D, Walkey A, Berkowitz D, et al. The relationship of pleural pressure to symptom development during therapeutic thoracentesis. Chest 2006; 129:1556–1560

Baumann MH, Strange C. Treatment of spontaneous pneumothorax: a more aggressive approach? Chest 1997; 112:789–804

94. D. Fixed, large airway obstruction.

The patient developed subglottic stenosis as a complication of her intubation. The combination of inspiratory and expiratory flow abnormalities (see Figure 94-A) is characteristic of a fixed obstruction (choice D is correct and choices A and C are incorrect). Variable inspiratory airflow obstruction may be present in vocal cord dysfunction, but expiratory flow is unaffected (see Figure 94-B). Severe obstruction, characteristically manifest in constrictive bronchiolitis, results in primarily expiratory airflow limitation (see Figure 94-C). In restrictive disease, supranormal airflow occurs, likely a result of "stenting" of airways and altering the natural closing point (see Figure 94-D). The significant reduction in airflow and lack of normal-supranormal airflow are not consistent with restrictive lung disease (choice B is incorrect).

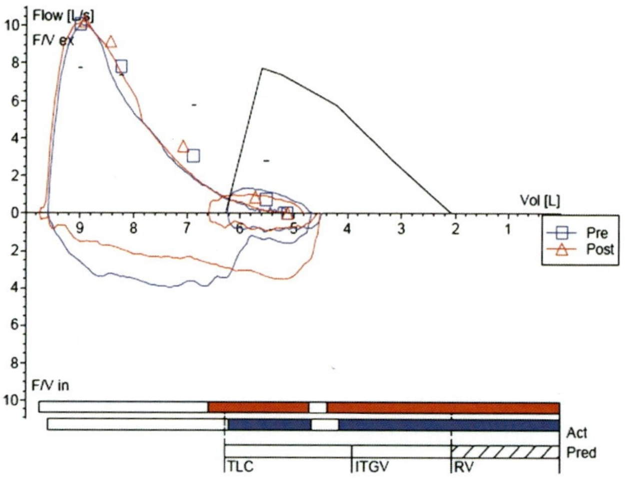

Figure 94-B

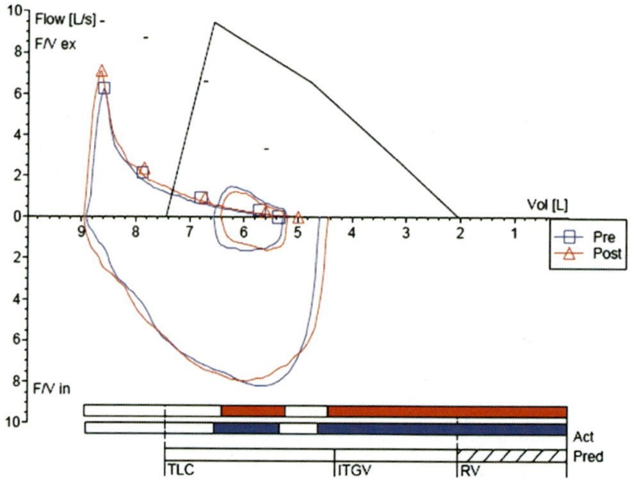

Figure 94-C

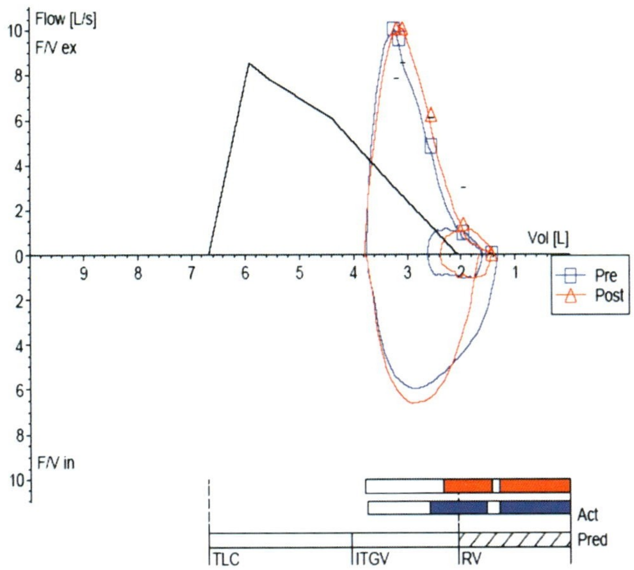

Figure 94-D

Bronchoscopy findings in the current patient revealed concentric narrowing of the trachea 1 inch (2.5 cm) below the vocal cords and extending for 1.4 cm. A CT scan confirmed the presence of subglottic narrowing (see Figure 94-E). The patient was taken to the operating room where rigid bronchoscopy and dilatation of tracheal stenosis were carried out.

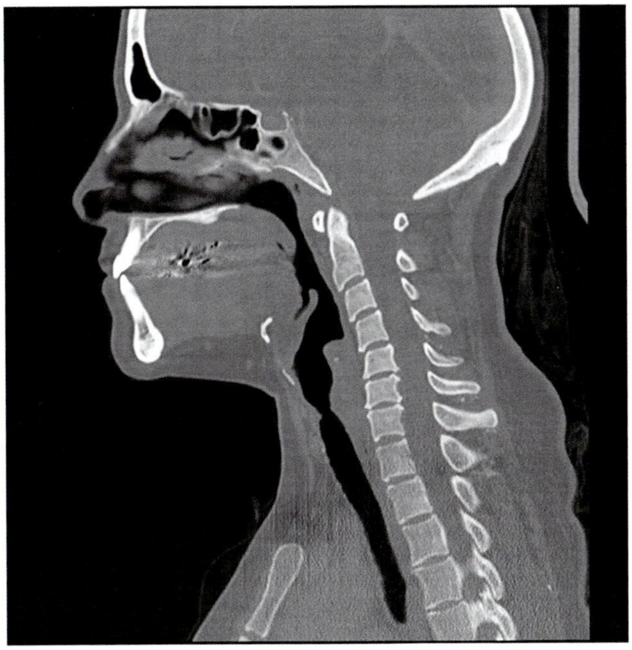

Figure 94-E

The most common cause of tracheal stenosis is trauma, particularly after intubation or tracheostomy. Other disorders that cause tracheal stenosis include relapsing polychondritis, Wegener granulomatosis, benign and malignant neoplasms, and, rarely, sarcoidosis and amyloidosis.

Affected individuals often are seen with dyspnea, which is worse on exertion, and are frequently misdiagnosed with asthma. Most patients are asymptomatic at rest until the airway is narrowed by more then 70%. They may have stridor. The flattening of the inspiratory and expiratory flow-volume loops is characteristic of a fixed obstruction to a large airway (see Figure 94-A).

Definitive treatment is usually surgical, with resection of the involved segment and end-to-end anastomosis. Serial dilatations can be successful, but there is a high rate of restenosis. This effect may be mitigated with the use of adjunctive therapy with laser or mitomycin-C, an alkylating agent that inhibits fibroblast production. Finally, stents may be used as an adjunctive measure during endoscopy or for patients who are not surgical candidates.

Mark EJ, Meng F, Kradin RL, et al. Idiopathic tracheal stenosis: a clinicopathologic study of 63 cases and comparison of the pathology with chondromalacia. Am J Surg Pathol 2008; 32:1138–1143

Terra RM, de Medeiros IL, Minamoto H, et al. Idiopathic tracheal stenosis: successful outcome with antigastroesophageal reflux disease therapy. Ann Thorac Surg 2008; 85:1438–1439

Ashiku SK, Mathisen DJ. Idiopathic laryngotracheal stenosis. Chest Surg Clin N Am 2003; 13:257–269

Lorenz RR. Adult laryngotracheal stenosis: etiology and surgical management. Curr Opin Otolaryngol Head Neck Surg 2003; 11:467–472

Nouraei SA, Murphy K, Nouraei SM, et al. Diagnosis of laryngotracheal stenosis during routine spirometry using the "Expiratory Disproportion Index" [abstract]. Clin Otolaryngol 2008; 33:644

95. D. Perform bronchoscopy with central airway inspection.

This patient's bilateral pneumothoraces are the result of a partial dehiscence of the bronchial anastomosis performed for lung transplantation. Identifying this process so that immunosuppressive treatment can be reduced, if possible, and surgical repair can be undertaken, if necessary, is important (choice D is correct).

Airway complications occur in about 10 to 15% of lung transplant recipients and include anastomotic dehiscence, bronchial stenosis, bronchomalacia, and bronchopleural fistula. These complications usually begin to develop within several weeks to months after transplantation. Although these anatomic complications were a common cause of mortality in the early posttransplant period in the past, improvements in surgical technique and immunosuppressive regimens appear to have reduced the frequency of mortality and significant morbidity. Risk factors for anastomotic complications include prolonged ischemic injury to the graft exacerbated by disruption of the bronchial circulation because the bronchial artery is not typically reconnected to the donor artery. As a result, perfusion of the anastomotic site depends on retrograde blood from the pulmonary arterial circulation, which flows at a lower pressure and partial pressure of oxygen. Extensive postoperative hypotension is also a likely contributor to anastomotic complications. Many surgeons attempt to ameliorate these risks by using a short donor mainstem bronchus and long recipient bronchus. Telescoping anastomoses are associated with reduced risk of anastomotic dehiscence but increase stricture risk. Prolonged high doses of steroids may impair wound healing, and rapamycin (sirilimus) in particular has been associated with early fatal bronchial dehiscence. These drugs can be used safely after anastomotic healing has occurred. Finally, bacterial and fungal infection of the ischemic airway may increase inflammation and further impair healing. A right-sided dehiscence may lead to bilateral pneumothoraces, as is seen in this case. This is more common in patients whose operation is done via bilateral anterior thoracotomies with a transverse sternotomy ("clamshell" incision). This incision severs the anterior pleural reflections and can result in a persistent intrapleural communication and, hence, a predisposition to bilateral pneumothoraces despite dehiscence isolated to the right.

In this case, bronchoscopy revealed a dehiscence of the right mainstem anastomosis. Immunosuppressive therapy was reduced for a 3-week period, facilitating healing, and surgical intervention was not required.

Some intervention is needed for bronchial dehiscence, so simply observing the patient would not be advisable (choice A is incorrect). Increasing immunosuppressive therapy, if not needed to preserve transplant function, would be ill-advised in the setting of bronchial dehiscence given the adverse effects on wound healing (choice B is incorrect). Bilateral chest tube placement would be unnecessarily aggressive and would not correct this patient's underlying problem (choice C is incorrect).

Weder W, Inci I, Korom S, et al. Airway complications after lung transplantation: risk factors, prevention, and outcome. Eur J Cardiothoracic Surg 2009; 5:293–298

Murthy SC, Blackstone EH, Gildea TR, et al. Impact of anastomotic airway complications after lung transplantation. Ann Thorac Surg 2007; 84:401–409

96. C. Hamartoma.

This patient has a left lower lobe 4-cm solitary lung mass that has all the characteristics of a hamartoma (choice C is correct). Hamartomas are benign tumors of the lung characterized by the presence of both areas of fat and calcification (in a popcorn pattern in 30% of cases) on chest radiograph or chest CT as shown in these scans (see Figures 96-D [sagittal] and 96-E [coronal]). On CT, the presence of fat can be found by comparing areas of the lesion with the fat in the chest wall or, more accurately, by assessing density units (Hounsfield units) by CT scan. Hounsfield units < 25 U are consistent with fat (see Figure 96-F, arrow).

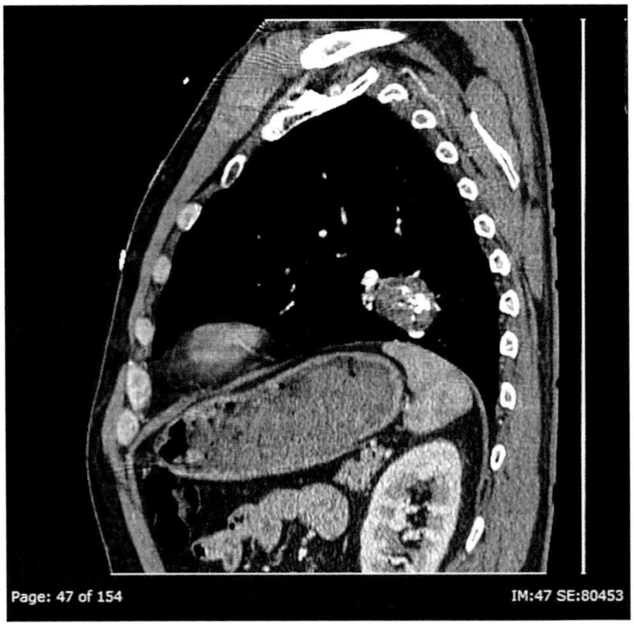

Figure 96-D

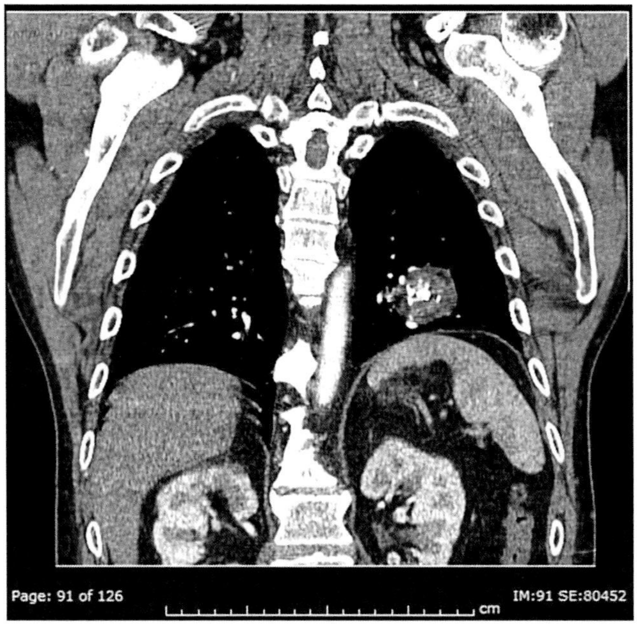

Figure 96-E

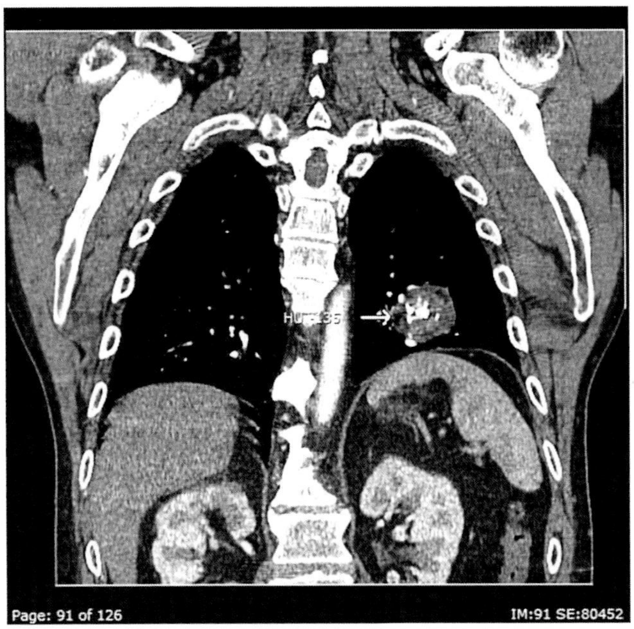

Figure 96-F

The point of the arrow in Figure 96-F indicates a region of the lesion with a Hounsfield unit of −135, consistent with fat.

Hamartomas are one of the most common benign, noninfectious causes of lung nodules and masses, accounting for 10% of benign lung nodules. The diagnosis can be nearly definitively made if CT shows a mixture of low-attenuation fat and high-attenuation calcification. Intranodular fat density is more sensitive for identifying a hamartoma than popcorn calcification. High-resolution scans may be needed to better define the diagnostic characteristics of a hamartoma.

The typical age in which hamartomas are found is 40 to 60 years, with a ratio of 3:1 in men to women. They are most often located peripherally but can also occur endobronchially in 20% of cases. Nearly all patients with the lesion are asymptomatic. Histologically, hamartomas are characterized by a heterogeneous mixture of cartilage with calcification, fat, muscle, and fibrous and myxomatous tissue. They can continue to grow slowly and can range from 2 to 8 cm in size. Occasional reports of massive-sized hamartomas have been reported. In general, no further evaluation of a lesion with these classic characteristics is required, although conservative follow-up may be indicated. This is a fairly large hamartoma, and, if the patient developed symptoms of cough or chest pain, resection could be considered on that basis.

Granulomas would typically have central or more diffuse calcification and would not contain fat (choice B is incorrect). In addition, the patient has a negative PPD test result. This patient is a heavy smoker, so bronchogenic carcinoma must also be of concern; however, again, the characteristic hamartoma appearance makes this diagnosis less likely (choice A is incorrect). Lipomas can develop in the lung but generally contain more homogenous fat, although calcification can occasionally develop (choice D is incorrect).

Although strictly defined as a lesion < 3 cm in size—and this lesion exceeds that size—benign patterns of calcification that should be considered when evaluating a solitary pulmonary nodule include diffuse, central, laminated, and popcorn (as in the case of hamartoma). All other patterns of calcification, such as stippled or eccentric, need further evaluation.

Ost D, Fein AM, Feinsilver SH. Clinical practice: the solitary pulmonary nodule. N Engl J Med 2003; 348:2535–2542
Gjevre JA, Myers JL, Prakash UB. Pulmonary hamartomas. Mayo Clin Proc 1996; 71:14–20
Siegelman SS, Khouri NF, Scott WW, et al. Pulmonary hamartoma: CT findings. Radiology 1986; 160:313–317
Gould MK, Fletcher J, Iannettoni MD, et al. Evaluation of patients with pulmonary nodules: when is it lung cancer? ACCP evidence-based clinical practice guidelines, 2nd edition. Chest 2007; 132(suppl):108S–130S
Ost D, Fein A. Evaluation and management of the solitary pulmonary nodule. Am J Respir Crit Care Med 2000; 162:782–787

97. A. The subsequent increase in PEEP setting.

In the patient with acute lung injury, alveolar collapse is common. Many of these alveoli can be opened with application of positive-pressure breaths. However, these opened alveoli are prone to collapsing again during expiration. To prevent this collapse, PEEP is often added. This will serve to maintain the patency of alveoli opened by the tidal breath.

An expansion of this concept is to apply an RM. An RM takes the lung above the set tidal excursion to total lung capacity in an effort to open as many alveoli as possible. This can be done by applying high-level (*eg,* 40 cm H_2O) CPAP, by elevating PEEP settings to 30 to 40 cm H_2O, or by applying "sigh breaths" of 1.5 to 2 times the set tidal volume. Each of these approaches is used for up to a minute.

Many studies have shown that RMs have the potential to open more alveoli than those recruited during a standard tidal volume, especially in patients receiving smaller tidal volumes. A critical point to remember, however, is that this recruitment will be short-lived if an appropriate increase in the PEEP setting is not present to prevent derecruitment. Thus, choice A is correct. Indeed, many authorities recommend only using recruitment maneuvers when either PEEP has been lost (*eg,* a ventilator disconnect) or if there is a clinical assessment that additional PEEP is necessary to improve ventilation-perfusion mismatching. RMs can also be used when performing a decremental PEEP trial, maneuvers that titrate PEEP down from high levels to levels just sufficient to prevent substantial derecruitment.

Choice B is incorrect because the RM is not dependent on the FIO_2 setting. Choice C is incorrect because, as noted previously, the recruitment attained with an RM is often lost fairly quickly, and thus waiting 3 to 6 h will clearly

not maintain the recruitment desired. Finally, the RM strategy of immediately reapplying 50 cm H_2O without an accompanying PEEP increase will also likely provide only short-term recruitment. In addition, this high pressure could excessively overdistend many lung units. Choice D is thus incorrect.

Another point to remember about RMs is that they are uncomfortable and can have important hemodynamic effects. Heavy sedation and/or paralysis may therefore be necessary. Moreover, hypotension and arrhythmias could occur in patients who are particularly volume sensitive and, thus, susceptible to the effects of high intrathoracic pressure.

Gattinoni L, Caironi P, Cressoni M, et al. Lung recruitment in patients with the acute respiratory distress syndrome. New Engl J Med. 2006; 354:1775–1786

Lim SC, Adams AB, Simonson DA, et al. Intercomparison of recruitment maneuver efficacy in three models of acute lung injury. Crit Care Med 2004; 32:2371–237

Crotti S, Mascheroni D, Caironi P, et al. Recruitment and derecruitment during acute respiratory failure. Am J Respir Crit Care Med 2001; 164:131–140

Benito S, LeMaire F. Pulmonary pressure volume relationships in acute respiratory distress syndrome in adults: role of positive end-expiratory pressure. J Crit Care 1990; 5:27–34

98. B. Cyclophosphamide.

Data best support the use of oral cyclophosphamide for the treatment of scleroderma-associated ILD with active alveolitis (choice B is correct). A randomized, double-blind, placebo-controlled trial of 158 patients with scleroderma, restrictive lung physiology, dyspnea, and evidence of inflammatory ILD in which participants received either oral cyclophosphamide (< 2 mg/kg/day) or placebo for 12 months found that, among patients treated with cyclophosphamide, 49% improved vs only 26% in the placebo group. Modest improvements in lung function, dyspnea, and health-related quality of life were noted in the treatment group. However, hematuria, leukopenia, anemia, and pneumonia were also more common in the treatment group.

It should be noted, however, that most of these benefits were not sustained over time. When these patients were observed for an additional 12 months, almost all of the improvements observed in the cyclophosphamide-treated group had waned and were no longer apparent. Thus, although cyclophosphamide is the best validated treatment option for active ILD associated with scleroderma, its effects are modest and transient; better therapies are clearly needed.

Although some small trials support the use of azathioprine in the setting of scleroderma-related lung disease, these data are less robust than those supporting the use of cyclophosphamide (choice A is incorrect). Cyclosporine does not have an established role in the treatment of ILD in this setting (choice C is incorrect). Glucocorticoids such as prednisone have been used to treat ILD associated with scleroderma, but their efficacy is unclear, and they should generally not be used because of concerns about increasing the risk of scleroderma renal crisis (choice D is incorrect).

Nadashkevich O, Davis P, Fritzler M, et al. A randomized unblinded trial of cyclophosphamide versus azathioprine in the treatment of systemic sclerosis. Clin Rheumatol 2006; 25:205–212

Strange C, Bolster MB, Roth MD, et al. Bronchoalveolar lavage and response to cyclophosphamide in scleroderma interstitial lung disease. Am J Respir Crit Care Med 2008; 177:91–98

Tashkin DP, Elashoff R, Clements PJ, et al. Cyclophosphamide versus placebo in scleroderma lung disease. N Engl J Med 2006; 354:2655–2666

Tashkin DP, Elashoff R, Clements PJ, et al. Effects of 1-year treatment with cyclophosphamide on outcomes at 2 years in scleroderma lung disease. Am J Respir Crit Care Med 2007; 176:1026–1034

White B, Moore WC, Wigley FM, et al. Cyclophosphamide is associated with pulmonary function and survival benefit in patients with scleroderma and alveolitis. Ann Intern Med 2000; 132:947–954

99. B. Prescribe a regular exercise program or refer him to a pulmonary rehabilitation program.

The results of exercise testing reveal a physiologically submaximal effort, with maximal workload, oxygen uptake, minute ventilation, and heart rate not even nearly achieved. The anaerobic threshold also apparently was not achieved,

and there is no evidence of arterial oxygen desaturation. Although the response of the flow-volume curves is abnormal and typical of COPD (*ie,* flow limitation associated with an increase in end-expiratory lung volume), there is still significant inspiratory reserve volume and expiratory flow available, suggesting that further increases in ventilation are achievable. The results are consistent with features often clinically attributed to deconditioning, but in the setting of submaximal physiologic effort. Patients with COPD and other conditions frequently limit their activity as a means of reducing the adverse symptoms they experience. As a result, over time, they often become limited for reasons other than their underlying disease process. In this instance, the results of exercise testing suggest that participation in a regular exercise program would allow the patient to experience meaningful and achievable benefit (choice B is correct).

Further attempts to enhance this patient's pharmacologic therapy would be the preferred option if he were primarily limited by his respiratory system during exercise (*ie,* either mechanical or gas exchange abnormalities), but this did not occur (choice C is incorrect). Although supplemental oxygen would provide some benefit by reducing ventilation for a given exercise workload, its effect would be minimal in the absence of significant oxygen desaturation (choice D is incorrect). Although underlying cardiac disease must always be considered in this setting, the clinical history is not highly suggestive of cardiac disease. Moreover, the absence of arrhythmias, significant ST segment or T-wave changes, and a normal BP response during exercise are reassuring at this stage in excluding a significant underlying cardiac etiology (choice A is incorrect).

O'Donnell DE, Aaron S, Bourbeau J, et al. Canadian Thoracic Society Recommendations for management of chronic obstructive pulmonary disease: 2007 update. Can Resp J 2007; 14:5B–32B

Rabe KF, Hurd S, Anzueto A, et al. Global strategy for the diagnosis, management, and prevention of chronic obstructive pulmonary disease: GOLD executive summary. Am J Respir Crit Care Med 2007; 176:532–555

Hamilton AL, Killian KJ, Summers E, et al. Symptom intensity and subjective limitation to exercise in patients with cardiorespiratory disorders. Chest 1996; 110:1255–1263

Weisman IM, Beck K, Casaburi R, et al. American Thoracic Society/American College of Chest Physicians joint statement on cardiopulmonary exercise testing. Am J Resp Crit Care Med 2003; 167:211–277

100. D. Azithromycin.

Patients with cystic fibrosis have a neutrophil-predominant inflammation in the airways. These neutrophils perpetuate the inflammatory cycle through the release of cytokines, chemotactants, and proteolytic enzymes. Thus, many patients with cystic fibrosis with more advanced lung disease will benefit from chronic antiinflammatory medications. The Cystic Fibrosis Foundation currently recommends azithromycin (500 mg po 3 days/week) for patients chronically infected with Pseudomonas (choice D is correct). Macrolide therapy was found to be beneficial in patients with panbronchiolitis, which led to empiric use by some physicians in patients with cystic fibrosis. Several well-conducted clinical trials have now shown that long-term use of azithromycin, which appears to act primarily as an antiinflammatory agent, is associated with improved lung function and a reduction in the number of exacerbations. In a large randomized trial, patients treated with azithromycin for 24 weeks had a statistically significant improvement in FEV_1 and fewer pulmonary exacerbations than a group receiving placebo. Prior to initiation, some experts recommend that sputum be examined for nontuberculous mycobacteria because macrolides would be an essential part of treatment, but, if used alone, there is a high incidence of emergent resistance and treatment failure.

Oral corticosteroids have been shown to improve pulmonary function in children with cystic fibrosis but are associated with an unacceptable rate of side effects, such as growth retardation, cataracts, and glucose intolerance, and not routinely used. Therefore, systemic glucocorticoids are only recommended for patients with asthma or allergic bronchopulmonary aspergillosis (ABPA) complicating their disease (choice A is incorrect). Inhaled steroids have been studied, with controversial results, and there are no large, well-designed clinical trials of inhaled corticosteroids in patients with cystic fibrosis. Therefore, inhaled corticosteroids also are only routinely recommended in cystic fibrosis patients with asthma (or significant airway hyperreactivity) or ABPA (choice B is incorrect). Ibuprofen also has been studied because of its ability to inhibit migration and activation of neutrophils. In high doses, ibuprofen does appear to slow the progressive decline in lung function, particularly in younger patients with more mild disease. Data on long-term safety are lacking; however, so it is not used routinely in patients with cystic fibrosis (choice C is incorrect).

Another consideration in this patient (which was not offered as a choice) would be the addition of hypertonic saline. Decreased airway surface liquid is an important factor in the underlying pathophysiology of cystic fibrosis. Osmotically drawing water onto the airway surface via inhalation of a hypertonic substance might help clear secretions and restore mucociliary transport. Inhaled hypertonic saline has been used for this purpose in patients with cystic fibrosis and has been associated with increased mucus clearance and improvement in lung function. In one long-term study, it has been associated with fewer exacerbations requiring antibiotic therapy. Inhaled mannitol has also been used for this purpose in patients with cystic fibrosis. There have been no randomized controlled trials comparing dornase alfa with hypertonic saline, but considering that the mechanism of action differs somewhat between the two, it is reasonable to assume that they may be complimentary. Twice-daily treatments (4 mL of 7% saline) in patients with chronic cough and sputum production can be considered. New treatment strategies for cystic fibrosis in development include gene therapy, correction of the abnormal folding of the CFTR protein, improvement in the ion channel function, induction of alternative ion channels, alternative means of suppressing the inflammatory responses, and newer antibiotics such as inhaled ciprofloxacin.

Davis JC, Alton E, Bush A. Clinical review: cystic fibrosis. Br Med J 2007; 335:1255–1259

Elkins MR, Robinson M, Rose BR, et al. A controlled trial of long-term inhaled hypertonic saline in patients with cystic fibrosis. N Engl J Med 2006; 354:229–240

Ratjen F. New pulmonary therapies for cystic fibrosis. Curr Opin Pulm Med 2007; 13:541–546

Flume PA, O'Sullivan BP, Robinson KA, et al. Cystic fibrosis pulmonary guidelines: chronic medications for maintenance of lung health. Am J Respir Crit Care Med 2007; 176:957–969

Saiman L, Marshall BC, Mayer-Hamblett N, et al. Azithromycin in patients with cystic fibrosis chronically infected with *Pseudomonas aeruginosa*: a randomized controlled trial. JAMA 2003; 290:1749–1756

101. D. Linezolid and ceftriaxone.

This patient was admitted with rapid-onset respiratory failure and pneumonia approximately 10 days after an influenza-like illness. The results of a chest radiograph and CT scan show a dense necrotizing pneumonia with signs of early mediastinitis consistent with a postinfluenza *Staphylococcus aureus* infection. Given his frequent contact with children and the increase in community-associated methicillin-resistant *S aureus* (MRSA), appropriate coverage for MRSA should be included in the antibiotic regimen, as well as coverage for community-acquired pneumonia (choice D is correct).

S aureus pneumonia classically occurs after influenza when the respiratory epithelium is damaged and ciliary function is altered, leading to difficulty removing pulmonary secretions. Subsequent aspiration of oral secretions colonized with *S aureus* leads to pneumonia. This effect is most profound in elderly patients, although younger adults and children are also susceptible to this type of infection. *Streptococcus pneumoniae* and *Haemophilus influenzae* can also cause postinfluenza pneumonia; therefore; the addition of appropriate coverage with ceftriaxone should be provided.

Over the last 8 years, the incidence of MRSA has increased in the community and has become increasingly associated with postinfluenza pneumonia. Given this patient's history of contact with children with impetigo, the likelihood of MRSA colonization is high, and antibacterial therapy should reflect this accordingly (choices A and C are incorrect). Community-associated MRSA pneumonia is severe, rapidly causing pulmonary necrosis with a high associated morbidity and mortality. From 2006 to 2007, the Centers for Disease Control and Prevention determined that 73% of the cases of postinfluenza *S aureus* pneumonia were caused by MRSA. Eighty-four percent of patients were hospitalized, and of the patients that were followed, 51% died. These community-associated strains also carried a leukocidin (Panton-Valentine leukocidin [PVL]) that appears to increase the development of necrosis and abscess formation in the lung and may be a large factor behind the severity of illness seen with these cases. Additionally, recent *in vitro* studies have shown that PVL production decreases dramatically when linezolid or clindamycin, protein synthesis inhibitor antibiotics, are administered. Conversely, the administration of nafcillin at low and high doses was shown to increase PVL production, but vancomycin had no effect. Thus, the addition of a protein synthesis inhibitor, such as clindamycin or linezolid, may be warranted in these cases.

The recent community-acquired pneumonia guidelines from the Infectious Diseases Society of America suggest considering MRSA pneumonia in an ICU patient with postinfluenza or severe necrotizing pneumonia with Gram-positive cocci on Gram stain of the sputum. Given that vancomycin has poor lung penetration, recommended dosing is

weight-based, with a dosing of 30 mg/kg divided twice daily for a normal creatinine clearance. Although vancomycin provides coverage for MRSA, the inadequate dose, along with poor lung penetration and the theoretical disadvantage of its poor activity against a PVL-producing strain of MRSA in this patient, makes it a poor choice (choice B is incorrect). Subsequent dosing should be directed toward a goal trough of 15 to 20 mg/L and adjusted accordingly.

Kallen AJ, Brunkard J, Moore Z, et al. *Staphylococcus aureus* community-acquired pneumonia during the 2006 to 2007 influenza season. Ann Emerg Med 2009; 53:358–365. Available at www.annemergmed.com/article/PIIS0196064408007737/fulltext. Accessed December 11, 2008

Severe methicillin-resistant *Staphylococcus aureus* community-acquired pneumonia associated with influenza: Louisiana and Georgia, December 2006–January 2007. MMWR 2007; 56:325–329

Mandell LA, Wunderink RG, Anzueto A, et al. Infectious Diseases Society of America/American Thoracic Society consensus guidelines on the management of community-acquired pneumonia in adults. Clin Infect Dis 2007; 44(suppl):S27–S72

Boucher HW, Corey GR. Epidemiology of methicillin-resistant *Staphylococcus aureus*. Clin Infect Dis 2008; 46(suppl):S344–S349

Stevens DL, Ma Y, Salmi DB, et al. Impact of antibiotics on expression of virulence-associated exotoxin genes in methicillin-sensitive and methicillin-resistant *Staphylococcus aureus*. J Infect Dis 2007; 195:202–211

102. B. Autotriggering.

Autotriggering is recognized by frequent (often > 1/s) rhythmic breaths that are caused by drops in airway pressure below the threshold for initiating a breath or inspiratory flow exceeding the flow-triggering threshold (choice B is correct) that is not related to breathing efforts. Although common causes include a leak in the ventilator circuit or a chest tube with air leak, autotriggering can occur as a result of water in the circuit or from cardiogenic oscillations. Autotriggering is more likely when the trigger threshold (flow or pressure) is set at an overly sensitive level, and autotriggering can often be eliminated by resetting the threshold. Autotriggering caused by cardiogenic oscillation is best studied in patients who had cardiac surgery. In one study, patients with frequent cardiogenic oscillation-induced autotriggering had larger cardiogenic oscillations, higher cardiac output, and larger heart size. Cardiogenic oscillations are noted in the airway flow tracing (arrows) of Figure 102-B. The change in volume of the beating heart causes changes in intrathoracic pressure, as well as cyclic compression and expansion of adjacent lung, producing low-level air flow.

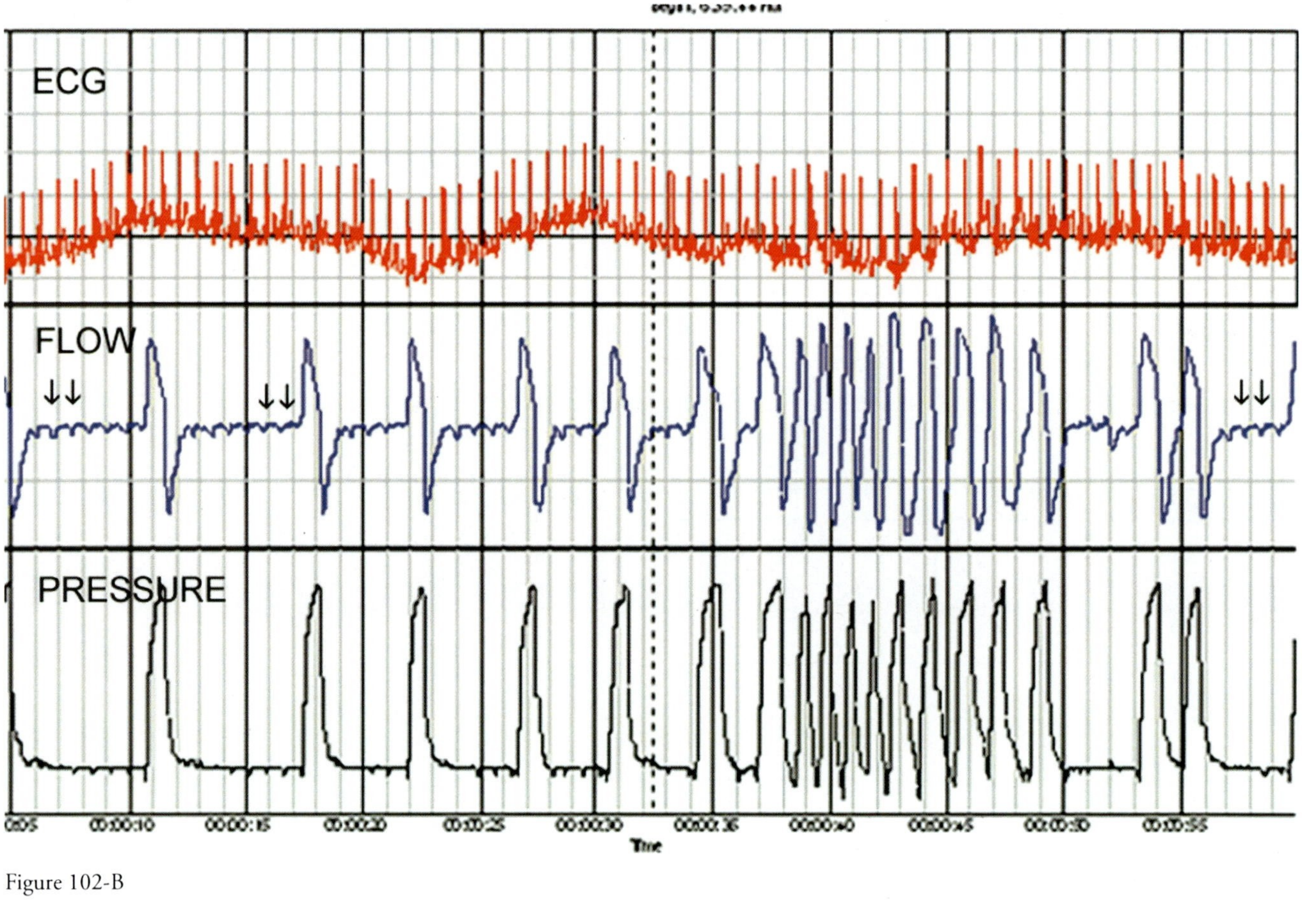

Figure 102-B

Double triggering is a form of patient ventilator asynchrony that can be recognized by the presence of two positive pressure breaths separated by a very brief (*ie,* less than one-half of the preceding inspiratory time) expiratory phase, as depicted at the arrow in Figure 102-C (choice A is incorrect). This is often the result of a patient's continued inspiratory effort beyond the relatively short duration of set inspiratory time, producing a drop in airway pressure early in exhalation that quickly triggers a second positive-pressure breath. Double triggering is generally regarded as the second most frequent asynchrony.

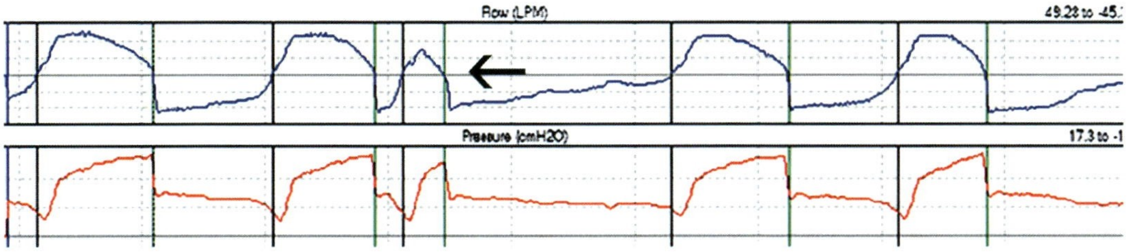

Figure 102-C

Ineffective triggering, the most common form of patient ventilator asynchrony, occurs when a patient's inspiratory effort to trigger a ventilator breath is unsuccessful. The patient's inspiratory effort produces a brief dip in airway pressure and small upward deflection in flow but does not elicit a full positive-pressure breath, as shown at the arrows in Figure 102-D (choice C is incorrect). The presence of auto-PEEP is a common cause of ineffective triggering.

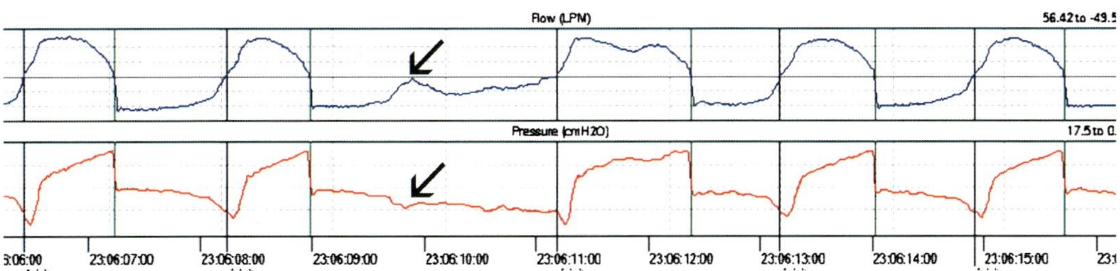

Figure 102-D

Flow asynchrony occurs when the ventilator flow is insufficient to match the patient's inspiratory flow and is recognized by a "scooped" or concave upward contour to the inspiratory phase of the pressure curve, as shown at the arrow in Figure 102-E (choice D is incorrect). When flow asynchrony is recognized, flow should be increased to meet the patient's demand.

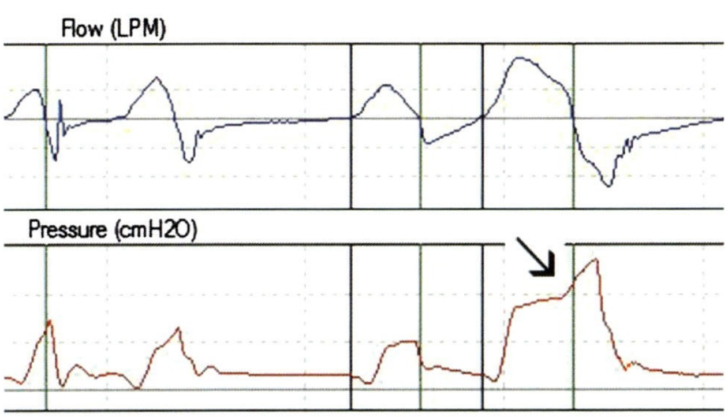

Figure 102-E

Thille AW, Rodriguez P, Cabello B, et al. Patient-ventilator asynchrony during assisted mechanical ventilation. Intensive Care Med 2006; 32:1515–1522

Nilsestuen JO, Hargett KD. Using ventilator graphics to identify patient-ventilator asynchrony. Respir Care 2005; 50:202–234
Georgopoulos D, Prinianakis G, Kondili E. Bedside waveforms interpretation as a tool to identify patient-ventilator asynchronies. Intensive Care Med 2006; 32:34–47
Imanaka H, Nishimura M, Takeuchi M, et al. Autotriggering caused by cardiogenic oscillation during flow-triggered mechanical ventilation. Crit Care Med 2000; 28:402–407
Imanaka H, Takeuchi M, Tachibana K, et al. Exhaled tidal volume overestimation in mechanically ventilated patients with large cardiogenic oscillation. Crit Care Med 2004; 32:1546–1549

103. C. Varenicline and behavioral therapy.

The correct answer is choice C, varenicline and behavioral therapy. Due to the potent CNS stimulant properties of nicotine, nicotine addiction and dependence has become a chronic relapsing disease, with tobacco-related illness remaining one of the most significant health problems in the world. Although 40% of tobacco users attempt to quit each year, more than 50% relapse within 1 year, and only 10% maintain permanent abstinence. The use of pharmacologic agents has been shown to improve abstinence rates.

Varenicline is the first approved drug in a relatively new class of agents for smoking cessation. Varenicline is unique in that it is a selective $\alpha_4\beta_2$ partial agonist active at the nicotinic acetylcholine receptor in the ventral tegmentum in the midbrain. The result is stimulation of release of dopamine that counteracts the common nicotine withdrawal symptoms (cognitive impairment, dysphoria, depression, mood fluctuations), while also serving as a partial antagonist by blocking further nicotine binding to the receptors. In two large (total $>$ 2,400 patients) randomized, placebo-controlled, double-blind, multicenter trials comparing varenicline for 12 weeks, bupropion for 12 weeks, and placebo for 12 weeks (all in combination with behavioral therapy), the varenicline arm was found to have superior 4-week (weeks 9 to 12) continuous abstinence rates of 44%, 30%, and 18%, respectively. A secondary endpoint of these studies was continuous abstinence rate from weeks 9 through 52, and varenicline was found to be superior to bupropion and placebo (statistically significant in one of the two studies) at 23%, 16%, and 8%, respectively (choice C is correct and choices B and D are incorrect). The major side effects reported with varenicline are nausea and insomnia. A 52-week follow-up, randomized, double-blind, placebo-controlled study examined an additional 12 weeks of drugs in those patients who had achieved successful abstinence in a 12-week open-label varenicline trial. In this study, continuous abstinence rates at weeks 13 through 24 were 71% for varenicline and 50% for placebo and, for weeks 13 through 52, 44% for varenicline and 37% with placebo. Other drugs with a similar action are currently under study, as are studies with nicotine vaccines.

Behavioral therapy (a smoking cessation class, individual or group counseling, telephone therapy, self-help materials, or a combination of these) by itself has not been shown to achieve comparable abstinence rates to patients receiving pharmacologic therapy (choice D is incorrect). Nicotine replacement therapy is more successful than placebo in achieving abstinence, but results are still not as favorable as when other pharmacologic agents are employed in combination or alone (choice A is incorrect). In a study comparing bupropion plus nicotine replacement therapy with bupropion alone, abstinence rates at 12 months were not significantly different than those achieved with bupropion alone but were well above those achieved in the placebo group.

Gonzales D, Rennard SI, Nides M, et al. Varenicline, an $\alpha_4\beta_2$ nicotinic acetylcholine receptor partial agonist vs sustained-release bupropion and placebo for smoking cessation: a randomized controlled trial. JAMA 2006; 296:47–55
Henningfield JE, Fant RV, Buchhalter AR, et al. Pharmacotherapy for nicotine dependence. CA Cancer J Clin 2005; 55:281–299
Jorenby DE, Hays JT, Rigotti NA, et al. Efficacy of varenicline, an $\alpha_4\beta_2$ nicotinic acetylcholine receptor partial agonist vs placebo or sustained-release bupropion for smoking cessation: a randomized controlled trial. JAMA 2006; 296:56–63
Nides M, Oncken C, Gonzales D, et al. Smoking cessation with varenicline, a selective $\alpha_4\beta_2$ nicotinic receptor partial agonist: results from a 7-week, randomized, placebo- and bupropion-controlled trial with 1-year follow-up. Arch Intern Med 2006; 166:1561–1568
Oncken C, Gonzales D, Nides M, et al. Efficacy and safety of the novel selective nicotinic acetylcholine receptor partial agonist, varenicline, for smoking cessation. Arch Intern Med 2006; 166:1571–1577
Ranney L, Melvin C, Lux L, et al. Systematic review: smoking cessation intervention strategies for adults and adults in special populations. Ann Intern Med 2006; 145:845–856
Tonstad S, Tonnesen P, Hajek P, et al. Effect of maintenance therapy with varenicline on smoking cessation: a randomized controlled trial. JAMA 2006; 296:64–71

104. B. It will overdiagnose obstruction in older subjects and underdiagnose obstruction in younger subjects.

The spirometric measurement of lung function is a key component of making a diagnosis of airflow obstruction. The Global Obstructive Lung Disease (GOLD) consortium criterion for airflow obstruction is an FEV_1/FVC ratio less than 0.70, regardless of age. While this value is appealing because it is simple to apply to all patients, the recent National Health and Nutrition Examination Survey III (NHANES III) data on spirometry in normal subjects demonstrate clearly that the FEV_1/FVC ratio declines with age. Moreover, the 95% CI reflecting the lower limit of normal begins to fall below this 0.70 threshold in subjects entering their sixth decade, and it is substantially below this value in subjects in their eighth and ninth decades.

Several large spirometry databases of adult patients have been analyzed retrospectively to document the magnitude of the discrepancies in the two approaches. One reported overall discordance in 11.7% of all tests and up to 35% overdiagnosis of obstruction using the fixed 0.70 cutoff in certain older age groups. Another revealed up to 20% overdiagnosis in older subjects and up to 60% underdiagnosis in the youngest subjects when using a fixed cutoff of 0.70 (choice B is correct; choices A, C, and D are incorrect).

Because of these observations, many authorities advocate using a lower limit of normal cutoff for the FEV_1/FVC ratio to diagnose obstruction, rather than 0.70. However, recently reported data have examined the long-term outcomes of adults whose FEV_1/FVC ratio was less than 0.70 but above the lower limit of normal. Interestingly, this group had a similar mortality to those with an FEV_1/FVC ratio above 0.70, but they did have a higher hospitalization rate. These data suggest that subjects in this group have airway dysfunction, even though their values are above the lower limit of normal. These results also argue for incorporating outcome data in selecting diagnostic thresholds for tests.

Aggarwal AN, Gupta D, Behera D, et al. Comparison of fixed percentage method and lower confidence limits for defining limits of normality for interpretation of spirometry. Respir Care 2006; 51:737–743

Hankinson JL, Odencrantz JR, Fedan KB. Spirometric reference values from a sample of the general US population. Am J Respir Crit Care Med 1999; 159:179–187

Hansen JE, Sun XG, Wasserman K. Spirometric criteria for airway obstruction: use percentage of FEV_1/FVC ratio below the fifth percentile, not <70%. Chest 2007; 131:349–355

Roberts SD, Farber MO, Knox KS, et al. FEV_1/FVC ratio of 70% misclassifies patients with obstruction at the extremes of age. Chest 2006; 130:200–206

Quadrelli S, Roncoroni A, Montiel G. Assessment of respiratory function: influence of spirometry reference values and normality criteria selection. Respir Med 1999; 93:523–535

105. C. Switch to liposomal amphotericin B.

The histologic specimen reveals the characteristic nonseptated, wide-angle branching hyphae of Mucor. Mucormycosis is an invasive fungal disease seen most commonly in patients with an underlying immunodeficiency. Patients with hematologic malignancies are at risk, particularly when they are neutropenic. In these patients, the lungs are the most frequent site of infection, with sinus being the second most common. Recent reports suggest that there may be a rise in the number of cases of mucormycosis in the era of empiric or prophylactic voriconazole use.

Mucormycosis is almost uniformly fatal without treatment. Mortality is significant even with therapy, but survival rates averaging 60% can be seen when some form of antifungal therapy is used. The best response rates have been documented with the use of liposomal amphotericin B (choice C is correct). Although voriconazole has been shown to be superior to amphotericin B in the treatment of invasive aspergillosis, this azole has no activity against Mucor (choice A is incorrect).

Posaconazole is a newer generation oral extended-spectrum triazole agent, structurally similar to itraconazole. Although itraconazole is not active against Mucor (choice D is incorrect), *in vitro* studies, animal models, and case reports indicate that posaconazole has activity against this pathogen and may play a role in the treatment of

patients with invasive infections. As the data are still limited, it should be reserved for patients who fail therapy with amphotericin B (choice B is incorrect).

Combination antifungal therapies have been studied in an attempt to improve the high mortality of invasive fungal infections in these patients. Most studies have been conducted in patients with invasive aspergillosis, and although the initial reports appear promising, they are limited to small numbers of patients and typically involve salvage therapy only. Therefore, larger randomized trials of patients are needed before combination therapy can be recommended.

Whenever possible, surgical debridement or resection should be considered, as this improves survival. Other options to consider are endobronchial antifungal therapy (either inhaled or instilled bronchoscopically) and immune augmentation strategies (colony-stimulating factors, granulocyte transfusions, and interferon-γ).

Kontoyiannis DP, Lionakis MS, Lewis RE, et al. Zygomycosis in a tertiary-care cancer center in the era of aspergillus-active antifungal therapy: a case-control observational study of 27 recent cases. J Infect Dis 2005; 191:1350–1360
Roden MM, Zaouitis TE, Buchanan WL, et al. Epidemiology and outcome of zygomycosis: a review of 929 reported cases. Clin Infect Dis 2005; 41:634–653
Raad II, Graybill JR, Bustamante AB, et al. Safety of long-term posaconazole use in the treatment of refractory invasive fungal infections. Clin Infect Dis 2006; 42:1726–1734
Shao P, Huang L, Hsueh P. Invasive fungal infection: laboratory diagnosis and antifungal treatment. J Microbiol Immunol Infect 2006; 39:178–188

106. A. Lung cancer is the most common non–AIDS-defining malignancy.

Patients with HIV infection have a several-fold increased risk of developing lung cancer compared with matched control populations, and lung cancer is the most common non–AIDS-defining malignancy in HIV-infected people (choice A is correct). With increasing use of combination ART around the world, the incidence of opportunistic infections and AIDS-defining neoplasms (Kaposi sarcoma and non-Hodgkin lymphoma) has declined, but the incidence of other cancers in patients with HIV infection has remained stable or increased. Although most cohorts with HIV infection are current or former smokers, their risk of developing lung cancer appears to be increased even when incidence ratios are adjusted for smoking. The prevalence of microsatellite alternations reflecting genomic instability occurs with greatly increased frequency in HIV-associated lung cancers, possibly playing a role in the pathogenesis.

The risk of developing lung cancer does not seem to be related to the severity of immunosuppression because most patients with lung cancer and HIV do not have severely reduced CD4+ lymphocyte counts (choice B is incorrect). In contrast with the general population, where the incidence of lung cancer has declined steadily over the last decade, the incidence among patients with HIV has not decreased, despite the introduction of ART in 1996 (choice C is incorrect). It is also unlikely that HIV itself is oncogenic, at least for lung cancer. The potential roles of increased susceptibility to carcinogens or even oncogenicity of ART remain unexplored.

Patients with lung cancer in the setting of HIV infection tend to be relatively young at presentation (mean age 45 years), and the majority present with stage III or IV disease, similar to age-matched HIV-uninfected control patients. As in the general population, adenocarcinoma is the most common histologic type, but the prognosis appears to be worse in patients with HIV infection (choice D is incorrect). Until further studies are performed, the diagnostic and therapeutic approaches to HIV-associated lung cancer are the same as for other patients, although the efficacy and toxicity of chemotherapy and radiotherapy may be different.

Lavolé A, Wislez M, Antoine M, et al. Lung cancer, a new challenge in the HIV-infected population. Lung Cancer 2006; 51:1–11
Wistuba II, Behrens C, Milchgrub S, et al. Comparison of molecular changes in lung cancers in HIV-positive and HIV-indeterminate subjects. JAMA 1998; 279:1554–1559
Engels EA, Brock MV, Chen J, et al. Elevated incidence of lung cancer among HIV-infected individuals. J Clin Oncol 2006; 24:1383–1388
Patel P, Hanson DL, Sullivan PS, et al. Incidence of types of cancer among HIV-infected persons compared with the general population in the United States, 1992–2003. Ann Intern Med 2008; 148:728–736

107. A. A 27-year-old man is treated for pneumococcal bacteremic pneumonia with clarithromycin. A sputum culture produces a macrolide-resistant strain (erythromycin MIC_{90} = 2 µg/mL).

Breakpoints for antimicrobial susceptibility have been developed to guide physicians in the treatment of serious bacterial infections. They were initially devised for closed space infections such as meningitis but have been extended to other therapeutic areas such as pneumonia. The relationship between clinical failure and *in vitro* resistance is clear in meningitis but rather obscure in pneumonia. Macrolide resistance generally falls into two categories: low-level resistance (90% minimum inhibitory concentration [MIC_{90}] ranges from 0.5 to 8 µg/mL), thought to be mainly related to a bacterial efflux pump mechanism (*mefE* gene, M phenotype), and high-level resistance ($MIC_{90} \geq 16$ µg/mL), most often related to alteration of the macrolide-binding site (*ermAM* gene, MLSB phenotype). In a 5-year surveillance study, among 1,696 episodes of pneumococcal bacteremia, 60 (3.5%) were failures of outpatient macrolide therapy. Macrolide failures were significantly more common among cases of pneumococcal bacteremia: isolates exhibiting an erythromycin MIC_{90} of 1 µg/mL (resistant strains) and isolates exhibiting an $MIC_{90} \leq 0.25$ µg/mL (susceptible strains; choice A is correct). Low-level resistance conferred by *mefA* and high-level resistance conferred by *ermB* were equally overrepresented among macrolide failures. This is the best evidence presented to date that confirms macrolide resistance of any mechanism is associated with clinical failure if discordant therapy is given.

In a prospective, international, observational study of 844 hospitalized patients with blood culture results positive for *Streptococcus pneumoniae*, 15% of isolates had *in vitro* intermediate susceptibility to penicillin (MIC, 0.12 to 1 µg/mL), and 9.6% of isolates were resistant (MIC $\geq$ 2 µg/mL). Age, severity of illness, and underlying disease with immunosuppression were significantly associated with mortality; penicillin resistance was not a risk factor for mortality. Discordant therapy (inactive *in vitro*) with penicillins, cefotaxime, and ceftriaxone (but not cefuroxime) did not affect mortality rate. Similarly, the time required for defervescence and frequency of suppurative complications was not associated with concordance of β-lactam antibiotic therapy (choices B and C are incorrect).

Reduction in *S pneumoniae* susceptibility to fluoroquinolones can result from spontaneous mutations in the quinolone resistance–determining regions (QRDRs) of genes encoding subunits of topoisomerase IV (*parC*) or DNA gyrase (*gyrA*), the targets for these agents. Resistance occurs in a stepwise fashion, with first-step mutations in one target gene (either *parC* or *gyrA*) resulting in low-level resistance and second-step mutations in the other target gene (either *parC* or *gyrA*) leading to higher levels of resistance. Resistance to fluoroquinolones can also be the result of an active efflux mechanism. The ratio of the area under the serum concentration-time curve (AUC) of a given antibiotic to the MIC of the patient's infecting pathogen (*ie*, the AUC/MIC ratio), has been directly linked to the probability of a successful clinical or microbiological outcome. For Gram-positive microorganisms, an AUC/MIC ratio of > 35 has been associated with bacterial eradication and good clinical outcome. Resistance can emerge more readily for antimicrobial agents that have AUC/MIC ratios of < 35, such as ciprofloxacin and levofloxacin, than for more active agents that have AUC/MIC ratios of > 80, such as moxifloxacin, gatifloxacin, and gemifloxacin. Although there have been well-documented clinical failures in pneumococcal-infected patients treated with levofloxacin or ciprofloxacin related to preexisting resistance or the development of resistance during therapy, there has not been a single report of a clinical failure that was the result of resistance following therapy with moxifloxacin, gatifloxacin, or gemifloxacin (choice D is incorrect).

Vanderkooi OG, Low DE, Green K, et al. Predicting antimicrobial resistance in invasive pneumococcal infections. Clin Infect Dis 2005; 40:1288–1297

Daneman N, McGeer A, Green K, et al. Macrolide resistance in bacteremic pneumococcal disease: implications for patient management. Clin Infect Dis 2006; 43:432–438

Yu VL, Chiou CCC, Feldman C, et al. An international prospective study of pneumococcal bacteremia: correlation with *in vitro* resistance, antibiotics administered, and clinical outcome. Clin Infect Dis 2003; 37:230–237

Tleyjeh IM, Tlaygeh HM, Hejal R, et al. The impact of penicillin resistance on short-term mortality in hospitalized adults with pneumococcal pneumonia: a systematic review and meta-analysis. Clin Infect Dis 2006; 42:788–797

Fuller JD, Low DE. A review of *Streptococcus pneumoniae* infection treatment failures associated with fluoroquinolone resistance. Clin Infect Dis 2005; 41:118–121

108. B. Discontinue interferon/ribavirin therapy.

The CT scan reveals subcarinal and hilar lymphadenopathy (see Figure 108-A) and peribronchovascular opacities with mild beading of vascular bundles (see Figure 108-B). This, combined with the well-formed noncaseating granulomas seen on transbronchial biopsy (see Figure 108-C), is diagnostic of sarcoidosis. However, given the onset of symptoms after initiation of interferon/ribavirin therapy, the possibility of interferon-induced sarcoidosis should be considered, and the initial approach should be discontinuation of interferon/ribavirin therapy (choice B is correct).

There have been numerous reports of sarcoidosis complicating either interferon or interferon/ribavirin therapy but no reports of ribavirin alone causing the disease. The mechanism is most likely related to an imbalance of T_H1 to T_H2 cells. Interferon-α given as part of hepatitis C therapy increases interferon-γ production by CD4+ T cells, upregulating the T_H1 response thought to be key to granuloma formation in sarcoidosis. This may be more likely to occur as a complication of interferon therapy in individuals with an interferon-α17 polymorphism.

The clinical disease caused by interferon mimics sarcoidosis, with pulmonary and cutaneous involvement being most common, but reports of parotid swelling and eye, neurologic, and joint involvement are well described. In almost all cases reported, the disease went into remission with withdrawal or, in some cases, with reduction in the dose of interferon. Cutaneous involvement may respond to topical steroid treatment even with continued interferon therapy and, similarly, there have been responses reported to systemic steroid therapy. However, if possible, primary therapy should involve discontinuation of interferon treatment.

There are case reports of interferon-induced sarcoidosis responding to oral corticosteroids. However, corticosteroids may increase the burden of hepatitis C virus, both *in vivo* and *in vitro*; thus, caution should be used if contemplating therapy (choice A is incorrect). Patients with hepatitis C are at increased risk of developing hepatic malignancies that may rarely metastasize to the lungs, but there is no increased risk of bronchogenic carcinoma and nothing in the biopsy to suggest malignancy (choice C is incorrect). Chronic hepatitis C infection and TB infection are both more common in HIV-positive individuals and/or IV drug users, and hepatitis might be a risk factor for the development of TB in chronically immunosuppressed renal transplant patients. However, there is no evidence that hepatitis C infection increases the risk for TB in immunocompetent individuals, and there is nothing to suggest this disease in the current case (choice D is incorrect).

Doyle MK, Berggren R, Magnus JH. Interferon-induced sarcoidosis. J Clin Rheumatol 2006; 12:241–248

Yan KKL, Dinihan I, Freiman J, et al. Sarcoidosis presenting with granulomatous uveitis induced by pegylated interferon and ribavirin therapy for hepatitis C. Intern Med J 2008; 38:207–210

Hurst EA, Mauro T. Sarcoidosis associated with pegylated interferon alfa and ribavirin treatment for chronic hepatitis C: a case report and review of the literature. Arch Dermatol 2005; 141:865–868

Goldberg HJ, Fiedler D, Webb A, et al. Sarcoidosis after treatment with interferon-alpha: a case series and review of the literature. Respir Med 2006; 100:2063–2068

109. B. Chest physiotherapy.

This patient has bronchiectasis, as evidenced by his high-resolution CT showing a "signet ring" (bronchus larger than accompanying airway; see Figure 109-D, arrow) and markedly dilated and thickened airways (see Figure 109-E, arrows). These CT findings are radiographically diagnostic of bronchiectasis. The patient's chest radiograph shows bilateral cystic changes (see Figure 109-F, small arrows) and tram tracks (enlarged bronchi with thickened parallel walls; see Figure 109-F, large arrow), findings diagnostically supportive of bronchiectasis. Of the therapies offered, chest physiotherapy is the most appropriate (choice B is correct). Chest physiotherapy may be accomplished by a variety of interventions including chest percussion, vibration, and postural drainage and is used to facilitate mucus mobilization.

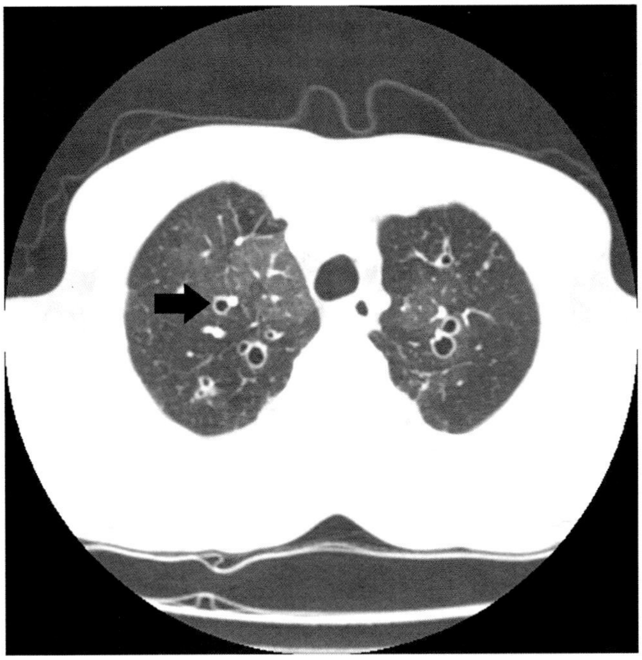

Figure 109-D

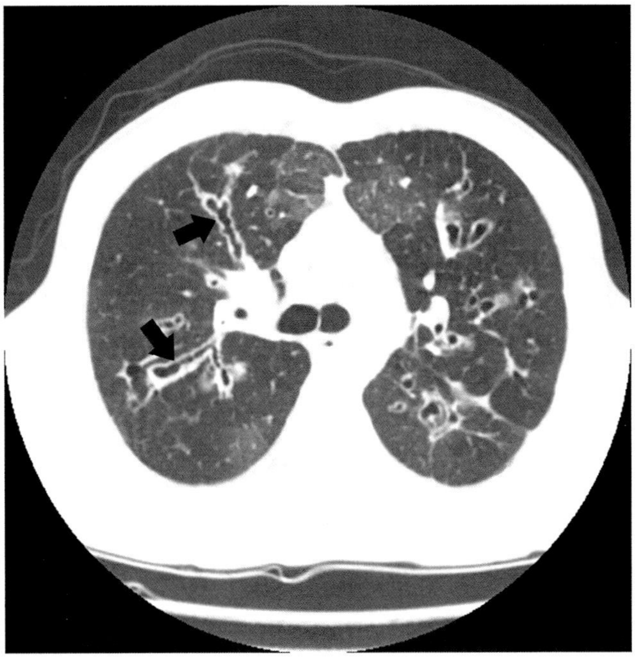

Figure 109-E

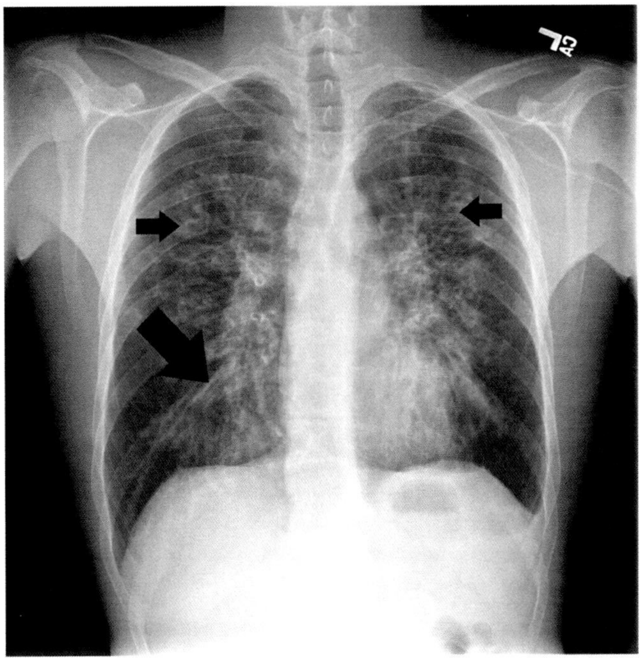

Figure 109-F

Bronchiectasis is the abnormal and irreversible dilation of the bronchi manifest by chronic coughing (productive of mucoid sputum), airway obstruction, and recurrent infections. Multiple etiologies are possible, and evaluation is necessary to rule out potentially causative and treatable diseases (as pursued in this patient). Most often in the adult population, the etiology is either idiopathic (as in this patient; roughly 50 to 80%) or occurs after infection. CF, ruled out in this patient as a cause of bronchiectasis, is the most common genetically inherited disorder in the white population.

Treatment of non-CF bronchiectasis, in addition to focusing on any discovered precipitating cause, should be individualized. Included in the patient care is a microbiological examination of the sputum for routine bacterial

and nontuberculous mycobacterium. Although rotating antibiotics is commonly used and may have small benefits in reducing sputum volume and purulence, evidence from well-controlled trials is forthcoming. Chronic antibiotic use may promote the emergence of resistant organisms. (However, in an acute exacerbation of bronchiectasis, antibiotics should be used and tailored to the sputum microbiology findings.) Similarly, mobilization of secretions (bronchopulmonary hygiene), by chest physiotherapy, is a mainstay of bronchiectasis management. Chest physiotherapy (choice B is correct) has modest effects on increasing sputum volume, but the long-term impact is unknown and, compared with the other treatment choices, has the least potential negative impact. Although beneficial in patients with CF, inhaled tobramycin in non-CF patients with bronchiectasis is not recommended and appears to increase bronchospasm (choice A is incorrect). Similarly, recombinant human DNase, a mucolytic, produces no improvement in non-CF patients with bronchiectasis; has adverse effects, including FEV_1 decline; and should not be a mainstay of therapy (choice C is incorrect). Although inhaled corticosteroids and oral macrolides may reduce airway inflammation, additional trials are needed. One series in patients with bronchiectasis not caused by CF showed that administration of azithromycin was associated with a decrease in infective exacerbations and chronic symptoms, including sputum volume. Systemic steroids have not been studied in a controlled fashion in non-CF bronchiectasis, and chronic systemic corticosteroids have significant side effects and are not recommended (choice D is incorrect). Short-acting inhaled bronchodilators and anticholinergic agents in patients with airflow obstruction and/or bronchial hyperreactivity may be of some benefit, but to our knowledge, no randomized trials exist.

O'Donnell AE. Bronchiectasis. Chest 2008; 134:815–823

Rosen MJ. Chronic cough due to bronchiectasis: American College of Chest Physicians evidence-based clinical practice guidelines. Chest 2006; 129(suppl):122S–131S

King P. Is there a role for inhaled corticosteroids and macrolide therapy in bronchiectasis? Drugs 2007; 67:965–974

Rubin B. Aerosolized antibiotics for non-cystic fibrosis bronchiectasis. J Aerosol Med Pulm Drug Deliv 2008; 21:71–76

Davies G, Wilson R. Prophylactic antibiotic treatment of bronchiectasis with azithromycin. Thorax 2004; 59:540–541

110. D. Potassium chloride.

This patient has an alkalemic pH and elevated serum bicarbonate level consistent with the presence of an alkalosis. This patient likely has a chloride-responsive alkalosis due to the vomiting and volume contraction. IV sodium chloride and potassium chloride should be administered at this time (choice D is correct).

The decreased $Paco_2$ indicates a concurrent respiratory alkalosis. The increased anion gap indicates the presence of a metabolic acidosis. This represents a "triple acid-base disorder." The vomiting generated the metabolic alkalosis by eliminating hydrogen ions and maintained the alkalosis through extracellular volume depletion; decreased chloride concentration resulted in hypokalemia, preventing the kidney from excreting the excess bicarbonate.

The treatment of metabolic alkalosis in all cases involves correction of the underlying disorder that has generated the disturbance. If this condition has already been resolved, other factors that maintain the alkalosis should be investigated and treated.

Acetazolamide can be beneficial by increasing renal bicarbonate excretion; however, it is not necessary in this instance because the normal saline will likely help to resolve this problem, and the patient is able to tolerate the volume expansion (choice C is incorrect). H2 blockers can prevent the loss of hydrogen ions (as can occur through nasogastric suctioning); however, that would not be the next step in management of this patient (choice B is incorrect). IV infusion of hydrochloric acid can rapidly lower the blood pH. This patient has no significant sequellae (*eg*, cardiac dysrhythmias or tetany) from the severe alkalosis, and the risk of providing hydrochloric acid potentially outweighs the benefits (choice A is incorrect).

Smith JD, Bia MJ, DeFronzo RA. Clinical disorders of potassium metabolism. In: Arieff AI, DeFronzo RA, eds. Fluid, electrolyte and acid based disorders. New York, NY: Churchill Livingstone, 1985; 413–510
Sabatini S, Kurtzman NA. Metabolic alkalosis. In: Narins RG, ed. Clinical disorders of fluid and electrolyte metabolism. 5th ed. San Francisco, CA: McGraw-Hill Book Company, 1993; 933–956
Androgue HG, Madias NE. Management of life-threatening acid-base disorders. N Engl J Med 1998; 338:107–111

111. C. Argatroban.

This patient has a high likelihood of having developed heparin-induced antiplatelet antibodies, and if so, she is at risk for progressive clotting. Accordingly, she needs ongoing treatment with a nonheparin anticoagulant that will be safe in the context of her new renal dysfunction. Argatroban would be the drug of choice under these circumstances (choice C is correct).

Heparin-induced thrombocytopenia (HIT) is a well-recognized adverse reaction to unfractionated heparin and low-molecular-weight heparin (LMWH) therapy. HIT may occur with exposure to any type of heparin therapy, including infusions, subcutaneous injections, and even low-dose IV flushes. HIT represents a prothrombotic state arising from the development of antibodies to the heparin–platelet factor 4 (PF4) complex. Despite the thrombocytopenia that often signals the evolution of HIT, the patient is clinically prothrombotic. Rates of both arterial and venous thrombosis are increased in the initial days following the onset of HIT and gradually decrease over 30 days when heparin is discontinued. Given the high associated rate of arterial and venous thrombosis with HIT and associated morbidity, it is recommended to immediately discontinue all heparin products and provide anticoagulation therapy with an alternative medication while awaiting confirmatory laboratory tests.

The choice of alternative anticoagulants should include patient-related factors (associated organ failure, need for intervention and reversing anticoagulation, and risk of bleeding) and drug-related factors (pharmacokinetic properties of the drug, immunogenicity of the alternative drug, and availability). LMWH agents such as enoxaparin should not be considered as an alternative, given the high cross-reactivity to the PF4-heparin antibody (choice D is incorrect).

Current treatment recommendations do not include the use of the synthetic factor 10a inhibitor fondaparinux for the treatment of HIT (choice A is incorrect). Experience with fondaparinux for the treatment of HIT is limited to case reports and retrospective analyses, and one report associated fondaparinux with the development of HIT.

Warfarin should not be used as an initial alternative anticoagulant agent for the management of the patient with acute HIT. Initial use of warfarin has been causally linked with warfarin-associated ischemia and necrosis. Initiation of warfarin therapy for the treatment of a thrombosis is deferred until the platelet count has recovered. Additionally, the need for urgent intervention in the ICU environment may preclude the use of warfarin and its sustained anticoagulant effect.

The remaining alternative agents are the direct thrombin inhibitor (DTI) agents: lepirudin, bivalirudin, and argatroban. Bivalirudin use is largely limited to procedures, such as cardiac catheterization. All of the direct thrombin inhibitors exert their anticoagulant effect by inhibition of thrombin. There are some important distinguishing characteristics for each of the DTI agents that may make a specific agent ideal more suitable for a given patient.

Lepirudin is excreted primarily renally, and the dosing needs to be adjusted for patients with renal impairment. Importantly, there are no current recommendations on dosing adjustments for lepirudin for patients receiving

continuous renal replacement therapy. There are different dosing recommendations for lepirudin therapy depending on whether treatment is for isolated HIT by laboratory criteria alone (0.1 mg/kg/h infusion) or HIT with thrombosis (0.4 mg/kg bolus and 0.15 mg/kg/h adjusted for renal impairment). Additionally, the titration parameter of activated partial thromboplastin time (aPTT) is 1.5 to 2.5 times baseline, which is different than for argatroban. Additionally, lepirudin has been associated with inducing an immunogenic reaction and anaphylaxis in a small number of patients. For these reasons and because this patient is exhibiting significant renal dysfunction, lepirudin would not be a good choice for this patient (choice B is incorrect).

Argatroban is primarily cleared through the liver, necessitating dose adjustments for patients with liver impairment. Anecdotally, a lower dose is recommended for critically ill patients, although there is no official recommendation. To further differentiate argatroban from lepirudin, the aPTT goal for argatroban is 1.5 to 3 times the baseline value. There are no reported cases of immunogenic or anaphylactic reactions with argatroban therapy.

Warkentin TE, Greinacher A, Oster A, et al. Treatment and prevention of heparin-induced thrombocytopenia: American College of Chest Physicians evidence-based practice guidelines (8th edition). Chest 2008; 133(suppl):340S–380S

Warkentin TE. Heparin-induced thrombocytopenia: pathogenesis and management. Br J Haematol 2003; 121:535–555

Dager WE, Dougherty JA, Nguyen PH, et al. Heparin-induced thrombocytopenia: treatment options and special considerations. Pharmacotherapy 2007; 27:564–587

Warkentin TE, Maurer BT, Aster RH. Heparin-induced thrombocytopenia associated with fondaparinux. New Engl J Med 2007; 356:2653–2655

112. B. Schedule a repeat polysomnography with adaptive servoventilation titration.

Baseline polysomnographic data demonstrate the presence of sleep-disordered breathing, with respiratory events consisting mostly of obstructive apneas and hypopneas. Increasing numbers of central apneas develop during CPAP titration, suggesting the diagnosis of complex sleep apnea. Adaptive servoventilation has been shown to be an effective positive airway pressure modality for this disorder (choice B is correct).

APAP devices, which provide variable pressures using device-specific diagnostic and therapeutic algorithms, are not indicated for the therapy of complex sleep apnea (choice A is incorrect). Unless the emerging central apneas are postarousal in nature secondary to significant sleep disruption, hypnotic agents are unlikely to be of benefit (choice C is incorrect). Finally, supplemental oxygen is not recommended as a primary therapy for obstructive sleep apnea (OSA). Although oxygen therapy can potentially improve nocturnal oxygen saturation, there is a risk of possibly increasing apnea duration (choice D is incorrect).

Complex sleep apnea is considered by many clinicians as a distinct form of sleep-related breathing disorder that is characterized by the development of central apneas or Cheyne-Stokes respiration with acute application of CPAP therapy in people who initially have predominantly obstructive or mixed apneas. Thus, CPAP successfully eliminates obstructive respiratory events, but apnea-hypopnea indices remain significantly elevated, and sleep disruption persists because of central apneas and hypopneas.

Central apneas are postulated to occur when application of CPAP leads to a reduction of $Paco_2$ below the apneic threshold and persists until $Paco_2$ has risen above eupneic levels (see Table 112-1). The probability of central apneas developing is, thus, greater in patients with a narrow difference between baseline $Paco_2$ and the apneic threshold (CO_2 reserve) and increased respiratory sensitivity to $Paco_2$ (controller gain). In complex sleep apnea, the application of CPAP decreases $Paco_2$ below the apneic threshold, in part by improving physiologic shunt and decreasing work of breathing. Changes in baroreflex sensitivity during CPAP therapy may also contribute to the development of complex sleep apnea.

Table 112-1. Pathophysiology of Complex Sleep Apnea

Application of CPAP
⇓
Reduction of $Paco_2$ below apneic threshold
⇓
Development of central apnea
⇓
Increase in $Paco_2$ above apneic threshold
⇓
Cessation of central apnea/Resumption of breathing
⇓
Hyperventilatory overshoot
⇓
Reduction of $Paco_2$ below apneic threshold

Complex sleep apnea is estimated to develop in about 15% of patients with OSA who are undergoing CPAP titration. Complex sleep apnea shares many of the clinical features of OSA, including habitual snoring, witnessed apneas, insomnia, and nocturnal dyspnea, none of which reliably distinguishes the two syndromes from each other. Patients with complex sleep apnea have been reported to have a slightly lower BMI than those with OSA but a higher BMI, more frequent snoring, less congestive heart failure, and higher left ventricular ejection fraction than those with central sleep apnea (CSA). Compared with OSA, there is a greater occurrence of complex sleep apnea in men. The mean age at presentation is similar to that of OSA.

During polysomnography, CSA, periodic breathing, or Cheyne-Stokes respiration develops during application of CPAP in patients with initially predominant obstructive respiratory events and results in clinically significant sleep disruption with frequent arousals. CSAs persist despite additional pressure increases, whereas obstructive or mixed apnea reemerges with lowering of CPAP pressures. Residual CSAs appear to be more prevalent during nonrapid eye movement sleep compared with rapid eye movement (REM) sleep. Oxygen desaturation, if present, is generally less severe compared with that accompanying obstructive or mixed apneas.

Although the long-term clinical response to CPAP therapy is not well characterized, persistence of CSAs over time during CPAP therapy has been described. CSAs also tend to persist during multiple attempts at CPAP retitration. Adaptive servoventilation (ASV) uses an automatic minute ventilation-targeted device. Using breath-to-breath analysis, it provides constant pressure and airflow readjustment to maintain steady minute ventilation. In one retrospective study involving 100 subjects who underwent ASV titration (63% for complex sleep apnea), this device demonstrated superior effectiveness for complex sleep apnea compared with CPAP and bilevel positive airway pressure therapy, with greater improvements in apnea-hypopnea indices, % REM sleep, and arousal indices.

Morgenthaler TI, Gay PC, Gordon N, et al. Adaptive servoventilation versus noninvasive positive pressure ventilation for central, mixed, and complex sleep apnea syndromes. Sleep 2007; 30:468–475

Morgenthaler TI, Kagramanov V, Hanak V, et al. Complex sleep apnea syndrome: is it a unique clinical syndrome? Sleep 2006; 29:1203–1209

Snigdha S, Pusalavidyasagar SS, Olson EJ, et al. Treatment of complex sleep apnea syndrome: a retrospective comparative review. Sleep Med 2006; 7:474–479

Allam JS, Olson EJ, Gay PC, et al. Efficacy of adaptive servoventilation in treatment of complex and central sleep apnea syndromes. Chest 2007; 132:1839–1846

Pusalavidyasagar SS, Olson EJ, Gay PC, et al. Treatment of complex sleep apnea syndrome: a retrospective comparative review. Sleep Med 2006; 7:474–479

113. B. Functional residual capacity.

The major changes in pulmonary function testing in pregnancy are a progressive decrease in the expiratory reserve volume by 8 to 40% and a decrease in residual volume by 7 to 22%, both of which are due to the enlarging uterus and diaphragmatic elevation. Because of these changes, functional residual capacity, in turn, decreases by 10 to 25% by the third trimester of pregnancy (choice B is correct). Total lung capacity may decrease slightly, inspiratory capacity increases, and vital capacity does not change significantly during pregnancy (choice C is incorrect). The decrease in residual volume with a relatively maintained total lung capacity results in a low ratio of residual volume to total lung capacity.

Tidal volume increases significantly during pregnancy by 150 mL to a final value of 450 to 600 mL, or a 30 to 50% increase in the average patient (choice D is incorrect). This is most likely due to a direct progesterone-mediated increase in central respiratory drive and enhancement of the hypercapnic ventilatory drive. There is little or no change in the respiratory rate during pregnancy, and tachypnea is an unusual finding. Because of the increase in tidal volume, there is a significant increase in resting minute ventilation from 6 L in the nonpregnant state to 9 L at full term (or 20 to 50% above baseline).

There are no significant changes in peak flow rates, FEV_1, airway resistance, or maximum voluntary ventilation during pregnancy (choice A is incorrect). Although lung compliance does not change significantly during pregnancy, there is a reduction in total respiratory compliance because of a reduction in chest wall compliance as a result of an elevated diaphragm caused by uterine enlargement by the third trimester. Diffusing capacity of the lung for carbon monoxide may increase slightly in the first trimester followed by a slight decrease later in pregnancy, likely due to alterations in pulmonary vascular volume.

Elkus R, Popovich JL. Respiratory physiology in pregnancy. Clin Chest Med 1992; 13:555–565
Unterborn J. Pulmonary function testing in obesity, pregnancy, and extremes of body habitus. Clin Chest Med 2001; 22:759–767

114. D. Uninterpretable values because of system leak.

One of the hallmarks of obstructive lung disease is air trapping or the inability to empty the lungs in the available expiratory time. This leads to lung hyperinflation and places the diaphragm at a mechanical disadvantage. With exercise and an increased minute ventilation, air trapping can increase, which further limits function.

To assess air trapping, measurements of FRC and RV can be done. Common techniques include whole body plethysmography, inert gas equilibration techniques, and nitrogen washout. In this patient, the nitrogen washout technique is being used. This involves breathing 100% oxygen starting at the FRC. Over time, the oxygen completely washes out the nitrogen in the lung and, knowing that the fractional concentration of nitrogen in inspired gas is 0.8 in the initial room air, the lung volume at the beginning of the maneuver can be calculated.

In this patient, the high RV suggests air trapping and hyperinflation. However, the washout curve shows several instances where the nitrogen concentration suddenly increases (see Figure 114-B, panel a). This is a reflection of intermittent leaks in the system, allowing nitrogen in the room air to enter the breathing circuit. This will lead to a much slower-appearing washout and, thus, gross overestimation of the lung volumes. Therefore, the patient's data are uninterpretable because of these leaks. Choice D is thus correct, and choices A, B, and C are incorrect.

In addition to washing out the lungs and calculating the FRC, the pattern of the washout can also be instructive. In healthy lungs with even gas mixing, the washout curve is essentially a straight line (see Figure 114-B, panel b).

In contrast, where gases are poorly mixed (often the case in obstructive lung disease), the washout curve is curvilinear (see Figure 114- B, panel c).

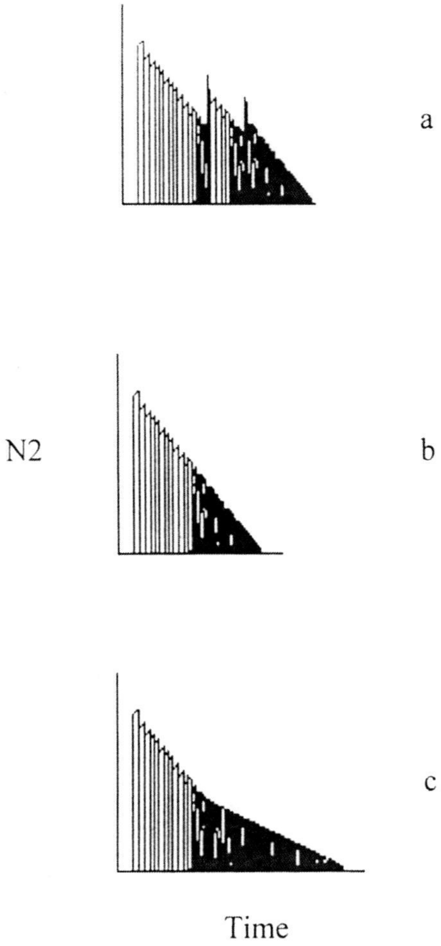

Figure 114-B

ATS-ERS Task Force. Standardization of the measurement of lung volume. Eur Respir J 2005; 26:511–522
Macklem PT. Relationship between lung mechanics and ventilation distribution. Physiology 1973; 16:580–588
Fleming GM, Chester EH, Sanii J, et al. Ventilation inhomogeneity using multibreath nitrogen washout. Am Rev Resp Dis 1980; 121:789–794
Bouhuys A. Pulmonary nitrogen clearance in relation to age in healthy males. J Appl Physiol 1963; 18:297–300
Fowler WS, Cornish ER, Kety SS. Lung function studies VIII: analysis of alveolar ventilation by pulmonary nitrogen clearance curves. J Clin Invest 1952; 31:40–50

115. A. Ganglioneuroma.

Neurogenic tumors, such as ganglioneuromas, are the most common masses in the posterior mediastinum (choice A is correct). On the posteroanterior chest radiograph, one can recognize that this mass is located in the posterior mediastinum by noting the location of the mass above the clavicles (see Figure 115-B, arrow). Use of a T1-weighted MRI (see Figure 115-C) is helpful in determining vertebral column and spinal cord involvement (the arrow is directed at the mass). Other entities that can appear as posterior mediastinal masses include aortic aneurysm, enteric cyst, hiatal hernia, esophageal tumor, bronchogenic tumor, paraspinal abscess, or extramedullary hematopoiesis.

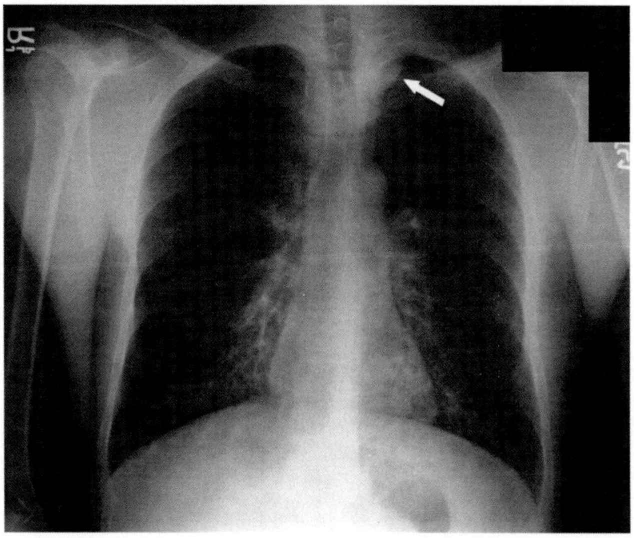

Figure 115-B

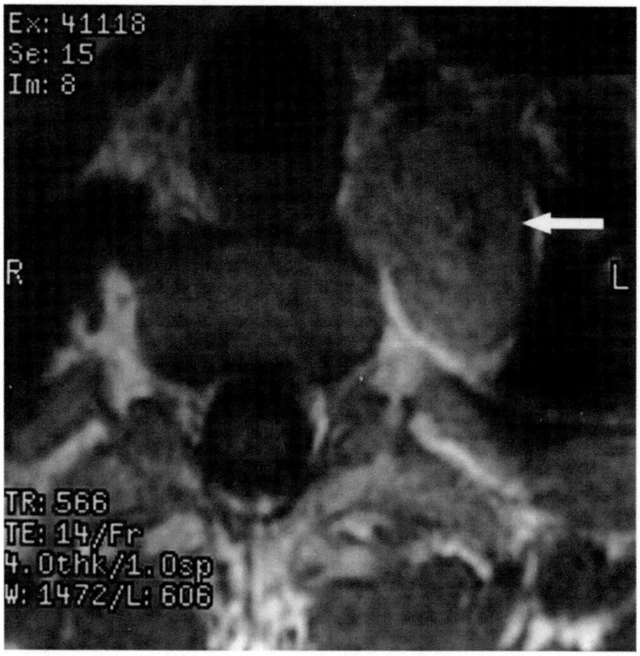

Figure 115-C

Ganglioneuromas are benign tumors that may grow very slowly over a number of years. Along with other neurogenic tumors that may develop in this area, such as ganglioneuroblastoma and neuroblastoma, they develop from mediastinal peripheral nerves, sympathetic and parasympathetic ganglia, and embryonic remnants of the neural tube. Ganglioneuromas can be asymptomatic or cause pain or Horner syndrome by compression of neurologic structures. Excision of the neoplasm is usually curative.

Lymphoma, parathyroid adenoma, and teratoma typically occur in the anterior, rather than the posterior, compartment of the mediastinum (choices B, C, and D are incorrect). In addition, thymoma, goiter, ascending aortic aneurysm, esophageal tumor, angiomatous tumor, lipoma, Morgagni hernia, or pericardial cyst are commonly found in the anterior compartment. Masses in the middle mediastinum are most commonly lymphoma, lymph node hyperplasia, bronchogenic tumor, or bronchogenic cyst.

Duwe BV, Sterman DH, Musani AI. Tumors of the mediastinum. Chest 2005; 128:2893–2909
Marchevsky AM. Mediastinal tumors of peripheral nervous system origin. Semin Diagn Pathol 1999; 16:65–78
Strollo DC, Rosado-de-Christenson ML, Jett JR. Primary mediastinal tumors: Part 2. Tumors of the middle and posterior mediastinum. Chest 1997; 112:1344–1357

116. D. Inform the patient of the diagnosis of primary hyperventilation syndrome and explore possible contributing factors.

The results of exercise testing are characteristic of primary hyperventilation syndrome. The cardinal finding in this condition is the abnormal breathing pattern during exercise, an impressive increase in ventilation, minute ventilation ($\dot{V}_E$)/carbon dioxide output ($\dot{V}CO_2$), and respiratory frequency, accompanied by decreases in $PaCO_2$ and/or end-tidal CO_2 ($PETCO_2$). Breathing pattern is very erratic, with striking tachypnea (see Figure 116-C, arrow), and excessive for the simultaneous metabolic stress.

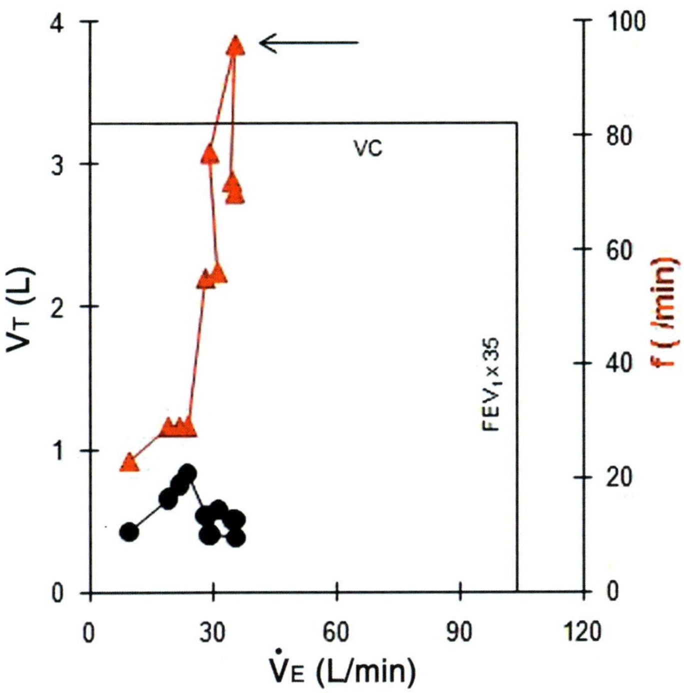

Figure 116-C
VT = tidal volume; f = respiratory frequency; V̇E = expired volume per unit time.

The flow-volume curves during exercise in this case also are typical because, although the behavior of operational lung volumes is markedly abnormal, they are uncharacteristic for any physiologic abnormality such as obstructive or restrictive lung disease. Exercise is typically terminated in the absence of cardiopulmonary abnormality, and patients with this condition may report exertional dyspnea, chest pain, and light-headedness, often due to anxiety and stress, and occasionally with no apparent psychopathology. Once the diagnosis is established, a careful search for these symptoms and stressors should be undertaken (choice D is correct).

There are no findings from the physical examination, chest radiograph, resting pulmonary function testing, or cardiopulmonary exercise testing to suggest interstitial lung disease or a connective tissue disease (choices A and B are incorrect). Moreover, the clinical presentation and the findings from cardiopulmonary exercise testing do not infer pulmonary vascular disease (choice C is not correct). Although these conditions often are causes of unexplained dyspnea and should be considered, a thoughtful and systematic approach to exclude these conditions (and others such as asthma) should always be undertaken. Unexplained dyspnea is one of the most common reasons for referral for cardiopulmonary exercise testing.

Waraich S, Seitsema KE. Clinical cardiopulmonary exercise testing: patient and referral characteristics. J Cardiopulm Rehabil Prev 2007; 27:400–406

Weisman IM, Zeballos RL. Clinical evaluation of unexplained dyspnea. Cardiologia 1996; 41:621–34

Weisman IM, Beck K, Casaburi R, et al. American Thoracic Society/American College of Chest Physicians joint statement on cardiopulmonary exercise testing. Am J Respir Crit Care Med 2003; 167:211–277

117. A. A serum IgE level.

The patient has poorly controlled asthma despite fairly aggressive medical therapy. In addition, he has a marked peripheral eosinophilia. His CT scan (see Figure 117-B) reveals multifocal tree-in-bud opacities (thick white arrows), peribronchial dilatation and thickening, and endobronchial plugging in the right upper lobe (thin white arrow). The two conditions to consider in patients with asthma who have worsening symptoms and eosinophilia are allergic

bronchopulmonary aspergillosis (ABPA) and Churg-Strauss syndrome. Although the parenchymal abnormalities are consistent with either condition, the likely bronchial mucus plug and central bronchiectasis noted on the CT, the lack of extrapulmonary symptoms, and the normal C-reactive protein level and sedimentation rate make ABPA more likely than Churg-Strauss syndrome (choice A is correct and choice B is incorrect). In patients with asthma, the diagnosis of ABPA is based on a combination of clinical, biological, and radiologic criteria (asthma, sinusitis, immediate cutaneous reaction to *Aspergillus fumigatus*, total serum IgE level > 1,000 ng/mL [1 mg/L], elevated *A fumigatus* serum IgE levels, precipitating antibodies to *A fumigatus* in the serum, peripheral eosinophilia, fleeting parenchymal infiltrates, and central bronchiectasis). The serum IgE level test is thought to be the most useful laboratory test for ABPA because it also correlates with disease activity. Although IgE levels can be elevated in patients with the Churg-Strauss syndrome, they are not usually elevated to the same degree as in ABPA and almost never > 1,000 µg/L (1 mg/L).

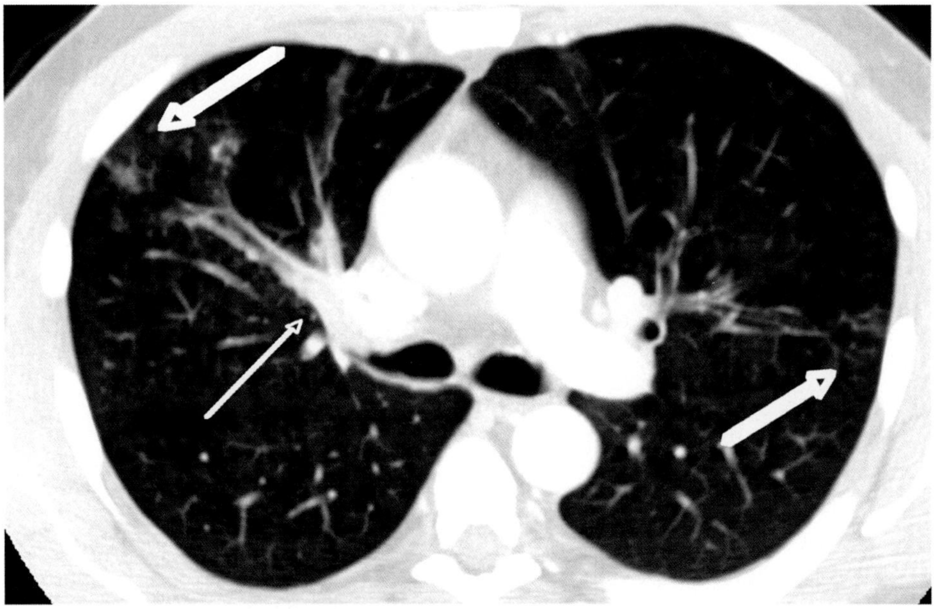

Figure 117-B

In patients with poorly controlled asthma, it is also prudent to assess for conditions known to complicate the management of the disease, such as gastroesophageal reflux disease or sinusitis. Nothing in the patient's history is strongly supportive of either condition, and the eosinophilia would be uncommon in these conditions (choice C is incorrect). In addition, although patients with Churg-Strauss syndrome often have paranasal sinus abnormalities, obtaining a sinus CT would not be specific in differentiating this condition from ABPA.

The presence of the endobronchial abnormality is initially concerning for an endobronchial mass. However, mucus impaction has been shown to have a very high attenuation on CT scanning (the plug is visually more dense than the normal skeletal muscles). This finding, which is present in this patient, is very characteristic, if not pathognomonic, of ABPA. Given the patient's fairly classic presentation, which is consistent with ABPA, an endobronchial mass is unlikely, and bronchoscopy would not be necessary (choice D is incorrect).

ABPA is caused by a hypersensitive reaction to *A fumigatus,* which results in immune activation, worsening asthma, recurrent pulmonary infiltrates, and bronchiectasis. The disease occurs in 1 to 2% of patients with persistent asthma and 2 to 15% of patients with cystic fibrosis. The diagnostic criteria already have been discussed. The mainstay of therapy for patients with ABPA remains oral corticosteroids. The recommended dose for the acute phase is 0.5 mg/kg/day for the first 2 weeks, followed by a progressive decrease over the next 6 to 8 weeks. Itraconazole

appears to be effective adjunctive therapy. Studies suggest that, when used in combination with oral corticosteroids, itraconazole can reduce airway inflammation, the number of acute exacerbations, and disease progression. It may also allow for lower effective dosing of the corticosteroids. Metaanalysis suggests that itraconazole modifies the immunologic activation associated with ABPA and improves clinical outcome.

Tillie-Leblond I, Tonnel AB. Allergic bronchopulmonary aspergillosis. Allergy 2005; 60:1004–1013

Agarwal R, Gupta D, Aggarwal AN, et al. Allergic bronchopulmonary aspergillosis: lessons from 126 patients attending a clinic in North India. Chest 2006; 130:442–448

Wark P, Gibson PG, Wilson A. Azoles for allergic bronchopulmonary aspergillosis associated with asthma. Cochrane Database Syst Rev 2004; 3: CD001108

Feong YF, Kim K, Seo IF, et al. Eosinophilic lung diseases: a clinical, radiologic, and pathologic overview. Radiographics 2007; 27:617–639

118. B. If her interferon-γ release assay is negative, her reactive TST is from the BCG or non-TB mycobacteria exposure.

As a health-care worker, she is considered reactive to the TST at ≥ 10 mm. Therefore, on the basis of the TST, she is considered reactive. However, the purified protein derivative (PPD) used in the TST may react with the *Mycobacterium bovis* BCG proteins or other environmental mycobacteria, thus producing a reactive test. With an interferon-γ release assay (IGRA), *Mycobacterium tuberculosis* RD1 proteins are used that are absent from *M bovis* BCG or environmental bacteria. Thus, discordance between the TST and IGRA occurs when TST reactivity is due to BCG vaccination or environmental mycobacterial exposure with a negative IGRA. With a negative IGRA and a reactive TST, her reaction is from her BCG vaccination prior to immigration (choice B is correct).

Health-care workers and immigrants from areas of high TB disease (within 5 years of immigration) are considered to be reactive at ≥ 10-mm induration. Administration of the TST is usually performed by the intradermal Mantoux method, with administration of 0.1 mL PPD. When administered intradermally, a small wheal and flare should arise. Subcutaneous administration leads to false-negative, not false-positive results, and the TST should be repeated (choice D is incorrect). When assessing the TST, induration, not erythema, is measured at 48 to 72 h after testing. Prior BCG or environmental mycobacterial exposure can lead to a reactive TST (choice A is incorrect). Prior history of BCG vaccination has no impact on reactivity reading when evaluating individuals with intermediate-to-high risk. In individuals who have received BCG and are at low risk (areas of low endemicity and no exposure or travel), high false-positive rates can occur with TST, and thus, IGRA may be useful in determining latent TB from BCG or environmental exposure. In addition, a false-negative TST can be boosted by a reaction to the test itself. This is usually seen in individuals with a TB infection from many years ago and whose delayed hypersensitivity reaction has diminished with time. In order to differentiate a new infection from a boosting effect, an initial test is given, and if negative, a repeat TST is done 2 to 3 weeks later. Reactivity is measured. This procedure is usually done in the first testing of individuals who will undergo routine screening, such as a new health-care worker. However, in this case, the patient has no history of TB or recent TST, so a boosting effect is unlikely (choice C is incorrect).

The IGRA may be a more specific test in certain circumstances: 93 to 99% in BCG-naive populations compared with 59 to 97% for patients who had a TST. An IGRA is an *ex vivo* T-cell–based assay where exposure to a TB-specific protein, such as RD1, occurs. T cells exposed to TB will produce interferon-γ when reexposed to these proteins. The sensitivity ranges from 60 to 80%, depending on study population, cutoff values, and the antigen used. A metaanalysis showed that the pooled T-SPOT.TB test (Oxford Immunotec; Marlborough, MA) had a higher sensitivity (90%, range 86 to 93%) than the two QuantiFERON assays (QuantiFERON-TB Gold; Cellestis, Ltd; Carnegie, Victoria, Australia: 78%, range 73 to 82%; QuantiFERON-TB Gold In-Tube; Cellestis, Ltd; Carnegie, Victoria, Australia: 70%, range 63 to 78%). Although this observation is factually correct, the studies were not all head-to-head trials.

Among trials that directly compared these tests, the T-SPOT.TB test was still more sensitive (7%, range 0 to 25%). The sensitivity was higher among non–BCG-vaccinated populations (97%, range of 95 to 99%) when compared with BCG-vaccinated populations (59%, range of 46 to 73%).

Concordance between TST and IGRA varies but is roughly 50 to 80%, depending on the study. Discordance can occur with BCG sensitization or environmental bacteria in areas of lower endemicity of TB. However, in areas of high TB rates, many individuals with BCG vaccination and a reactive TST also had a positive IGRA, suggesting a high rate of latent TB infections in these individuals (IGRA results were negative in the BCG-vaccinated control patients from the United Kingdom).

Brock I, Weldingh K, Lillebaek T, et al. Comparison of tuberculin skin test and new specific blood test in tuberculosis contacts. Am J Respir Crit Care Med 2004; 170:65–69

Lalvani A, Nagvenkar P, Udwadia Z, et al. Enumeration of T cells specific for RD1-encoded antigens suggests a high prevalence of latent *Mycobacterium tuberculosis* infection in healthy urban Indians. J Infect Dis 2001; 183:469–477

Hill PC, Brookes RH, Fox A, et al. Large-scale evaluation of enzyme-linked immunospot assay and skin test for diagnosis of *Mycobacterium tuberculosis* infection against a gradient of exposure in The Gambia. Clin Infect Dis 2004; 38:966–973

American Thoracic Society and the Infectious Diseases Society of America. Targeted tuberculin testing and treatment of latent tuberculosis infection. Official Statement of the American Thoracic Society and the Infectious Diseases Society of America. Am J Respir Crit Care Med 2000; 161(suppl):S221–S247

Pai M, Zwerling A, Manzies D. Systemic review: T-cell based assays for the diagnosis of latent tuberculosis infection: an update. Ann Intern Med 2008; 149:177–187

119. C. Maximum exercise tests demonstrate cardiovascular limitation to exercise.

This patient has pectus excavatum, a congenital condition characterized by a concave depression of the anterior chest wall. It is usually noted in childhood, although symptoms, such as dyspnea with exertion, chest pain at the site of the pectus deformity, and being easily fatigued, typically become apparent in adolescence or adulthood. Interestingly, dyspnea is largely related to impaired cardiovascular performance. Evidence from maximum exercise tests demonstrates cardiovascular limitation, rather than ventilatory limitation (choice C is correct).

Pulmonary function test results are typically normal or reveal only a mild restrictive ventilatory defect (choice A is incorrect). During exercise testing, some patients experience restriction of ventilation, as indicated by limitations in the increase in tidal volume that usually accompany exercise. In studies of maximal incremental exercise testing performed in active individuals who have severe pectus excavatum, however, patients exhibited prominent cardiovascular limitation, with significantly reduced maximum oxygen uptake and oxygen-pulse, whereas no ventilatory limitation was observed. Imaging and physiologic studies show that pectus excavatum can reduce cardiac output and stroke volume, primarily as the result of compression of the right ventricular outflow tract and the right ventricle, not of the left ventricle or outflow (choice D is incorrect). These findings are accentuated during exercise. The pectus severity index (PSI), which is calculated as the inner width of the chest divided by the distance between the posterior surface of the sternum and the anterior surface of the spine on CT scan or standard posteroanterior and lateral radiographs of the chest, is a common measure of deformity. Our patient's PSI is about 3.0 because chest width is about 300 mm (see Figure 119-C), and the sternal-spine distance is 100 mm (see Figure 119-D). In one study, patients with higher PSIs (*ie*, > 4.0) were eight times more likely to have impaired aerobic capacity on formal exercise testing.

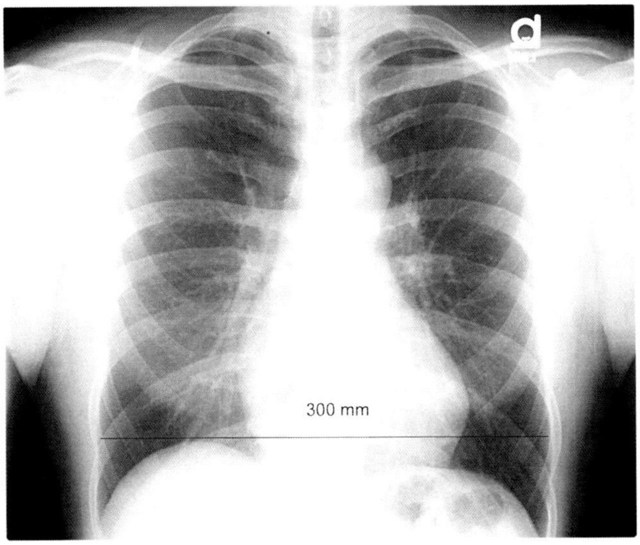

Figure 119-C

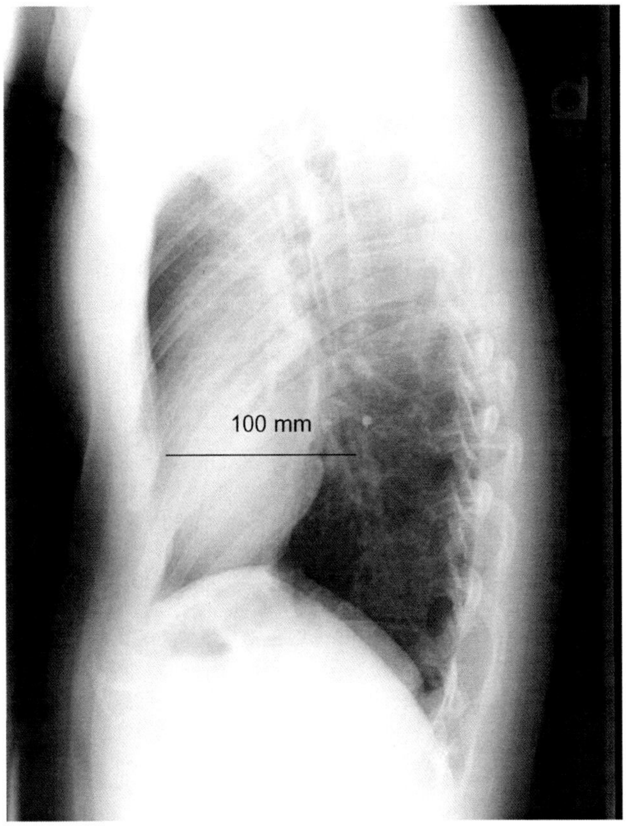

Figure 119-D

Surgical repair is generally performed using the "highly modified Ravitch repair"—an open operation with a transverse inframammary incision—or the minimally invasive (or Nuss) repair. Most surgery is performed in children and adolescents, although there is a sizeable incidence in adults. In many instances, the indication for surgery is primarily cosmetic, with good success toward this goal. However, in symptomatic patients, it is commonplace for surgery to result in symptomatic improvement, with improved exercise tolerance and endurance, as well as reduction in chest pain. The effect of surgery on pulmonary function has been variable among studies, but a metaanalysis demonstrates no significant impact of surgery on pulmonary function (choice B is incorrect). Although less well studied, improved cardiac function is commonly noted after surgery.

Castile RG, Staats BA, Westbrook PR. Symptomatic pectus deformities of the chest. Am Rev Respir Dis 1982; 126:564–568
Malek MH, Fonkalsrud EW, Cooper CB. Ventilatory and cardiovascular responses to exercise in patients with pectus excavatum. Chest 2003; 124:870–882
Fonkalsrud EW. Current management of pectus excavatum. World J Surg 2003; 27:502–508
Guntheroth WG, Spiers PS. Cardiac function before and after surgery for pectus excavatum. Am J Cardiol 2007; 99:1762–1764
Fonkalsrud EW, DeUgarte D, Choi E. Repair of pectus excavatum and carinatum deformities in 116 adults. Ann Surg 2002; 236:304–312

120. A. Patent foramen ovale.

High-altitude pulmonary edema (HAPE) is a form of pulmonary edema that generally occurs 2 to 3 days after rapid ascent to altitudes >8,500 feet (2,590 m) and at lower altitudes in people with increased susceptibility to the disorder. Some people are clearly at increased risk of developing HAPE compared with others. The risk is increased in those with agenesis of a pulmonary artery and increased fourfold in patients with patent foramen ovale; it is present in around 25% of the population (choice A is correct). Patients who have experienced an episode of HAPE are clearly at risk of developing the condition again after ascending to high altitudes. The pathophysiology of HAPE is complex, but common findings in those who are susceptible include blunted ventilatory responses and increased pulmonary vasoconstrictive responses to hypoxia, decreased nitric oxide synthesis, and increased sympathetic tone.

Hypoxic pulmonary hypertension at altitude may lead to capillary stress failure in overperfused areas with formation of alveolar edema. In addition, susceptible people appear to have deficient clearance of alveolar edema fluid. Exaggerated pulmonary vasoconstriction at altitude increases right-to-left shunt through a patent foramen ovale, exacerbating hypoxemia and edema formation.

There is genetic predisposition to developing HAPE in those with the human leukocyte antigen-DR6 phenotype, but there is no increased risk in people with asthma or advanced age (choices B and C are incorrect). Administration of salmeterol before ascent was shown to *decrease* the incidence of HAPE in susceptible subjects (*ie*, those with a prior episode) by more than 50% compared with placebo (74% with placebo, 33% with salmeterol) (choice D is incorrect). This may occur through β-adrenergic agonist-mediated upregulation of transepithelial sodium clearance and enhanced alveolar edema clearance. Nifedipine also reduces the risk of developing HAPE, perhaps by reducing pulmonary artery pressure. People susceptible to developing HAPE should be counseled against travel to high altitude or, if they must go, to use one or both of these preventive measures. It is not possible to counsel people whose risk of HAPE is unknown on how to best prevent the disorder.

Treatment of HAPE centers on descent, while maintaining oxygenation with supplemental oxygen. Nifedipine accelerates recovery during descent, but the effectiveness of salmeterol in treating established HAPE is unproven. A portable hyperbaric chamber consisting of an airtight bag pressurized by a manual pump is also available in mountaineering expeditions.

Allemann Y, Huter D, Lipp E, et al. Patent foramen ovale and high-altitude pulmonary edema. JAMA 2006; 296:2954–2958
Barry PW, Pollard AJ. Altitude illness. BMJ 2003; 326:915–919
Hackett PH, Roach RC. High-altitude illness. N Engl J Med 2001; 345:107–114
Sartori C, Allemann Y, Duplain H, et al. Salmeterol for the prevention of high-altitude pulmonary edema. N Engl J Med 2002; 346:1631–1636

121. B. Pulmonary and spinal TB.

The syndrome of inappropriate antidiuretic hormone secretion (SIADH) is defined as the following: (1) hyponatremia with corresponding hypoosmolality of the serum and extracellular fluid; (2) continued renal excretion of sodium; (3) absence of clinical evidence of fluid volume depletion (*ie*, normal skin turgor and BP); (4) osmolality of the urine greater than appropriate for the tonicity of the plasma (*ie*, urine less than maximally dilute); (5) normal renal function; and (6) normal adrenal function. SIADH has been described in a variety of conditions, including respiratory disorders, such as pulmonary TB, pneumonias, and bronchogenic carcinoma. The basic management of SIADH is restriction of water intake, in addition to the treatment of the primary disorder. Our patient clearly has SIADH, and the differential diagnosis should include disorders associated with this syndrome.

Our patient has had weight loss, flank pain, a chest radiographic abnormality showing a right lung density, and evidence on CT scan and MRI of an epidural abscess. While many entities can cause thoracic spine destruction, intervertebral disc destruction strongly suggests an infectious process. In this patient, a nonsmoking Indian immigrant, the most likely diagnosis is TB of the spine (tuberculous spondylitis, or "Pott disease") (choice B is correct). A needle aspiration of the epidural abscess confirmed the diagnosis. Assessment by an orthopedic surgeon or neurosurgeon is appropriate, because there may be cord compression, even if there are no clinical features to suggest it. Most patients respond to routine antituberculous chemotherapy without surgical intervention. In most series of skeletal TB, Pott disease makes up 50 to 70% of cases reported. In adults, the lower thoracic and upper lumbar vertebrae are most commonly involved, whereas, in children, the upper thoracic vertebrae predominate. Evidence of previous or current pulmonary TB is found in about 50% of patients. Most patients present with pain, with or without systemic signs of infection.

While the patient has SIADH, she is not receiving any medication that has been associated with this syndrome (choice C is incorrect). Common medications associated with SIADH are chlorpropamide, carbamazepine, cyclophosphamide, vincristine, vinblastine, amitriptyline, haloperidol, the selective serotonin reuptake inhibitors,

and the monoamine oxidase antidepressants. Metastatic lung cancer can be associated with SIADH but would not account for the epidural abscess visualized on MRI (choice A is incorrect). Histoplasmosis, while rarely associated with SIADH, would be unlikely to cause the destruction of the vertebrae and the epidural abscess (choice D is incorrect).

Adrogue HJ, Madias NE. Hyponatremia. N Engl J Med 2000; 342:1581–1589
Chung DK, Hubbard WW. Hyponatremia in untreated active pulmonary tuberculosis. Am Rev Respir Dis 1969; 99:595–597
Moorthy S, Prabhu NK. Spectrum of MR imaging findings in spinal tuberculosis. AJR Am J Roentgenol 2002; 179:979–983

122. D. Mortality best correlates with degree of cardiac involvement.

This patient has primary amyloidosis, and mortality best correlates with cardiac involvement (choice D is correct). Patients with cardiac amyloidosis have a mean survival of 6 months from the time of diagnosis The typical findings on echocardiography include a nondilated left ventricle with thickened and hyperrefractile walls and a mild diffuse hypokinesis. The right ventricle, interatrial septum, and atrioventricular valves can also be thickened. Prognosis is also very poor after pulmonary disease is diagnosed, with median survivals reported between 12 and 16 months (choice B is incorrect). However, pulmonary disease significantly contributes to mortality in only around 10% of cases (choice C is incorrect).

Amyloidosis is a disorder of protein folding in which normally soluble proteins are deposited as abnormal, insoluble fibrils that disrupt tissue structure and cause disease. The biopsy specimen (see Figure 73-A in the stem) shows pulmonary amyloid deposition, vascular and interstitial involvement, and focal alveolar hemorrhage and hemosiderin-laden macrophages. A Congo Red stain shows organophilic deposits and, under polarized light, an appearance of apple-green birefringence.

Amyloidosis is classified based on the subtype of protein that forms the amyloid fibril. The most common proteins are amyloid L (AL), seen in primary amyloidosis, and amyloid A (AA), seen in secondary amyloidosis. AL protein is composed of monoclonal light chains and is associated with multiple myeloma and plasma cell dyscrasias (as in this patient). The AA protein is an acute phase reactant of hepatic origin associated with a variety of chronic inflammatory conditions. Primary amyloidosis tends to be a more aggressive disease with a shorter survival than secondary/reactive amyloidosis.

The incidence of pulmonary involvement associated with secondary (AA) amyloidosis is low. In contrast, primary amyloidosis commonly involves the respiratory tract, with several autopsy series estimating the incidence to be above 85%. Pulmonary disease in primary amyloidosis can be isolated solely to the respiratory tract, or more commonly, as part of a systemic disease. The localized form can present with upper airway involvement in the form of endobronchial amyloid tumors or pulmonary nodules. Endobronchial tumors may produce cough, wheezing, dyspnea, and hemoptysis and can be mistaken for asthma. Diffuse interstitial or alveolar-septal amyloid infiltration is the most common pattern. Rarely, pleural and hilar/mediastinal adenopathy are seen. Severe pulmonary hypertension can develop secondary to vascular wall involvement.

The diagnosis of amyloidosis is usually established by tissue biopsy. However, a high success rate can be achieved with abdominal fat pad aspirate (85%) or rectal biopsy (65%). Once a positive biopsy result is obtained, the type of amyloidosis must be determined. Monoclonal light chains are detected by serum/urine immunofixation, a technique more sensitive than simple protein electrophoresis. Immunofluorescence microscopy to protein A is typically positive in secondary amyloidosis, while incubation with permanganate will cause the fibrils in secondary, but not primary, amyloidosis, to lose their affinity for the Congo Red stain. Pulmonary amyloidosis can be diagnosed with either a surgical or transbronchial biopsy.

There is no known treatment in amyloidosis that mobilizes the amyloid deposits (choice A is incorrect). The goal of therapy is to reduce the amyloid precursor proteins, but there are little data supporting efficacious treatment of AA amyloidosis, with the exception of colchicine. One trial demonstrated prolonged survival in a few patients with AL amyloidosis treated with melphalan and prednisone. Also, 4-iodo-4-deoxydoxorubicin has been reported to provide clinical benefit in AL amyloidosis. This new class of drug is postulated to act by binding to amyloid fibrils, thus blocking deposition of new amyloid.

Berk J, O'Regan A, Skinner M. Pulmonary and tracheobronchial amyloidosis. Semin Respir Crit Care Med 2002; 23:155–165
Comenzo RL. Amyloidosis. Curr Treat Options Oncol 2006; 7:225–236
Lachmann HJ, Booth DR, Booth SE, et al. Misdiagnosis of hereditary amyloidosis as AL amyloidosis. N Engl J Med 2002; 346:1786–1791

123. A. There is a correlation between this disorder and decreased left ventricular ejection fraction and lower awake $Paco_2$.

There is a correlation between left ventricular ejection fraction and occurrence of central sleep apnea (CSA) in patients with congestive heart failure (CHF) (choice A is correct). CSA is characterized by episodes of apnea lasting at least 10 s during sleep without associated ventilatory effort. The 2-min polysomnographic tracing (see Figure 123-B) demonstrates episodes of central apneas with absence of airflow (FLOW), thoracic (THO), and abdominal (ABD) respiratory efforts accompanied by significant oxygen desaturations (Spo_2). Patients with CSA may present with complaints of insomnia, daytime hypersomnolence, repetitive nighttime awakenings, nocturnal sensations of dyspnea, and morning headaches, but many remain asymptomatic.

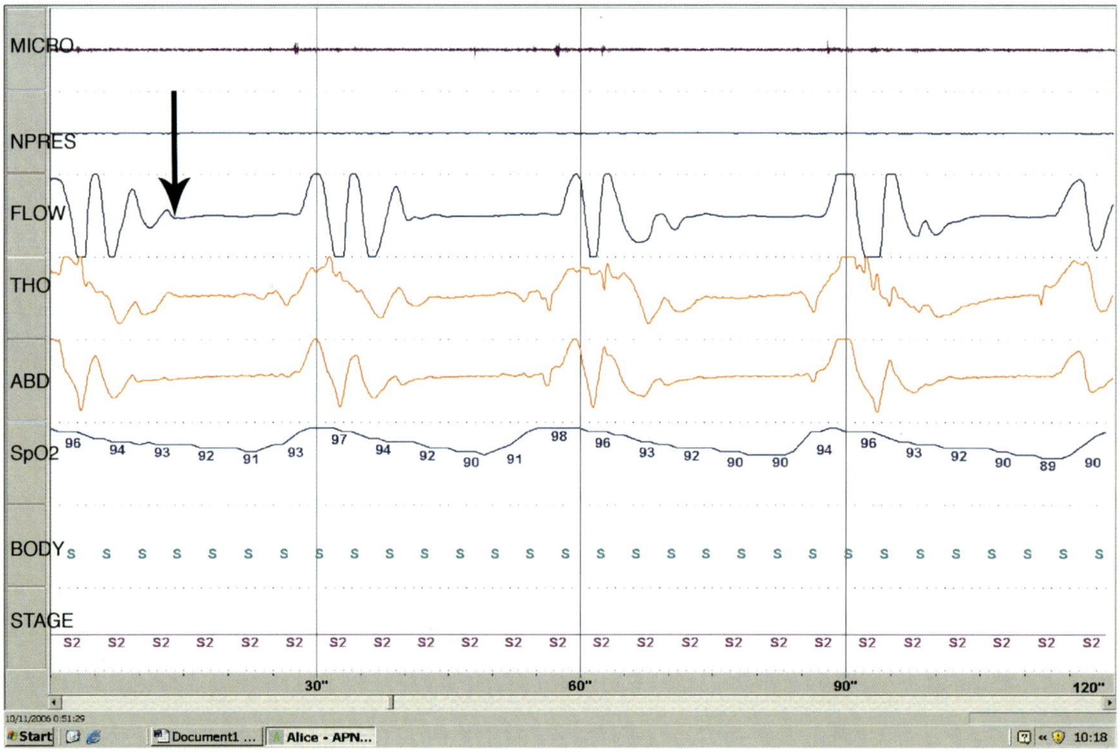

Figure 123-B

MICRO = microphone; NPRES = nasal pressure; FLOW = airflow; THO = thoracic; ABD = abdominal; Spo_2 = oxygen saturation as measured by pulse oximetry.

CSA can be idiopathic (resulting from a failure of ventilatory drive), secondary (due to CHF, neurologic/neuromuscular disorders), or chronic (due to use of long-acting opioids), related to sleep following ascent to high altitudes or associated with sleep onset in otherwise healthy individuals. The true incidence of idiopathic CSA is

not known but appears to be rare. Secondary causes of CSA are more common than the idiopathic form. Factors that increase the risk of developing CSA include a high CO_2 ventilatory drive, increased frequency of sleep-wake transitions, male gender, and increasing age. Men are more likely to have central apneas than women due to a higher hypocapnic apneic threshold during nonrapid eye movement (NREM) sleep.

CSA can be classified into hypercapnic and nonhypercapnic forms (see Table 123-1), based on the level of ventilation while awake. Hypercapnic CSA is associated with daytime hypoventilation (high waking $Paco_2$) and diminished response to hypercapnia. Hypoventilation persists during sleep. Hypercapnic CSA involves ventilatory impairment due to neuromuscular diseases affecting the respiratory apparatus or due to diminished chemoresponsiveness. In contrast, nonhypercapnic CSA is associated with normal or low waking $Paco_2$ due to increased ventilatory response to hypercapnia. Patients with idiopathic CSA or central apnea related to CHF are included in the nonhypercapnic group (choice B is incorrect).

Table 123-1. Types of CSA

Classifications	Features	Etiology
Hypercapnic	High waking $Paco_2$; diminished response to hypercapnia	Neuromuscular diseases; diminished chemoresponsiveness
Nonhypercapnic	Normal or low waking $Paco_2$; increased ventilatory response to hypercapnia	Idiopathic CSA; central apnea related to CHF

Relative hypoventilation occurs normally during sleep. Ventilation is stimulated if $Paco_2$ rises above the apneic threshold and may lead to a ventilatory overshoot with a subsequent fall in $Paco_2$ below this threshold, leading to a central apnea that continues until $Paco_2$ increases and once again exceeds the apneic threshold. This cycle repeats itself until both sleep and ventilation become regular during deeper stages of NREM sleep.

Polysomnography is necessary for the diagnosis of CSA. Central apneas occur more frequently at sleep onset and during NREM stages 1 and 2 sleep, and less commonly during NREM stages 3 and 4 sleep and REM sleep. Compared with obstructive sleep apnea, CSA is associated with milder oxygen desaturation and fewer hemodynamic changes.

Therapy involves treating the underlying causes of apnea along with supplemental therapy, positive airway pressure therapy, nocturnal noninvasive ventilation, or respiratory stimulants. Supplemental oxygen therapy may reduce nonhypercapnic CSA by stabilizing respiratory control centers, but not in all patients. Oxygen therapy in some patients with hypercapnic CSA can result in worsening hypercapnia. Patients with CSA, especially CSA secondary to CHF, may benefit from positive airway pressure therapy, and some may require mechanical ventilation support during sleep (choice C is incorrect). Acetazolamide, theophylline, and hypnotic agents have also been used to treat CSA. Acetazolamide is effective in improving high-altitude periodic respiration but has not been found to be effective for CSA secondary to CHF (choice D is incorrect). Theophylline has been used in CSA and Cheyne-Stokes respiration related to CHF, while medroxyprogesterone can stimulate ventilation in patients with obesity-hypoventilation syndrome.

Bradley T, Holloway RM, McLaughlin PR, et al. Cardiac output response to continuous positive airway pressure in congestive heart failure. Am Rev Respir Dis 1992; 145:377–382

Hanly PJ, Millar TW, Steljes DG, et al. The effect of oxygen on respiration and sleep in patients with congestive heart failure. Ann Intern Med 1989; 111:777–782

Javaheri S. A mechanism of central sleep apnea in patients with heart failure. N Engl J Med 1999; 341:949–954

McNicholas W, Carter JL, Rutherford R, et al. Beneficial effect of oxygen in primary alveolar hypoventilation with central sleep apnea. Am Rev Respir Dis 1982; 125:773–775

Naughton MBD, Rutherford R, Bradley TD. Effect of continuous positive airway pressure on central sleep apnea and nocturnal Pco_2 in heart failure. Am J Respir Crit Care Med 1994; 150:1598–1604

124. A. Obstructive impairment.

This patient has a reduced FEV_1 and FEV_1/FVC, with a normal total lung capacity (TLC), indicating an obstructive ventilatory defect (choice A is correct). Proper interpretation of spirometry depends first on reliable equipment that has been calibrated against a standard (usually a syringe) and a patient who is prepared, capable of, and willing to perform FVC maneuvers. Patients should maintain an upright posture, inhale completely and rapidly to TLC, pause for < 1 s, and exhale maximally until no more air can be expelled. Patients and technicians must terminate the maneuver if the patient experiences undue discomfort or if there is < 0.025 L change in volume for at least 1 s. In general, adults should be able to maintain a forced exhalation for > 6 s, and FEV_6 is often used as a surrogate for FVC in patients who cannot exhale for more than that time. The maneuver with the largest value of $FVC + FEV_1$ should be selected as the best effort.

Measurements derived from the patient are then compared with a reference population, and predicted normal values generally are adjusted for age, gender, height, and race. Values below the fifth percentile of normal distribution of predicted values are considered abnormal. When the FVC is normal, obstructive defects are defined by a reduced FEV_1/slow vital capacity (VC). VC is preferred to FVC because the latter value may be reduced in patients who have dynamic airway collapse during forced exhalation. In this case, VC and FVC are nearly identical, and the FVC and FEV_1/FVC are both reduced, usually reflecting failure of the patient to inhale or exhale completely. Nevertheless, a reduced FEV_1/FVC indicates the presence of airflow obstruction. Measurement of TLC is helpful to distinguish whether there is a concomitant restrictive disorder; in this case the TLC is normal, so there is no restrictive ventilatory defect (choice B is incorrect). Rather, a pure restrictive defect is characterized by a reduced TLC, FVC, and VC and a normal FEV_1/FVC. A mixed restrictive and obstructive defect is identified when both the TLC and FEV_1/FVC are reduced. Although this patient had a TLC that was 92% of predicted, this was not below the lower 5% value for the reference group (choice C is incorrect). Finally, this patient did not exhale for a full 6 s, which, by definition, was an "unacceptable" effort. However, even suboptimal tests can sometimes be interpreted with confidence. In this case, the FEV_1 would not change even if the patient exhaled longer, and the FEV_1/FVC would only decline. Therefore, the conclusion that the patient has obstructive dysfunction is still valid (choice D is incorrect).

Hankinson JL, Odencrantz JR, Fedan KB. Spirometric reference values from a sample of the general U.S. population. Am J Respir Crit Care Med 1999; 159:179–187

Miller MR, Hankinson J, Brusasco F, et al. Standardisation of spirometry. Eur Respir J 2005: 26:319–338

Pellegrino R, Viegi G, Brusasco V. Interpretive strategies for lung function tests. Eur Respir J 2005; 26:948–968

125. D. A written action plan should be offered.

Patients, as well as the parents and caregivers of children with peanut allergy, must be educated to avoid accidentally ingesting peanuts, learn to recognize early signs of an allergic reaction, and learn to medicate themselves as soon as symptoms develop. All patients with peanut allergy should be given a written emergency plan and adequate doses of liquid diphenhydramine and self-injectable epinephrine for use in case they accidentally ingest peanuts (choice D is correct). Patients offered comprehensive management that includes a written action plan have fewer acute attacks and require parenteral therapy with adrenalin and corticosteroids less often. Patients who have had unequivocal symptoms of allergy after the isolated ingestion of a peanut product (especially if they occur on more than one occasion) and who have evidence of peanut-specific IgE antibodies (a positive skin-prick test or radioallergosorbent test result) do not usually need to undergo oral peanut challenges to establish the diagnosis (choice A is incorrect). A role for an oral food challenge is present when the history of peanut allergy is unclear and the specific peanut IgE level is < 2 kU/L. Negative test results for IgE do not necessarily exclude the diagnosis, particularly in the face of a highly suggestive clinical history. Peanuts are legumes and are therefore related to soybeans, green beans, and lentils. Positive IgE reactions may be found to other beans (tree nuts and seeds, such as sesame seeds) if peanut allergy is present. Despite the presence of *in vitro* cross-sensitization, clinical cross-reactions are uncommon (5% at most; choice B is incorrect). Traditional subcutaneous allergen immunotherapy with crude peanut extract is associated with an unacceptable

risk of severe systemic side effects, including life-threatening anaphylaxis (choice C is incorrect). A number of novel approaches to immunotherapy are being investigated, but none is currently available.

Burks AW. Peanut allergy. Lancet 2008; 371:1538–1546
Ewan PW, Clark AT. Long-term prospective observational study of patients with peanut and nut allergy after participation in a management plan. Lancet 2001; 357:111–115
Sampson HA. Clinical practice: peanut allergy. N Engl J Med 2002; 346:1294–1299

126. D. Bronchoscopy.

The finding of a focal wheeze in any individual, including a patient with asthma, should raise the possibility of a localized endobronchial lesion. The CT scan (see Figures 126-A and 126-B) suggests an endobronchial lesion with loss of volume in the lingula so that bronchoscopy would be the next step (choice D is correct). In this patient, bronchoscopy confirmed a left lower lobe lesion (see Figure 126-C). Biopsy results revealed cells consistent with a carcinoid tumor that was subsequently resected with a left lower lobectomy.

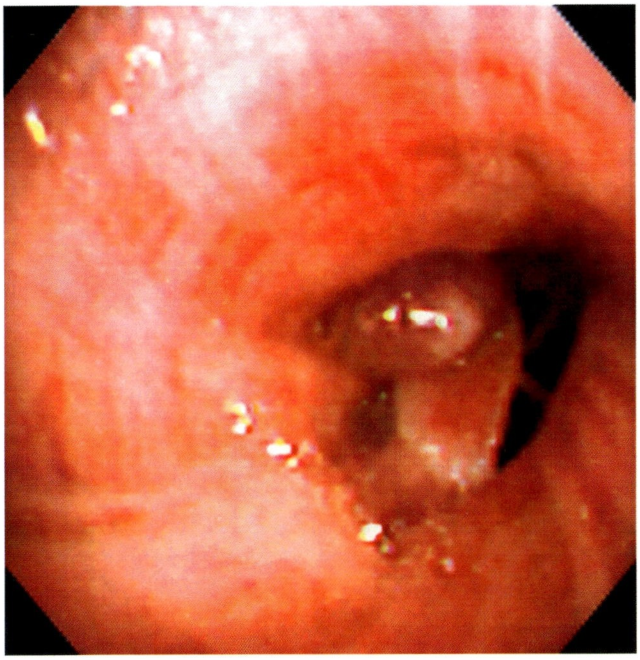

Figure 126-C

The approach to poorly controlled asthma includes assessment of the environment in an attempt to identify contributing irritant and allergic factors. However, allergy skin testing would not be recommended as the first step in a patient with a focal wheeze and deteriorating asthma control (choice A is incorrect). The finding of a focal wheeze in an asthmatic patient may be due to a complication of the disease, such as a mucous plug that perhaps is related to allergic bronchopulmonary aspergillosis (ABPA), or may be unrelated (foreign body, recurrent aspiration, tumor). ABPA is a well-recognized complication of asthma, leading to poor disease control and frequent need for oral corticosteroid therapy. Criteria for the diagnosis include the presence of asthma, a positive immediate skin test for *Aspergillus fumigatus*, peripheral eosinophilia, an elevated IgE level, fixed or transient pulmonary infiltrates, precipitating antibodies against Aspergillus, and central bronchiectasis. This can lead to mucoid impaction, but the current CT scan does not show central bronchiectasis, and the endobronchial lesion does not show the characteristic branching ("finger in glove") associated with mucous plugging. In addition, his serum IgE and eosinophil concentrations were normal, so a workup for ABPA would not be warranted at this time (choice B is incorrect). Doubling the dose of inhaled steroids has not been shown to be beneficial during asthma flares, although quadrupling of the dose of inhaled steroids might be beneficial (choice C is incorrect). However, in the presence of a focal wheeze, attention should turn toward ruling out more sinister causes of clinical worsening.

Bronchial carcinoids are considered a low-grade malignant tumor composed of neuroendocrine cells. They account for 1 to 5% of all pulmonary neoplasms. Symptoms include cough, hemoptysis, or evidence of focal bronchial obstruction, as in this patient. Although the carcinoid syndrome associated with nonpulmonary carcinoid tumors can cause wheezing suggestive of asthma, bronchial carcinoids rarely cause the carcinoid syndrome. Treatment usually involves surgical resection, although recently there have been some successful attempts using interventional bronchoscopic techniques. The finding of a focal wheeze in any patient, including a person with asthma, should lead to a search for an endobronchial lesion using bronchoscopy.

Dipaolo F, Stull MA. Bronchial carcinoid presenting as refractory asthma. Am Fam Physician 1993; 48:785–789

Brokx HA, Risse EK, Paul MA, et al. Initial bronchoscopic treatment for patients with intraluminal bronchial carcinoids. J Thorac Cardiovasc Surg 2007; 133:973–978

Morandi U, Casali C, Rossi G. Bronchial typical carcinoid tumors. Semin Thorac Cardiovasc Surg 2006; 18:191–198

Martinez S, Heyneman LA, McAdams HP, et al. Mucoid impactions: finger-in-glove sign and other CT and radiographic features. Radiographics 2008; 28:1369–1382

FitzGerald JM, Becker A, Sears MR, et al. A randomized controlled trial of doubling the dose of inhaled steroids versus placebo in acute asthma exacerbations. Thorax 2004; 59:550–556

127. C. Omalizumab.

This man with asthma has had multiple exacerbations despite the use of a β-agonist, leukotriene modifier, and inhaled corticosteroid therapy. He is compliant with his regimen but has had a recent escalation of his symptoms prompting several acute-care visits. He has a positive skin test result and has a normal IgE level. Omalizumab is approved for patients with moderate or severe persistent asthma who are not achieving the goals of asthma management on inhaled corticosteroids, who exhibit a wheal-flare reaction to a perennial allergen, and whose IgE level is in the range of 30 to 700 μg/L (0.03 to 0.7 mg/L) (choice C is correct).

Omalizumab is a recombinant, monoclonal anti-IgE antibody that binds to the IgE at the same crystallizable fragment site as the high-affinity IgE receptor. Its primary mechanism of action is the binding of free IgE in the circulation, forming biologically inert, small complexes that do not activate complement. It has been associated with a clinically significant benefit in randomized, double-blind, placebo-controlled clinical trials.

Tiotropium is not indicated in the maintenance treatment of asthma (choice D is incorrect). Although theophylline may be helpful, little additional benefit can be expected in this instance (choice B is incorrect). Oral corticosteroids are beneficial during the acute exacerbation, but attempts should be avoided to use this agent on a chronic basis, particularly given this patient's age (choice A is incorrect).

National Heart, Lung, and Blood Institute, National Asthma Education and Prevention Program. Expert Panel Report 3: guidelines for the diagnosis and management of asthma. Available at www.nhlbi.nih.gov/guidelines/asthma. Accessed March 6, 2009

Busse W, Corren J, Lanier B, et al. Omalizumab, anti-IgE recombinant humanized monoclonal antibody for the treatment of severe allergic asthma. J Allergy Clin Immunol 2001; 108:184–190

128. C. Granulocyte-macrophage colony-stimulating factor (GM-CSF).

This patient has idiopathic pulmonary alveolar proteinosis (PAP), and the best treatment option of those offered is GM-CSF (choice C is correct). Restoration of lung function is achieved with whole lung lavage to remove the accumulated lipoproteinaceous material. This remains the standard therapy for patients with PAP. The identification of neutralizing antibodies to GM-CSF has led to observational series that suggest efficacy of GM-CSF, both by subcutaneous and inhaled administration, for patients with PAP. From these series, there is a suggestion of a more durable response and less frequent recurrences. In contrast to whole-lung lavage, where an immediate clinical benefit is experienced, the response to therapy is delayed with GM-CSF administration.

PAP may occur in association with underlying lymphoproliferative or myeloproliferative disorders, but the majority of patients with PAP present with idiopathic PAP. Opportunistic infections, such as *Pneumocystis jirovecii* or Nocardia sp, may complicate the course of patients with PAP in 10 to 15% of patients because of impaired macrophage function. Trimethoprim-sulfamethoxazole is appropriate therapy for *P jirovecii* pneumonia or nocardiosis but is not effective in isolation in patients with PAP (choice A is incorrect). Neutralizing antibodies to GM-CSF result in impaired macrophage function and clearance of lipoproteinaceous surfactant, which then accumulates within the lung. Corticosteroids and cyclophosphamide do not have a role in the treatment of PAP and may further impair clearance of surfactant from the lung and increase the risk of opportunistic infections (choices B and D are incorrect).

PAP is a rare disease with a worldwide prevalence of 3.7 cases per million people. It is more common in men than in women. Congenital forms of PAP exist with mutations in surfactant protein B having been identified, although they are rare. The majority of patients are previously healthy and acquire a neutralizing antibody to GM-CSF. The median age at the time of diagnosis is 39 years. Dyspnea on exertion and a cough are the most common symptoms. Characteristic radiographic features include a diffuse, bilateral alveolar filling process in a midlung zone distribution that may spare the lower lung zones (see Figure 128-C). CT imaging further characterizes a unique radiographic pattern with ground-glass opacities superimposed on interlobular thickening, termed "crazy paving," which is identified in Figure 128-B. Similar infiltrates may be seen in silica inhalation, lipoid pneumonia, and bronchoalveolar carcinoma. A diagnosis is suggested by the presence of dense, opaque periodic acid-Schiff–positive lipoproteinaceous material identified during BAL, as noted in Figure 128-D, or present on a surgical lung biopsy sample. The presence of anti-GM-CSF antibodies in serum or BAL fluid is highly specific and appears to be a sensitive marker of disease.

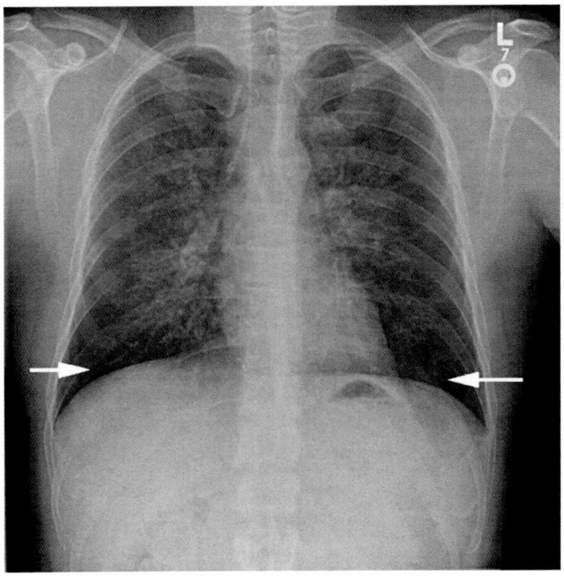

Figure 128-C

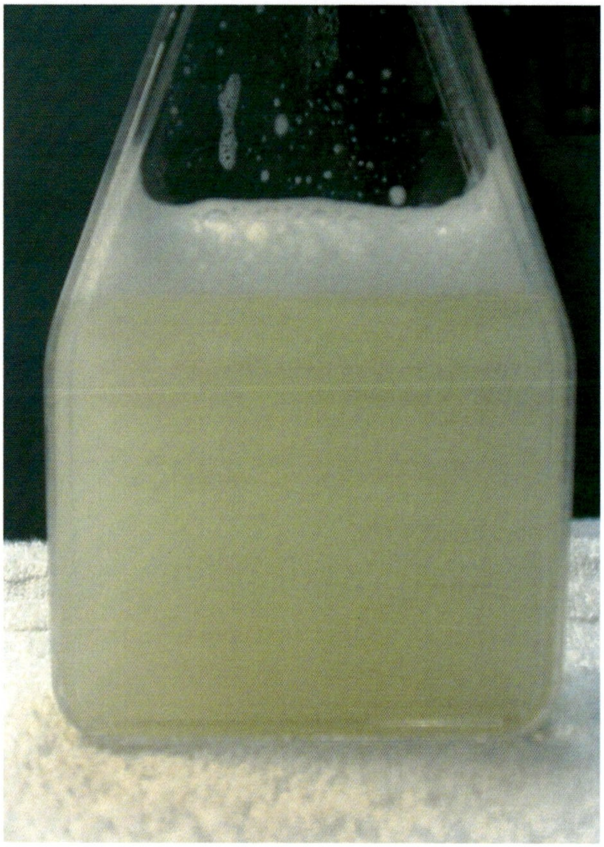

Figure 128-D

Presneill JJ, Nakata K, Inoue Y, et al. Pulmonary alveolar proteinosis. Clin Chest Med 2004; 25:593–613
Seymour JF, Doyle IR, Nakata K, et al. Relationship of anti-GM-CSF antibody concentration, surfactant protein A and B levels, and serum LDH to pulmonary parameters and response to GM-CSF therapy in patients with idiopathic alveolar proteinosis. Thorax 2003; 58:252–257
Kitamura T, Uchida K, Tanaka N, et al. Serological diagnosis of idiopathic pulmonary alveolar proteinosis. Am J Respir Crit Care Med 2000; 162:658–662
Uchida K, Nakata K, Trapnell BC, et al. High-affinity autoantibodies specifically eliminate granulocyte-macrophage colony-stimulating factor activity in the lungs of patients with idiopathic pulmonary alveolar proteinosis. Blood 2004; 103:1089–1098

129. B. Acute rejection of the allograft.

Given the chest radiographic findings of a diffuse interstitial infiltrate in the allograft, a lack of history or findings suggesting infection, and the time course of the appearance of this abnormality, acute rejection of the allograft is the most likely diagnosis (choice B is correct). Nonetheless, the possibility of infection and other possibilities exist, and prompt bronchoscopy is indicated with escalation of immunosuppressive therapy if rejection is confirmed. This patient underwent bronchoscopy and transbronchial biopsy that revealed a perivascular infiltrate that did not extend into the interstitium or alveolar spaces and, hence, was graded as mild acute rejection at an A2 level. The patient received high-dose methylprednisolone, 10 mg/kg/day for 3 days, and a repeat chest radiograph on the fourth day showed significant clearing (see Figure 129-B).

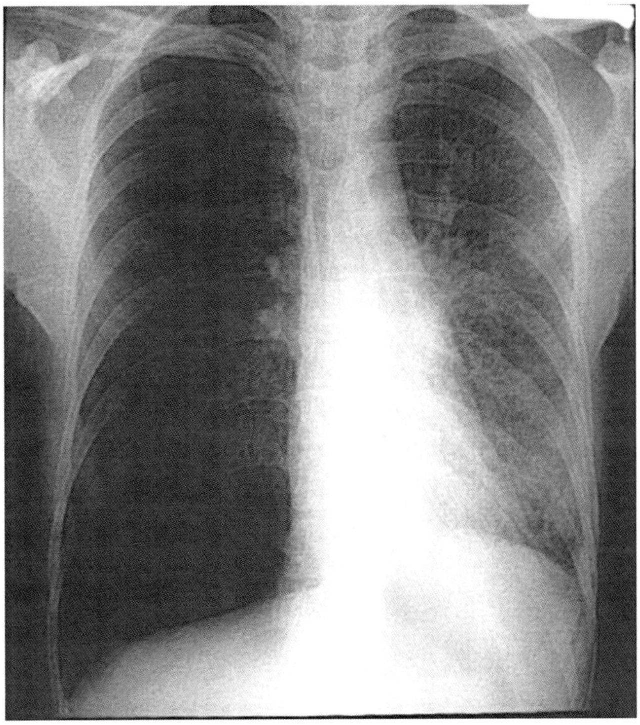

Figure 129-B

Lung rejection results when the recipient's immune system recognizes donor antigens as being foreign and mounts an immune response against the allograft. Acute rejection of the lung is orchestrated primarily by the cell-mediated arm of the immune system, although there is increasing evidence that the innate and humoral immune systems also play a role.

Despite use of potent immunosuppressive drugs, acute rejection still occurs in > 50% of lung recipients in the first posttransplant year. Presenting symptoms include dyspnea, particularly with exertion, and low-grade fever, but it is important to note that patients may present with no symptoms or findings, as in this case, so surveillance for rejection is conducted apart from the clinical profile. Exertional desaturation and radiographic abnormalities are useful clues to rejection, and the chest radiograph may show a diffuse interstitial infiltrate or pleural effusions. Rejection may be accompanied by normal findings on chest radiograph, however, especially later in the postoperative period. Most patients are sent home with a microspirometer and are asked to document daily FEV_1 and FVC measurements because rejection may be signaled by declining spirometric values, as in this patient.

Transbronchial biopsy, if at least five adequate specimens are obtained, has a sensitivity of approximately 90% for diagnosing acute rejection. The classic pathologic finding is that of a lymphocytic vasculitis. When this extends beyond the perivascular space into the interstitium and alveolar spaces (see Figure 129-C), the rejection is moderate (A3) or severe (A4).

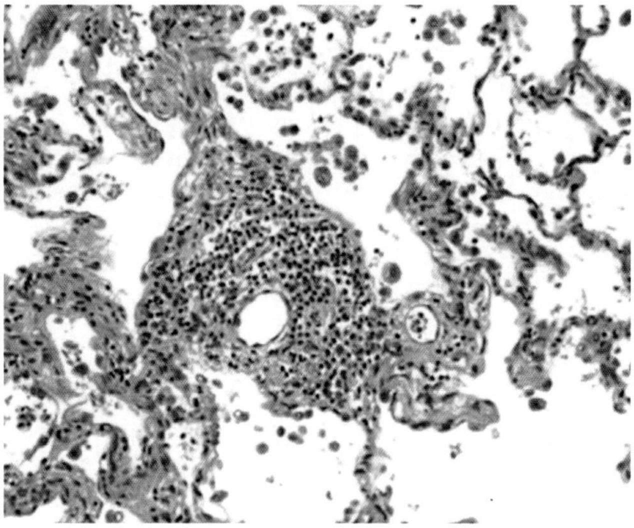

Figure 129-C
Hematoxylin-eosin

Other causes of lung infiltrates in these patients include infectious agents and effects of immunosuppressive agents themselves, particularly rapamycin (sirilimus), which can produce an interstitial pneumonitis. Bacterial infections such as staphylococcal pneumonia certainly occur in these patients, but the diffuse infiltrate without fever or sputum in this patient speaks against this diagnosis (choice A is incorrect). CMV pneumonitis is a common problem in these patients, but it would be atypical to have the infiltrate isolated to the allograft (choice C is incorrect), as would be true of cardiogenic pulmonary edema (choice D is incorrect).

Kotloff RM, Ahya VN. Medical complications of lung transplantation. Eur Respir J 2004; 23:334–342
Granton J. Update of early respiratory failure in the lung transplant recipient. Curr Opin Crit Care 2006; 12:19–24

130. D. Stage R.

The American Academy of Sleep Medicine proposed new criteria for scoring sleep stages in 2007. The presence of low-amplitude, mixed-frequency EEG activity and rapid eye movements in this epoch identifies it as stage R (REM) (choice D is correct; choices A, B, and C are incorrect).

Using data obtained from EEG, electrooculography (EOG), and chin electromyography (EMG), adult sleep can be classified into nonrapid eye movement (NREM) or REM sleep. NREM sleep can be further subdivided into stages N1, N2, and N3. Recommended electrode placements are F4M1, C4M1, and O2M1 for EEG, and E1M2 and E2M1 for EOG (F, frontal; C, central; O, occipital; M, mastoid; E, outer canthus; odd numbers are left-sided electrodes; even numbers are right-sided electrodes).

Three locations are recommended for chin EMG electrodes, namely midline, 1 cm above the inferior edge of the mandible; 2 cm to the right of midline and 2 cm below the inferior edge of the mandible; and 2 cm to the left of midline and 2 cm below the inferior edge of the mandible.

Sleep stages are scored in 30-s epochs; each epoch is assigned a sleep stage that comprises the greatest percentage of the epoch. Stage Wake is present if > 50% of epoch has either alpha EEG waves (8 to 13 Hz) over the occipital region with eye closure, *or* if alpha waves are absent or if there is a presence of conjugate vertical eye blinks, reading eye movements (conjugate slow movement followed by a rapid movement in the opposite direction), or voluntary rapid open eye movements.

A sleep stage is considered N1 if alpha EEG waves are replaced by low-amplitude, mixed-frequency (4 to 7 Hz) waves occupying > 50% of the epoch *or* the start of 4- to 7-Hz waves with slowing of background activity by at least 1 Hz compared with stage Wake, vertex sharp waves, or slow eye movements (see Figure 130-B). Stage N2 is identified by the presence of low-amplitude, mixed-frequency EEG rhythms and K complexes (not associated with arousals) or sleep spindles during the first half of the epoch or during the last half of the previous epoch, if criteria for stage N3 are absent. Sleep spindles are brief oscillations with a frequency of 12 to 14 Hz, lasting 0.5 to 1.5 s, and generally have an amplitude < 50 μV. A K complex is a high-amplitude, biphasic wave that consists of an initial sharp negative deflection followed by a positive high-voltage slow wave, with a duration of ≥ 0.5 s (see Figures 130-C and 130-D).

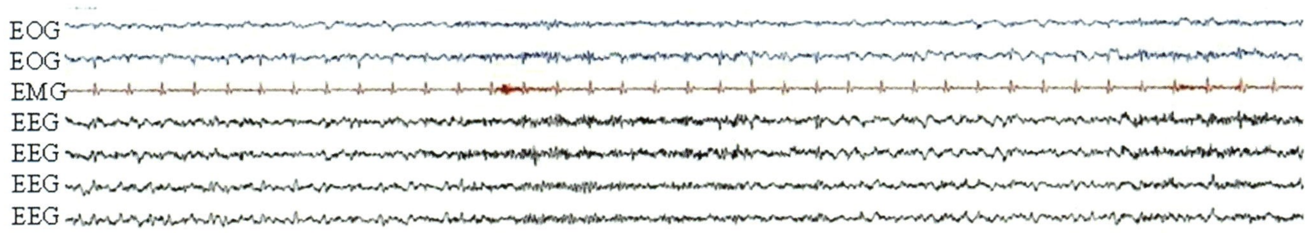

Figure 130-B

Stage NREM N1 sleep. In this sleep stage, alpha EEG waves are replaced by low-amplitude, mixed-frequency (4 to 7 Hz) waves occupying > 50% of the epoch. Slow eye movements can be seen in the EOG. Chin EMG tone remains high. Electrocardiographic artifacts are present on the EMG tracing.

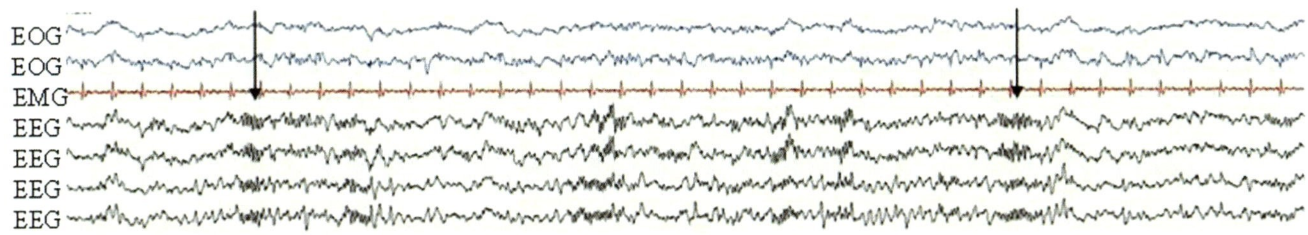

Figure 130-C

Stage NREM N2 sleep. This sleep epoch demonstrates the presence of sleep spindles (arrows), which are brief oscillations with a frequency of 12 to 14 Hz lasting 0.5 to 1.5 s and an amplitude generally < 50 μV. No movements are present in the EOG tracings, and there is low chin EMG activity. Electrocardiographic artifacts are present on the EMG tracing.

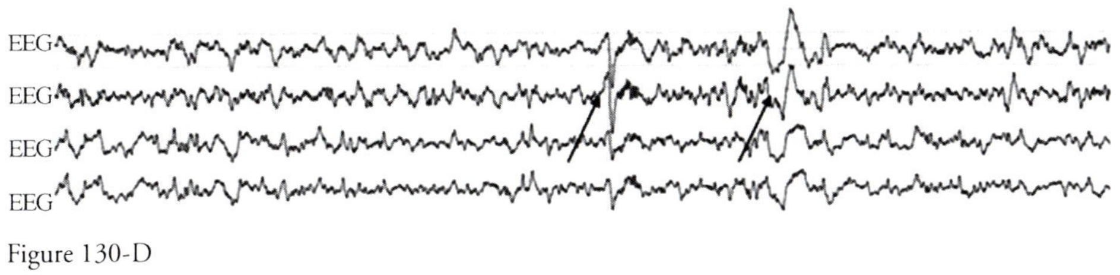

Figure 130-D

Stage NREM N2 sleep. K complexes (arrows) are evident in this epoch, stage N2 sleep. K complexes are high-amplitude, biphasic waves with an initial sharp negative deflection followed by a positive high-voltage slow wave and a duration of ≥ 0.5 s that is generally maximal over the vertex.

In stage N3, at least 20% of the epoch is occupied by slow delta wave (0.5 to 2 Hz and > 75 μV) EEG activity over the frontal regions (see Figure 130-E). Finally, stage R is scored if the epoch consists of low-amplitude, mixed-frequency EEG activity, rapid eye movements, and low chin EMG tone (lowest level in the study or at least no higher than the other sleep stages; see Figure 130-F).

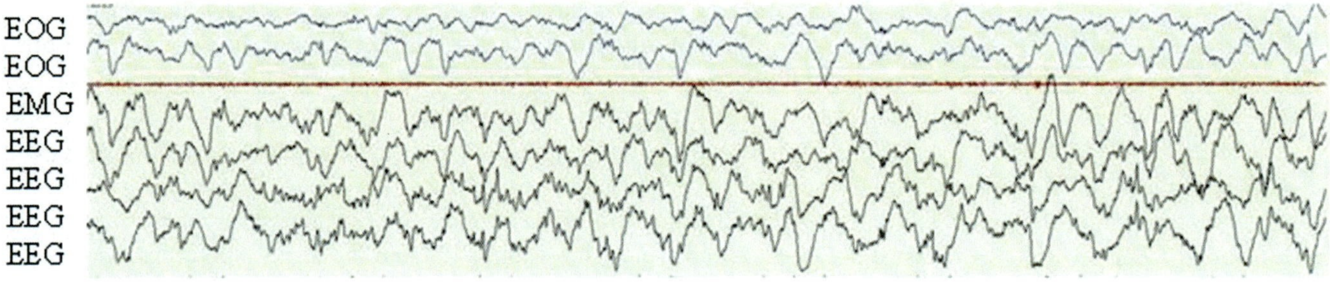

Figure 130-E

Stage NREM N3 sleep. Increased slow delta wave activity is readily apparent in this epoch. Stage N3 is scored when ≥ 20% of the epoch is occupied by slow-wave (0.5 to 2 Hz and > 75 μV) EEG activity over the frontal regions. Chin EMG activity is low.

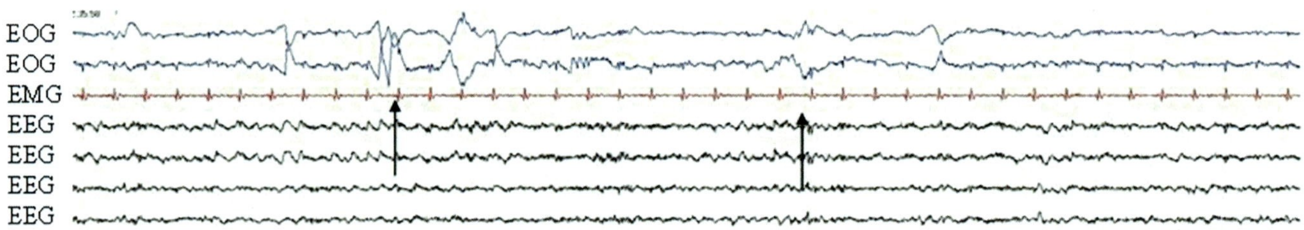

Figure 130-F

Stage REM sleep. This epoch of REM sleep demonstrates low-amplitude, mixed-frequency EEG activity, REMs (arrows) on the EOG, and low chin EMG tone. ECG artifacts are present on the EMG tracing.

Iber C, Ancoli-Israel S, Chesson A, et al. American Academy of Sleep Medicine: the AASM manual for the scoring of sleep and associated events: rules, terminology and technical specifications. 1st ed. Westchester, IL: American Academy of Sleep Medicine, 2007

131. A. A 60-year-old man with upper lobe emphysema and an exercise capacity of 30 W following rehabilitation. FEV_1 is 30% of predicted, and DLCO is 28% of predicted.

LVRS may provide benefit to select patients with COPD by allowing an increase in lung elastic recoil, improving expiratory airflow, allowing an improvement in mechanical function of the diaphragm, and decreasing functional residual capacity.

Patient A is the best candidate to undergo LVRS. In the large National Emphysema Treatment Trial (NETT) of 1,218 patients, patients with the combination of upper lobe predominant emphysema and low exercise capacity following rehabilitation were the best candidates for LVRS, resulting in a reduced risk of death and improved exercise capacity and respiratory quality of life compared with a similar medically managed group (choice A is correct).

Early in the NETT trial, the highest risk patients were identified by interim analysis and excluded from further study enrollment. This included patients with FEV_1 < 20% of predicted and a DLCO < 20% of predicted or diffuse changes with CT (choice D is incorrect). The patient in choice D is at high risk of death and will have little benefit from LVRS and might be a better candidate for lung transplantation.

The overall results of the trial concluded that LVRS can improve exercise capacity but does not result in a survival advantage over medical therapy. However, when different subsets were analyzed on the basis of the presence of upper lobe-predominant vs diffuse emphysema and high exercise capacity, vs low exercise capacity, interesting results were found. In the subgroup with upper lobe-predominant emphysema and low baseline exercise capacity, LVRS did result in a survival advantage, as discussed earlier. Patients with diffuse emphysema and high exercise capacity had increased mortality following LVRS without improvements in exercise capacity or quality of life (choice B is incorrect). The other two subgroups, upper lobe-predominant emphysema with high exercise capacity (choice C is incorrect) and diffuse emphysema with low exercise capacity, had similar mortality with LVRS, and the former subset had some functional improvement with LVRS.

Exercise capacity, as defined in the study, was determined following a period of 6 to 10 weeks of pulmonary rehabilitation and defined by a gender-specific 40% percentile as 25 W for women and 40 W for men (all testing was performed with a FIO_2 of 0.3). Below these values, a patient was classified as having low exercise capacity and, above these values, as having high exercise capacity.

Fishman A, Martinez F, Naunheim K, et al. A randomized trial comparing lung-volume-reduction surgery with medical therapy for severe emphysema. N Engl J Med 2003; 348:2059–2073

Kim V, Criner GJ, Abdallah HY, et al. Small airway morphometry and improvement in pulmonary function after lung volume reduction surgery. Am J Respir Crit Care Med 2005; 171:40–47

Miller JD, Berger RL, Malthaner RA, et al. Lung volume reduction surgery vs medical treatment for patients with advanced emphysema. Chest 2005; 127:1166–1177

Geddes D, Davies M, Koyama H, et al. Effect of lung-volume-reduction surgery in patients with severe emphysema. N Engl J Med 2000; 343:239–245

National Emphysema Trial Research Group. Patients at high risk of death after lung-volume-reduction surgery. N Engl J Med 2001; 345:1075–1083

Lederer DJ, Thomashow BM, Ginsburg ME, et al. Lung-volume reduction surgery for pulmonary emphysema: improvement in body mass index, airflow obstruction, dyspnea, and exercise capacity index after 1 year. J Thorac Cardiovasc Surg 2007; 133:1434–1438

132. B. Noninvasive ventilation.

This patient is clearly failing the extubation attempt. Generally speaking, extubation failures are of two broad types: (1) a failure to protect the airways and/or (2) abnormal respiratory mechanics (resistance and/or compliance) that exceed the respiratory muscles' capabilities. In this case, it appears to be the latter in that his cough is strong and his breath sounds are clear, but his muscles are clearly tiring.

Under these conditions, reinstitution of some positive-pressure ventilatory support is warranted. Although this could be done with reinsertion of the endotracheal tube and reapplication of the positive-pressure device, in the COPD population, it appears that providing the support through a noninvasive mask system can be quite effective and avoid the complications of an endotracheal tube. Choice B is thus correct.

Choice A is incorrect because, as noted, endotracheal intubations can often be avoided in COPD patients under these circumstances. It is important to note, however, that this may not be the case in other forms of respiratory failure. Thus, patients with acute lung injury or other forms of respiratory failure who have failed an extubation attempt probably should be promptly reintubated. Choice C is incorrect because this patient is failing the extubation attempt, and it would be inappropriate to wait an additional 60 min and hope that medications can reverse things. Choice D is incorrect because it does not appear that this patient has upper airway obstruction and/or bronchospasm.

Ferrer M. Non-invasive ventilation in the weaning process. Minerva Anestesiol 2008; 74:311–314

Epstein SK. Using non-invasive ventilation to shorten the duration of mechanical ventilation. Respir Care 2009; 54:150–155

MacIntrye NR. Evidence-based guidelines for weaning and discontinuing mechanical ventilatory support. Chest 2001; 120(suppl):375S–396S

Esteban A, Frutos-Vivar F, Ferguson ND, et al. Noninvasive positive-pressure ventilation for respiratory failure after extubation. N Engl J Med 2004; 350:2452–2460

133. C. 2 weeks.

A 15-day course of glucocorticoids is the preferred duration of treatment for most individuals with an acute exacerbation of COPD requiring hospitalization (choice C is correct). Although glucocorticoids have been used for decades to treat acute exacerbations of COPD, high-quality studies of their optimal use in this setting have unfortunately been scarce. The largest trial randomized 271 patients with acute exacerbations requiring hospitalization to receive placebo or glucocorticoids; the duration of treatment in the glucocorticoid group was randomized to either 2 or 8 weeks. The patients who received glucocorticoids had a shorter hospital stay than those receiving placebo (8.5 vs 9.7 days), showed more rapid improvement with spirometry, and were less likely to have treatment failure at 30 and 90 days. Interestingly, there was no apparent advantage to an 8- vs a 2-week course of glucocorticoids (choice D is incorrect). Hyperglycemia was more common with glucocorticoid treatment, also arguing for a 2-week course.

A smaller trial found better outcomes among hospitalized patients treated with oral prednisolone for 14 days than those treated with placebo. A different trial found lower rates of relapse in outpatients who received a prescription for a 10-day course of prednisone vs placebo in the ED when evaluated, but not admitted, for a COPD exacerbation. Oral glucocorticoids donot appear to be inferior to IV treatment.

Thus, although there remains significant practice variation in the type, dose, and duration of glucocorticoid used for acute exacerbations of COPD, data are strongest for a tapering schedule of oral prednisone for a total of approximately 2 weeks of treatment. Data do not support the general use of significantly shorter courses (choices A and B are incorrect).

Aaron SD, Vandemheen KL, Hebert P, et al. Outpatient oral prednisone after emergency treatment of chronic obstructive pulmonary disease. N Engl J Med 2003; 348:2618–2625

Davies L, Angus RM, Calverley PM. Oral corticosteroids in patients admitted to hospital with exacerbations of chronic obstructive pulmonary disease: a prospective randomised controlled trial. Lancet 1999; 354:456–460

de Jong YP, Uil SM, Grotjohan HP, et al. Oral or IV prednisolone in the treatment of COPD exacerbations: a randomized, controlled, double-blind study. Chest 2007; 132:1741–1747

Niewoehner DE, Erbland ML, Deupree RH, et al. Effect of systemic glucocorticoids on exacerbations of chronic obstructive pulmonary disease. Department of Veterans Affairs Cooperative Study Group. N Engl J Med 1999; 340:1941–1947

Sayiner A, Aytemur ZA, Cirit M, et al. Systemic glucocorticoids in severe exacerbations of COPD. Chest 2001; 119:726–730

134. B. A transthoracic needle biopsy.

This 31-year-old patient has a 2.3-cm solid lung nodule that has objectively increased in size over the past 6 months. An increase in size from 2.0 to 2.3 cm represents an increase in volume of 50%. This is the defining concern in this patient, and even though she is a nonsmoker, a tissue diagnosis should be obtained unless specifically contraindicated (choice B is correct). The best method for confirming the diagnosis depends on the patient's preference and the techniques available to the attending physician. Options would include transthoracic needle aspiration biopsy, bronchoscopy (including with various CT or fluoroscopic guidance techniques), and excisional surgery with initial frozen-section determination. Surgery is the diagnostic "gold standard" and the definitive treatment for malignant nodules, but it would be desirable to avoid surgery in patients with benign nodules. Similarly, biopsy results commonly establish a specific benign or malignant diagnosis, but biopsy is still invasive and frequently nondiagnostic. It is also important to emphasize this is a difficult clinical problem, and approaches to management are constantly evolving, but it is important to ensure that all potentially malignant nodules are removed, recognizing that this will lead to resection of some benign nodules. In this instance, surgical resection was undertaken, establishing the diagnosis of malignancy (adenocarcinoma).

The lung nodule has already been demonstrated to increase in size (a 50% increase in 6 months), and therefore, further observation or watchful waiting would be inappropriate (choice A is incorrect). In the absence of a demonstrated increase in size, a PET scan might yield meaningful information, as it has high sensitivity for malignancy in nodules of this size. While false-positive results are documented as the result of infective or inflammatory conditions, the

PET scan can also be helpful in assessing hilar and mediastinal lymph nodes, as well as involvement of chest wall and mediastinal structures. False-negative findings on PET scan can be seen in patients with bronchioalveolar cell carcinoma, carcinoid tumors, mucinous adenocarcinomas, and potentially, uncontrolled hyperglycemia. Most importantly, in this patient with a documented enlarging lung nodule, a negative PET scan result would still not reliably exclude malignancy or obviate the need for tissue confirmation or resection (choice C is incorrect). At the very least, it would be recommended that a needle biopsy be performed in high-probability patients with negative PET scan results; thus, the PET scan would not alter further management. Despite the extensive travels of this patient, it is important to recognize that the lesion is not cystic and that parasitic agents are not common causes of solid lung nodules (choice D is incorrect). Moreover, serologic findings for the various parasitic agents are not diagnostic and often take months to obtain; significantly delaying further management while awaiting the results of these investigations would not be desirable.

Gould MK, Fletcher J, Iannettoni MD, et al. Evaluation of patients with pulmonary nodules: when is it lung cancer? Chest 2007; 108S–130S

135. A. Administer IV unfractionated heparin (UFH).

The CT scan reveals a saddle embolus (see Figure 135-C, arrow). The radiologist also noted large right and left main pulmonary thrombi and more distal thrombi bilaterally on the full examination. Evidence-based guidelines recommend short-term treatment with either IV UFH, subcutaneous low-molecular-weight heparin (LMWH), fixed-dose UFH, or subcutaneous fondaparinux for patients with objectively confirmed pulmonary embolism (PE; choice A is correct). Given the intracranial mass in this patient, IV UFH would be preferred over LMWH because it can be more rapidly and reliably reversed should she develop intracranial bleeding. This patient's hypotension and right ventricle dysfunction characterize this as a massive PE. For patients with massive PE and evidence of hemodynamic compromise, the recommended treatment is systemically administered thrombolytic therapy, in the absence of major contraindications. Major contraindications include intracranial disease (such as tumor, as in this patient, or recent [within 6 months] stroke), uncontrolled hypertension, and recent major surgery or trauma (choice B is incorrect).

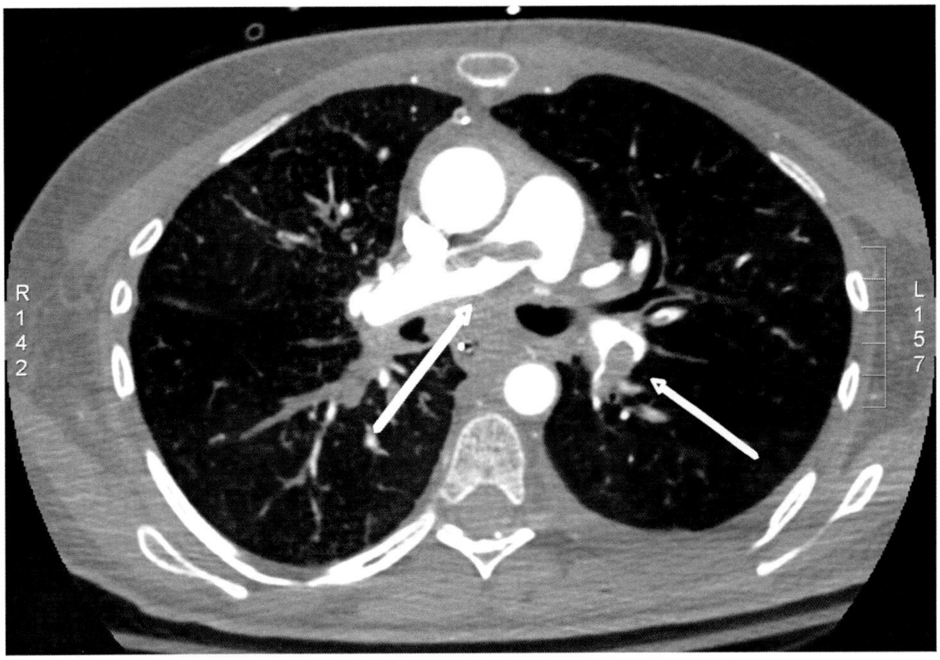

Figure 135-C

The guidelines specifically recommend against the routine use of inferior vena cava (IVC) filters. IVC filters are recommended only in patients thought to have an absolute contraindication to anticoagulant therapy because of an unacceptable risk of bleeding. Patients with intracranial metastases are often thought to be at high risk of bleeding because of the vascularity of the tumors and anecdotal reports of bleeding. However, most reports of intracranial

bleeding in patients with cerebral metastases suggest that this occurs predominantly in the setting of supratherapeutic anticoagulation. Most experts believe that, in the absence of a primary tumor that is known to be significantly vascular (renal, melanoma, and choriocarcinoma), patients with cerebral metastases can be safely treated with anticoagulant therapy, provided they are monitored closely. In addition, patients with brain tumors who are treated with IVC filters are much more likely to develop complications due to the filter and recurrent thromboembolism. No prospective clinical trials have directly compared anticoagulation and IVC filters in this population. At the present time, then, patients with metastatic tumors without a propensity for bleeding should be treated with anticoagulation therapy rather than IVC filters (choice C is incorrect).

Interventional catheter techniques include mechanical fragmentation of the thrombus, clot pulverization, and catheter embolectomy. There are no randomized clinical trials that have evaluated these techniques in patients with massive PE, and thus, the guidelines do not currently recommend these as first-line therapy (choice D is incorrect). Should this patient's clinical status continue to deteriorate despite anticoagulation, interventional catheter techniques or surgical embolectomy could be considered.

Kearon C, Kahn SR, Agnelli G, et al. Antithrombotic therapy for venous thromboembolic disease: American College of Chest Physicians evidence-based clinical practice guidelines, 8th edition. Chest 2008; 133(suppl):454S–545S
Walsh DC, Kakkar AK. Thromboembolism in brain tumors. Curr Opin Pulm Med 2001; 7:326–331
Wen PY, Marks PW. Medical management of patients with brain tumors. Curr Opin Oncol 2002; 14:299–307

136. C. Symptoms usually persist for months after exposure and can persist for years.

After exposure to a single agent in high concentrations as occurs with RADS, bronchial hyperresponsiveness and airflow obstruction will occur within 24 h. These symptoms will usually last for a few months, when some individuals become asymptomatic. However, two out of three patients will still have some symptoms at 1 year after exposure, with some having symptoms lasting 2 years (choice C is correct).

RADS falls under a larger umbrella of irritant-induced asthma, which is considered an occupational asthma from exposure to a household or occupational agent. RADS is traditionally defined as exposure to high concentrations of an irritant gas, aerosol, or particle, with respiratory symptoms occurring minutes to hours later. This exposure at high concentrations is followed by asthma-like symptoms and hyperresponsiveness for an extended period of time of months to years. In addition to a single high-level event, exposure can occur repeatedly and at low levels ("low-dose RADS"). A delayed response of a few days can be seen as well. However, this repeated exposure and delayed response variant does not fit the RADS definition but falls under the more general category of irritant-induced asthma. Finally, exposure with a latency period, usually of months to years, is common in workplace-associated asthma, thus distinguishing it from RADS and irritant-induced asthma variants. However, in many situations, distinguishing between RADS and workplace-associated asthma can be difficult.

Many products and chemicals, including chlorine, detergents, and concrete dust, can cause RADS. Risk factors for the development of RADS include wet or vapor aerosol exposure, high-concentration exposure, and chlorine exposure when working in a paper mill. Atopy is a risk factor for the variant irritant-induced asthma, has a delayed response of days, and is not seen in individuals with RADS (choice A is incorrect). Additionally, a history of airway hyperresponsiveness is also not a risk factor for RADS development. Reexposure to the agent in a clinical setting or at low levels will not reproduce symptoms in RADS and irritant-induced asthma. However, reproduction of symptoms with reexposure is classic with workplace-associated asthma and has a latency period (choice D is incorrect).

With a single high-concentration exposure or repeated lower concentration exposures, mucosal injury ensues that leads to mucosal denudation and fibrinohemorrhagic exudates in the submucosa. Polymorphonuclear cells are found predominantly in the inflammation and are largely found on BAL. RADS and irritant-induced asthma can be differentiated from workplace-associated asthma because RADS has a more significant mucosal and submucosal injury

with basement membrane thickening when compared with workplace-associated asthma. Additionally, lymphocytes and eosinophils are seen predominantly in the bronchial-alveolar fluid in workplace-associated asthma, whereas polymorphonuclear cells *are* predominant in RADS (choice B is incorrect).

Brooks SM, Weiss MA, Bernstein IL. Reactive airways dysfunction syndrome (RADS): persistent asthma syndrome after high level irritant exposures. Chest 1985; 88:376–384
Lemière C, Malo JL, Gautrin D. Nonsensitizing causes of occupational asthma. Med Clin North Am 1996; 80:749–774
Brooks SM, Hammad Y, Richards I, et al. The spectrum of irritant-induced asthma: sudden and not-so-sudden onset and the role of allergy. Chest 1998; 113:42–49
Kern, DG. Outbreak of the reactive airways dysfunction syndrome after a spill of glacial acetic acid. Am Rev Respir Dis 1991; 144:1058–1064
Tarlo SM, Balmes J, Balkissoon R, et al. Diagnosis and management of work-related asthma: American College of Chest Physicians consensus statement. Chest 2008; 134(suppl):1S–44S

137. B. Morphine sulfate is metabolized in the liver to active metabolites that accumulate in renal failure.

Many critically ill patients supported by mechanical ventilation receive opioid analgesic medications in order to provide pain relief and as cosedation to improve tolerance of mechanical ventilation and the ICU environment. Each agent has advantages and disadvantages, including different pharmacokinetic properties, metabolism, and potential adverse effects. Morphine sulfate has an onset of action of 5 to 10 min and duration of 2 to 4 h. It is metabolized in the liver to active compounds such as morphine 6-glucuronide, which is as active as the parent drug and accumulates in renal failure or with very high doses, leading to prolonged sedation (choice B is correct). Morphine is also associated with histamine release, possibly increasing the likelihood of bradycardia, hypotension, and/or bronchospasm, although clinically important effects are uncommon. Fentanyl is a synthetic compound that has high lipophilicity and a rapid onset of action (choice C is incorrect). It is rapidly redistributed, accounting for a short duration of action, but may have progressively delayed elimination with prolonged use because of its large volume of distribution. Fentanyl and related agents have a propensity to produce muscle rigidity, including chest wall rigidity that can interfere with ventilation. Hydromorphone has an onset of action of 5 to 10 min and is eliminated by demethylation in the liver. It is highly potent and addictive. Of note, hydromorphone may provide effective analgesia in patients who have become tolerant of other agents. Hydromorphone is not associated with prolonged QT syndrome (choice D is incorrect); however, methadone is associated with prolonged QT syndrome that can produce tachyarrhythmias such as torsade de pointes. Remifentanil is a newer, more expensive agent that undergoes metabolism in a unique fashion—via tissue esterases. Metabolites are not active; thus, this drug may offer advantages for the patient with hepatic or renal failure (choice A is incorrect). Remifentanil may cause bradycardia, hypotension, and/or rigidity. In addition to drug-specific adverse effects, opioids as a general class of drugs can produce dose-dependent respiratory depression, delayed GI transit, nausea, pruritus, and urinary retention.

Erstad B, Puntillo K, Gilbert H, et al. Pain management principles in the critically ill. Chest 2009; 135:1075–1086
Sessler CN, Varney K. Patient-focused sedation and analgesia in the ICU. Chest 2008; 133:552–565

138. B. Urine toxicology screen.

This man presents with rapidly progressive lung injury and expectoration of black material (melanoptysis). In addition, he has burns on this fingers, the telltale sign of crack cocaine smoking. While the clinical presentation is quite characteristic, the final diagnosis rests on documenting cocaine in the urine (choice B is correct). The cocaine epidemic has plagued many hospitals. Pure crystalline cocaine is expensive and is usually snorted into the nasal passages; however, when crystalline cocaine is boiled with baking soda and water and the precipitated material is then filtered or extracted with ether or alcohol, a stable lipid-soluble free-base is formed, which forms small, hard pellets that crackle when they are smoked—so-called "crack." This material can be smoked in a pipe, either alone or with tobacco or other substances. Smoked cocaine reaches the brain very quickly after it is absorbed by the lungs.

Cocaine causes lung disease by several mechanisms. The drug has direct toxicity by producing intense vasoconstriction leading to direct lung injury. Expectoration of the black material is quite suggestive of crack cocaine use. This material is caused by inhalation of the combustible materials used in smoking crack. While there are well-recognized causes of melanoptysis, such as coal miner's pneumoconiosis or silicosis with submassive fibrosis, there is no past history to suggest this etiology in our patient.

The agitation and severe shortness of breath are compatible with pulmonary embolism but fail to account for the expectoration of the black material or the burned fingers (choice A is incorrect). It is highly unlikely that bronchoscopy will be helpful because melanoptysis has been confirmed (choice C is incorrect). The rapid development of the shortness of breath and the diffuse radiographic picture does not suggest a bacterial infection (choice D is incorrect).

Catof D, Albert RK. Bilateral thumb burns leading to the diagnosis of crack lung. Chest 2002; 121:289–291

Haim DY, Lippmann MI, Goldberg SK, et al. The pulmonary complications of crack cocaine: a comprehensive review. Chest 1995; 107:233–240

Klinger JR, Bensadoun E, Corrao WM. Pulmonary complications from alveolar accumulation of carbonaceous material in a cocaine smoker. Chest 1992; 101:1171–1173

Thadani PV. NIDA conference report on cardiopulmonary complications of "crack" cocaine use: clinical manisfestations and pathophysiology. Chest 1996; 110:1072–1076

139. B. Discontinue clopidogrel for 7 days before performing bronchoscopy.

This patient is at increased risk for bleeding complications from flexible bronchoscopy with transbronchial biopsy because of the use of clopidogrel, and the procedure should be delayed until after clopidogrel has been discontinued for 5 to 7 days (choice B is correct). In a recent prospective study, 28 of 30 patients (93%) who continued clopidogrel (with or without aspirin) and underwent transbronchial biopsy had significant bleeding, whereas only 20 of 574 (3.4%) not receiving clopidogrel had bleeding. In contrast, in a prospective cohort study of 1,217 patients who had transbronchial biopsy performed, there was no difference in bleeding rates for those who received aspirin compared with those who did not. Therefore, discontinuation of aspirin for transbronchial biopsy is not necessary (choice A is incorrect). Despite this, a 2001 survey showed that 61.3% and 71.5% of pulmonologists indicated they would hold clopidogrel and aspirin, respectively, before proceeding with a bronchoscopic biopsy.

The safety of flexible bronchoscopy and transbronchial biopsy in the setting of coronary artery disease has not been studied in detail. Although myocardial ischemia can occur during or after bronchoscopy, a study of 21 patients who underwent bronchoscopy during hospitalization for myocardial infarction, but who had no evidence of ongoing ischemia, suffered no procedure-related adverse cardiovascular events. Similarly, no patients out of 20 coronary care unit patients had chest pain or evidence of cardiac ischemia with bronchoscopy. By contrast, in a prospective British study of elderly patients undergoing elective bronchoscopy, a subset of patients (7 of 45) had transient ST segment depression and/or bundle branch block that accompanied significant tachycardia (average of 152 beats/min) and hypertension (average of 238/131 mm Hg). However, all of these patients received intratracheal topical anesthesia with 2.5% cocaine, a well-known inducer of coronary vasoconstriction. Lidocaine is the safest local anesthetic for flexible bronchoscopy, has no vasoconstrictive properties, and can be administered safely (choice C is incorrect). There are no firm guidelines for timing of elective flexible bronchoscopy after myocardial infarction. Relying on expert opinion, the British Thoracic Society recommends that bronchoscopy be delayed for 6 weeks after myocardial infarction, if possible. Twelve weeks have passed since our patient had a myocardial infarction, and there is no evidence that delaying bronchoscopy for 6 months after myocardial infarction is necessary (choice D is incorrect).

Ernst A, Eberhardt R, Wahidi M, et al. Effect of routine clopidogrel use on bleeding complications after transbronchial biopsy in humans. Chest 2006; 129:734–737

Herth FJ, Becker HD, Ernst A. Aspirin does not increase bleeding complications after transbronchial biopsy. Chest 2002; 122:1461–1464

Wahidi MM, Rocha AT, Hollingsworth JW, et al. Contraindications and safety of transbronchial lung biopsy via flexible bronchoscopy. A survey of pulmonologists and review of the literature. Respiration 2005; 72:285–295

Dweik RA, Mehta AC, Meeker DP, et al. Analysis of the safety of bronchoscopy after recent acute myocardial infarction. Chest 1996; 110:825–828

Dunagan DP, Burke HL, Aquino SL, et al. Fiberoptic bronchoscopy in coronary care unit patients: indications, safety, and clinical implications. Chest 1998; 114:1660–1667
Davies L, Mister R, Spence DP, et al. Cardiovascular consequences of fibreoptic bronchoscopy. Eur Respir J 1997; 10:695–698
Osula S, Stockton P, Abdelaziz MM, et al. Intratracheal cocaine induced myocardial infarction: an unusual complication of fibreoptic bronchoscopy. Thorax 2003; 58:733–734
British Thoracic Society guidelines on diagnostic flexible bronchoscopy. Thorax 2001; 56 (suppl 1):i1–i21

140. D. Adenocarcinoma.

Figure 84-A (in the stem) shows an abnormal opacity in the lingula and enlargement of the left hilum, and the CT scan images (see Figures 84-B and 84-C in the stem) show mass lesions in the lingula, hilum, and mediastinum, with encasement of the left upper lobe bronchus. These findings are most consistent with advanced lung cancer (choice D is correct). Although Kaposi sarcoma, non-Hodgkin lymphoma, and cervical cancer are recognized as AIDS-defining diseases in people who are HIV-seropositive, the incidence of lung cancer is now recognized to be increased in persons with HIV infection, especially in the years following the use of combination antiretroviral therapy as the standard of care. Although members of most populations with HIV infection are current or former smokers, their risk of developing lung cancer appears to be increased, even when incidence ratios are adjusted for smoking. The prevalence of microsatellite alternations reflecting genomic instability also occurs with greatly increased frequency in HIV-associated lung cancers, possibly playing a role in their pathogenesis.

Patients with lung cancer in the setting of HIV infection tend to be relatively young at presentation (mean age 45 years) and have mild or moderate immunosuppression. Similar to age-matched control subjects, 75 to 90% present with stage III or IV disease. Adenocarcinoma is the most common histologic type, and the prognosis appears to be worse in patients with HIV infection. Until further studies are performed, the diagnostic and therapeutic approaches to HIV-associated lung cancer are the same as for other patients, although the efficacy and toxicity of chemotherapy and radiotherapy may be different.

Pneumocystis pneumonia is the most common opportunistic infection in patients with HIV infection but would neither be expected to present with lung and mediastinal masses nor be present in a patient with a CD4+ lymphocyte count $> 200/\mu L$ ($> 0.200 \times 10^9/L$) (choice A is incorrect). Kaposi sarcoma may present with multiple pulmonary nodules, pleural effusions, and intrathoracic lymphadenopathy, but this pattern of a single large lung mass with unilateral lymphadenopathy would be distinctly unusual with this neoplasm (choice B is incorrect). Invasive pulmonary aspergillosis occurs in patients with HIV infection but usually presents with invasive and cavitary disease, without hilar and mediastinal lymphadenopathy, and only in the setting of severe immunosuppression (CD4+ lymphocyte count usually $< 50/\mu L$ [$< 0.050 \times 10^9/L$]) (choice C is incorrect).

Cadranel J, Garfield D, Lavolé A, et al. Lung cancer in HIV infected patients: facts, questions, and challenges. Thorax 2006; 61:1000–1008
Engels EA, Brock MV, Chen J, et al. Elevated incidence of lung cancer among HIV-infected individuals. J Clin Oncol 2006; 24:1383–1388
Wistuba II, Behrens C, Milchgrub S, et al. Comparison of molecular changes in lung cancers in HIV-positive and HIV-indeterminate subjects. JAMA 1998; 279:1554–1559

141. C. Residual volume (RV) increases.

Lung function generally peaks in the third decade in life and then declines progressively with age. Because of structural changes associated with aging, progressive loss of recoil forces of the lung exceed the effects of increasing chest wall stiffness, resulting in an increase in RV and functional residual capacity (FRC) (choice C is correct).

Chest wall compliance decreases with age because of structural changes of the intercostal muscles and joints and may be further decreased with kyphosis (choice B is incorrect). Although lung collagen increases with age, elastic fibers are decreased, and changes in cross-linking and the spatial arrangement of elastic tissues lead to an increase in lung

compliance and progressive enlargement of air spaces, an increase in diameter of alveolar ducts, and a reduction of alveolar surface area. Loss of elastic recoil also increases airway resistance through reduction of bronchiolar diameter, leading to premature airway closure with exhalation and air trapping (choice A is incorrect). Overall, this pattern may functionally resemble emphysema but without histologic evidence of alveolar destruction. Aging populations typically show progressive reductions in FVC and FEV_1, with the latter often declining more rapidly. Measurements of FEV_1/FVC < 0.7 are common in otherwise healthy, asymptomatic elderly subjects, and defining airflow obstruction using this calculation in the absence of other data is problematic.

The net effect of reduced lung recoil and increased chest wall stiffness in the aging lung is an increase in RV and FRC, whereas TLC remains unchanged (choice D is incorrect). RV/TLC increases from 0.25 at 20 years of age to about 0.4 at age 70 years. With progressively premature airway closure, the closing volume begins to exceed the supine FRC at about 44 years and the sitting FRC at about age 65 years; airway closure in dependent terminal bronchi eventually occurs during tidal breathing, contributing to progressively reduced Pao_2 in elderly people. Because respiratory muscle strength declines progressively with age, while the work of breathing increases because of reduced chest wall compliance and increased airway resistance, ventilatory capacity and exercise tolerance decline.

Sprung J, Gajic O, Warner DO. Review article. Age related alterations in respiratory function: anesthetic considerations. Cardiothorac Anesth 2006; 53:1244–1257

Chan ED, Welsh CH. Geriatric respiratory medicine. Chest 1998; 114:1704–1733

Aalami OO, Fang TD, Song HM, et al. Physiologic features of aging persons. Arch Surg 2003; 138:1068–1076

142. C. Cytomegalovirus infection.

Figure 142-A reveals lung tissue with lymphoplasmacytic inflammatory infiltrates and occasional markedly enlarged (cytomegalic) cells with large amphophilic (purple) intranuclear inclusions and multiple small basophilic (blue) intracytoplasmic inclusions. (Two of these cells are at the center of the picture, with surrounding inflammatory infiltrates.) These changes are pathognomonic for cytomegalovirus (CMV) infection (choice C is correct). An example of intranuclear inclusion bodies with the classic "owl eyes" appearance characteristic of CMV is shown in Figure 142-C (see arrows).

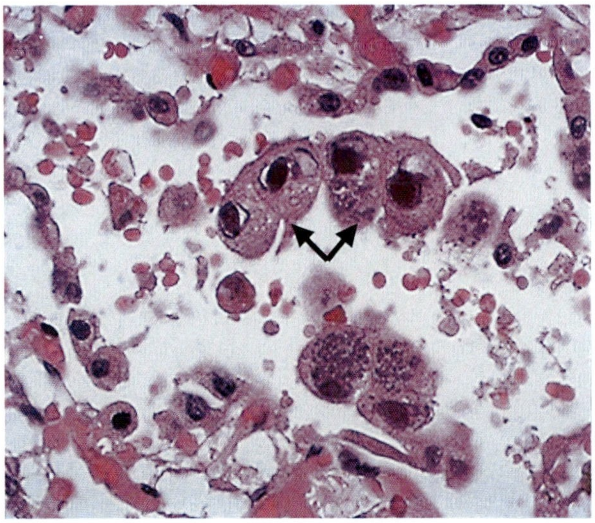

Figure 142-C
Hematoxylin-eosin

The CT scan (see Figure 142-B) reveals numerous tiny nodules in the left lower lobe with thickening of the interlobular septi in a micronodular configuration. These findings may be seen secondary to infection but are also suggestive of posttransplant lymphoproliferative disease (PTLD), the second most common neoplasm after

nonmelanoma skin cancers, and lung transplantation complications. The incidence of PTLD is highest within the first posttransplantation year and is a consequence of B-cell proliferation caused by the Epstein-Barr virus (EBV) in the immunocompromised host. Acute graft rejection usually occurs within the first 3 months after transplant but can occur up to 2 years after initial transplantation. Clinical features are nonspecific and include dyspnea, fever, leukocytosis, nonproductive cough, hypoxemia, or malaise, but patients with midler cases may be asymptomatic. Diagnosis is made on transbronchial lung biopsy, which reveals perivascular lymphocytic infiltrates. These aggregates of lymphocytes may be confused with PTLD on small biopsies. The current case results clearly show viral inclusion bodies and no evidence for lymphocytic aggregates (choices A and B are incorrect).

The level of immunosuppression peaks at 1 to 6 months after transplant, and it is at this time that opportunistic infections are most common. Opportunistic infections from *P jirovecii,* Aspergillus or Candida sp, and *Clostridium difficile* are most commonly seen. This patient was receiving appropriate prophylaxis for pneumocystis, and neither the CT scan nor biopsy findings are characteristic of this infection (choice D is incorrect). Viral infections also are common during the first 6 months and include CMV, EBV, and human herpes viruses.

Infection with CMV is of particular concern after lung transplant because early infection has been associated with subsequent development of bronchiolitis obliterans and chronic allograft dysfunction. The risk of infection is higher in recipient-positive, donor-negative and recipient-positive, donor-positive transplants. The most severe infections occur due to primary infections in donor-positive, recipient-negative recipients. Secondary CMV infection occurs with reactivation of latent disease, which is unmasked with immunosuppression. CMV most commonly causes pneumonitis, but it may also present as retinitis, hepatitis, colitis, or gastroenteritis. Monitoring for viral proliferation is done with serial measures of CMV polymerase chain reaction (PCR) or antigenemia in the blood. This case is unusual because the patient's CMV antigenemia assay remained negative, yet clear evidence of infection was seen on biopsy.

The treatment for CMV infection is IV ganciclovir or oral valganciclovir. The latter is only approved for prophylaxis in the United States but is widely used for preemptive treatment of antigenemia or less severe infections in other countries and appears efficacious. Many transplant centers routinely administer CMV prophylaxis. However, the exact duration of prophylaxis remains contentious because of a combination of costs and concerns over rising resistance rates. Most commonly, recipient-negative individuals receive 6 months of valganciclovir prophylaxis, recipient-positive individuals (including the current patient) receive 3 months of therapy, whereas donor- and recipient-negative patients receive 3 months of acyclovir therapy.

Lyu DM, Zamora MR. Medical complications of lung transplantation. Proc Am Thorac Soc 2009; 6:101–107
Remund KF, Best M, Egan JJ. Infections relevant to lung transplantation. Proc Am Thorac Soc 2009; 6:94–100
Lee P, Minai OA, Mehta AC, et al. Pulmonary nodules in lung transplant recipients: etiology and outcome. Chest 2004; 125:165–172
Kotloff RM, Ahya VN. Medical complications of lung transplantation. Eur Respir Dis 2004; 23:334–342
Fishman JA, Emery V, Freeman R, et al. Cytomegalovirus in transplantation-challenging the status quo. Clin Transplant 2007; 21:149–158
Len O, Gavalda J, Aguado JM, et al. Valganciclovir as treatment for cytomegalovirus disease in solid organ transplant recipients. Clin Infect Dis 2008; 46:20–27

143. B. Choice of transplantation conditioning regimen influences the risk of developing this disorder.

The patient's histologic findings of bronchiolar-centric changes of near complete obliteration of the bronchiolar lumen by concentric submucosal and adventitial scarring, with near complete destruction of the bronchiolar epithelium and sparing of the surrounding alveoli/interstitium (see Figures 143-A and 143-B), are diagnostic of obstructive bronchiolitis (OB; also known as constrictive bronchiolitis). Many risk factors have been associated with the development of OB in the setting of bone marrow transplantation (BMT), including some immunosuppressive medications such as busulfan (choice B is correct). Other risks for developing OB include human leukocyte antigen (HLA) mismatch, unrelated donor, hypogammaglobulinemia, and methotrexate prophylaxis against GVHD. The most common risk factor is chronic GVHD (as in this patient). OB has been described in autologous BMT, but the

absence of GVHD after these transplantations makes OB a rare event (compared with allogeneic BMT) (choice A is incorrect). Additional significant risk factors for OB identified from analysis of the International Bone Marrow Transplant Registry data in patients with allogeneic hematopoietic stem cell transplantation include long duration to transplantation, female donor to male recipient, and a prior episode of interstitial pneumonitis.

Clinically recognized OB usually develops 6 to 12 months after transplantation (choice C is incorrect) but may occur as early as 30 days and as late as 2 years after transplant. More than 80% of patients developing OB symptoms do so within 12 months. The average rate of posttransplant OB is 9%, with a range of 0 to 48%. Nonproductive cough, progressive dyspnea, new-onset obstructive changes in lung function (as in this patient), and high-resolution CT (HRCT) findings of "mosaic attenuation" enhanced on expiration (areas of differing attenuation based on obstructive airway abnormalities of OB prompting air trapping; not seen in this patient's HRCT, even in expiratory films) are consistent with a presumptive diagnosis of OB. Definitive diagnosis requires a tissue examination (most often not successfully accomplished by bronchoscopy) requiring surgical lung biopsy. Often, bronchoscopy is performed first to rule out concomitant infectious complications. Therapy consists of reinitiating or augmenting immunosuppression, with corticosteroids being the mainstay of therapy. Mortality ranges from 40 to 100% (median of 65%) (choice D is incorrect), with rates of improvement or stabilization ranging from 0 to 60% (median of 35%). Earlier diagnosis may be central to success. Unfortunately, pulmonary complications of BMT, both infectious and noninfectious (including OB), are often not correctly identified before death.

Marras TK, Chan CKN. Obliterative bronchiolitis complicating bone marrow transplantation. Semin Respir Crit Care Med 2003; 24:531–542

Tomas LHS, Loberiza FR, Klein JP, et al. Risk factors for bronchiolitis obliterans in allogeneic hematopoietic stem-cell transplantation for leukemia. Chest 2005; 128:153–161

Sharma S, Nadrous HF, Peters SG, et al. Pulmonary complications in adult blood and marrow transplant recipients: autopsy findings. Chest 2005; 128:1385–1392

144. A. Transesophageal echocardiography (TEE).

The patient's presentation and chest radiograph (see Figure 144-A) are highly suggestive of an aortic dissection. The chest radiograph reveals diffuse aortic dilation with a widened mediastinum. The presence of hypotension and bradycardia, in combination with enlargement of the cardiac silhouette, suggests a type A acute aortic dissection with extension into the pericardium, resulting in hemorrhagic tamponade. Because of hemodynamic instability, TEE is the best choice because it can be done quickly and at the bedside (choice A is correct). Subsequent transesophageal echocardiography confirmed the clinical suspicion for an acute aortic dissection with physiologic findings of tamponade leading to surgical repair of the dissection.

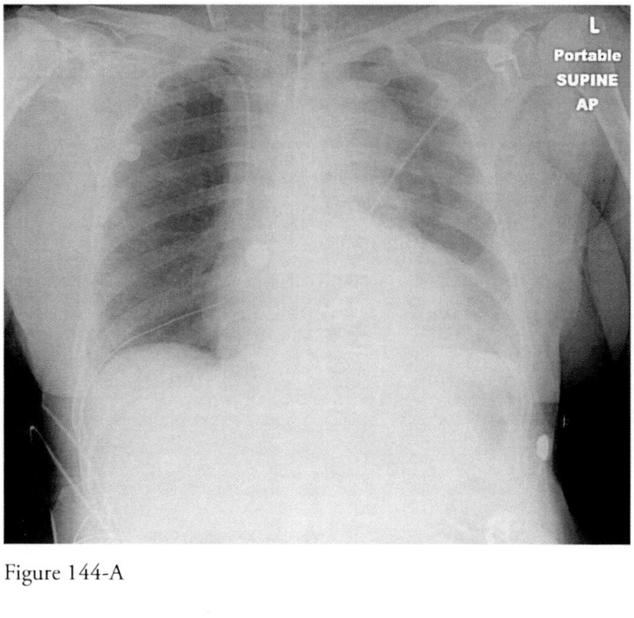

Figure 144-A

Echocardiography, MRI, and angiography are all sensitive tests to accurately make a diagnosis of acute aortic dissection, with a collective mean sensitivity and specificity >95%. Although the performance characteristics are similar in all three diagnostic tests, additional factors such as availability of experienced echocardiographers, side effects from either CT or MRI IV contrast, and hemodynamic instability affecting the safety of transportation need to be considered. CT angiography would have been an option for our patient but was not pursued because of her hemodynamic instability and the requirement for her to be transported to the radiology suite. The use of IV contrast also would have increased the risk for contrast nephropathy given the patient's history of chronic kidney disease (choice B is incorrect). Similarly, MRI with angiography was not considered for evaluation of an aortic dissection in the patient because of her hemodynamic instability and the duration required to perform the study (choice C is incorrect). Diagnostic biomarkers, such as d-dimer, elastin fragments, and smooth-muscle myosin heavy-chain protein, are currently under investigation to facilitate an accurate diagnosis of aortic dissection but have not been validated (choice D is incorrect). The clinical suspicion for an aortic dissection obviated further risk stratification and required a definitive evaluation.

The management of acute aortic dissections is based on society-based consensus guidelines given the inherent emergency of the disorder and the limited ability to conduct randomized, controlled clinical trials. Type A acute dissections are treated with surgical resection of the ascending aorta and replacing it with a prosthetic graft. Surgical repair/replacement of the aorta may be necessary as well. In patients with multiple comorbidities, medical management alone may be necessary but is associated with 50% in-hospital mortality at 30 days compared with 24% for those treated with surgical repair.

The mainstay of the management of a type B acute aortic dissection is strict BP control. Surgical repair is reserved for patients with progressive dissection, aortic rupture, or secondary complications such as mesenteric, renal, or peripheral artery hypoperfusion.

The success of endovascular stent in the treatment of other vascular disease has lead to interest in using aortic stent in the treatment of aortic dissection, namely type B dissections. The in-hospital mortality approaches 5%, with a complication rate of 11%. Long-term follow-up is necessary to guide the ongoing use of endovascular stents.

Golledge J, Eagle KA. Acute aortic dissection. Lancet 2008; 372:55–66

Shiga T, Wajima Z, Apfel CC, et al. Diagnostic accuracy of transesophageal echocardiography, helical computed tomography, and magnetic resonance imaging for suspected thoracic aortic dissection: systematic review and meta-analysis. Arch Intern Med 2006; 166:1350–1356

Shinohara T, Suzuki K, Okada M, et al. Soluble elastin fragments in serum are elevated in acute aortic dissection. Arterioscler Thromb Vasc Biol 2003; 23:1839–1844

145. B. The disease-free interval.

This patient has a hematogenous metastasis from colorectal carcinoma. Colon cancer is one of the common tumors to metastasize to the lungs, forming solitary or multiple pulmonary nodules. Other tumors that metastasize in this fashion are sarcoma, melanoma, testicular carcinoma, and renal cell carcinoma. Some factors that portend a favorable outcome from metastasectomy include control of the original cancer, a single or smaller number of lesions, the cell type, complete resection of the metastases, and a prolonged disease-free interval (defined as the time from diagnosis of the primary cancer to the appearance of pulmonary metastases). Data from the International Registry of Lung Metastases for patients who had undergone metastasectomy indicate that patients with a single metastasis have a significantly better 5-year survival than those with two to three or more than three metastases (43% vs 34 and 27%, respectively). In this case, the short disease-free interval portends a poor prognosis but does not preclude an attempt at metastasectomy (choice B is correct).

When specifically examining colon cancer, 5- and 10-year survival rates after metastasectomy can approach 45 and 30%, respectively. Favorable prognostic factors include a small number of pulmonary metastases (particularly solitary metastases), a normal carcinoembryonic antigen (choice A is incorrect), and a disease-free interval > 36 months.

Solitary and multiple metastatic nodules tend to occur in the periphery of the lungs presumably because they spread hematogenously. The lower and middle lung fields tend to be involved more commonly because these are the zones of greatest blood flow. Often the metastatic lesions are bilateral and well circumscribed and occur in varying sizes. Chest CT is understandably superior to plain chest radiography for detecting small metastases involving the subpleural, apical, and costophrenic angle regions, as well as in assessing mediastinal lymphadenopathy.

In a large series of patients undergoing metastasectomy for varying histologic diagnoses, 2-, 5-, and 10-year survival rates are 50 to 69%, 36 to 48%, and 26 to 35%, respectively, but vary widely by the tumor histologic findings. Patients with metastasectomy for teratomas and other germ cell tumors have the best prognosis (10-year survival rates approaching 70%), whereas metastasectomies for melanomas have the worse prognosis (5-year survival rates of 11 to 25%). Survival rates following resection for colon cancers fall between these rates, and colon cancers are one of the most common tumors to be treated with metastasectomy.

When contemplating a metastasectomy, most thoracic oncologic surgeons agree on the following criteria: (1) the primary tumor must be controlled; (2) there is no other evidence of extrathoracic metastatic disease; (3) the metastatic lung disease must be amenable to complete resection; (4) the patient must be physiologically able to tolerate the proposed surgery; and (5) there is no other effective systemic therapy. More controversial issues regarding the potential success of metastasectomies include tumor doubling time, smaller sized nodules (some studies have suggested a worse prognosis if lesions are > 3 cm in size; choice D is incorrect), and unilateral vs bilateral metastatic disease. Location of the lesion (right vs left lung) has not been found to be a prognostic factor (choice C is incorrect). Surgical approaches for metastasectomy include wedge resections, segmentectomy, and only rarely lobectomy. The surgery can be done via either open thoracotomy or video-assisted thoracoscopic surgery. The completeness of the resection is a key factor in survival.

Pastorino U, Buyse M, Friedel G, et al. Long-term results of lung metastasectomy: prognostic analyses based on 5,206 cases. The International Registry of Lung Metastases. J Thorac Cardiovasc Surg 1997; 113:37–49

van Halteren HK, van Geel AN, Hart A, et al. Pulmonary resection for metastases of colorectal origin. Chest 1995; 107:1526–1531

Yedibela S, Klein P, Feuchter K, et al. Surgical management of pulmonary metastases from colorectal cancer in 153 patients. Ann Surg Oncol 2006; 13:1538–1544

Gould MK, Fletcher J, Iannettoni MD, et al. Evaluation of patients with pulmonary nodules: when is it lung cancer? ACCP evidence-based clinical practice guidelines (2nd edition). Chest 2007; 132(suppl):108S–130S

Warwick R, Page R. Resection of pulmonary metastases from colorectal carcinoma. Eur J Surg Oncol 2007; 33(suppl):S59–S63

Rena O, Papalia E, Oliaro A, et al. Pulmonary metastases from epithelial tumours: late results of surgical treatment. Eur J Cardiothorac Surg 2006; 30:217–222

Iizasa T, Suzuki M, Yoshida S, et al. Prediction of prognosis and surgical indications for pulmonary metastasectomy from colorectal cancer. Ann Thorac Surg 2006; 82:254–260

146. C. Dyspnea score, BMI, and 6MWD.

The degree of airway obstruction as measured by the FEV_1 has been known for decades to correlate with survival in COPD. Other important factors that correlate with survival include poor oxygenation and impaired right heart function. However, assessing these parameters requires invasive and/or expensive testing procedures. More recently, simpler assessments that can be done in many settings have been incorporated into the BODE score and have been shown to have strong correlations with survival.

The BODE score has four components: B = BMI; O = obstruction (FEV_1); D = dyspnea (Medical Research Council [MRC] four-point scale that ranges from "not troubled with breathlessness" to "too breathless to leave house or breathless with dressing/undressing"); and E = exercise (6MWD). Therefore, answer C is correct, and the others are incorrect.

The values used to calculate the four components of the BODE score are shown in Table 146-1.

Table 146-1. Values for Calculating the Four Components of the BODE Score

Variable	**BODE Score**			
	0	1	2	3
FEV_1, % predicted	>65	50–65	35–49	<35
Dyspnea: MRC 4-point scale	0–1	2	3	4
6MWD, m	>350	250–349	150–249	<149
BMI	>21	<21		

The scores of the four component are then added together for the final BODE score.

Table 146-2 shows how the BODE score is related to the likelihood of 4-year mortality.

Table 146-2. Relationship of BODE Score and 4-Year Mortality

BODE Score	**4-Year Mortality**
0–2	20–30%
3–4	50–60%
5–6	70–80%
>7	80–90%

Because BODE scores are easy to obtain, they have potential utility in assessing risk and changes in that risk from various interventions.

Celli B, Cote C, Marin J, et al. The body mass index, airflow obstruction, dyspnea, and exercise capacity index in chronic obstructive pulmonary disease. New Engl J Med 2004; 350:1005–1012
Celli BR, Cote CG, Lareau SC, et al. Predictors of survival in COPD: more than just the FEV_1. J Respir Med 2008; 102(suppl 1):s27–s35
Martinez FJ, Han MK, Andre AC, et al. Longitudinal change in the BODE index predicts mortality in severe emphysema. Am J Respir Crit Care Med 2008; 178:491–499
Imfeld S, Bloch KE, Weder W, et al. The BODE index after lung volume reduction surgery correlates with survival. Chest 2006; 129:873–878

147. A. Add a long-acting β-agonist to her current dose of inhaled fluticasone.

In this patient whose asthma is no longer well controlled by a low-dose inhaled corticosteroid alone (step 2 treatment), the preferred treatment option is the addition of a long-acting β-agonist to the low-dose inhaled corticosteroid (step 3 treatment); thus, choice A is correct. Addition of a long-acting β-agonist in this setting has been shown in multiple studies to produce better symptomatic and spirometic results than increasing the dose of inhaled corticosteroids to medium- or high-dose range or combining inhaled corticosteroids with other agents.

A long-acting β-agonist should not be used in the absence of a controller medication because an increased risk of death has been observed in such circumstances. However, safety concerns are less acute when a long-acting β-agonist is used in conjunction with an inhaled corticosteroid, and prescribing a preparation that combines the two drugs in a single inhaler should be considered to minimize the possibility that the patient will take a long-acting β-agonist alone.

Although the 2007 National Asthma Education and Prevention Program: Expert Panel Report 3 gives equal preference to the option of low-dose inhaled corticosteroids plus an inhaled long-acting β-agonist or the use of medium-dose inhaled corticosteroids as monotherapy, the use of high-dose inhaled corticosteroids would not be appropriate in this setting (choice D is incorrect). For reference, dose ranges for commonly used inhaled corticosteroids from the 2007 National Heart, Lung, and Blood Institute, National Asthma Education and Prevention Program Expert Panel Report 3 are shown in Table 147-1.

Addition of either a leukotriene receptor antagonist such as montelukast or the addition of theophylline to low-dose inhaled corticosteroids does tend to result in improvement, but these effects are generally less impressive than those obtained by the addition of a long-acting β-agonist (choice B is incorrect).

Omalizumab is a recombinant, humanized IgG1 monoclonal antibody that binds IgE with high affinity. It is approved for treatment of asthma as a subcutaneous dose administered every 2 to 4 weeks. However, because of its cost and safety profile, it should be considered only in patients as part of step 5 or step 6 therapy, *ie,* when the patient remains symptomatic despite trigger avoidance, high-dose inhaled corticosteroids, and a long-acting β-agonist ± systemic corticosteroids (choice C is incorrect).

Table 147-1. Dose Ranges for Commonly Used Inhaled Corticosteroids*

Drug	Low Dose	Medium Dose	High Dose
Beclomethasone dipropionate CFC	168–504 µg	504–840 µg	> 840 µg
42 µg/puff	(4–12 puffs)	(12–20 puffs)	(> 20 puffs)
84 µg/puff	(2–6 puffs)	(6–10 puffs)	(> 10 puffs)
Beclomethasone HFA	80–240 µg	240–480 µg	> 480 µg
40 µg/dose	(2–6 puffs daily)	(6–12 puffs daily)	(> 12 puffs daily)
80 µg/dose	(1–3 puffs daily)	(3–6 puffs daily)	(> 6 puffs daily)
Budesonide inhalation powder (Pulmicort Flexhaler; AstraZeneca Pharmaceuticals; Wilmington, DE)	90–360 µg	360–540 µg	> 540 µg
90 µg/dose	(1–4 inhalations)	(4–6 inhalations)	(> 6 inhalations)
180 µg/dose	(1 inhalation)	(1–2 inhalations)	(> 2 inhalations)
Flunisolide	500–1,000 µg	1,000–2,000 µg	> 2,000 µg
250 µg/puff	(2–4 puffs)	(4–8 puffs)	(> 8 puffs)
Fluticasone	88–264 µg	264–660 µg	> 660 µg
MDI: 44, 110, 220 µg/puff	(2–6 puffs, 44 µg) or (2 puffs, 110 µg)	(2–6 puffs, 110 µg)	(> 6 puffs, 110 µg) or (> 3 puffs, 220 µg)
DPI: 50, 100, 250 µg/dose	(2–6 inhalations, 50 µg)	(3–6 inhalations,100 µg)	(> 6 inhalations, 100 µg) or (> 2 inhalations, 250 µg)
Mometason: 20 µg/dose	(1–2 inhalations)	(2–3 inhalations)	(> 3 inhalations)
Triamcinolone acetonide	400–1,000 µg	1,000–2,000 µg	> 2,000 µg
100 µg/puff	(4–10 puffs)	(10–20 puffs)	(> 20 puffs)

* From the 2007 National Heart, Lung, and Blood Institute, National Asthma Education and Prevention Program Expert Panel Report 3.
DPI = dry powder inhaler; MDI = metered-dose inhaler.

Ernst P, McIvor A, Ducharme FM, et al. Safety and effectiveness of long-acting inhaled beta-agonist bronchodilators when taken with inhaled corticosteroids. Ann Intern Med 2006; 145:692–694
Global Initiative for Asthma (GINA). 2008 global strategy for management and prevention. Available at www.ginasthma.org. Accessed April 18, 2009
Greenstone IR, Ni Chroinin MN, Masse V, et al. Combination of inhaled long-acting β_2-agonists and inhaled steroids versus higher dose of inhaled steroids in children and adults with persistent asthma. Cochrane Database Syst Rev 2005; Oct 19:CD005533
National Asthma Education and Prevention Program: Expert Panel Report 3: Guidelines for the diagnosis and management of asthma. Bethesda, MD: National Heart, Lung, and Blood Institute, 2007 (NIH publication no. 08-4051)
Nelson HS, Weiss ST, Bleecker ER, et al. The Salmeterol Multicenter Asthma Research Trial: a comparison of usual pharmacotherapy for asthma or usual pharmacotherapy plus salmeterol. Chest 2006; 129:15–26
Woolcock A, Lundback B, Ringdal N, et al. Comparison of addition of salmeterol to inhaled steroids with doubling of the dose of inhaled steroids. Am J Respir Crit Care Med 1996; 153:1481–1488

148. A. Arrange for diagnostic bronchoscopy.

This patient has a 10-day history of nonspecific clinical deterioration and diffuse pulmonary infiltrates in the setting of a prior diagnosis of secondary pulmonary alveolar proteinosis. His symptoms of increasing shortness of breath, cough, chest heaviness, low-grade fever, and lassitude could be related to worsening of his underlying disease or potentially to infection. His lung function tests are abnormal and have worsened since his last assessment but, importantly, do not demonstrate severe impairment. His chest radiograph is markedly abnormal, showing bilateral patchy airspace infiltrates with confluence, characteristic of pulmonary alveolar proteinosis but also potentially superimposed infection. As is often the case in patients with this disease, the magnitude of radiographic abnormalities is disproportionate to the severity of symptoms and physical findings. Unfortunately, this patient is not producing sputum.

Patients with pulmonary alveolar proteinosis are at risk of secondary infection from a variety of pathogens, including opportunistic organisms such as Nocardia, but also from common respiratory pathogens. In patients dying from the disease, approximately 20% of deaths are attributable to infections. Mild self-limiting respiratory infections would not lead to progressive 10-day worsening, and, as such, serious consideration of significant infection must be undertaken. In the absence of a readily obvious etiology, a diagnostic bronchoscopy would be indicated to obtain appropriate specimens to rule out associated infection (choice A is correct). Initiating therapy with broad-spectrum antibiotic therapy pending the bronchoscopy might be appropriate, depending on the clinical impression at the time.

Starting GM-CSF would assume the underlying cause of this patient's clinical deterioration was pulmonary alveolar proteinosis, and this has not yet been established. Moreover, GM-CSF has shown effectiveness largely in patients with primary pulmonary alveolar proteinosis and not in secondary causes such as in this patient (choice B is incorrect). Similarly, because whole-lung lavage is the gold standard for management of the patient's underlying condition, it would not be appropriate therapy if an infective etiology was deemed to be responsible (choice C is incorrect). Finally, systemic corticosteroid therapy has not demonstrated effectiveness in this disease and may be associated with increased mortality (choice D is incorrect).

Juvet SC, Hwang D, Waddell TK, et al. Rare lung disease II: pulmonary alveolar proteinosis. Can Respir J 2008; 15:203–210
Presneill JJ, Nakata K, Inoue Y, et al. Pulmonary alveolar proteinosis. Clin Chest Med 2004; 25:593–613
Trapnell BC, Whitsett JA, Nakata K. Pulmonary alveolar proteinosis. New Engl J Med 2003; 349:2527–2539

149. D. Have a better overall prognosis.

Nodular sarcoidosis is an uncommon manifestation of the disease that is seen in 2 to 4% of patients. The chest radiograph and chest CT scan characteristically reveal multiple pulmonary nodules or masses. These nodules are often described as "fluffy" or as having a "snowball" appearance. The masses can vary in size and are sometimes as large as

8 cm in diameter. Air bronchograms and cavitation are not uncommon. Despite the dramatic radiographic appearance, however, patients with nodular sarcoidosis typically have a benign clinical course (choice D is correct). Most patients have complete or nearly complete resolution of radiologic findings, either spontaneously or with corticosteroid treatment.

Case series findings suggest that the majority of patients with nodular sarcoidosis are young, African-American women (choice A is incorrect). Extrapulmonary involvement is noted in approximately 40% of patients, which is similar to the other forms of sarcoid disease (choice B is incorrect). The radiologic features are interesting. As noted above, patients will have multiple pulmonary nodules and/or masses. There is a tendency toward upper lobe predominance. The nodules are often peripheral, with pleural-based lesions seen in almost two-thirds of patients. Approximately 60% of the masses will contain air bronchograms. Pleural involvement (thickening and effusions) is more common than in other forms of sarcoidosis and can be seen in up to one-third of patients. Mediastinal lymphadenopathy is seen in the majority of patients (up to 90% in one series), which is similar to other forms of sarcoidosis (choice C is incorrect).

Malaisamy S, Dalal B, Bimenyuy C, et al. The clinical and radiologic features of nodular sarcoidosis. Lung 2009; 187:9–15
McCullough PC, McCullough AE. Nodular sarcoidosis. New Engl J Med 2002; 346:1970
Lynch JP, Ma YL, Koss MN, et al. Pulmonary sarcoidosis. Semin Resp Crit Care Med 2007; 28:53–74

150. A. Increased for malignant mesothelioma.

Malignancy is one of the major complications from prolonged exposure to asbestos. Most commonly, exposure is through occupational sources (*eg,* cement, friction materials, textiles, insulation, and shipbuilding) or the mining of fibers. Exposure can also occur in a natural setting, such as environmental exposure in the neighborhood of industrial sources or natural environmental exposure to geologic sources. When occurring through natural or industrial environmental exposure, only the risk of malignant mesothelioma is increased (choice A is correct). Additionally, the risk appears to increase in proportion to the proximity of an individual's location to the source of the environmental asbestos.

Asbestos exposure can lead to nonmalignant disease, such as pleural plaques and asbestosis. However, malignant disease is the major complication of asbestos exposure. The following malignancies have been linked to asbestos: mesothelioma, bronchogenic carcinoma, laryngeal and oropharyngeal malignancies, renal carcinoma, and esophageal and biliary carcinoma. Asbestos is one of the few risk factors for malignant mesothelioma (along with medical radiation exposure and certain other minerals, such as erionite from volcanic emissions). A genetic predisposition, as seen with the erionite exposure in the Anatolian plateau of Turkey, may also play a role. The relative risk for malignancy depends on the length of exposure, magnitude of the exposure, and amount of cigarette use. Thus, casual exposure through environmental emissions presents a significantly lower risk than high levels of exposure seen with asbestos mining. In addition, the type of asbestos fiber affects the risk of lung cancer because the risk is considerably higher for workers exposed to amphibole fibers than for those exposed to chrysotile fibers. The increased risk of lung cancer associated with asbestos is greatly increased by the additional exposure to tobacco smoke. In one study, the risk of dying from bronchogenic carcinoma in asbestos workers increased 16-fold if they smoked more than 20 cigarettes per day and ninefold for less than 20 cigarettes per day when compared with asbestos workers with no smoking history. Asbestos workers with no smoking history had a sixfold increase in bronchogenic carcinoma, illustrating that the risk is more than additive.

The studies evaluating these risks have been performed in individuals with a significant occupational exposure to asbestos. Environmental exposure through industrial or natural means has been shown to increase only the likelihood

of malignant mesothelioma, not the other malignancies (choices B and C are incorrect). At low levels of exposure, a small risk remains (choice D is incorrect).

Reid A, Berry G, de Klerk N, et al. Age and sex differences in malignant mesothelioma after residential exposure to blue asbestos (crocidolite). Chest 2007; 131:376–382

Pan XL, Day HW, Wang W, et al. Residential proximity to naturally occurring asbestos and mesothelioma risk in California. Am J Respir Crit Care Med 2005; 172:1019–1025

Kurumatani N, Kumagai S. Mapping the risk of mesothelioma due to neighborhood asbestos exposure. Am J Respir Crit Care Med 2008; 178:624–629

Hammond EC, Selikoff IJ, Seidman H. Asbestos exposure, cigarette smoking and death rates. Ann NY Acad Sci 1979; 330:473–490

Dickensoy O. Mesothelioma due to environmental exposure to erionite in Turkey. Curr Opin Pulm Med 2008; 14:322–325

151. A. Anion gap metabolic acidosis + non-anion gap metabolic acidosis + respiratory acidosis.

Acid-base status can be evaluated by examining the mathematical relationship of pH, Pco_2, and HCO_3^- within the context of the clinical circumstances. A number of tools, including various equations of the relationship of pH, Pco_2, and HCO_3^-, can be used to identify acid-base disorders as well as determine if a mixed acid-base disturbance is present. These strategies consider the primary change in Pco_2 or HCO_3^- as well as the expected compensations that occur in an attempt to normalize pH. When a metabolic acidosis is present, additional calculations can be made to determine if unmeasured anions are present—thus, an anion gap–positive metabolic acidosis. Finally, comparison of the change (Δ) in the anion gap to the change (Δ) in bicarbonate can be used to determine the likelihood of a second metabolic disturbance. In this case, a triple acid-base disturbance is present with an anion gap metabolic acidosis + a non-anion gap metabolic acidosis + a mild respiratory acidosis (choice A is correct).

A four-step strategy can be used to identify primary acid-base disorders and differentiate a simple disorder with expected compensation from a mixed acid-base disturbance:

Step 1. Is pH, Pco_2, or HCO_3^- out of the normal range (normal range 7.35 to 7.45, 35 to 45 mm Hg, and 21 to 28 mEq/L [mmol/L], respectively)? If so, an acid-base disorder is present. In our case, both pH and HCO_3^- are out of range.

Step 2. Is pH $>$ or $<$ 7.40? If $>$ 7.40, then an alkalosis is a primary disorder. If $<$ 7.40, then an acidosis is a primary disorder. In this case, pH is 7.10; thus, an acidosis is present.

Step 3. Is a primary disorder metabolic or respiratory? In this case, HCO_3^- is lower than the normal range; thus, a metabolic acidosis is present.

Step 4. Is the compensation consistent with a simple compensated acid-base disorder, or is a mixed disorder present? The compensation moves in the same direction as the primary change. The magnitude of compensation is different for each of the primary acid-base disturbances and differs for primary respiratory disorders depending on the duration (acute vs chronic). Conversion factors represent an approximate mean value, and most cases should be within 20% of these values. Table 151-1 is based on standard equations for each disorder and displays relative change in HCO_3^- for a change of 10 mm Hg in Pco_2. It is easier to memorize the table by considering the logical HCO_3^- change progression of 1, 2, 3, and 5, 10, 15 and that the acid-base disorders are listed in alphabetical order. The change in HCO_3^- is relative to the center of the normal range (25 mEq/L [mmol/L]), and the change in Pco_2 of 10 mm Hg is compared with normal, 40 mm Hg.

Table 151-1. Example of HCO_3^- Change Progression

Primary Acid-Base Disorder	Change in Pco_2, mm Hg	Change in HCO_3^-, mEq/L
Acute respiratory acidosis	**10***	1
Acute respiratory alkalosis	**10**	2
Chronic respiratory acidosis	**10**	3
Chronic respiratory alkalosis	**10**	5
Metabolic acidosis	10	**10**
Metabolic alkalosis	10	**15**

* Primary change is in boldface.

In our patient, metabolic acidosis is the primary disorder. HCO_3^- is 12 mEq/L (mmol/L), which is 13 mEq/L (mmol/L) less than the middle of the normal range (25 mEq/L [mmol/L]); thus a decrease of 13 mm Hg in Pco_2 would be expected as compensation. However, the Pco_2 is not 27 mm Hg (*ie,* 40 to 13 mm Hg), but is higher at 35 mm Hg, indicative of another primary acid-base disorder (*ie,* respiratory acidosis) in addition to metabolic acidosis (choices B, C, and D are incorrect).

The anion gap can be calculated as follows: $AG = Na - (Cl + HCO_3^-)$ and has a normal range of 8 to 16 mEq/L. In our case, $AG = 140 - (112 + 12) = 16$ mEq/L, which is at the upper limits of the normal range. However, the majority of "unmeasured anions" are composed of albumin and inorganic phosphorus, and a corrected anion gap can be calculated as follows: $cAG = Na - (Cl + HCO_3^-) - [2 \times (\text{albumin}) + 0.5 \times (\text{phosphate})]$, with a "normal" range of 0 to 5. For our patient, the corrected anion gap is $140 - (112 + 12) - [2 \times (2.5) + 0.5 \times (4)]$, or 9, which is increased and is consistent with an anion gap acidosis. An additional metabolic acidosis or metabolic alkalosis could be present. The ratio of the difference between measured anion gap and the middle of the anion gap range (Δ AG) to the difference between normal HCO_3^- and measured HCO_3^- ($\Delta\ HCO_3^-$) can help identify such a case. If the ratio is > 1, metabolic alkalosis is likely to be present (or pure lactic acidosis) and if < 1, then a hyperchloremic non-anion gap metabolic acidosis is probably present. In our case, $\Delta\ AG/\Delta\ HCO_3^- = (16 - 12)/(25 - 12) = 4/13$. This is < 1 and is consistent with the additional presence of a non-anion gap metabolic acidosis.

Kellum JA. Disorders of acid-base balance. Crit Care Med 2007; 35:2630–2636

Adrogue HJ. Mixed acid-base disturbances. J Nephrol 2006; 19(suppl):S97–S103

152. B. Isoniazid, rifampin, and ethambutol.

This patient receiving treatment with corticosteroids for his myelodysplastic syndrome developed a disseminated disease characterized by small upper lobe pulmonary infiltrates, bilateral pleural effusions, and mediastinal lymphadenopathy. The mediastinal lymph node biopsy shows a granuloma with central necrosis and numerous acid-fast bacilli, and a DNA probe of organism culture confirms *Mycobacterium kansasii* as the causative pathogen. There are no randomized trials of treatment for disseminated *M kansasii,* but the recommended treatment regimen for disseminated disease with this organism, based on *in vitro* resistance patterns and case series, includes rifampin, ethambutol, and isoniazid (choice B is correct) for at least 18 months, and 12 months after negative culture results. A regimen of three times weekly clarithromycin, ethambutol, and rifampin is recommended for nodular/bronchiectatic pulmonary disease caused by *Mycobacterium avium* complex (MAC), but not for disseminated *M kansasii* (choice A is incorrect). Isolates of *M kansasii* are usually resistant to pyrazinamide (choice C is incorrect). Isolates of *M kansasii* may be less sensitive to isoniazid, and streptomycin might be considered as an alternative. However, in the absence of prior treatment with antituberculous drugs, isoniazid would be preferred (choice D is incorrect).

The incidence of TB has declined in recent years in the United States, with only 14,097 cases reported in 2005. Of these, 55% were in foreign-born people and only 20% had extrapulmonary disease. These numbers indicate that

extrapulmonary TB in a person born in the United States is unusual. Consequently, nontuberculous mycobacteria should also be considered as possible pathogens. MAC and *M kansasii* are the nontuberculous mycobacteria most often associated with human disease. Information on the incidence of human disease caused by nontuberculous mycobacteria is limited because they are not reportable pathogens. However, there were approximately 9,500 isolates of MAC reported to the Centers for Disease Control and Prevention in the mid-1990s, suggesting that the number of cases of nontuberculous mycobacterial disease in the United States might be comparable with those caused by TB. Both MAC and *M kansasii* cause disseminated disease in patients with AIDS, but they can also cause disease in patients who do not have AIDS. Cancer, hematologic malignancies, underlying COPD, and immunosuppression seem to be predisposing factors for human disease with MAC and *M kansasii*, but infection may occur in people who are otherwise immunocompetent. In patients who do not have AIDS, MAC and *M kansasii* cause upper lobe pulmonary disease and both cavitating and nodular bronchiectasis, but are infrequently associated with either pleural effusions or mediastinal lymphadenopathy.

Griffith DE, Aksamit T, Brown-Elliott BA, et al. An official ATS/IDSA statement: diagnosis, treatment, and prevention of nontuberculous mycobacterial diseases. Am J Respir Crit Care Med 2007; 175:367–416

Han XY, Tarrand JJ, Infante R, et al. Clinical significance and epidemiologic analyses of *Mycobacterium avium* and *Mycobacterium intracellulare* among patients without AIDS. J Clin Microbiol 2005; 43:4407–4412

Kanathur N, Shataveerapa HN, Byrd RP, et al. Nontubercular mycobacterial pulmonary infection in immunocompetent men. South Med J 2001; 94:719–723

Maliwan N, Zvetina JR. Clinical features and follow up of 302 patients with *Mycobacterium kansasii* pulmonary infection. Postgrad Med J 2005; 81:530–533

Shitrit D, Baum GL, Priess R, et al. Pulmonary *Mycobacterium kansasii* infection in Israel, 1999-2004. Chest 2006; 129:771–776

153. B. A 63-year-old man with tobacco-related COPD who stopped smoking 12 months ago. He has an FEV_1 of 0.8 L (20% of predicted), a BODE score of 8, and no other significant medical history. He is being treated with prednisone, 20 mg po qd.

The original consensus-based guidelines for selection of lung transplant candidates were revised recently. The newer guidelines are also consensus-based, consider a greater body of evidence and transplant experience since the 1999 version, and have several important modifications outlined in Tables 153-1 and 153-2. The patient in choice B meets age criteria and disease criteria, has the FEV_1 and BODE index score suggesting the need for transplantation, and is the most appropriate candidate to undergo lung transplantation (choice B is correct).

Table 153-1. Relative and Absolute Contraindications to Lung Transplantation

Relative contraindications	• Age > 65 years • Critical or unstable clinical condition • Systemic or untreated extrapulmonic disease • Colonization with resistant fungus, atypical mycobacteria, or bacteria • Severe or symptomatic osteoporosis • Severely limited functional status • Mechanical ventilation • Ideal body weight < 70% or > 130% (BMI > 30 kg/m^2) • Significant pleural disease from prior thoracic procedures
Absolute contraindications	• Extrapulmonic disease, *ie*, renal (Creatinine clearance < 50 mL/min/1.73 m^2 [0.835 mL/s/m^2]) • HIV infection • Malignancy within prior 2 years • Hepatitis B antigen positivity • Hepatitis C biopsy-proven liver disease • Severe musculoskeletal disease • Substance addiction in prior 6 months (including tobacco use) • Absence of a reliable support system • Untreatable psychosocial problems • Medical noncompliance

Table 153-2. Disease-Specific Criteria for Lung Transplantation*

COPD	BODE index > 7 <u>or</u> at least one of the following: • FEV_1 < 20% of predicted (nonreversible) <u>and</u> diffusing capacity < 20% <u>or</u> homogenous emphysema on high-resolution CT scan • Hospitalization with $Paco_2$ > 50 mm Hg • Cor pulmonale • O_2-dependent patients with hypercapnia (refer early)
IPF	Diagnosis of usual interstitial pneumonitis with any of the following: • DLCO < 39% of predicted • A decrease in FVC of > 10% in 6 months of follow-up • A decrease in pulse oximetry below 88% on a 6-min walk test • Honeycombing on high-resolution CT scan
CF	• FEV_1 < 30% of predicted • Clinical deterioration with FEV_1 > 30% of predicted (exacerbation, hemoptysis, pneumothorax) • $Paco_2$ > 50 mm Hg • Pao_2 while receiving room air < 55 mm Hg • Pulmonary hypertension • Young, female patients (refer early)
PPH	• NYHA III–IV, despite vasodilator treatment, including an epoprostenol agent • Cardiac index < 2 L/min/m^2 • Right atrial pressure > 15 mm Hg • Low (< 350 m) or declining 6-min walk

*CF = cystic fibrosis; IPF = idiopathic pulmonary fibrosis; NYHA = New York Heart Association; PPH = primary pulmonary hypertension; VC = vital capacity.

The major modifications have been in the areas of age (now 65 years is generally, but not firmly, suggested as the upper limit regardless of procedure type) and the inclusion of the BODE index (derived from measurements of BMI, degree of airway obstruction, dyspnea score, and exercise capacity) when evaluating patients with COPD.

The patient in choice A meets age and severity criteria for transplantation for cystic fibrosis but is infected with a particular strain of resistant bacteria that is considered a strong relative contraindication to transplantation (choice A is incorrect). The patient in choice D has several relative contraindications to lung transplantation. She is older than 65 years and, in addition, has significant osteoporosis that can pose a problem with rehabilitation following lung transplantation and could be further worsened by the corticosteroids used for post-lung-transplantation immunosuppression (choice D is incorrect). The patient in choice C meets age criteria and is approaching severity criteria but has not received a trial of epoprostenol therapy (choice C is incorrect).

Aris RM, Routh JC, LiPuma JJ, et al. Lung transplantation for cystic fibrosis patients with *Burkholderia cepacia* complex: survival linked to genomovar type. Am J Respir Crit Care Med 2001; 164:2102–2106

Celli BR, Cote CG, Marin JM, et al. The body-mass index, airflow obstruction, dyspnea, and exercise capacity index in COPD. N Engl J Med 2004; 350:1005–1012

Orens JB, Estenne M, Arcasoy S, et al. International guidelines for the selection of lung transplant candidates: 2006 update—a consensus report from the Pulmonary Scientific Council of the International Society for Heart and Lung Transplantation. J Heart Lung Transplant 2006; 25:745–755

154. B. Assessment of sperm motility.

The high-resolution CT scan reveals bronchiectasis in the middle lung fields on the right and left, as well as total situs inversus (right-sided heart, spleen, stomach, left-sided liver) (see Figure 154-C). The triad of sinusitis, bronchiectasis, and situs inversus is highly suggestive of Kartagener syndrome, now called *primary ciliary dyskinesia* (PCD). The next step would be to assess mucociliary clearance. Historically, the saccharin test was used as an inexpensive and noninvasive way to screen older children and adults. A properly performed test excluded the diagnosis and precluded

the need for more sophisticated or invasive testing (such as tracheal or nasal biopsy for ciliary function studies). However, the test requires a patient to sit still for an hour without sniffing, sneezing, or coughing. Therefore, it was not useful in children and uncooperative patients. Another noninvasive test of ciliary function in men is the assessment of sperm motility (choice B is correct).

More recent literature suggests that measurement of exhaled nitric oxide (NO) is also a useful screening test for PCD. NO is produced from the upper and lower respiratory tract. Exhaled levels are increased in uncontrolled asthma and some forms of bronchiectasis, but normal in cystic fibrosis. In patients with PCD, exhaled NO is abnormally low. A low level of exhaled NO or an abnormal saccharin test result, however, should be followed by an assessment of both ciliary structure and function.

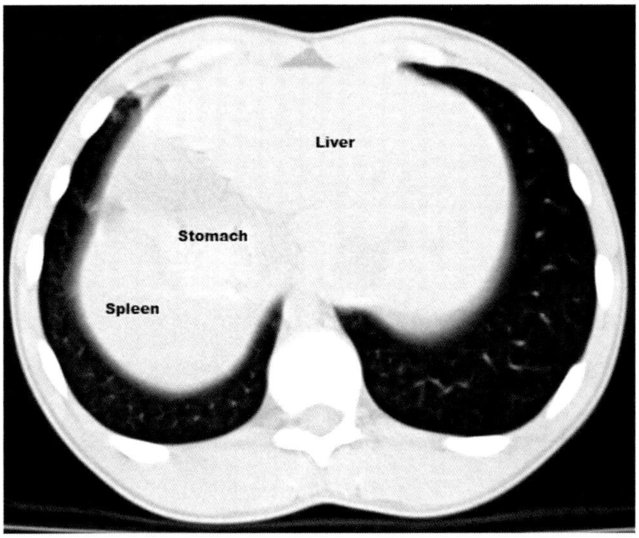

Figure 154-C

Although the situs inversus in our patient makes PCD the most likely diagnosis, newly discovered bronchiectasis in a young adult should also raise the possibility of cystic fibrosis, a primary immunodeficiency, previous infection with *Mycoplasma pneumoniae* or adenovirus, allergic bronchopulmonary aspergillosis, and α_1-antitrypsin deficiency. These could be assessed with a sweat chloride or cystic fibrosis genotype, quantitative immunoglobulins, antibodies to *M pneumoniae*, serum IgE levels and total eosinophils, or an α_1-antitrypsin level. Given our patient's classic presentation, these would all be considered only if the diagnosis of PCD is excluded (choices A, C, and D are incorrect).

Bush A, Cole P, Hariri M, et al. Primary ciliary dyskinesia: diagnosis and standards of care. Eur Respir J 1998; 12:982–988
Carlen B, Stenram U. Primary ciliary dyskinesia: a review. Ultrastruct Pathol 2005; 29:217–220
Corbelli R, Bringolf-Isler B, Amacher A, et al. Nasal nitric oxide measurements to screen children for primary ciliary dyskinesia. Chest 2004; 126:1054–1059
Van's Gravesande KS, Omran H. Primary ciliary dyskinesia: clinical presentation, diagnosis, and genetics. Ann Med 2005; 37:439–449

155. D. Clarithromycin.

Starting clarithromycin treatment in a patient already taking theophylline can lead to a rapid increase in plasma theophylline concentrations and toxic effects by reducing plasma clearance (choice D is correct). Although the use of theophylline has declined in the last decade in North America, it is still used widely. Theophylline is a phosphodiesterase inhibitor and causes an increase of intracellular concentration of cyclic adenosine monophosphate (cAMP) in various cells, including cells in the lung. Increased cAMP concentrations eventually lead to smooth muscle relaxation and airway dilatation. When combined with other classes of inhaled bronchodilators, such as anticholinergics and β_2-agonists, theophylline may afford a modest improvement in airflow and gas exchange. It is

recommended that if a macrolide is going to be administered during COPD exacerbation, then the theophylline dose should be decreased by 50%.

Theophylline is metabolized by hepatic cytochrome P450, and only a small fraction is excreted in the urine. Theophylline clearance is slow, and it is slowed further by chronic administration because the clearance pathway is saturated.

Many factors affect theophylline clearance, and these factors need be considered when theophylline toxicity develops.

Factors increasing theophylline clearance
- Drugs (phenobarbital, rifampin)
- Smoking (tobacco, marijuana)
- High-protein, low-carbohydrate diet
- Young age

Factors decreasing theophylline clearance
- Enzyme inhibition (macrolides, fluoroquinolones, cimetidine, allopurinol)
- Viral infections
- Chronic liver disease or congestive heart failure
- Pneumonia
- High-carbohydrate diet
- Old age

Omeprazole, low-molecular-weight heparin, and prednisone have no effect on theophylline clearance (choices A, B, and C are incorrect).

Duffy N, Walker P, Diamantea F, et al. Chronic obstructive pulmonary disease: intravenous aminophylline in patients admitted to hospital with nonacidotic exacerbations of chronic obstructive pulmonary disease: a prospective randomized controlled trial. Thorax 2005; 60:713–717
Pea F, Furlanut M. Pharmacokinetic aspects of treating infections in the intensive care unit: focus on drug interactions. Clin Pharmacokinet 2001; 40:833–868
Periti P, Mazzei T, Mini E, et al. Pharmacokinetic drug interactions of macrolides. Clin Pharmacokinet 1992; 23:106–131
Town GI. Aminophylline for COPD exacerbations? Not usually. Thorax 2005; 60:709

156. D. Malignant thymoma.

This patient has a soft tissue lobulated mass in the anterior mediastinum and bilateral pleural-based masses (see Figures 156-A and 156-B). In the absence of other radiographic abnormalities suggesting alternative diagnoses, the most likely diagnosis is malignant thymoma with "drop metastases" to the pleura (choice D is correct). Thymoma is the most common neoplasm of the anterior mediastinum, with a peak incidence from age 40 to 60 years. Malignancy is defined by invasive behavior, rather than by histologic features. Thymoma rarely metastasizes through the bloodstream or lymphatics; rather, it spreads locally or seeds the pleural or pericardial surfaces, as in this case. It may also spread through the diaphragm into the abdomen. Thymoma can be classified as encapsulated, invasive (invading into and beyond the capsule), and metastasizing, with pleural and pulmonary parenchymal seeding but no extrathoracic involvement. In this case, tumor invaded into and through the mediastinal pleura and later led to "drop metastases" with migration and proliferation of malignant cells in the lower recesses of the pleura. When thymoma invades through the capsule, it may proceed to invade local mediastinal structures and vessels and may cause obstruction to the airway and superior vena cava. Extensive chest wall invasion may encase the lung and resemble malignant mesothelioma.

Although TB can involve mediastinal lymph nodes and pleura, especially in patients with immune deficiencies, tuberculous lymph nodes would probably have a wider distribution than a single mediastinal mass, show necrosis (not the homogeneous density that is exhibited in this case), and be associated with systemic symptoms. For these reasons, TB is unlikely (choice A is incorrect). Mediastinal involvement with non-Hodgkin lymphoma is usually in the middle mediastinum, and extrathoracic lymph nodes are involved in the great majority of cases. Hodgkin disease usually involves the anterior mediastinum, but most patients with this disease also have involvement of other lymph nodes; in this case, the coincidental finding of pleural-based masses makes that diagnosis unlikely (choice B is incorrect). Small cell carcinoma also may present with prominent mediastinal lymphadenopathy and pleural involvement, but the large anterior mediastinal mass and pleural masses in the absence of a discernable lung mass and pleural effusion make that diagnosis unlikely (choice C is incorrect).

Tecce PM, Fishman EK, Kuhlman JE. CT evaluation of the anterior mediastinum. Radiographics 1994; 14:973–990

Duwe BV, Sterman DH, Musani AI. Tumors of the mediastinum. Chest 2005; 128:2893–2909

Strollo PC, de Christenson MLR, Jett JR. Primary mediastinal tumors: Part 1. Tumors of the anterior mediastinum. Chest 1997; 112:511–522

157. B. Levofloxacin.

The admission chest radiograph demonstrates extensive left lung consolidation on the CT scan that progresses to involve the contralateral lung by the next day. With the positive urinary antigen test, the diagnosis of severe Legionnaires disease is confirmed. Legionnaires disease is an acute bacterial infection generally caused by *Legionella pneumophila*, primarily involving the lower respiratory tract. Outbreaks have been described related to a common source of contamination. Erythromycin has been the treatment of choice ever since a retrospective study of the original outbreak in Philadelphia indicated a lower mortality rate with this antibiotic. Because Legionella is an intracellular pathogen, antibiotics that penetrate intracellularly are likely to be active against this pathogen. Both fluoroquinolones and macrolides penetrate cells well, and both classes demonstrate good *in vitro* activity. Fluoroquinolones achieve high intracellular levels and have a lower minimum inhibitory concentration against Legionella than erythromycin. They are more active than erythromycin in inhibiting *L pneumophila* in different intracellular models. Three observational studies with a total of 458 patients have indicated that that fluoroquinolones (mainly levofloxacin) are associated with a superior clinical response when compared with that of macrolides (erythromycin and clarithromycin), as evidenced by a shorter time to apyrexia, shorter hospital stay, and fewer drug-related complications (choice B is correct and choice D is incorrect). However, randomized clinical trials have not been performed. Mortality appears to be the same. Although it has been traditional to add rifampin to erythromycin to treat severe legionellosis, an observational cohort study revealed that the addition of rifampin to clarithromycin was associated with more side effects and a longer hospital stay than erythromycin alone (choice A is incorrect). Ceftriaxone is not active against Legionella sp and should not be used in this setting (choice C is incorrect). In all cases of severe, life-threatening pneumonia, prompt administration of appropriate antibiotics is associated with improved outcomes.

Grau S, Mateu-de Antonio J, Ribes E, et al. Impact of rifampicin to clarithromycin in *Legionella pneumophila* pneumonia. Intern J Antimicrob Agents 2006; 28:249–252

Sabrià M, Pedro-Botet ML, Gómez J, et al. Fluoroquinolones vs macrolides in the treatment of Legionnaires disease. Chest 2005; 128:1401–1405

Mykietiuk A, Carratalà J, Fernández-Sabé N, et al. Clinical outcomes for hospitalized patients with *Legionella* pneumonia in the antigenuria era: the influence of levofloxacin therapy. Clin Infect Dis 2005; 40:794–799

Pedro-Botet L, Yu VL. *Legionella*: macrolides or quinolones? Clin Microbiol Infect 2006; 12(suppl 3):25–30

Yu VL, Greenberg RN, Zadeikis N, et al. Levofloxacin efficacy in the treatment of community-acquired legionellosis. Chest 2004; 125:2135–2139

158. A. Leukemic infiltrates.

The BAL results shown in Figure 158-C shows numerous large cells with a high nuclear/cytoplasmic ratio and irregular nuclear contours, consistent with blasts and confirming the presence of leukemic infiltrates (choice A is correct). The stable hemoglobin, lack of pinkish color to the BAL return, and the presence of blast cells argue against alveolar hemorrhage (choice B is incorrect). The finding of blast cells in BAL fluid does not rule out concomitant infection, as there may be more than one etiology to explain the pulmonary infiltrates in this type of patient. Neutropenic patients with leukemia are certainly at risk of developing fungal infections, and the patchy ground-glass infiltrates with some nodular components seen on CT scan (see Figures 158-A and 158-B) are consistent with this, but no fungal organisms were seen on the silver stain (choice C is incorrect). Virtually any chemotherapeutic agent can lead to lung toxicity, but etoposide has rarely been associated with such a complication and has led to interstitial pneumonitis rather than airspace or nodular disease (choice D is incorrect).

The most common pulmonary complications in patients with leukemia are caused by infection or hemorrhage. The reported incidence of leukemic pulmonary infiltrates at autopsy in patients who die of leukemia ranges from 24 to 64%, but the percentage with an abnormal chest radiograph attributable to these infiltrates is much smaller, around 5%. A common misconception is that these infiltrates only occur with extremely high peripheral WBC counts, but leukemic infiltrates have been found in a patient with a peripheral WBC count as low as 800/μL (0.8×10^9/L). BAL is very helpful in making the diagnosis, although the yield is lower in the presence of alveolar hemorrhage. In those cases, transbronchial biopsies are very helpful in making the diagnosis but frequently are not possible because of associated thrombocytopenia.

Our patient seemed to deteriorate after starting etoposide chemotherapy. A syndrome called acute lysis pneumopathy has been used to describe worsening of respiratory status within hours of initiating chemotherapy in patients with acute myelomonocytic leukemia, presumably due to the release of proinflammatory cytokines from destroyed blast cells in the pulmonary circulation. A similar phenomenon has not been reported in acute lymphoblastic leukemia, which was the diagnosis for our patient.

There are no characteristic clinical or radiologic findings to definitively diagnose leukemic infiltrates, and it must always be kept in the differential diagnosis of new infiltrates in this group of patients. The risk may be higher when there is a high peripheral leukocytosis, particularly with a high percentage of blast cells. A consistent finding on CT scan has been interlobular septal thickening, although only minor septal thickening in the middle lobe was noted in the current patient. Nodular and ground-glass opacities, as demonstrated in our patient, have frequently been described but are completely nonspecific, as they may also be seen in drug toxicity, alveolar hemorrhage, pulmonary edema, and infection, all of the other entities that are usually possible in this group of patients.

Heyneman LE, Johkoh T, Ward S, et al. Pulmonary leukemic infiltrates: high-resolution CT findings in 10 patients. Am J Roentgenol 2000; 174:517–521

Valentino DJ III, Gelfand MC, Nava VE, et al. Hypoxemic respiratory failure in a 57-year-old woman with acute monocytic leukemia. Chest 2005; 128:3629–3633

Azoulay E, Fieux F, Moreau D, et al. Acute monocytic leukemia presenting as acute respiratory failure. Am J Respir Crit Care Med 2003; 167:1329–1333

Gurjal A, An T, Valdivieso M, et al. Etoposide-induced pulmonary toxicity. Lung Cancer 1999; 26:109–112

159. C. Distant metastases are unlikely.

This patient's CT scan and pathology findings are most compatible with a solitary fibrous tumor of the pleura (SFTP). These tumors may be either benign or malignant, with the frequency of malignancy varying from 7 to 60%. Up to 80% of SFTP may be benign. The variability is likely accounted for by different applications of criteria for malignancy. Even in malignant SFTP, distant metastases are uncommon. Even with recurrence after surgical excision, the

definitive treatment is usually local (choice C is correct). Surgical resection is generally needed for a definitive diagnosis and differentiation between malignant and benign SFTP, although needle biopsy has been found to be successful in ≤ 43% of cases. As in this patient, immunohistochemical stain results are distinctive, being positive for vimentin and CD34 and negative for keratin; malignant mesothelioma is generally just the opposite—negative for vimentin and CD34 and positive for keratin.

SFTPs arise from the submesothelial mesenchymal layer of the pleura, with roughly two-thirds arising from the visceral pleura. Extrathoracic solitary fibrous tumors have been reported in locations including the meninges, nose, oral cavity, breast, and bladder. SFTPs occur primarily in the sixth and seventh decade of life with equal frequency in men and women. Asbestos exposure plays no role in SFTP (choice B is incorrect), compared with the most common primary tumor of the pleura, malignant mesothelioma. Smoking is not an identified risk factor for the development of SFTP (choice A is incorrect). Roughly half of patients are asymptomatic on presentation, with symptomatic patients being more common if the diagnosis is malignant SFTP. Hypertrophic pulmonary osteoarthropathy (HPO) is the most common paraneoplastic syndrome in SFTP, occurring in up to 22% of patients (choice D is incorrect), compared with a 5% incidence with lung cancer. Hypoglycemia (Doege-Potter syndrome) due to high levels of insulin-like growth factor occurs in 3 to 4% of cases and tends to be associated with larger tumors. Both HPO and hypoglycemia tend to resolve after tumor removal. Radiographically these tumors vary in size, may be lobulated, tend to be well circumscribed (as in this patient), and are usually located peripherally. Two thirds of tumors may be enhanced with contrast because of their hypervascularity. PET and MRI scanning currently add little to the management of SFTP.

Histologic findings, rather than tumor size, appear to be the primary indicator of clinical outcome. Surgical resection with negative surgical margins is the treatment of choice but can be challenging, particularly in SFTP arising from the visceral pleura, given the need for lung tissue resection and even lobectomy. A staging system to predict outcome notes that malignant sessile tumors have a 63% recurrence rate and a 30% mortality rate, with most deaths occurring within 24 months, as opposed to benign pedunculated tumors that have only a 2% recurrence rate. Long-term follow-up is necessary given late recurrences, usually local, even with benign lesions, which may undergo malignant transformation. Aggressive surgery is the preferred treatment for recurrence.

Robinson LA. Solitary fibrous tumor of the pleura. Cancer Control 2006; 13:264–269
De Perrot M, Fischer S, Bründler MA, et al. Solitary fibrous tumors of the pleural. Ann Thorac Surg 2002; 74:285–293
Sung SH, Change JW, Kim J, et al. Solitary fibrous tumors of the pleura: surgical outcome and clinical course. Ann Thorac Surg 2005; 79:303–307
Perna V, Rivas F, Morera R, et al. Localized (solitary) fibrous tumors of the pleura: an analysis of 15 patients. Int J Surg 2008; 6:298–301

160. C. Continue current therapy.

This man developed an acute upper airway obstruction following extubation from orotracheal intubation. With relief of the obstruction, he developed acute pulmonary edema. Maintaining mechanical ventilation support, supplemental oxygen therapy, and supportive care is usually all that is necessary (choice C is correct).

The mechanism behind the development of acute pulmonary edema in this situation is likely multifactorial. Patients with upper airway obstruction compensate by increasing inspiratory pressure, leading to highly negative pleural and alveolar pressures. This leads to an increase in venous return and increase in capillary pressure. Expiratory pressures are also increased, leading to highly positive pleural and alveolar pressure, with a subsequent decrease in venous return and increase in interstitial pressure. With relief of the obstruction, airway pressure is suddenly decreased and venous pressure is quickly decreased. The pulmonary capillary pressure remains high, injuring the alveolar-capillary membrane. This increases capillary permeability and the transudation of fluid into the interstitial and alveolar spaces.

Pulmonary thromboembolism should be considered; however, the time course for its development, the rapid development of symptoms following surgery in an otherwise healthy, ambulatory man, would be unusual; thus, the CT angiogram would not be helpful (choice A is incorrect). Aspiration of oropharyngeal or gastric contents is also a consideration here, although the radiographic infiltrates would likely be in the lower lung fields and not have a bat wing appearance. The use of IV antibiotics is not indicated at this time (choice B is incorrect). Given the improvement in the patient's oxygenation at the current ventilator settings, an increase in PEEP is not necessary at this time. High-level PEEP has not been shown to improve outcome in instances of acute noncardiogenic pulmonary edema (choice D is incorrect).

Cascade PN, Alexander GD, Mackie DS. Negative pressure pulmonary edema after endotracheal intubation. Radiology 1993; 186:671–678
Kallet RH, Daniel BM, Gropper M, et al. Acute pulmonary edema following upper airway obstruction: case reports and brief review. Respir Care 1998; 43:476–480
Fremont RD, Kallet RH, Matthay MA, et al. Postobstructive pulmonary edema: a case for hydrostatic mechanisms. Chest 2007; 131:1742–1746

161. A. Despite the relatively large size of the nodule and her long smoking history, the negative PET scan result makes the likelihood of lung cancer quite low and likely < 5%.

Although this nodule abuts the aorta and chest wall, its appearance resembles a solitary pulmonary nodule. Scanning techniques that couple assessment of metabolic characteristics of the nodule to its physical characteristics and the patient's demographic risk factors are available. A negative PET scan result is a strong predictor of a benign lesion despite other patient or CT characteristics that would otherwise yield a high posttest probability of lung cancer (choice A is correct). This is fortunate because the proliferation of CT scanning for evaluation of acute chest pain and other processes often identifies abnormalities, as in this patient.

From the era of solitary pulmonary nodule (SPN) evaluation by chest radiograph alone, it was known that the patient's age, cigarette exposure, and prior history of malignancy are important patient characteristics that influence the prior probability of lung cancer when an SPN is identified. The patient in this case has a significant smoking history and age risk for cancer. The characteristics found on chest radiograph that are important in determining the likelihood of malignancy include the location of the nodule (upper lobe higher risk than lower lobe; hence, choice B is incorrect), the size of the nodule, and evidence of spiculation. Chest CT has made the determination of these characteristics more precise, and given this patient's demographic characteristics and the specific findings by CT scan, in the absence of other information, the posttest (post-CT scan) probability of this SPN being malignant is likely about 50%. Accordingly, with this information alone, many would recommend surgical resection, given the unacceptable risk of observation.

PET scanning has provided additional information to assess risk. This scanning modality assesses the metabolic activity of the nodule, with threshold levels identified that suggest either the hypermetabolic state of malignant tissue or tissue with active inflammation vs benign processes such as granulomata. In one recent metaanalysis evaluating 22 retrospective and prospective published studies of PET scan evaluation of SPNs, the positive likelihood ratio of the studies taken in combination was 5.4, suggesting that a positive PET scan finding was additional valuable evidence for malignancy in addition to information forthcoming from patient characteristics and CT scan findings. Equally, if not more important, was the negative likelihood ratio of 0.06 in this analysis, suggesting that a negative PET scan finding was a powerful predictor of a benign lesion. This metaanalysis provided tables to compute risk based on patient characteristics, CT, and PET findings, and if these are applied to the patient in this question, the risk of malignancy is < 5%. Accordingly, it would be incorrect to counsel this patient that the PET scan findings do not substantially impact interpretation of the significance of the CT scan findings in isolation (choice C is incorrect).

Unfortunately, a negative PET scan finding does not take the posttest risk of malignancy to zero, presumably because some very slow-growing tumors may not have enhancement by this imaging modality. Accordingly, in most circumstances, some form of serial imaging is needed to accumulate greater assurance that an SPN is benign after

negative findings on PET imaging. This serial imaging, however, should determine whether the SPN is growing by assessing a change in size and not a change in metabolic activity (choice D is incorrect).

Even with these additional prognostic data, decision making for the individual patient remains complex and needs to be modified by factors such as the risk of surgical removal of a lesion, comorbid conditions, and even patient preference. In this particular circumstance, the patient was counseled that observation of the lesion was acceptable as long as serial imaging was conducted. Unfortunately, this plan was attended by almost paralyzing anxiety on her part, and she sought a surgical extirpation. She underwent a successful wedge resection of the lesion without complication. Fungal stains identified coccidioidomycosis (see Figure 161-B) that she likely contracted during her time spent in the Southwest.

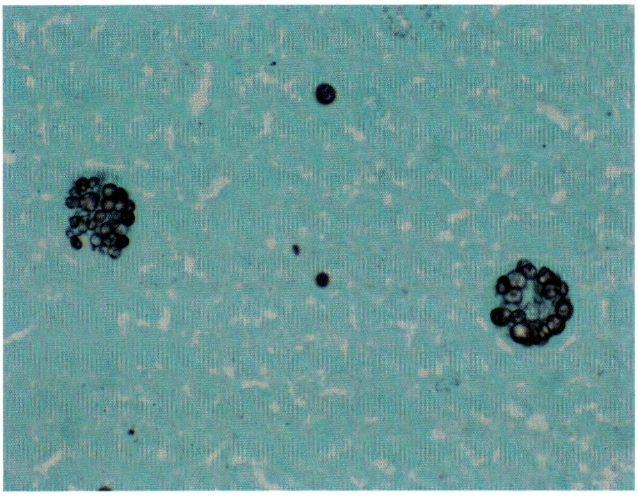

Figure 161-B
Gomori-Grocott methenamine silver

Cronin P, Dwamena BA, Kelly AM, et al. Solitary pulmonary nodules and masses: a meta-analysis of the diagnostic utility of alternative imaging tests. Eur Radiol 2008; 18:1840–1856
Girvin F, Ko JP. Pulmonary nodules: detection, assessment, and CAD. Am J Roentgenol 2008; 191:1057–1069

162. A. Provision of heated humidification.

Adherence to continuous positive airway pressure (CPAP) therapy for obstructive sleep apnea (OSA) is less than optimal. Airway humidification has been shown to improve CPAP use (choice A is correct) and may be particularly important in patients older than 60 years, those using drying medications, those with chronic mucosa disease, or those who have a history of uvulopalatopharyngoplasty. The use of CPAP with pressure relief technology, autotitrating positive airway pressure (APAP), or bilevel positive airway pressure (BPAP) does not consistently influence PAP acceptance or use (choices B, C, and D are incorrect).

CPAP therapy, which provides a constant pressure throughout the respiratory cycle, is the treatment of choice for most patients with OSA. It is generally indicated for all people with an AHI of at least 15 events/h and for patients with symptoms such as excessive sleepiness, insomnia, impaired cognition, mood disorder, hypertension, coronary artery disease or stroke, and an AHI between 5 and 30 events/h.

Among the different published studies, therapeutic adherence (*ie,* use of CPAP for ≥ 4 h nightly on 70% of monitored nights) has varied from 46 to 80%. Self-report, unfortunately, typically overestimates actual CPAP use. Patterns of CPAP can often be discerned by the first few days of initiating treatment. Reported reasons for nonadherence to CPAP therapy include perception of lack of benefit, inconvenience, discomfort with its use, claustrophobia, nasal congestion, or intolerance of the prescribed mask or delivered pressure.

Some CPAP devices are equipped with pressure relief technology (C-Flex; Respironics; Murrysville, PA) that permits a transient reduction in pressure during expiration and a subsequent return of pressure to the baseline setting before the initiation of the next inspiration. With BPAP devices, two pressure levels are delivered during the respiratory cycle, with a higher level during inspiration (inspiratory positive airway pressure) and a lower pressure during expiration (expiratory positive airway pressure). Both C-Flex and BPAP may benefit patients who complain of difficulty exhaling against the delivered CPAP pressure or who develop gastric distention from aerophagia.

APAP technology uses device-specific diagnostic and therapeutic algorithms to deliver variable pressures required to maintain upper airway patency. Pressure is progressively increased in the presence of upper airway obstruction or gradually reduced if no obstructive respiratory event is detected. Compared with CPAP, average mean airway pressure throughout the entire sleep period may be lower with APAP; although this may theoretically decrease air leaks and pressure intolerance, it has not been shown to enhance therapeutic adherence.

Kushida CA, Littner MR, Hirshkowitz M, et al. American Academy of Sleep Medicine: practice parameters for the use of continuous and bilevel positive airway pressure devices to treat adult patients with sleep-related breathing disorders. Sleep 2006; 29:375–380

Nilius G, Happel A, Domanski U, et al. Pressure-relief continuous positive airway pressure vs constant continuous positive airway pressure: a comparison of efficacy and compliance. Chest 2006; 130:1018–1024

163. B. Calretinin staining of the tissue will be positive.

This patient has developed a mesothelioma related to asbestos exposure during his occupation as a brake liner. Calretinin has become a useful marker to distinguish adenocarcinoma from mesothelioma (choice B is correct). The chest CT (see Figure 163-A) shows diffuse concentric pleural soft tissue thickening encasing the left hemithorax and a pleural effusion on the right, which also proved to be due to mesothelioma.

Mesothelioma is an aggressive neoplasm of serosal surfaces, in particular, the parietal pleura and peritoneum. Asbestos exposure is the major risk factor for the development of mesothelioma. Tobacco is not a risk factor for mesothelioma and is not synergistic with its development, as asbestos is with bronchogenic carcinoma (choice A is incorrect). Typically, the delay between asbestos exposure and development of mesothelioma is 30 years. Mesothelioma has also been reported to develop following radiation treatment for lymphoma, breast cancer, and lung cancer.

In the United States, the incidence of mesothelioma is 15 per 1 million people. The number of annual cases, approximately 2,500, is thought to have peaked in 2000 and may show a decline in the future. Patients are usually in the 50- to 70-year age range, and 80% are men. Malignant mesothelioma can arise from the pleura, peritoneum, or pericardium, but most cases are of pleural origin. The most common presenting symptoms are dyspnea and, in 60% of patients, chest pain that is usually nonpleuritic and can be severe. Often, these symptoms have been present for 2 to 3 months before the patient seeks treatment. Later symptoms include weight loss and fatigue. Radiographically, patients usually have a large pleural effusion and/or unilateral pleural masses. Diffuse concentric pleural thickening and encasing tumor (as seen in this patient) may also develop. Contralateral disease develops in 10 to 20% of patients.

Diagnosis can be made by pleural fluid cytologic findings, needle biopsy, or open biopsy, but with cytologic findings alone, it may be difficult to distinguish mesothelioma from adenocarcinoma, and usually tissue biopsy is required. Special immunohistochemical stains can be helpful in this differential diagnosis. Calretinin, cytokeratin 5 and 6, and Wilms tumor antigen are positive in mesothelioma, but only rarely in adenocarcinoma. The pleural fluid tends to be a bloody, viscous exudate with a high content of hyaluronic acid.

Paraneoplastic findings associated with malignant mesothelioma include hypoglycemia in approximately 1% (not as common as that seen with benign fibrous tumors of the pleura, an unrelated process formally called benign mesothelioma; choice C is incorrect), hypercalcemia, and thrombocytosis.

Recently, serum biomarkers have been evaluated for the screening and diagnosis of mesothelioma. Levels of the glycoprotein osteopontin have been shown to be elevated in patients with malignant mesothelioma vs those exposed to asbestos without mesothelioma. Soluble mesothelin-related peptide (SMRP) is another biomarker that looks promising for screening, diagnosis, and monitoring of treatment and is now commercially available. In the study validating this biomarker, 84% of patients with malignant mesothelioma exhibited an elevated SMRP, whereas only 2% of patients with other cancers or pulmonary disease did so. Individuals exposed to asbestos without malignant mesothelioma who exhibit an elevated SMRP level are more likely to develop malignant mesothelioma over time than asbestos-exposed individuals lacking this biomarker.

The prognosis for the patient with malignant mesothelioma is dismal, with progressive local invasion and less often dissemination. Combined modality treatment with radiation, chemotherapy, and surgery is palliative and rarely curative. Surgical treatment in selected cases for palliation and occasional cure is with extrapleural pneumonectomy. Mean survival is 6 to 12 months following diagnosis (choice D is incorrect).

Pistolesi M, Rusthoven J. Malignant pleural mesothelioma: update, current management, and newer therapeutic strategies. Chest 2004; 126:1318–1329

Robinson BWS, Lake RA. Advances in malignant mesothelioma. N Engl J Med 2005; 353:1591–1603

Pass HI, Lott D, Lonardo F, et al. Asbestos exposure, pleural mesothelioma, and serum osteopontin levels. N Engl J Med 2005; 353:1564–1573

Schwartz AM, Henson DE. Diagnostic surgical pathology in lung cancer: ACCP evidence-based clinical practice guidelines, 2nd edition. Chest 2007; 132(suppl):78S–93S

Sterman DH, Albelda SM. Advances in the diagnosis, evaluation, and management of malignant pleural mesothelioma. Respirology 2005; 10:266–283

Ray M, Kindler H. Malignant pleural mesothelioma: an update on biomarkers and treatment. Chest 2009 (in press)

Robinson BW, Creaney J, Lake R, et al. Mesothelin-family proteins and diagnosis of mesothelioma. Lancet 2003; 362:1612–1616

Scherpereel A, Lee YC. Biomarkers for mesothelioma. Curr Opin Pulm Med 2007; 13:339–443

164. A. Increase PEEP and accept higher plateau pressure.

The patient is severely hypoxemic because of poor ventilation-perfusion abnormalities and shunts induced by the obesity-related restrictive lung disease and the superimposed aspiration. Given that the FIO_2 is maximal, this can only be addressed by improving alveolar recruitment. Of the choices given to accomplish this, adding expiratory pressure will best improve and maintain alveolar recruitment.

Although the airway plateau pressure will almost certainly rise with an increase in PEEP, in this very obese patient, a significant amount of this increased airway plateau pressure could actually reflect only obesity-related chest wall stiffness pressure, not the potentially injurious transpulmonary pressure. This is important because the National Institutes of Health (NIH) ARDS Network ventilator management recommendation of limiting airway plateau pressure to < 30 cm H_2O assumes a near normal chest wall compliance, a situation in which the airway plateau pressure is an approximation of transpulmonary pressure.

This assumption, however, does not hold true in an obese patient, such as ours, where the stiffer chest wall can add as much as 15 cm H_2O or more to the airway plateau pressure. Thus, in our patient, airway plateau pressures approaching 40 cm H_2O would likely still represent a transpulmonary pressure < 30 cm H_2O, and our patient's settings could still be considered "compliant" with NIH ARDS Network recommendations. There is thus no need to reduce the tidal volume, especially given the respiratory acidosis (choice A is correct and choice B is incorrect).

If an esophageal pressure measurement is available, the actual transpulmonary pressure can be calculated (airway plateau pressure minus esophageal pressure). This can allow the clinician to be confident that settings are indeed in accordance with the NIH ARDS Network approach.

Choice C is incorrect for three reasons. First, as noted earlier, there is no need to be concerned about the levels of airway plateau pressure in this obese patient. Second, a higher tidal volume strategy, although potentially increasing the number of lung units that open, will not maintain that recruitment if the PEEP is lowered. Third, increasing the tidal volume to > 8 mL/kg ideal body weight violates the NIH ARDS Network recommendations for lung protection.

Choice D is incorrect because, although an increased ventilatory rate may compensate for the reduced tidal volume in terms of maintaining minute ventilation, faster breathing rates will not affect lung recruitment. Moreover, the reduction in tidal volume and PEEP will clearly worsen lung recruitment and further worsen oxygenation.

Harris RS. Pressure volume curves of the respiratory system. Respir Care 2005; 50:78–98

Pelosi P, Croci M, Ravagnan I, et al. Total respiratory system, lung and chest wall mechanics in sedated, paralyzed postoperative morbidly obese patients. Chest 1996; 109:144–151

Benditt JO. Esophageal and gastric pressure measurements. Respir Care 2005; 50:68–75

DeLorey DS, Wyrick BL, Babb TG. Mild to moderate obesity: implications for respiratory mechanics at rest and during exercise in young men. Int J Obesity 2005; 29:1039–1047

Talmor D, Sarge T, Malhotra A. Mechanical ventilation guided by esophageal pressure measurements in acute lung injury. New Engl J Med 2008; 359:2095–2104

165. A. Etomidate.

Etomidate is an imidazole sedative that is frequently used in rapid-sequence intubation and can reversibly inhibit the enzyme 11-β-hydroxylase (which converts 11-deoxycortisol to cortisol), decreasing circulating cortisol concentrations for up 24 h after a single dose and attenuating corticotropin responsiveness for even longer (choice A is correct). The clinical significance of this adrenal effect is unclear, although several small studies have suggested an association between the receipt of etomidate and inferior outcomes in some subsets of critical care patients. Some authors have suggested that patients who have received etomidate should receive a single dose of 100 mg of hydrocortisone, but this practice is not widespread or based on firm evidence. Others have suggested that the drug be avoided when possible in patients who are septic or in those being treated for trauma. Regardless, continuous infusion or multiple boluses of etomidate should be avoided.

It should also be noted that etomidate offers a number of advantages that account for its continued popularity. It has a rapid and dependable onset of action, is short acting, does not produce hypotension as severely as other sedatives, and does not stimulate histamine release.

Ketamine is a dissociative anesthetic agent that is related to phencyclidine. It results in the release of catecholamines, producing increases in heart rate, contractility, mean arterial pressure, and cerebral blood flow, and also has been associated with reemergence phenomena, in which patients experience disturbing dreams as they emerge from ketamine-induced anesthesia. It has no known effect on adrenal function (choice B is incorrect). Midazolam is a short-acting benzodiazepine, and propofol is a short-acting alkylphenol derivative; both can produce significant hypotension, but neither depresses adrenal function (choices C and D are incorrect).

Bergen JM, Smith DC. A review of etomidate for rapid sequence intubation in the emergency department. J Emerg Med 1997; 15:221–230

den Brinker M, Joosten KF, Liem O, et al. Adrenal insufficiency in meningococcal sepsis: bioavailable cortisol levels and impact of interleukin-6 levels and intubation with etomidate on adrenal function and mortality. J Clin Endocrinol Metab 2005; 90:5110–5117

Hildreth AN, Mejia VA, Maxwell RA, et al. Adrenal suppression following a single dose of etomidate for rapid sequence induction: a prospective randomized study. J Trauma 2008; 65:573–579

Jackson WL Jr. Should we use etomidate as an induction agent for endotracheal intubation in patients with septic shock? A critical appraisal. Chest 2005; 127:1031–1038

Marik PE. Critical illness-related corticosteroid insufficiency. Chest 2009; 135:181–193

Schenarts CL, Burton JH, Riker RR. Adrenocortical dysfunction following etomidate induction in emergency department patients. Acad Emerg Med 2001; 8:1–7

166. B. She should undergo a cerebral MRI prior to getting pregnant.

A cerebral MRI should be obtained prior to pregnancy in any patient with HHT to exclude cerebral AV malformations (even though this patient had a normal cerebral MRI 7 years previously). If an MRI is not performed before the patient becomes pregnant (*ie,* unplanned pregnancy), then close follow-up throughout pregnancy would be mandatory. If a serious headache or neurologic abnormality developed, then appropriate diagnostic assessment and potential therapeutic intervention would be immediately undertaken at any stage in pregnancy. It is also recommended that in those patients in whom cerebral AV malformations have not been excluded, a prolonged second stage of labor should be avoided (choice B is correct).

In stable patients, and with appropriate forethought and follow-up, pregnancy may be successfully undertaken in patients with HHT (choice A is incorrect). Antibiotic prophylaxis would be indicated for any appropriate procedures during pregnancy and also at the time of delivery but would not be administered throughout pregnancy because it is unnecessary (choice C is incorrect). All pregnancies in patients with HHT should be considered "high-risk," carrying a maternal death rate of 1% in some series (choice D is incorrect). These risks, however, can be minimized with appropriate prepregnancy assessment, close follow-up during pregnancy and after delivery, and prompt intervention at the first sign of potential complications.

Cottin V, Dupuis-Girod S, Lesca G, et al. Pulmonary vascular malformations of hereditary hemorrhagic telangiectasia (Rendu-Osler disease). Respiration 2007; 74:361–378

Gershon AS, Faughnan ME, Chon KS, et al. Transcatheter embolotherapy of maternal pulmonary arteriovenous malformations during pregnancy. Chest 2001; 119:470–477

Mandzia J, Henderson K, Faughnan M, et al. Compelling reasons to screen brain in HHT. Stroke 2001; 32:1957–1958

Shovlin CL, Sodhi V, McCarthy A, et al. Estimates of maternal risks of pregnancy for women with hereditary haemorrhagic telangiectasia (Osler-Weber-Rendu syndrome): suggested approach for obstetric services. Br J Obstet Gynecol 2008; 115:1108–1115

167. C. Clarithromycin, ethambutol, and rifampin three times weekly.

The patient meets the diagnostic criteria for MAC lung disease: pulmonary symptoms, nodular or cavitary opacities on chest radiograph or high-resolution CT with multifocal bronchiectasis with multiple small nodules (tree-in-bud), and positive culture results from at least two expectorated sputum samples. Evidence-based treatment recommendations for nontuberculous mycobacterial disease were updated and are outlined in an official American Thoracic Society/ Infectious Diseases Society of America statement published in 2007. The recommended initial regimen for most patients with nodular or bronchiectatic MAC lung disease (as seen in this patient) is a three times weekly regimen including clarithromycin (1,000 mg) or azithromycin (500 mg), ethambutol (25 mg/kg), and rifampin (600 mg; choice C is correct). The major advance over the past few decades in the care of patients with MAC has been the introduction of the newer macrolides, which have significant *in vitro* and clinical activity against the organism. This class of drugs is the most important element of multidrug treatment regimens, but they should never be used without companion antituberculous drugs (even drugs with less activity against MAC) in order to prevent the emergence of macrolide resistance. There have been no studies evaluating the effectiveness of two- vs three-drug regimens. However, there is some concern about increased risk of resistance even with two drugs, and thus three-drug regimens are preferred. Given the relatively narrow therapeutic window and significant risk of adverse effects of these medications, intermittent therapy has the advantage of lowering these risks and reducing overall costs. Daily therapy is recommended as first-line treatment only in patients with fibrocavitary disease or severe nodular/bronchiectatic disease (choice A is incorrect). A more aggressive approach includes the addition of amikacin or streptomycin for the first 2 or 3 months of therapy. This treatment is very poorly tolerated, so it is recommended only for patients with severe, multilobar, fibrocavitary disease (choice B is incorrect). Intermittent therapy is not recommended for such patients (choice D is incorrect).

A regimen of daily clarithromycin and ethambutol might be appropriate for select patients, such as those with very mild disease, those who have not tolerated the three-drug regimen, or those in whom disease suppression rather

peculiar pattern in which a sustained inspiration with a 2- to 3-s pause occurs followed by expiration (choice C is incorrect). Central neurogenic hyperventilation results in sustained hyperventilation (choice D is incorrect) with >40 breaths/min and marked respiratory alkalosis. This pattern may be found in patients with a lesion of the pons, midbrain, or medulla.

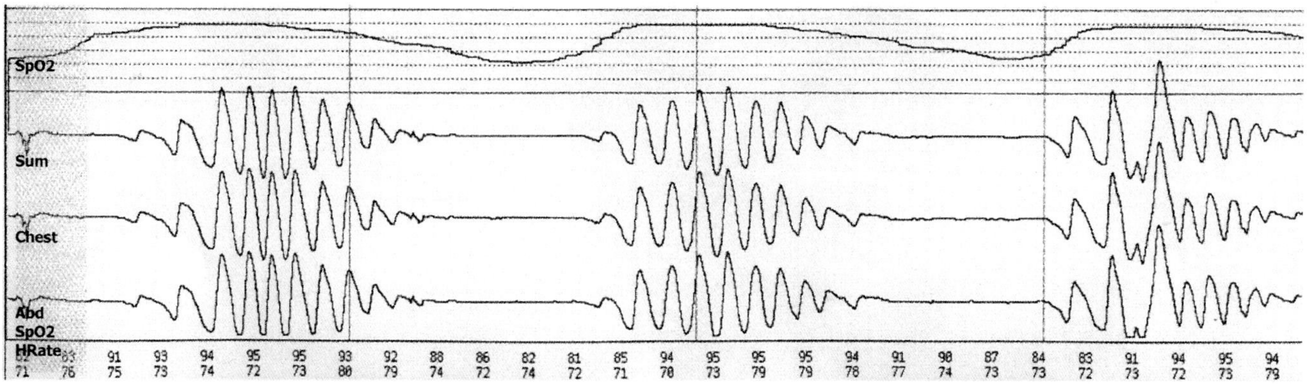

Figure 169-B

Posner JB, Saper CB, Schiff ND, et al. Plum & Posner's diagnosis of stupor and coma. 4th ed. Oxford, England: Oxford University Press, 2007

Freeman WD, Sen S, Roy TK, et al. Cluster breathing associated with bihemispheric infarction and sparing of the brainstem. Arch Neurol 2006; 63:1487–1490

North JB, Jennett S. Abnormal breathing patterns associated with acute brain damage. Arch Neurol 1974; 31:338–344

Nogues MA, Benarroch E. Abnormalities of respiratory control and the respiratory motor unit. Neurologist 2008; 14:273–288

170. D. Thyroid function tests.

This patient has a substernal goiter that is producing obstructing symptoms and tracheal deviation seen on radiograph. Additionally, she has subtle clinical evidence of possible hyperthyroidism, and the first test to be performed should be thyroid function testing (choice D is correct). Further imaging of the goiter is needed to further define the findings seen on chest radiograph, but there are a number of important considerations. Although CT scanning of the chest is useful, administration of an iodinated contrast agent as used in routine CT scanning can produce hyperthyroidism, including in patients with multinodular goiter. It can also lead to life-threatening airway compromise in thyrotoxic patients. Therefore, patients should be pretreated with an antithyroid drug prior to contrast administration (choice A is incorrect). Additionally, a patient who receives iodinated contrast cannot be treated effectively with radioactive iodine for 3 months or more because "cold" iodine has been incorporated into the gland and must be cleared by the kidneys before the gland would take up the contrast material. MRI is a useful alternative to define cervical and thoracic anatomy but is more expensive, whereas thyroid ultrasound has limited utility with inability to image retrosternal anatomy (choice B is incorrect). Thyroid radionuclide imaging identifies functioning thyroid tissue, but has limited value in defining the extent of the nonfunctional components of the goiter and airway anatomy (choice C is incorrect).

Thyroid enlargement, or goiter, typically results in outward growth in the anterior neck, but growth of one or both lobes through the thoracic inlet into the upper mediastinum may produce a substernal goiter. Because the thoracic inlet has bony boundaries of the thoracic vertebrae, sternum, and first ribs, such thyroid growth may produce compression and/or displacement of the trachea, or less commonly, of the blood vessels or esophagus. Most substernal goiters are benign, the majority being multinodular goiters or large follicular adenomas, but thyroid cancer is found in as many as 16%. Most multinodular goiters grow very slowly with fibrosis, calcification, and degenerating cysts, but little functioning thyroid tissue, thus producing a gradual onset of symptoms. However, hemorrhage into the gland can result in rapid enlargement and abrupt clinical deterioration.

The most common presenting symptom is exertional dyspnea, which may also be accentuated by change in body position or actions that move the goiter into the thoracic inlet. Other symptoms include wheezing, stridor, cough, and choking. Most patients who have a symptomatic substernal goiter have a visible cervical goiter. While most patients with multinodular goiters have normal thyroid function, as many as 25% may have subclinical or overt hyperthyroidism, and thyroid function testing should be performed on all patients who have a goiter.

Treatment options include surgery, suppressive therapy with levothyroxine, and radioactive iodine therapy. Surgery is generally considered the treatment of choice for substernal goiter.

Torre G, Borgonovo G, Amato A, et al. Surgical management of substernal goiter: analysis of 237 patients. Am Surg 1995; 61:826–831
Kadhim AL, Sheahan P, Timon C. Management of life-threatening airway obstruction caused by benign thyroid disease. J Laryngol Otol 2006; 120:1038–1041
Rieu M, Bekka S, Sambor B, et al. Prevalence of subclinical hyperthyroidism and relationship between thyroid hormonal status and thyroid ultrasonographic parameters in patients with non-toxic nodular goitre. Clin Endocrinol (Oxf) 1993; 39:67–71

171. C. Stop mesalamine and consider prednisone therapy.

The chest radiograph indicates peripheral lung infiltrates, and the chest CT scan shows confluent airspace disease with a marked peripheral distribution. This radiographic pattern, in conjunction with blood eosinophilia, is highly suggestive of eosinophilic pneumonia. Mesalamine has been identified as a cause of eosinophilic pneumonia. The most appropriate action would be to stop the mesalamine and consider corticosteroid therapy (choice C is correct). There is no evidence of bacterial pneumonia, and the administration of broad-spectrum antibiotics is inappropriate (choice A is incorrect). This combination of eosinophilia and unique radiographic pattern is one of the few occasions where physicians can be comfortable not performing other diagnostic tests (choice D is incorrect). There is no evidence that this patient has TB and initiating antituberculous therapy is not indicated (choice B is incorrect).

The active ingredient, mesalamine (5-aminosalicylic acid, also referred to as 5-ASA), is the major active component of sulfasalazine for the treatment of inflammatory bowel disease. The available evidence suggests that mesalamine has a topical antiinflammatory effect on the colon, where it inhibits prostaglandin and leukotriene synthesis. Mesalamine tablets have a special acrylic-based resin coating that does not allow the drug to be released below a pH of 7. The coating delays release of mesalamine until the tablets reach the terminal ileum and colon. Once released in the colon, mesalamine is minimally absorbed, and plasma levels are similar to those found following rectal administration of mesalamine. Approximately 20% of the administered dose released in the colon is absorbed, and the remainder is available for colonic therapeutic activity and excretion in the feces.

Mesalamine is an unusual cause of pulmonary eosinophilia, and two patterns of disease have been identified. The first is simple pulmonary eosinophilia; these patients tend to have mild pulmonary symptoms of cough and dyspnea, and the chest radiographs show patchy segmental or subsegmental infiltrates. Discontinuation of the drug leads to resolution of signs and symptoms, and corticosteroids are not required. The second is a subacute presentation with cough, dyspnea, and systemic symptoms, including fever that persists for weeks or months. The radiographic pattern may be patchy or confluent, unilateral, or bilateral. This form improves promptly with corticosteroids and, unlike chronic eosinophilic pneumonia, is not associated with relapse once the corticosteroids are withdrawn.

Allen JN. Drug-induced eosinophilic lung disease. Clin Chest Med 2004; 25:77–88
Parry SD, Barbatzas C, Peel ET, et al. Sulphasalazine and lung toxicity. Eur Respir J 2002; 19:756–764
Souza CA, Muller NL, Johkoh T, et al. Drug-induced eosinophilic pneumonia: high-resolution CT findings in 14 patients. Am J Roentgenol 2006; 186:368–373
Tanigawa K, Sugiyama K, Matsuyama H, et al. Mesalazine-induced eosinophilic pneumonia. Respiration 1999; 66:69–72

172. C. Pulmonary venoocclusive disease.

Figure 172-A (see stem) reveals a right pleural effusion, minimal subpleural interstitial disease, and mild centrilobular ground-glass opacities. Figure 172-B (see stem) shows mediastinal adenopathy. It also shows food in the esophagus, consistent with esophageal dysmotility attributable to this patient's scleroderma. Radiographically, the presence of ground-glass opacities, particularly with a centrilobular distribution; septal lines; and adenopathy on a pretreatment CT scan is indicative of pulmonary venoocclusive disease in patients presenting with pulmonary hypertension. The presence of any of these features in a patient with pulmonary hypertension should prompt consideration of pulmonary venoocclusive disease (PVOD). In this condition, the pulmonary pressures are elevated. However, the pulmonary artery occlusion pressure is normal (in the absence of flow, there is no resistance-mediated pressure rise; the occlusion pressure purely reflects the left atrial/left ventricular end-diastolic pressure). Traditional vasodilators may exacerbate this condition because vasodilation of the precapillary blood vessels by agents such as prostanoids leads to an increase in pulmonary blood flow. In the presence of venous obstruction, worsening of pulmonary parenchymal, interstitial and alveolar edema develops with worsening of symptoms, chest radiograph, and oxygenation (choice C is correct). Despite this concern, however, some reports of the successful use of these agents in PVOD exist. Although PVOD was suspected from the pretreatment CT scan, the ground-glass changes are not specific and may have been due to the patient's scleroderma, so a trial of therapy was warranted.

The patient had underlying scleroderma complicated by the development of pulmonary arterial hypertension. There was no evidence for another cause for the pulmonary hypertension. His left ventricular function at the time of assessment was near normal, making left heart failure the cause of his worsening after the institution of therapy unlikely (choice A is incorrect). Although pulmonary fibrosis is a known complication of scleroderma, there was little evidence of parenchymal lung disease on the chest CT scan at baseline, and there was not significant lung restriction as assessed by spirometry. It would be unlikely for the interstitial disease that complicates scleroderma to progress so rapidly, making this an unlikely cause for his worsening (choice B is incorrect). Although micrometastatic disease has been reported to cause pulmonary hypertension, there was no evidence of malignancy (choice D is incorrect).

PVOD is a known cause of pulmonary hypertension, and it has been reported in patients with scleroderma. It is characterized by progressive obliteration of the small pulmonary veins. Histologically, one sees occlusion of small pulmonary veins and thickening of the media of the veins (see Figure 172-C), with attendant venous congestion and eventual interstitial and alveolar edema. In this section, the pulmonary venules demonstrate intimal fibrosis with congestion in the surrounding lung parenchyma. There is no treatment for this condition other than lung transplantation.

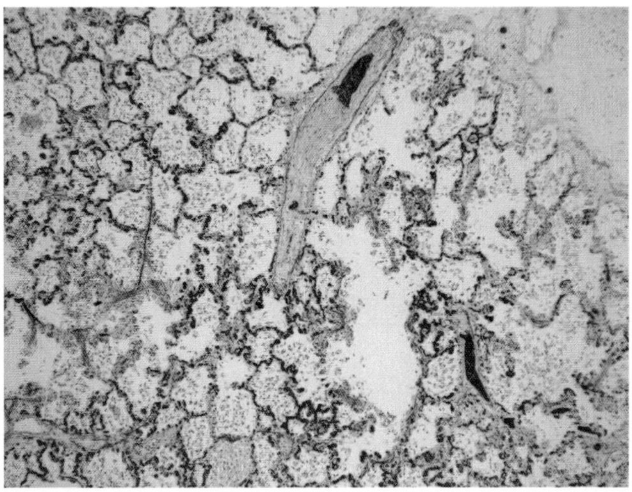

Figure 172-C
Movat elastin

Johnson SR, Patsios D, Hwang DM, et al. Pulmonary veno-occlusive disease and scleroderma associated pulmonary hypertension. J Rheumatol 2006; 33:2347–2350
Okumura H, Nagaya N, Kyotani S, et al. Effects of continuous IV prostacyclin in a patient with pulmonary veno-occlusive disease. Chest 2002; 122:1096–1098
Palmer SM, Robinson LJ, Wang A, et al. Massive pulmonary edema and death after prostacyclin infusion in a patient with pulmonary veno-occlusive disease. Chest 1998; 113:237–240
Resten A, Maitre S, Humbert M, et al. Pulmonary hypertension: CT of the chest in pulmonary venoocclusive disease. Am J Roentgenol 2004; 183:65–70
Simonneau G, Galie N, Rubin LJ, et al. Clinical classification of pulmonary hypertension. J Am Coll Cardiol 2004; 43(suppl S):5S–12S

173. B. Left upper lobe collapse.

The finding of increased opacity in the left chest on the PA image, with displacement of the major fissure anteriorly and parallel with the anterior chest wall on the lateral image (see Figure 173-B, arrows), indicates collapse of the left upper lobe (choice B is correct). The collapsed left upper lobe thus appears as a linear opacity behind the anterior chest wall, whereas loss of volume causes elevation of the left hemidiaphragm. As the apical segment of the upper lobe moves downward and anteriorly, the lower lobe inflates to fill the apex of the hemithorax.

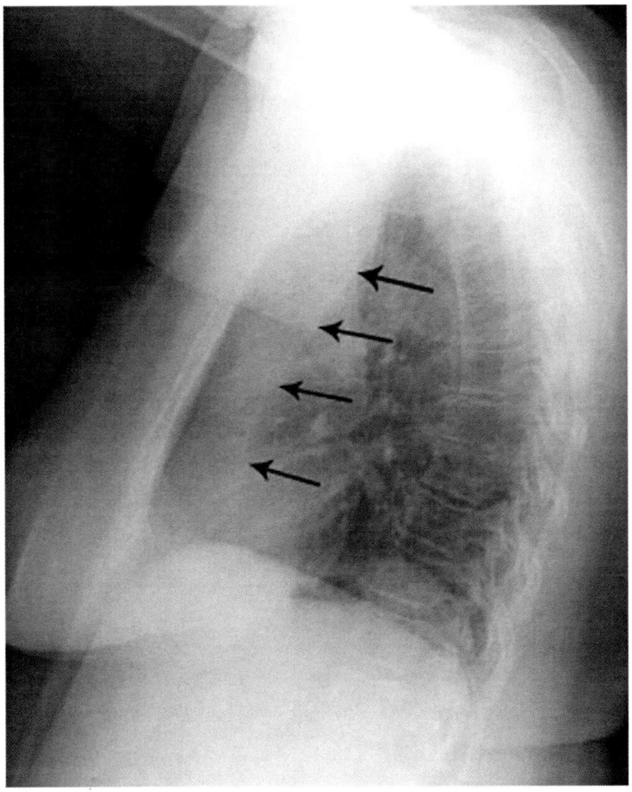

Figure 173-B

Although a large left pleural effusion could appear as opacity of the left hemithorax, the degree of aeration of the lung and the absence of a meniscus sign on both the PA and lateral views refute the possibility of a significant pleural effusion (choice A is incorrect). Unilateral pulmonary edema is also very unlikely because the lateral image shows normal left lung except for the atelectatic upper lobe (choice C is incorrect). Although weakness of the left hemidiaphragm would cause it to elevate, the anterior radiodensity indicates that the left upper lobe is collapsed (choice D is incorrect).

Woodring JH, Reed JC. Types and mechanisms of pulmonary atelectasis. J Thorac Imag 1996; 11:92–108
Mintzer RA, Sakowicz BA, Blonder JA. Lobar collapse: usual and unusual forms. Chest 1988; 94:615–620

174. D. Observation.

This patient's chest radiograph (see Figure 174-A) shows significant subcutaneous air and pneumoperitoneum. The CT scan (see Figure 174-B) reveals air within the mediastinum (possible pneumopericardium) and subcutaneous air. Additional scan sections showed air in the peritoneum, upper mediastinum, and neck. This presentation is compatible with the diagnosis of spontaneous pneumomediastinum (SPM). Given the patient's stability, observation is the most appropriate management option offered (choice D is correct). Observation may include hospital admission and close (expectant) monitoring for cardiopulmonary deterioration. Most patients are admitted and treated with analgesics. Additional diagnostic tests, including GI studies, are based on clinical suspicion. Supplemental oxygen has little effect, in contrast to cases of pneumothorax. The majority of patients have a benign course with hospital stays of 2 to 5 days; recurrence of SPM is rare.

SPM is a rare, largely self-limited and benign disease defined as the presence of interstitial air in the mediastinum without any clearly defined cause. Confounding this definition is the use of the terms "predisposing" and "precipitating/provoking/triggering" factors, perhaps making reports and the term "spontaneous" misleading. Predisposing factors (underlying diseases) commonly noted include asthma (8 to 59% of cases), COPD, and interstitial lung disease. Precipitating factors (events), found in 39 to 100% of cases, include illicit inhalational drug use, coughing (as in this patient), sneezing, defecation, vomiting, intense physical activity, and giving birth. Common to these factors is the Valsalva maneuver, reflecting the presumed pathophysiology: creation of a pressure gradient between the alveoli and the lung interstitium resulting in alveolar rupture and interstitial air (emphysema) that tracks to the mediastinum and points beyond, including the peritoneum, as in this patient. Patients are often young adult men (75% of cases) with a mean age of 20 years (in contrast to this patient) and with an age range of 3 to 71 years. The most common symptoms are chest discomfort, dyspnea, and neck pain or discomfort. Subcutaneous emphysema, especially of the neck, as in this patient, is found in 40 to 100% of cases. Results of a chest radiograph are normal in up to 30% of patients; CT of the chest should be performed in suspected cases with a normal chest radiograph. An elevated WBC count is found in 50% of cases. Boerhaave syndrome, a cause of pneumomediastinum, has a similar presentation of chest pain and subcutaneous emphysema but is often preceded by vomiting and the patient often has leukocytosis (neither seen in this patient). If Boerhaave syndrome is suspected, an esophagram and/or upper GI endoscopy may be indicated. With this patient's stable presentation and absent esophageal findings on CT, neither is indicated (choice C is incorrect). There is a question of pericardial air, but the patient is hemodynamically stable, and drainage of possible pericardial air is not indicated (choice A is incorrect); tension pneumopericardium is rare in SPM. Given the absence of fever, significant abdominal examination findings, and leukocytosis, surgical exploration is not indicated (choice B is incorrect).

Caceres M, Ali SZ, Braud R, et al. Spontaneous pneumomediastinum: a comparative study and review of the literature. Ann Thorac Surg 2008; 86:962–966

Macia I, Moya J, Ramos R, et al. Spontaneous pneumomediastinum: 41 cases. Eur J Cardiothorac Surg 2007; 31:1110–1114

Takada K, Matsumoto S, Hiramatsu T, et al. Management of spontaneous pneumomediastium based on clinical experience of 25 cases. Respir Med 2008; 102:1329–1334

Mondello B, Pavia R, Ruggeri P, et al. Spontaneous pneumomediastinum: experience in 18 adult patients. Lung 2007; 185:9–14

Newcomb AE, Clarke CP. Spontaneous pneumomediastium: a benign curiosity or a significant problem? Chest 2005; 128:3298–3302

175. B. ΔF508 *CFTR*.

This young person with recurrent respiratory tract infections and elevated sweat chloride values has cystic fibrosis. Approximately 70% of patients have the classic ΔF508 mutation in the cystic fibrosis transmembrane conductance regulator (*CFTR*) gene (choice B is correct).

Cystic fibrosis is a common autosomal recessive disease found in Caucasians in the United States, with an incidence of 1 in 35,000 births. The predicted median age of survival is 36 years, which has significantly improved over the past decades. The vast majority of patients receive the diagnosis in childhood, but an increasing number of patients now receive the diagnosis in adulthood, likely reflecting the heterogeneous phenotype of the disease and an increase in awareness in adults. An additional 23 mutations have been demonstrated to result in altered function in *CFTR* to

fulfill criteria for cystic fibrosis. In contrast to children who have cystic fibrosis, adults are rarely homozygous for the ΔF508 mutation, which occurs in up to 50% of children who have the disease.

Mutations in *hTERT* and *hTR* (human telomerase reverse transcriptase and human transferrin receptor), two genes essential to the catalytic activity of telomerase to enable it to add telomere repeats to the end of DNA, have been reported in patients with familial idiopathic pulmonary fibrosis but are not associated with bronchiectasis (choice A is incorrect). Sickle cell anemia is a common genetic disease in the United States but is not frequently found in Caucasians (choice C is incorrect). α_1-Antitrypsin deficiency is a well-characterized genetic disease, most commonly manifesting with hepatic and pulmonary dysfunction. Bronchiectasis, similar to that noted in patients with adult-onset cystic fibrosis, may occur with α_1-antitrypsin deficiency. In contrast to cystic fibrosis, mutations in *CFTR* are not present in α_1-antitrypsin deficiency, and the result of the sweat chloride test is normal (choice D is incorrect).

Rowe SM, Miller S, Sorscher EJ. Cystic fibrosis. N Engl J Med 2005; 352:1992–2001
Farrell PM, Rosenstein BJ, White TB, et al. Guidelines for diagnosis of cystic fibrosis in newborns through older adults: Cystic Fibrosis Foundation consensus report. J Pediatr 2008; 153:S4–S14
Nick JA, Rodman DM. Manifestations of cystic fibrosis diagnosed in adulthood. Curr Opin Pulm Med 2005; 11:513–518

176. D. Pleurobiliary fistula.

This patient has developed a fistulous tract complicating chemoembolization of the hepatic tumor mass, which is now resulting in accumulation of biliary drainage and consequent inflammatory fluid in the right pleural space (choice D is correct). The ratio of pleural fluid to serum bilirubin is used to make a diagnosis of the communication of the biliary tree with the pleural space, with a value > 2 highly suggestive of this disorder. In this patient, that ratio is well above 2 (18.4/5.5). The fluid collections within the liver substance, below the diaphragm and in the right pleural space, were well demonstrated by a CT scan performed several days after thoracentesis when fluid had once again accumulated (see Figure 176-C, arrows).

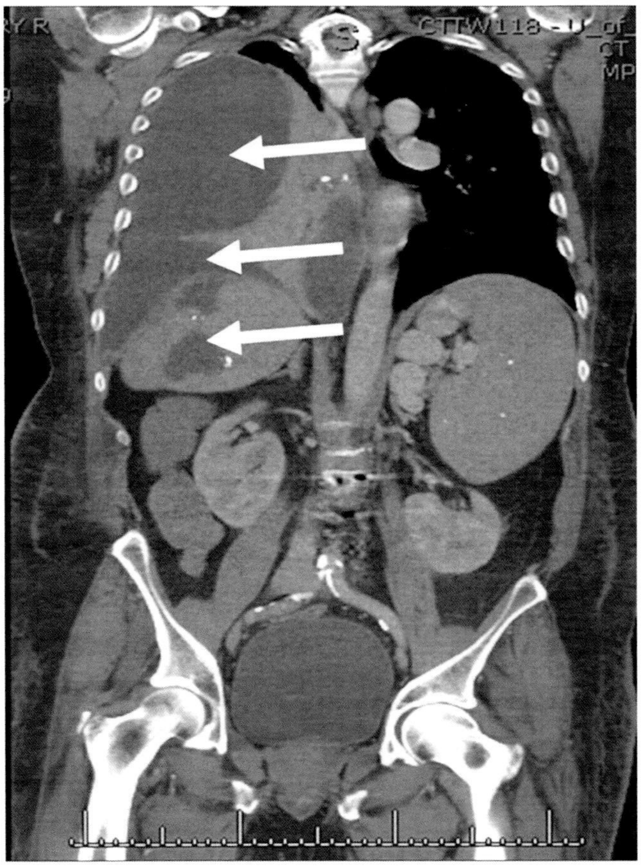

Figure 176-C

Apart from very rare congenital disorders with embryologic remnant communications between the biliary tree and airways, communications of the biliary tree with the thorax occurring in adults can arise from several different conditions, including trauma, posthepatic surgery or percutaneous biliary drainage, after chemo- or radiofrequency ablation of hepatic tumors, or complicating infectious processes (pyogenic, amoebic, hydatid, and mycobacterial). The fistulous tract may communicate with the pleural space (pleurobiliary fistula) or major bronchi (bronchobiliary fistula); in the latter case, the patient will often expectorate large quantities of bilious material ("biliptysis"). Fluid accumulations in the pleural space can be large, which is related to the negative pleural pressure favoring biliary flow to this space. Pleural fluid obtained in these patients will have high bilirubin levels, but the fluid will have a number of characteristics different from bile itself because of the marked inflammation resulting from bile salts and other constituents of the fluid draining into the pleural space. Inflammatory cells are typically seen, and the pH of the fluid is often much less than that of bile (usually 7.5 to 8.0). A very low pH was seen in this patient, which also raised a concern for secondary infection, and accordingly, antibiotics were given. Results of pleural fluid cultures and stains, however, were negative, and the findings of the pleural fluid in this patient are consistent with accumulation of sterile bile in the pleural space.

The management of these communications includes surgery repair, if feasible, because flow through the fistula tends to continue even if the biliary tree is patent. Surgery was not thought to be possible in this patient with complex anatomy and advanced chronic liver failure. Unfortunately, this complication of the treatment of her hepatocellular carcinoma resulted in her being denied liver transplantation. Medical management includes prophylactic antibiotics, efforts to favor biliary drainage to the bowel (this patient received a common bile duct stent for an area of moderate stenosis), intermittent thoracentesis or pleural drains, and octreotide to reduce bile flow.

The high bilirubin noted in the pleural fluid would not be seen in ascitic fluid accumulations in the chest, empyema, or pancreatic communications with the thorax (choices A, B, and C are incorrect). The lack of fever and purulent sputum speaks against a diagnosis of empyema complicating pneumonia and the lack of abdominal pain against pancreatic disease or spontaneous bacterial peritonitis. This patient did not have ascites by history or physical examination complicating her cirrhosis to support a diagnosis of spontaneous bacterial peritonitis. Finally, the low amylase level in the pleural fluid speaks against the finding of communication of the pleural space with the pancreas.

Akazama S, Omagari K, et al. Biliopleural fistula associated with intrahepatic biloma after transcatheter arterial chemoembolization for hepatocellular carcinoma. J Hepatol 2004; 40:1045–1046

Pisani RJ, Zeller FA. Bilious pleural effusion following liver biopsy. Chest 1990; 90:1545–1537

177. A. A 50-year-old man with rheumatoid arthritis with a purified protein derivative (PPD) result of 12-mm induration, being evaluated for infliximab therapy. His chest radiograph is clear.

Patient A should receive isoniazid (INH) prophylaxis for LTBI (choice A is correct). Tumor necrosis factor (TNF) inhibitors are used to treat patients with rheumatoid arthritis and Crohn disease, among others. Drugs in this category include infliximab, adalimumab, and etanercept. TNF is required to protect against mycobacterial disease and form granulomas to wall off infection. The use of TNF inhibitors has been associated with increased infections, particularly mycobacterial but also bacterial, viral, and fungal infections. These categories of drugs increase the risk of reactivation of LTBI and active disease. The risk appears to be greatest with infliximab. Recently, Centers for Disease Control and Prevention guidelines have recommended that patients being considered for this therapy be screened for LTBI and placed on prophylaxis if the reaction is ≥ 5 mm prior to beginning the agent (usually for ≥ 1 to 2 months). Patients with evidence of old TB on chest radiograph or evidence of TB exposure should also receive prophylaxis even if the skin test result is negative. If there is a diagnosis of active disease in a patient receiving a TNF inhibitor, the drug should be stopped.

Reviews of a large US Food and Drug Administration database reveal that the estimated rates of TB were 54/100,000 patients on infliximab and 28/100,000 patients on etanercept, much higher than that of the general population.

Cases typically developed on average 12 weeks following initiation of therapy, and extrapulmonary disease was not uncommon. LTBI was a risk factor for active disease. European databases have shown a similarly increased rate of TB infection in patients receiving these agents.

Patient B falls in a low-risk group and would only require prophylaxis if the PPD were ≥ 15 mm, and, even then, prophylaxis might be controversial. This type of patient with no or minimal risk factors should not undergo routine testing. A PPD convertor is defined as conversion of 10 mm over a 2-year time period. This patient's last PPD test was 5 years ago, so conversion cannot be documented (choice B is incorrect). Patient C has risk factors for TB but is HIV negative, so 10 mm of induration would be required to define positivity in this scenario (choice C is incorrect). Patient D may need INH prophylaxis but has an abnormal chest radiograph, and active disease must be excluded by sputum analysis prior to beginning single-drug prophylaxis. LTBI therapy should not be initiated until active disease is excluded (choice D is incorrect). Foundry workers are exposed to silica, which can reduce cell-mediated immunity and predispose them to the development of TB.

The most recent guideline for screening and treatment of latent LTBI outlines recommendations for screening, definition of a positive test, and treatment. The goals for LTBI testing should be to identify those patients at high risk of developing TB and those who would most benefit from prophylaxis. Patients who should be screened, and the PPD size that defines positivity and subsequent prophylaxis, include the following:

Induration of ≥ 5 mm

- Recent contacts of active cases
- Abnormal chest radiograph findings consistent with possible prior TB
- HIV-positive patients
- Recipients of organ transplants or other immunosuppression equivalent to prednisone ≥ 15 mg/d
- Patients being considered for anti-TNF therapy

Induration of ≥ 10 mm

- Recent immigrants from high-prevalence countries
- HIV-negative injection drug users
- Residents and employees of high-risk congregate settings (hospitals and other health-care facilities, prisons and jails, nursing homes, and homeless shelters)
- Medical illnesses resulting in increased risk of active disease such as malignancy, diabetes, silicosis, gastrectomy, chronic renal failure, hematologic malignancies, head and neck cancer, weight loss of ≥ 10% of body mass, and jejunal bypass
- Medically underserved and low-income groups

Induration of ≥ 15 mm (screening not indicated)

- Patients not listed in the above categories

The recommended prophylactic regimen is INH for 9 months.

Gardam MA, Keystone EC, Menzies R, et al. Anti-tumour necrosis factor agents and TB risk: mechanisms of action and clinical management. Lancet Infect Dis 2003; 3:148–155

Centers for Disease Control and Prevention. Tuberculosis associated with blocking agents against tumor necrosis factor-alpha: California, 2002–2003. MMWR Morb Mortal Wkly Rep 2004; 53:683–686

Carmona L, Gomez-Reino JJ, Rodriguez-Valverde V, et al. Effectiveness of recommendations to prevent reactivation of latent tuberculosis infection in patients treated with tumor necrosis factor antagonists. Arthritis Rheum 2005; 52:1766–1772

Wolfe F, Michaud K, Anderson J, et al. Tuberculosis infection in patients with rheumatoid arthritis and the effect of infliximab therapy. Arthritis Rheum 2004; 50:372–379

Wallis RS. Tumour necrosis factor antagonists: structure, function, and tuberculosis risks. Lancet Infect Dis 2008; 8:601–611

Targeted tuberculin testing and treatment of latent tuberculosis infection. Joint Statement of the American Thoracic Society (ATS) and the Centers for Disease Control and Prevention (CDC). Am J Respir Crit Care Med 2000; 161:S221–S247

Centers for Disease Control and Prevention (CDC). Trend in tuberculosis: United States, 1998–2003. MMWR Morb Mortal Wkly Rep 2004; 53:209–214

178. A. Mode change to pressure-assist control ventilation.

Several clinical trials have confirmed that using smaller tidal volumes (*eg,* 6 mL/kg IBW) can protect the lung from overdistention injury. One of the consequences of smaller tidal volumes, however, is that patients who have active respiratory drives may be uncomfortable and demand higher flows than are generally provided. This may be particularly true during volume-assist control ventilation where the flow setting is fixed by the clinician.

In our patient, volume-assist control ventilation is being delivered, and the flow setting is a decelerating pattern (see Figure 178-B, left panel). Note, however, that the graphic shows that the airway pressure is literally being sucked downward (solid arrow) because this flow pattern is inadequate for this patient's respiratory drive. This is the cause of the patient's discomfort.

In Figure 178-B, right panel graphic, the patient's airway pressure is seen to be more synchronous, being more convex, in an upward configuration. This reflects the ventilator's ability to provide inspiratory pressure more evenly during inspiration. This is due to a flow pattern that is delivering a higher flow earlier in the breath, which persists during the middle of the breath (broken arrow) and then tails off. This variable flow is characteristic of pressure-targeted ventilation, or in this example, pressure-assist control ventilation (choice A is correct). Note that the tidal volume and the inspiratory time settings are the same as during the original volume-assist control ventilation, so the 6 mL/kg IBW protective tidal volume is still being delivered. Choices B and C are incorrect in that the flow profile is variable, not a set constant or sine wave setting that is chosen by the clinician. Choice D is incorrect because the tidal volume has not increased.

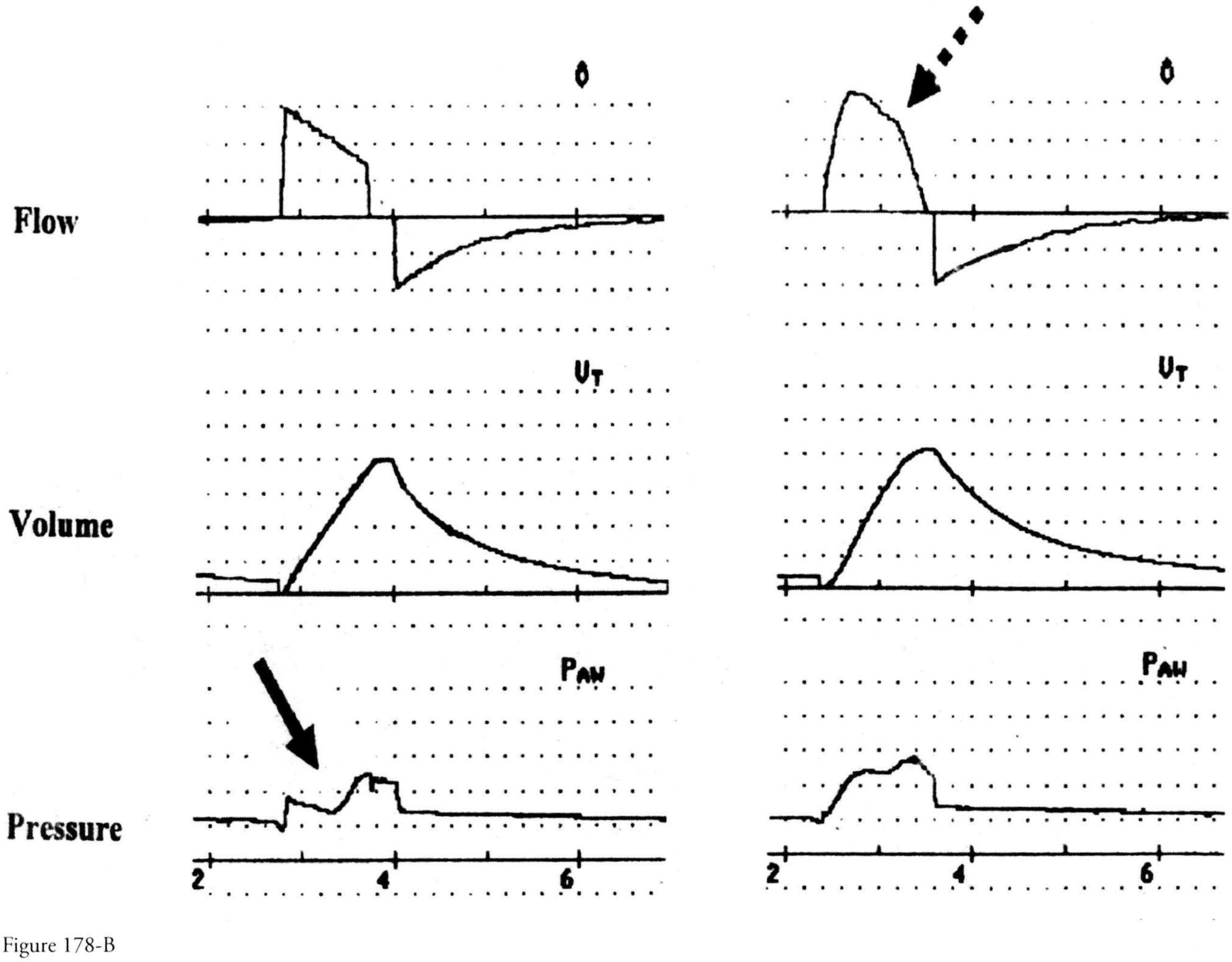

Figure 178-B

Other strategies to improve patient-ventilator synchrony include breath trigger sensitivity/responsiveness adjustments, inspiratory flow/timing adjustments, and breath cycling criteria adjustments. Newer approaches include proportional assist ventilation (adjusts support to patient flow demand) and neurally adjusted ventilatory assistance (controls assisted breaths according to diaphragmatic electromyographic measurements).

Yang LY, Huang YC, MacIntyre NR. Patient-ventilator synchrony during pressure-targeted versus flow-targeted small tidal volume assisted ventilation. J Crit Care 2007; 22:252–257

MacIntyre NR, McConnell R, Cheng KC, et al. Patient-ventilator flow dys-synchrony: flow limited vs pressure limited breaths. Crit Care Med 1997; 25:1671–1677

Leung P, Jubran A, Tobin MJ. Comparison of assisted ventilator modes on triggering, patient effort, and dyspnea. Am J Respir Crit Care Med 1997; 155:1940–1948

Prinianakis G, Kondili E, Georgopoulos D. Patient-ventilator interaction: an overview. Respir Care Clin N Am 2005; 11:201–224

179. C. Review the individual spirometry efforts.

Although the measured values for spirometry are within normal limits, the flow-volume curve reveals flattening of the expiratory flow, an absent inspiratory curve, and suspicion of a submaximal effort. Interpretation of pulmonary function test results first involves an assessment of the reliability of the data and then classification of the values compared with an appropriate reference population, followed by assimilation of the results into the diagnosis and management of the patient. Although experienced technicians will routinely communicate any potential factors that might affect test result reliability, this often does not occur in many clinical settings. In this case, appropriate consultation with the technician and review of the individual efforts would have revealed the following (see Figure 179-B):

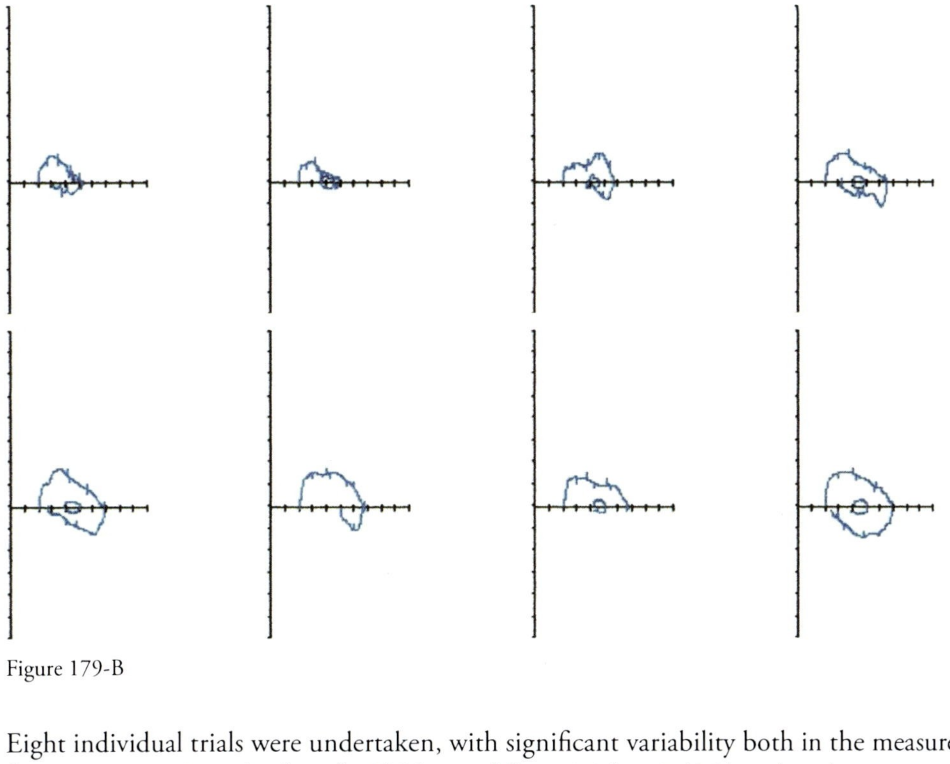

Figure 179-B

Eight individual trials were undertaken, with significant variability both in the measured values (values for FEV_1 varied from 1.2 to 2.8 L, and values for FVC varied from 2.04 to 3.43 L) and in the appearance of the flow-volume curves. These results reflect variable and submaximal efforts (choice C is correct) and would not confirm a clinical suspicion of central airway obstruction. After repeated testing, the following results were observed: an FEV_1 of 3.13 L (107% predicted), FVC of 3.48 L (113% predicted), and an FEV_1/FVC of 0.89 (see Figure 179-C).

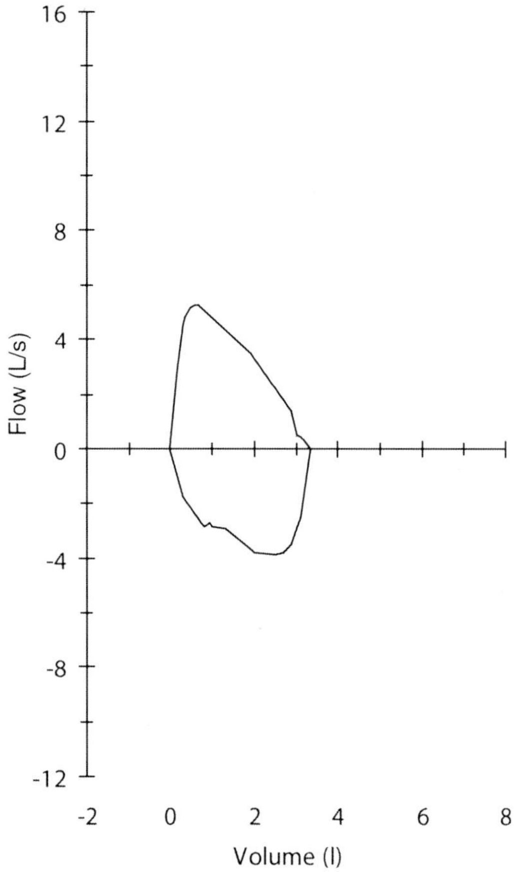

Figure 179-C

Difficult-to-control asthma is a diagnostic and management challenge. Central airway obstruction, from whatever underlying etiology, must be considered in any patient with this clinical presentation. However, with significant physiologic central airway obstruction excluded, there is no need to proceed with further investigations in this regard (choices A and B are incorrect). Increasing therapy might be appropriate in the setting of persistent symptomatic asthma, but in this instance, later methacholine challenge testing while the patient was symptomatic did not reveal any increase in bronchial hyperreactivity. As such, the diagnosis of asthma was excluded, and increasing therapy would not be appropriate (choice D is incorrect). This finding also highlights the importance of confirming the diagnosis of asthma in this setting.

Miller MR, Crapo R, Hankinson J, et al. General considerations for lung function testing. Series: ATS/ERS Task Force: standardisation of lung function testing. Eur Respir J 2005; 26:153–161

Miller MR, Hankinson J, Brusasco V, et al. Standardisation of spirometry. Series: ATS/ERS Task Force: standardisation of lung function testing. Eur Respir J 2005; 26:319–338

Pellegrino R, Viego G, Brusasco V, et al. Interpretative strategies for lung function tests. Series: ATS/ERS Task Force: standardisation of lung function testing. Eur Respir J 2005; 26:948–968

180. D. IV epoprostenol.

This patient has idiopathic pulmonary arterial hypertension (IPAH), functional class IV. Although all currently approved therapies can be used in patients with functional class IV, evidence indicates that IV epoprostenol is the treatment of choice for these patients (choice D is correct). This is based on evidence of improved exercise capacity, hemodynamics, quality of life, and mortality in this group of patients. Longer-acting prostacyclin analogs have been developed for IV, subcutaneous, inhaled, and oral use, but tolerability and effectiveness in patients with advanced PAH are variable. Therefore, these agents should be reserved for patients who refuse IV therapy or who are considered to be incapable of managing the IV delivery system of epoprostenol.

Patients with PAH are classified according to the World Health Organization functional assessment classification. Patients in functional class I are those who have PAH but in whom physical activity does not cause dyspnea or fatigue, chest pain, or other symptoms. Class II patients note a mild limitation of physical activity, although they are comfortable at rest. Class III patients experience marked limitation of physical activity. They are comfortable at rest, but even ordinary activity causes dyspnea, fatigue, chest pain, or near syncope. The most advanced patients are categorized as class IV. They note an inability to carry out any physical activity without symptoms. These symptoms are often present at rest, and many patients will demonstrate signs of right-heart failure (as seen in this patient).

Calcium channel blockers are used only in patients with a positive vasodilator challenge. The vasodilator challenge is done using a short-acting vasodilator, such as IV epoprostenol or adenosine or inhaled nitric oxide during cardiac catheterization. A positive challenge is defined as a decrease in mean PA pressure > 10 mm Hg to a value < 40 mm Hg, without a decrease in cardiac output. The decrease in cardiac output is an ominous sign because it reflects an inability of the right ventricle to compensate and to generate a significant pressure. Given the decrease in this patient's cardiac output, she would not be considered a responder, so she would not be a candidate for calcium channel blockers (choice A is incorrect). In addition, prostacyclins are considered first-line therapy in patients with advanced IPAH, given their overall low long-term response to calcium channel blockers and their poor prognosis.

Other agents approved for the treatment of PAH include endothelin receptor antagonists and phosphodiesterase inhibitors. Circulating endothelin-1 levels are increased in patients with PAH and correlate with disease severity. Bosentan is a nonspecific endothelin A and B receptor antagonist that has been demonstrated to improve exercise capacity and hemodynamics in patients with PAH. Sildenafil is a phosphodiestarase inhibitor that increases the effects of locally produced nitric oxide, resulting in pulmonary vasodilation and inhibition of smooth muscle growth. Benefits in patients with PAH include improvements in symptoms, 6-min walking distance, and hemodynamics. Given the lack of survival data in patients with more advanced class IV disease, however, these agents are also reserved for those who refuse or cannot tolerate IV therapy (choices B and C are incorrect).

Combination therapy has been suggested based on additive or synergistic effects. Improvements in surrogate outcomes are now being reported. However, the optimal combination of these agents is still unknown. Currently, combination therapy is suggested for patients with functional class III or IV disease who have persistent symptoms despite treatment with a single medication.

Chin KM, Rubin LJ. Pulmonary arterial hypertension. J Am Coll Cardiol 2008; 51:1527–1538

Badesch DB, Abman SH, Simoneau G, et al. Medical therapy for pulmonary arterial hypertension: updated ACCP evidence-based clinical practice guidelines. Chest 2007; 131:1917–1928

McGoon M, Gutterman D, Steen V, et al. Screening, early detection, and diagnosis of pulmonary arterial hypertension: ACCP evidence-based clinical practice guidelines. Chest 2004; 126(suppl):14S–34S

181. A. Morphine sulfate taken orally.

Breathlessness or dyspnea, defined as "a subjective experience of breathing discomfort that consists of qualitatively distinct sensations that vary in intensity," is a common and disabling symptom in advanced stages of a variety of malignant and nonmalignant diseases. This is particularly true for advanced COPD, particularly at the end of life. Management of breathlessness includes treatment directed at the underlying disease processes, as well as both pharmacologic and nonpharmacologic interventions designed to relieve the sensation of dyspnea. Considering the combinations of pharmacologic and nonpharmacologic interventions proposed to our patient, there is stronger evidence of effectiveness for morphine sulfate taken orally than for the other options (choice A is correct). Multiple systematic reviews cite high-quality evidence of benefit from systemic opioid use for relief of dyspnea in COPD, based on multiple positive results of randomized controlled trials (RCTs). Positive but weaker evidence of effectiveness is present for systemic opioids in cancer-related dyspnea. In contrast, however, analyses of RCT-based evidence reveal no benefit from nebulized morphine for relief of breathlessness in COPD or malignancy (choice B is incorrect). A wide variety of nonpharmacologic interventions directed at relief of dyspnea in COPD has been tested in RCTs and other

prospective controlled clinical trials. In a recent comprehensive systematic review of nonpharmacologic interventions for breathlessness in advanced stages of disease, chest wall vibration and neuroelectrical muscle stimulation gave strong evidence of effectiveness, and walking aids produced moderate evidence for relief of breathlessness in patients with COPD. In contrast, clinical trial findings for acupuncture and acupressure were found to yield mixed results, with low strength of evidence (choice C is incorrect). Similarly, interventions such as music, relaxation, and use of a fan (choice D is incorrect) were judged to have inadequate evidence to recommend their routine use. Some experts take a more liberal approach to use of nonpharmacologic interventions that are simple and safe, despite the lack of robust evidence.

Bausewein C, Booth S, Gysels M, et al. Non-pharmacological interventions for breathlessness in advanced stages of malignant and non-malignant diseases. Cochrane Database Syst Rev 2008; CD005623

Lorenz KA, Lynn J, Dy SM, et al. Evidence for improving palliative care at the end of life: a systematic review. Ann Intern Med 2008; 148:147–159

Viola R, Kiteley C, Lloyd NS, et al. The management of dyspnea in cancer patients: a systematic review. Support Care Cancer 2008; 16:329–337

Lanken PN, Terry PB, Delisser HM, et al. An official American Thoracic Society clinical policy statement: palliative care for patients with respiratory diseases and critical illnesses. Am J Respir Crit Care Med 2008; 177:912–927

182. C. Actinomycosis.

This patient has empyema necessitatis caused by *Actinomycosis israelii*, confirmed by culture of a repeat pleural fluid aspiration and a first-time aspiration of chest wall material. The histopathologic findings of both shows sulfur granules, consisting of colonies of organisms with an amorphous center surrounded by bacterial filaments (see Figure 182-D), indicative of actinomycosis (choice C is correct). Persistent pleural fluid, adjacent pulmonary parenchymal disease, and extension of the process through the chest wall to subcutaneous tissues constitute empyema necessitatis (see Figures 182-B and 182-C in the item stem). This patient has a bronchopleural cutaneous fistula explaining the variable skin lesion size with mechanical ventilation. In the preantibiotic era, *Streptococcus pneumoniae* was second only to TB as the leading cause of empyema necessitatis, but *S pneumoniae* is a reported rarely as a cause today. This patient received multiple antibiotics that should have successfully treated even penicillin-resistant *S pneumoniae* (choice B is incorrect). TB remains the leading cause of empyema necessitatis today, accounting for 50% of cases reported from 1966 to 2004. Multiple negative smear and culture results for TB make TB unlikely in this patient (choice D is incorrect). Actinomycosis is the second leading cause today. Actinomycosis is frequently initially misdiagnosed as cancer, which may also erode through the chest wall, but a baseline "normal" finding on chest radiograph in this nonsmoking patient makes cancer unlikely (choice A is incorrect).

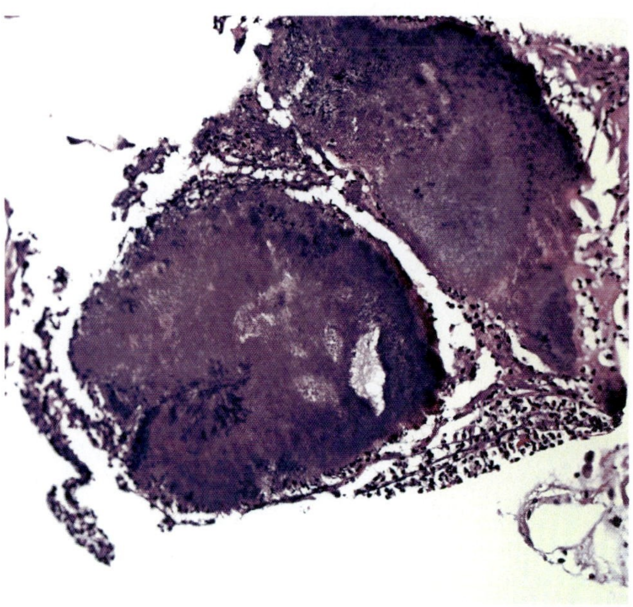

Figure 182-D
Hematoxylin-eosin

Pulmonary actinomycosis is a rare disease, primarily caused by *Actinomyces israelii* and not clearly associated with immunosuppression. Actinomyces are commensals of the oropharynx, GI tract, and female genitalia. The pulmonary form of actinomycosis constitutes about 15% of presentations with cervicofacial disease (50%), and abdominal disease (30%) is more common. Pulmonary disease occurs more commonly with underlying emphysema, chronic bronchitis, and bronchiectasis. Dental disease, as in this patient, and alcoholism may increase risk. Pulmonary actinomycosis probably starts with aspiration of oropharyngeal secretions, with acute inflammation followed by a chronic indolent phase. The diagnosis requires a high degree of suspicion and is often delayed until late in disease, as in this patient. Nocardia may resemble actinomycosis, but it does not form sulfur granules in visceral lesions. Actinomyces are facultative anaerobic Gram-positive bacteria, and any material obtained should be cultured anaerobically; semiselective media may increase the rate of isolation. The treatment of choice is penicillin for a prolonged course, although shorter courses may be successful. Tetracyclines, erythromycin, and clindamycin are alternatives.

Freeman A, Ben-Ami T, Shulman S. *Streptococcus pneumoniae* empyema necessitatis. Pediatr Infect Dis J 2004; 23:177–179

Heffner JE. Pleuropulmonary manifestations of actinomycosis and nocardiosis. Semin Respir Infect 1988; 3:352–361

Hooker TP, Hammond M, Corral K. Empyema necessitatis: a review of the manifestations of thoracic actinomycosis. Cleve Clin J Med 1992; 59:542–548

Yildiz O, Doganay M. Actinomycoses and Nocardia pulmonary infections. Curr Opin Pulm Med 2006; 12:228–234

183. C. Switch to a benzodiazepine at nighttime.

Restless legs syndrome (RLS) is defined as the presence of spontaneous, continuous leg movements at rest that are commonly associated with an uncomfortable sensation. Movement resolves these symptoms, and there is a common association with sleep disturbance and involuntary jerking leg movements, termed *periodic leg movements of sleep*. In some population surveys, symptoms have been noted in 5 to 15% of the population but are usually mild. The disorder may be idiopathic but is also associated with iron deficiency, end-stage renal disease, pregnancy, diabetes mellitus, and Parkinson disease.

Carbidopa/levodopa has become an accepted treatment for the symptoms of RLS and associated sleep disturbance. However, a common phenomenon noted in patients initially responding to treatment with levodopa is augmentation, which is a worsening of RLS symptoms earlier in the day after an evening dose, sometimes with spread of the symptoms to the upper extremities. Patients may present with total-body restlessness that is unrelenting, even when they are walking. The symptoms are indistinguishable from those of acute akathisia induced by neuroleptic drugs. Augmentation has been reported less frequently with dopamine agonists (in 20 to 30% of patients) than with levodopa (in 80% of patients). However, this difference may reflect the pattern of use of dopamine agonists in clinical studies, which have involved relatively low doses and short durations of treatment. It is possible that longer-term use and higher doses of dopamine agonists may result in rates of augmentation similar to those reported with levodopa.

Benzodiazepines are very effective to control symptoms of RLS and abort the progression of augmentation (choice C is correct). In most cases, a benzodiazepine can be administered for several weeks or longer with resolution of symptoms, and carbidopa/levodopa started again at a low dose. Maintenance of the same dose of carbidopa/levodopa when augmentation occurs will cause the symptoms to persist (choice B is incorrect). Increases in the dose of medication to cover the expanded symptomatic period relieves the symptoms in the short term, but, ultimately, symptoms begin to appear even earlier, accompanied by a noticeable decrease in the duration of action and the effectiveness of the drug (choice D is incorrect). RLS symptoms have been described to be more common in patients with iron deficiency and respond to iron replacement, but iron replacement would not be warranted in the absence of low ferritin levels (typically < 45 ng/mL [101 pmol/L]) (choice A is incorrect).

Earley CJ. Clinical practice: restless legs syndrome. N Engl J Med 2003; 348:2103–2109

Hogl B, Kiechl S, Willeit J, et al. Restless legs syndrome: a community-based study of prevalence, severity, and risk factors. Neurology 2005; 64:1920–1926

Silber MH, Ehrenberg BL, Allen RP, et al. An algorithm for the management of restless legs syndrome. Mayo Clin Proc 2004; 79:916–921

184. A. Inspiratory and expiratory vocal cord adduction with a posterior glottic chink.

The vocal cord dysfunction syndrome is not rare; it can account for up to 15% of patients referred to a tertiary care center for evaluation of exertional dyspnea. Nevertheless, the diagnosis is often missed because (1) it closely mimics asthma; (2) intermittent symptoms make endoscopic confirmation logistically difficult (confirmatory findings are present at the time of laryngoscopy approximately 50% of the time); and (3) the diagnostic laryngoscopic findings are not widely appreciated. Of the choices listed, only inspiratory and expiratory vocal cord adduction (*ie*, vocal cords move toward the midline) with a posterior glottic chink is specific for this condition (choice A is correct). Figure 184-A shows adduction of the true vocal cords during inspiration and narrowing of the glottis to a small diamond-shaped chink. An additional feature of vocal cord dysfunction syndrome also shown in Figure 184-A is adduction of the false vocal cords (the soft tissue bilateral bulging structures just above and posterior to the true vocal cords). Adduction by the false vocal cords obscures the laryngeal ventricles that are fusiform fossae bounded by the true and false vocal cords (Figure 184-B, arrows). Although not listed as a choice, vocal cord adduction with a posterior glottic chink limited to inspiration is also characteristic of this condition.

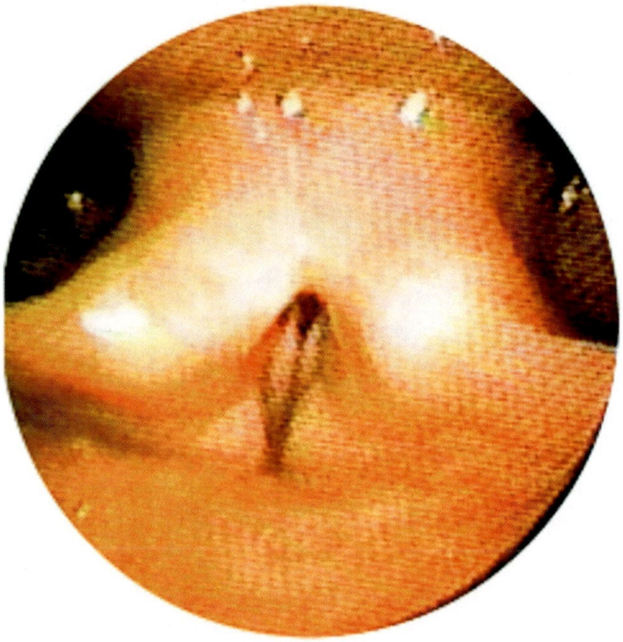

Figure 184-A

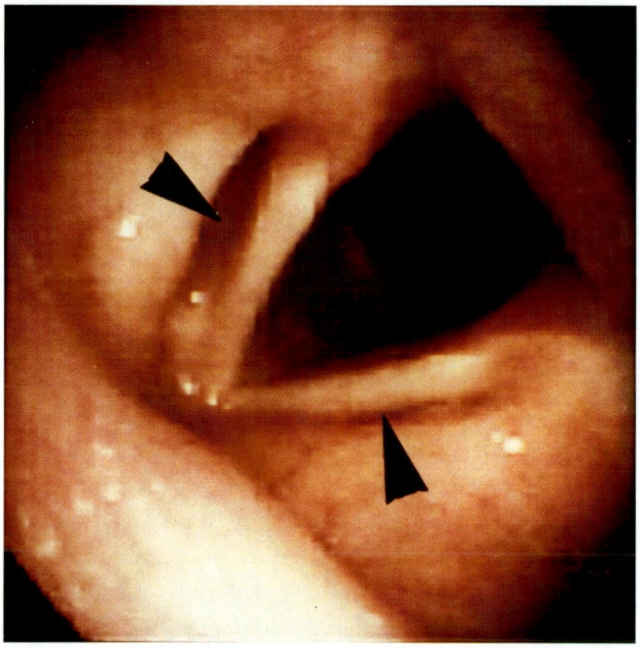

Figure 184-B

Isolated expiratory vocal cord (choice B) and false vocal cord adduction (choice D) are not specific for vocal cord dysfunction because these findings have been found (1) during early exhalation when healthy volunteers undergo histamine bronchoprovocation challenges and in patients with severe airflow obstruction, and (2) during mid-exhalation in asthmatic patients with experimentally induced bronchoconstriction. Therefore, choices B and C are incorrect. This effect in asthmatics was reversed with CPAP, suggesting that vocal cord adduction during expiration in these patients is a way of unloading inspiratory muscle activity.

Choice C is incorrect for two reasons: abduction of the vocal cords (*ie*, vocal cords move away from the midline) during inspiration is normal, and it is not possible to develop a posterior glottic chink when the vocal cords are open.

Christopher KL. Understanding vocal cord dysfunction: a step in the right direction with a long road ahead. Chest 2006; 129:842–843

Higenbottam T. Narrowing of glottis opening in humans associated with experimentally induced bronchoconstriction. J Appl Physiol 1980; 49:403–407

Higenbottam T, Payne J. Glottic narrowing in lung disease. Am Rev Respir Dis 1982; 125:746–750

Mikita J, Parker J. High levels of medical utilization by ambulatory patients with vocal cord dysfunction as compared to age- and gender-matched asthmatics. Chest 2006; 129:905–908

Wood RP, Milgrom H. Vocal cord dysfunction. J Allergy Clin Immunol 1996; 98:481–485

185. A. Upper-lobe-predominant disease with low exercise capacity.

In an updated report, the National Emphysema Treatment Trial defined the subgroups of patients with severe emphysema that would gain the most benefit from the operation. The group with upper-lobe-predominant disease with low exercise capacity gained the most benefit (choice A is correct). The intention-to-treat analysis of 1,218 patients showed an overall survival benefit for the surgically treated group, with a relative risk for death at 5 years of 0.86 ($p = 0.02$). The greatest benefit was demonstrated in the group with upper-lobe-predominant disease and low exercise tolerance, showing an improved survival at 5 years (relative risk, 0.67; $p = 0.003$). In addition, this same group exhibited improved exercise tolerance throughout 3 years ($p < 0.001$) and better health-related quality of life through 5 years ($p < 0.001$ for years 1 to 3) and at 5 years ($p = 0.01$).

The group with upper-lobe-predominant disease and high exercise tolerance also showed improved exercise capacity and an improved health-related quality of life but no survival advantage (choice D is incorrect). On the basis of this study, lung-volume-reduction surgery could be recommended for patients with upper-lobe-predominant emphysema and low exercise capacity and considered a palliative measure in patients with upper-lobe-predominant disease and high exercise tolerance. The procedure is not recommended for patients with non-upper-lobe-predominant emphysema, who have poor outcomes after surgery (choices B and C are incorrect).

Fishman A, Martinez F, Neunheim KS, et al. A randomized trial comparing lung-volume-reduction surgery with medical therapy for severe emphysema: the National Emphysema Treatment Trial Research Group. N Engl J Med 2003; 348:2059–2073

Naunheim KS, Wood DE, Mohsenifar Z, et al. Long-term follow-up of patients receiving lung-volume-reduction surgery vs medical therapy for severe emphysema by the National Emphysema Treatment Trial Research Group. Ann Thorac Surg 2006; 82:431–443

186. A. It is more accurate than mediastinoscopy in the diagnosis of lung cancer in subcarinal, posterior, and inferior mediastinal lymph nodes.

Histologic and microbiological sampling of the mediastinum is essential to properly stage lung cancer and make a diagnosis of infectious and neoplastic diseases that involve mediastinal structures. EBUS-TBNA allows access to most (but not all) mediastinal lymph node stations and is more likely than mediastinoscopy to yield diagnostic tissue samples in the subcarinal, posterior, and inferior mediastinal lymph node stations (choice A is correct). The mediastinoscope can reach these areas only with difficulty, if at all. In a prospective crossover trial comparing EBUS-TBNA with mediastinal lymph node dissection by cervical mediastinoscopy in the diagnosis of lung cancer, EBUS-TBNA had a higher diagnostic yield for these lymph node stations (91% vs 78%), with superior sensitivity and specificity and negative predictive value.

Endoscopic ultrasound (EUS) was first used by gastroenterologists for assessment and biopsy of structures outside the esophagus; EBUS uses an ultrasound probe passed through the bronchoscope to image and sample structures beyond the wall of the bronchus with real-time visualization. The two methods are, in fact, complimentary: EUS can effectively image and sample paraaortic and subaortic lymph nodes, whereas EBUS cannot (choice B is incorrect). Indeed, preliminary data show that combined EBUS and EUS procedures may be as (or more) accurate than mediastinoscopy in staging the mediastinum, and clinical trials to evaluate this hypothesis are in progress.

In addition to diagnosis of mediastinal disease, EBUS has been shown to increase the sensitivity of bronchoscopy in the diagnosis of solitary pulmonary nodules because imaging and real-time guided sampling are more accurate than older fluoroscopic methods. It also enhances the diagnostic yield of bronchoscopy and may replace mediastinoscopy in the diagnosis of other disorders, including lymphoma and sarcoidosis (choices C and D are incorrect).

Wallace MB, Pascual JMS, Raimondo, et al. Minimally invasive endoscopic staging of suspected lung cancer. JAMA 2008; 299:540–546

Ernst A, Anantham D, Eberhardt R, et al. Diagnosis of mediastinal adenopathy: real-time endobronchial ultrasound guided needle aspiration versus mediastinoscopy. J Thorac Oncol 2008; 3:577–582

Schulman L, Ost D. Advances in bronchoscopic diagnosis of lung cancer. Curr Opin Pulm Med 2007; 3:271–277
Kennedy MP, Jimenez CA, Bruzzi JF, et al. Endobronchial ultrasound-guided transbronchial needle aspiration in the diagnosis of lymphoma. Thorax 2008; 3:360–365
Garwood S, Judson MA, Silvestri G, et al. Endobronchial ultrasound for the diagnosis of pulmonary sarcoidosis. Chest 2007; 32:1298–1304

187. C. Dermatomyositis-associated interstitial lung disease (ILD).

The chest radiograph demonstrates bilateral lower lobe interstitial infiltrates that are confirmed by the CT scan. The biopsy results show an intraalveolar process with a proliferation of macrophages and fibroblasts, along with small amounts of fibrin, and some early collagen formation. There is no evidence of vasculitis or granuloma formation. The appearance is that of cryptogenic organizing pneumonia. Organizing pneumonia has been described with a variety of collagen vascular diseases affecting the lung, including rheumatoid arthritis and dermatomyositis-associated interstitial lung disease. In this case, the clinical clues identifying dermatomyositis-associated ILD as the correct diagnosis include the subungual telangiectasias, periorbital heliotrope rash, and the elevated creatine kinase level (choice C is correct). A negative anti-Jo-1 antibody is found in the majority of documented cases. Other antibody tests that suggest this disorder may be available in specialized centers. Although the patient has an inflammatory polyarthritis, there is no serologic evidence to support the diagnosis of rheumatoid arthritis (choice A is incorrect). The biopsy results are not consistent with IPF (choice D is incorrect), and there is no clinical or biopsy evidence for Pneumocystis infection (choice C is incorrect).

ILD has been reported to occur in 5 to 46% of patients with polymyositis (PM) and dermatomyositis (DM), depending on the criteria for diagnosis, and is a common cause of morbidity and mortality in these patients. Initial presentation is most commonly either musculoskeletal (arthralgias, myalgias, and weakness) or pulmonary (cough, dyspnea, and fever) symptoms alone. Pulmonary disease usually takes the form of acute to subacute antibiotic-resistant community-acquired pneumonia or aspiration pneumonia. The prognosis seems to differ between patients with different patterns of disease pathology. The histopathologic features of PM/DM include usual interstitial pneumonia (UIP), diffuse alveolar damage (DAD), bronchiolitis obliterans organizing pneumonia (BOOP), and cellular interstitial pneumonia. Patients with a histologic diagnosis of BOOP have a more favorable prognosis than do those with UIP, and patients with DAD generally have a poor prognosis. Treatment usually includes prednisone for initial control, followed by lower dose prednisone plus an immunosuppressive agent such as azathioprine or methotrexate for disease suppression. Survival is better than that observed for historical control subjects with idiopathic UIP and is more consistent with survival reported in idiopathic nonspecific interstitial pneumonia (NSIP). There is no difference in survival between Jo-1–positive and Jo-1–negative groups. In rheumatoid arthritis, unlike most other connective tissue diseases, the UIP pattern is more commonly seen on surgical lung biopsy than NSIP.

Douglas WW, Tazelaar HD, Hartman TE, et al. Polymyositis-dermatomyositis-associated interstitial lung disease. Am J Respir Crit Care Med 2001; 164:1182–1185
Arakawa H, Yamada H, Kurihara Y, et al. Nonspecific interstitial pneumonia associated with polymyositis and dermatomyositis: serial high-resolution CT findings and functional correlation. Chest 2003; 123:1096–1103

188. C. Advise him to be relocated to a cleaner area on a trial basis and add a long-acting β-agonist.

The patient has a history to suggest work-related asthma. He had childhood asthma and may have had continuing mild airway hyperresponsiveness with resulting asthma symptoms exacerbated by exposure to workplace airway irritants such as smoke and dust at work (work-exacerbated asthma/work-aggravated asthma). Alternatively, he could have occupational asthma from specific sensitization to mold on the logs or a specific wood dust that may have caused the recurrence of his asthma. He currently has poorly controlled asthma and requires optimization of asthma medications and asthma education, but he also needs to be investigated to determine whether he has occupational asthma (which would likely require a job change and compensation claim) or work-exacerbated asthma (which may be

controlled with a reduction in dust and smoke exposure at work and improved asthma management). Allergy testing may be helpful to identify a specific allergic response, for example, to a mold on the wood. Monitoring of serial peak flows (with recordings of symptoms and medications) and serial methacholine challenge tests can document the work-related changes. Peak flow changes may be suppressed if symptoms are completely controlled by increased medications, so the aim is to control asthma but not completely prevent symptoms during the testing period.

The best opportunity for diagnostic testing is while the patient is still working, and, therefore, he should not be advised to quit work until a diagnosis has been made. However, an initial trial transfer to a cleaner area at work and enhancing his therapy by the addition of a long-acting β-agonist may be sufficient to improve asthma control (choice C is correct). Monitoring of serial peak flow reading during that time followed by repeat recordings during a short trial in the initial work area would allow objective assessment of the work effects on his asthma. If feasible, a methacholine challenge toward the end of a period out of the usual area and another methacholine challenge at the end of a work week in the initial area would provide additional diagnostic assistance.

He should not leave work at this time because a diagnosis of work-related asthma is difficult once a patient has left work and may cause difficulty with a fair decision on any compensation claim he may later initiate (choice A is incorrect). He could be initially investigated in his current work area and then have a trial off work or in a cleaner area, but, because his asthma is poorly controlled, it would be safer to have a temporary relocation with the understanding that he can return again to the initial area on a trial basis once his asthma is controlled (choice B is incorrect). Although dust control at home may be part of the general management of his asthma, ignoring or failing to recognize the work contribution to asthma and failing to intervene with appropriate exposure changes as needed, is associated with increased morbidity (choice D is incorrect). In particular, ongoing exposure to a relevant work sensitizer is associated with ongoing asthma that may worsen over time and, after prolonged ongoing exposure, is likely to be associated with a failure to improve even after eventually leaving the exposure. Prognosis is best with early removal from exposure after confirming the diagnosis.

Fishwick D, Bradshaw LM, Henson M, et al. Occupational asthma: an assessment of diagnostic agreement between physicians. Occup Environ Med 2007; 64:185–190

Chan-Yeung M. Assessment of asthma in the workplace: American College of Chest Physicians consensus statement. Chest 1995; 108:1084–1117

Tarlo SM, Liss GM. Occupational asthma: an approach to diagnosis and management. Can Med Assoc J 2003; 168:867–871

Goe SK, Henneberger PK, Reilly MJ, et al. A descriptive study of work aggravated asthma. Occup Environ Med 2004; 61:512–517

Tarlo SM, Balmes J, Balkissoon R, et al. Diagnosis and management of work-related asthma: American College of Chest Physicians consensus statement. Chest 2008; 134(suppl):1S–41S

189. A. Not known to undergo malignant transformation.

The chest radiograph shows bilateral pleural plaques seen as irregular vague opacities; close scrutiny reveals calcification of the left hemi-diaphragm. The two CT scan images (see Figures 189-B and 189-C) show pleural plaques with calcification including diaphragm-based plaques bilaterally. All of these findings are compatible with pleural plaques because of the patient's history of asbestos exposure. As with mesothelioma, plaques may be associated with minimal asbestos exposure. Consequently, plaques, although having never been demonstrated to undergo malignant transformation, are associated with an increased risk of developing mesothelioma (choice A is correct). Pleural plaques are commonly associated with asbestos exposure (choice C is incorrect). Plaques develop slowly after asbestos exposure, with only 10% of exposed individuals having plaques 20 years after initial exposure, and > 50% after 40 years. Calcification, which makes plaques more readily visible on plain chest radiographs, rarely occurs before the first 20 years after asbestos exposure (choice D is incorrect). Pleural plaques are frequently bilateral and often symmetrically distributed, but with peripheral border irregularities, as seen in this patient's chest radiograph. The plaques involve the parietal pleura, thought to be related to their pathogenesis because of clearance of asbestos fibers by the lymphatic stomata found only on the parietal pleura. Most commonly, plaques are discrete raised gray-white to cream-colored

lesions separated by normal parietal pleural surfaces and found on the posterior wall of the chest and lower half of the pleural space including the hemi-diaphragms. The chest apices are generally spared.

Controversy exists as to whether pleural plaques cause symptoms or pulmonary function abnormalities. Causing this ambiguity is the confounding factor of potentially associated asbestosis (lung fibrosis from asbestos exposure). A commonly reported lung function abnormality in patients with pleural plaques is a decreased FVC. However, in a CT study of patients wherein asbestos-related changes were not present, no lung function abnormalities were found related to plaques. Generally, no pulmonary symptoms are clearly attributed to the presence of plaques.

Although pleural plaques are considered a marker of asbestos exposure, with asbestos the most likely cause of the majority of plaques, other factors may be associated with pleural plaques (choice B is incorrect). Several medical conditions including empyema, TB, rib fractures, and hemothorax have been reported to be associated with plaques. Various other occupational exposures have also been associated with pleural plaques, including vitreous fibers that include glass wool, glass filaments, rock and slag wool, and refractory ceramic fibers. Similarly, erionite, mica, and kaolin (china clay) exposures have been reported to be associated with pleural plaques.

Clarke CC, Mowat FS, Kelsch MA, et al. Pleural plaques: a review of diagnostic issues and possible nonasbestos factors. Arch Environ Occup Health 2006; 61:183–192

Cleemput JV, De Raeve H, Verschakelen JA, et al. Surface localized pleural plaques quantitated by computed tomography scanning: no relation with cumulative asbestos exposure and no effect on lung function. Am J Respir Crit Care Med 2001; 163:705–710

Hosoda Y, Hiraga Y, Sasagawa S. Railways and asbestos in Japan (1928–1987): epidemiology of pleural plaques, malignancies and pneumoconioses. J Occup Health 2008; 50:297–307

190. D. Further testing is not necessary.

Lung cancer typically manifests symptoms only after the disease has spread, making a cure unlikely. A screening technique that could detect lung cancer before it has spread might be helpful to decrease the mortality associated with the disease. No screening modality has been shown to alter the mortality outcomes to date (choice D is correct).

The risks of low-dose CT are observable, but the impact on mortality is unknown for patients who have no history of lung cancer. There are conflicting data regarding its use in this setting. Several randomized trials are currently underway in an attempt to address this topic. Therefore, low-dose CT should not be used to screen for lung cancer except in the context of a well-designed clinical trial (choice C is incorrect).

Sputum cytologic examination, primarily in the context of a supplement to a chest radiograph, was evaluated in the 1970s and 1980s. These trials were often underpowered and seldom concentrated on sputum cytologic studies alone. It appears to detect only a minority of all lung cancers. No mortality benefits were noted, and thus the discrete efficacy of sputum cytologic examination is unclear. The use of either single or serial sputum cytologies is not recommended to screen for the presence of lung cancer (choice B is incorrect). Chest radiographic screening every 4 or 6 months in combination with sputum cytologic examination has also been assessed in several randomized controlled trials. The power of these studies was limited, and in none was the control arm a "no-screening" intervention. Lung cancer screening using only chest radiographs has been evaluated in both randomized and observational studies, and although the identification rate was higher in the screened group, the mortality rate was similar in both groups (choice A is incorrect). Thus, neither obtaining chest radiographs nor sputum cytologic findings appear to prolong the life expectancy of an individual with the disease.

Bach PB, Silvestri GA, Hanger M, et al. Screening for lung cancer: American College of Chest Physicians evidence-based clinical practice guidelines, 2nd Edition. Chest 2007; 182(suppl):69S–77S

Bach PB, Kelley MG, Tate RC, et al. Screening for lung cancer: a review of the current literature. Chest 2003; 123(suppl):72S–82S

Patz EF, Goodman PC, Bepler G. Screening for lung cancer. N Engl J Med 2000; 343:1627–1633

191. D. Desquamative interstitial pneumonia (DIP).

DIP is a rare interstitial lung disease (ILD) characterized by a homogenous accumulation of pigment-laden macrophages within the alveolar spaces, as is present in this patient and is identified by the arrows in the image from her surgical lung biopsy (see Figure 191-E). Radiographically, this inflammatory process results in peripheral, basilar-predominant ground-glass opacities in 70% of patients. In 25 to 50% of patients, parenchymal cysts are present within the areas of ground-glass opacities and are identified in the patient's high-resolution CT of the chest (see Figure 191-F, arrows). Although similar accumulations of pigment-laden macrophages may be seen in respiratory bronchiolitis (RB), the spatial distribution is different. In RB-ILD, the pigment-laden macrophages are predominantly located adjacent to the bronchioles rather than accumulating with the alveoli. In contrast to pulmonary Langerhans histiocytosis, the cysts in DIP are within areas of ground-glass opacities. In PLH, the cystic structures are associated with nodules rather than ground glass (choice C is incorrect). The radiographic abnormalities in chronic obstructive lung disease are diverse but do not include ground-glass opacities with cysts. Pigmented macrophages are commonly present in patients who smoke and have COPD. In contrast to DIP, focal accumulation does not occur in COPD. In patients who have diffuse pulmonary hemorrhage, >90% have personal or immediate second-hand exposure to tobacco smoke, making it a tobacco-associated lung disease. In those patients, the lavage from bronchoscopy would be progressively hemorrhagic. The lavagate from our patient is caramel-brown from an accumulation of pigmented macrophages, characteristically seen in DIP (choice B is incorrect).

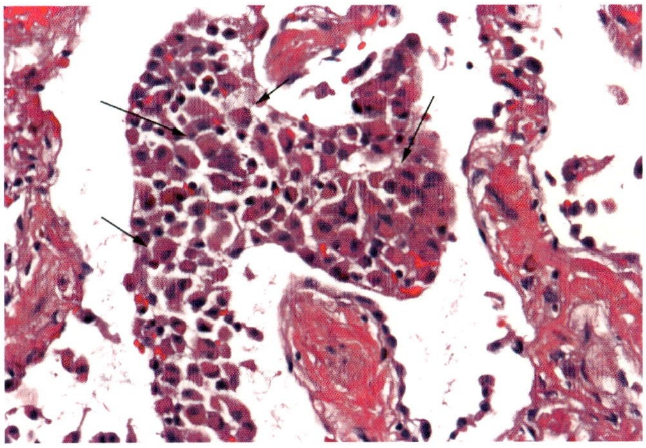

Figure 191-E
Hematoxylin-eosin

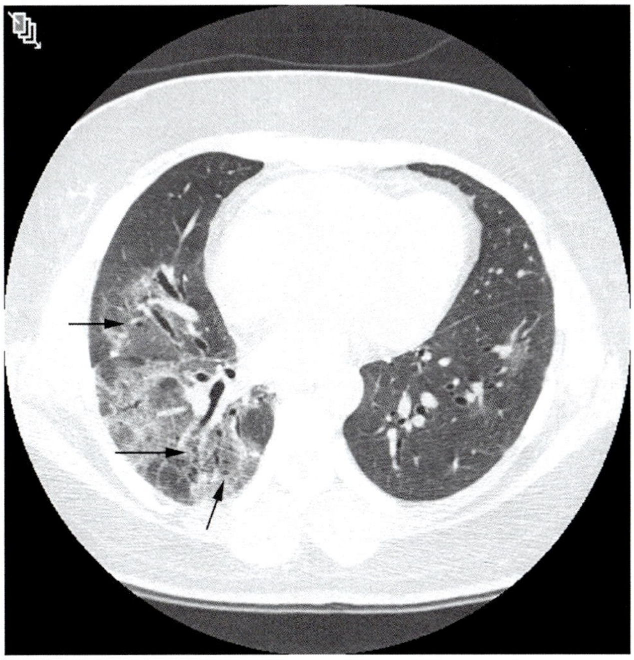

Figure 191-F

Ryu JH, Myers JL, Capizzi SA, et al. Desquamative interstitial pneumonia and respiratory bronchiolitis-associated interstitial lung disease. Chest 2005; 127:178–184

Davies G, Wells AU, du Bois RM. Respiratory bronchiolitis associated with interstitial lung disease and desquamative interstitial pneumonia. Clin Chest Med 2004; 25:717–726

Craig PJ, Wells AU, Doffman S, et al. Desquamative interstitial pneumonia, respiratory bronchiolitis and their relationship to smoking. Histopathology 2004; 45:275–282

192. B. Detection of antigen in BAL fluid is at least as sensitive as urinary antigen for identifying active infection.

In a number of studies comparing the detection of histoplasmosis antigen in urine and BAL fluid, the sensitivity in specimens collected directly by lung lavage were as good or better than urine-based assays (choice B is correct).

Histoplasmosis antigen radioimmunoassay was developed in the mid-1980s and modified several times to prevent false-positivity and improve performance. The assay has also been modified to permit quantification of antigen levels. Sensitivity of the assay in AIDS patients with progressive disseminated histoplasmosis (PDH) is not compromised, and in several studies, the sensitivity of urinary and serum antigen assay was $>90\%$ (choice D is incorrect). The sensitivity of these assays appears to be somewhat less, approximately 80%, in patients who have PDH but no identifiable immunosuppressed state. For active fungal infection, sensitivity seems lowest (approximately 30 to 40%) for patients with acute localized pulmonary histoplasmosis, a fairly rare process outside of conditions of disease outbreak.

Serologic testing assessing antibody responses to active histoplasmosis infection can be quite helpful, particularly for localized pulmonary disease. Methods employed include complement fixation, immunodiffusion, and enzyme immunoassay. The seropositivity of healthy subjects in the general population, even in endemic areas, is $<5\%$, making a positive assay significant for newly acquired infection (choice A is incorrect). Four to 6 weeks are required to mount a response; therefore, testing earlier than this significantly impairs the sensitivity of this test (choice C is incorrect).

The antibody response appears proportional to exposure to the infecting organisms and the severity of illness. In one study, significant antibody levels were positive in 18% of asymptomatic infections, 67% of mild infections, 86% of moderate infections, and 100% of severe infections requiring hospital admission. This makes the test useful to guide therapy in the most severely ill patients pending additional confirmatory tests if deemed necessary.

Cross reactions with other fungi complicate the interpretation of both antigen and antibody assays—particularly coccidiomycosis and blastomycosis. Thus, results should be interpreted in epidemiologic and clinical contexts to provide the best information for diagnosis.

Hage CA, Wheat LJ, Loyd J, et al. Pulmonary histoplasmosis. Semin Respir Crit Care Med 2008; 29:151–165
Wheat LJ. Current diagnosis of histoplasmosis. Trends Microbiol 2003; 11:488–494

193. A. *PHOX2B.*

Mutations in the *PHOX2B* gene have been described in patients with congenital central hypoventilation syndrome (CCHS) and associated autonomic dysfunction (choice A is correct). A majority of mutations involve five to nine alanine expansions within a 20-residue polyalanine tract (exon 3), with repeat mutation length correlating with severity of the CCHS phenotype.

A serine-to-glycine mutation in the CKIε-binding region of hPer2 (human Period 2) localized near the telomere of chromosome 2q is responsible for an autosomal dominant variant of familial advanced sleep-phase disorder. This mutation causes hypophosphorylation of the hPer2 protein by CKIε and results in shortening of the transcription-translation feedback loop cycle duration and phase advancement of the major sleep period (choice B is incorrect).

Fatal familial insomnia arises as an autosomal dominant single-point mutation at codon 178 of the prion protein gene on chromosome 20. Severity of the disease is influenced by codon 129, which can either be methionine homozygous (more severe disease) or methionine-valine heterozygous (milder disease; choice D is incorrect).

Type 2 hypocretin/orexin receptor gene mutation, transmitted in an autosomal recessive mode, has been demonstrated in canine models of narcolepsy. Other genetic variants of the narcolepsy phenotype include knockout mice for the precursor ligand for the hypocretin receptor and hypocretin ataxin-3 transgenic mice. A pre-prohypocretin gene mutation is responsible for a human case of early-onset narcolepsy (choice C is incorrect).

In CCHS, a dysfunction of central ventilatory responsiveness to hypoxia and hypercapnia gives rise to hypoventilation. This is a rare disorder with onset of symptoms, including apneic episodes, shallow breathing, cyanosis, and feeding difficulties, during the neonatal period. Hypoventilation is typically more severe during sleep, particularly in nonrapid eye movement sleep. Other features include tumors of neural crest derivatives (*eg*, ganglioneuromas and neuroblastomas), Hirschsprung disease, strabismus, growth impairment, hypotension, and arrhythmias.

Cognitive function is typically unaffected. Affected individuals require ventilatory support, either provided only during sleep or, in more severe disease, continuously. The course is chronic, with death usually due to respiratory failure or cor pulmonale.

Amiel J, Laudier B, Attié-Bitach T, et al. Polyalanine expansion and frameshift mutations of the paired-like homeobox gene *PHOX2B* in congenital central hypoventilation syndrome. Nat Genet 2003; 33:459–461

Medori R, Tritschler HJ, LeBlanc A, et al. Fatal familial insomnia, a prion disease with a mutation at codon 178 of the prion protein gene. N Engl J Med 1992; 326:444–449

Taheri S, Mignot E. The genetics of sleep disorders. Lancet Neurol 2002; 1:242–250

194. D. Rapamycin (sirolimus) may be therapeutic.

This patient has findings consistent with lymphangioleiomyomatosis (LAM). The chest CT shows irregular, thin-walled cysts (see Figure 194-A), and the abdominal CT shows a mass on the right kidney consistent with an angiomyolipoma (see Figure 194-B). Recently, sirolimus has been shown to effectively decrease the size of angiomyolipomas and also showed beneficial effect on pulmonary function in patients with LAM (choice D is correct).

LAM is a rare disease developing almost exclusively in women of reproductive age, with a prevalence of 1 to 2 per million people. The mean age at diagnosis is 36 years. The pathologic findings are characterized by atypical smooth muscle proliferation of the bronchioles, parenchyma, interstitium, vasculature, and lymphatics. Tissue in these patients stains positive for HMB-45 (a melanocytic marker) but not S-100, which is positive in eosinophilic granuloma (choice A is incorrect). The pathogenesis is thought to be a sporadic mutation in 85% of cases. Similar findings can be found in the disease tuberous sclerosis, which is an autosomal dominant disease characterized by seizures, brain tumors, cognitive impairment, sebaceous adenomas, angiomyolipomas, and pulmonary LAM in 1 to 25% of cases.

Clinical findings in LAM include progressive dyspnea, cough, and hemoptysis, often for 3 to 5 years before presentation. On examination, patients have crackles and decreased breath sounds and may have ascites and abdominal masses. Chest imaging shows diffuse thin-walled cyst formation (as seen on this chest CT), without nodules (as would be seen in eosinophilic granuloma) or fibrosis. Pneumothoraces, effusions, and hyperinflation may be present. Pulmonary function testing can show mixed restriction and/or obstruction or can be normal in one-third of patients. Effusions develop in one-third of patients with LAM and can be recurrent. They are chylous, defined by a high triglyceride (not cholesterol level; choice B is incorrect). Spontaneous, recurrent pneumothoraces can develop in 60 to 70% of patients. Nearly half of patients with LAM also have angiomyolipomas, tumors of the kidney that consist of blood vessels, muscle, and fat. These tumors can be large in size and often require surgical removal. Embolization of the tumor is often performed prior to surgical removal.

The diagnosis of LAM can be made by a compatible clinical course, classic high-resolution CT findings, and tissue biopsy for HMB-45.

The course of LAM is usually indolent but progressive, with a 10-year survival of 20 to 80%. The cause of death is respiratory failure. Treatment has included oophorectomy, medroxyprogesterone acetate, bronchodilators, and octreotide for recurrent effusions. Recently, sirolimus, which acts by suppressing smooth muscle proliferation and DNA synthesis of LAM cells *in vitro,* inactivating the mammalian target of rapamycin, has been used.

In studies, angiomyolipomas regressed during therapy (50% reduction in volume), but the size increased following discontinuation. A secondary outcome showed improved spirometric results (5 to 10% increase in FEV_1 and FVC). Patients are counseled to avoid estrogens or pregnancy. Lung transplantation has been successfully performed for LAM, with a 65% 5-year survival, but LAM is well documented to recur following lung transplantation (choice C is incorrect).

Bissler JJ, McCormack FX, Young LR, et al. Sirolimus for angiomyolipoma in tuberous sclerosis complex or lymphangioleiomyomatosis. N Engl J Med 2008; 358:40–151

McCormack FX. Lymphangioleiomyomatosis: a clinical update. Chest 2008; 133:507–516

Ryu JH, Moss J, Beck GJ, et al. The NHLBI Lymphangioleiomyomatosis Registry: characteristics of 230 patients at enrollment. Am J Respir Crit Care Med 2006; 173:105–111

Johnson SR. Lymphangioleiomyomatosis. Eur Respir J 2006; 27:1056–1065

Maurer JR, Ryu J, Beck G, et al. Lung transplantation in the management of patients with lymphangioleiomyomatosis: baseline data from the NHLBI LAM Registry. Heart Lung Transplant 2007; 26:1293–1299

Kpodonu J, Massad MG, Chaer RA, et al. The US experience with lung transplantation for pulmonary lymphangioleiomyomatosis. J Heart Lung Transplant 2005; 24:1247–1253

195. A. Conservative fluids, monitoring devices equivalent.

Patients with acute lung injury (ALI) and ARDS have noncardiogenic pulmonary edema as a hallmark of their disease process. IV fluid management in these patients thus poses important challenges. On the one hand, IV fluids are critical to maintain appropriate intravascular volume to ensure hemodynamic stability and vital organ perfusion in patients who have compromised gas exchange. On the other hand, excessive fluid administration can worsen the lung edema, further impairing gas exchange.

An associated challenge in managing fluids in patients with ALI/ARDS is the proper way to monitor fluid status. Some believe that a PAC with the ability to measure pulmonary vascular pressures (especially the pulmonary artery occlusion [PAOP] or "wedge" pressure) and cardiac output is required. Others argue that the PAC carries a significant mortality risk and that fluids can be properly managed with a CVC to measure central venous pressures (CVP) in conjunction with careful physical examinations.

Available data were inconclusive in supporting either a fluid-liberal or a fluid-conservative approach and are also inconclusive regarding the clinical value and risks of a PAC vs a CVC in ALI/ARDS, so the NIH ARDS Network launched the FACTT (Fluid and Catheter Therapy Trial) study. FACTT recruited 1,000 patients with ALI/ARDS and randomized them to one of four treatment strategies for 7 days:

1. Fluid conservative/CVC: Fluids were restricted, and diuretics were administered to maintain a CVP < 4 mm Hg.
2. Fluid conservative/PAC: Fluids were restricted, and diuretics were administered to maintain a PAOP < 8 mm Hg.
3. Fluid liberal/CVC: Fluids were used to maintain CVP between 10 and 14 mm Hg.
4. Fluid liberal/PAC: Fluids were used to maintain PAOP between 14 and 18 mm Hg.

Importantly, if patients were in shock, the fluid management rules were suspended, and clinicians were free to use fluids and pressors as needed.

The results showed no differences in important outcomes in patients with PAC monitoring vs patients with CVC monitoring, so the routine use of PAC monitoring is not needed (choices B and D are incorrect). Catheter use had no influence on results, so the data from the patients monitored by CVC and PVC in both fluid categories were combined.

Not surprisingly, the conservative fluid strategy required more than twice as much diuretic administration as the liberal fluid strategy and resulted in a nearly even fluid balance over the 7 study days in the conservative group vs a positive fluid balance of almost 1 L/day with the liberal fluid strategy. Although mortality was not affected by fluid strategy, the conservative strategy was associated with significant improvement in lung function and a significant increase in the number of ventilator-free days (14.6 ± 0.5 vs 12.1 ± 0.5; p = 0.0002) and ICU-free days (13.4 ± 0.4 vs 11.2 ± 0.4; p = 0.0003) to 28 days. Therefore, Choice A is correct and choice C is incorrect. Importantly, the conservative fluid approach in this trial was not associated with any adverse renal or cardiovascular effects.

Connors AF Jr, Speroff T, Dawson NV, et al. The effectiveness of right heart catheterization in the initial care of critically ill patients. JAMA 1996; 276:889–897
Matthay MA, Broaddus VC. Fluid and hemodynamic management in acute lung injury. Semin Respir Crit Care Med 1994; 15:271–288
Humphrey H, Hall J, Sznajder I, et al. Improved survival in ARDS patients associated with a reduction in pulmonary capillary wedge pressure. Chest 1990; 97:1176–1180
NIH ARDS Network. Comparison of two fluid-management strategies in acute lung injury. New Engl J Med 2006; 354:2564–2575
NIH ARDS Network. Pulmonary-artery versus central venous catheter to guide treatment of acute lung injury. New Engl J Med 2006; 354:2213–2224

196. C. Pulmonary edema secondary to terbutaline.

Approximately 0.3% of women treated with IV β-agonists to inhibit preterm labor develop tocolytic-induced pulmonary edema (choice C is correct). The pathophysiology of this complication is unclear, and a variety of contributors have been proposed, including decreased diastolic filling due to tachycardia, volume expansion due to stimulation of antidiuretic hormone release, and increased pulmonary capillary permeability. Treatment is supportive, with supplemental oxygen, diuretics, and discontinuation of the β-agonist comprising the mainstays of therapy. This complication may be less frequent in the future because magnesium sulfate is now used more commonly than β-agonist tocolytics.

Patients with amniotic fluid embolism generally have respiratory failure that is accompanied by circulatory collapse and disseminated intravascular coagulation, none of which was present in this patient (choice A is incorrect). Peripartum cardiomyopathy is unlikely because of the patient's acute onset of symptoms and the absence of jugular venous distension or significant lower extremity edema (choice B is incorrect). Pregnant women are clearly at increased risk for pulmonary embolism compared with the general population, particularly during the third trimester and the postpartum period, but the physical examination and radiographic findings of pulmonary edema would not be present if pulmonary embolism were the cause of her deterioration (choice D is incorrect).

Karetzky M, Ramirez M. Acute respiratory failure in pregnancy: an analysis of 19 cases. Medicine 1998; 77:41–49
Lamont RF. The pathophysiology of pulmonary oedema with the use of beta-agonists. Br J Obstet Gynaecol 2000; 107:439–444
Sciscione AC, Ivester T, Largoza M, et al. Acute pulmonary edema in pregnancy. Obstet Gynecol 2003; 101:511–515

197. A. They are free from artifacts, they have good starts, and they show satisfactory exhalation.

Spirometric quality is described by acceptability and reproducibility. Acceptability criteria are met if efforts are free from artifacts (cough, glottis closure, early termination, submaximal effort, leak, or obstructed mouthpiece), they have good starts (extrapolated volume is < 5% of the FVC or 0.15 L, whichever is greater), and they show satisfactory exhalation (duration of > 6 s or a plateau in the curve is noted; choice A is correct).

Spirometry testing requires appropriate equipment, calibration, testing procedures, assessment of within-maneuver acceptability, assessment of between-maneuver repeatability, interpretation, and integration with the patient's clinical presentation. Inherent in optimal quality control is the acceptability of each individual spirogram, as well as the

repeatability of a number of acceptable spirograms, recognizing that an adequate test requires at least three acceptable maneuvers. Repeatability criteria are only applied after the acceptability of individual spirograms has been met. The two largest values (from three acceptable individual spirograms) for both the FEV_1 and FVC must be within 0.15 L of each other in order to achieve repeatability criteria (choice B is incorrect). If FEV_1 and FVC repeatability criteria are not achieved, testing may be terminated after a total of eight acceptable individual maneuvers have been performed or if the patient cannot or should not continue. Both of these last criteria reflect repeatability and not individual acceptability criteria (choices C and D are incorrect).

Miller MR, Hankinson J, Brusasco V, et al. Standardisation of spirometry. Series: ATS/ERS Task Force: standardisation of lung function testing. Eur Resp J 2005; 26:319–338

Aaron SD, Vandemheen KL, Boulet L-P, et al. Overdiagnosis of asthma in obese and nonobese adults. Can Med Assoc J 2008; 179:1121–1131

198. B. Cohort study.

The hierarchy of levels of scientific evidence is based on causation and bias. The highest level of evidence is the RCT. Systematic review with metaanalysis (the synthesis of more than one RCT), when many high-quality RCTs exist, is also considered to be a high level of evidence (especially when several of the primary studies reveal consistent findings). These are followed by cohort studies, case-control studies, and case reports. Although each level may increase our understanding of diseases or disease processes, the actual hypothesis can often define the appropriate study design. Questions about causation generally require cohort studies (choice B is correct). In a cohort study, two groups are chosen based on their differences in exposure to a particular agent, such as tobacco products. The follow-up period is often measured in years because many of the conditions in question (such as cancer) take years to develop. After enough incident cases, statistical analyses can determine the relationship between the exposure (tobacco) and the disease (lung cancer).

In a case-control study, patients with the identified disease (*ie,* lung cancer) are matched with patients without the disease. Data are then collected on past exposures (such as tobacco use) to identify a possible causal agent. Although this design is useful for very rare diseases, the study design is not able to prove causality. These studies can only show an association (and the association of tobacco with lung cancer does not necessarily prove that tobacco causes lung cancer) and are, thus, scientifically inferior to cohort studies (choice C is incorrect). Case-control studies, because they are typically easy, quick, and inexpensive, are commonly used as a first step in testing a hypothetical association prior to undertaking a lengthier and more costly cohort study.

Although RCTs are felt to be one of the strongest methodologic designs, they usually involve people who already have the disease, not people who may or may not develop the disease (choice A is incorrect). In an RCT, participants are randomly allocated by a process equivalent to the flip of a coin to either an intervention (treatment) or placebo arm. The groups are then followed-up for a specified period of time for the occurrence of predetermined outcomes. The randomization process theoretically creates groups that are identical at the start of the study, so any differences in outcome are generally attributed to the intervention. Advantages of RCTs are that they allow evaluation of a single variable and for prospective collection of data. Disadvantages include time, cost, the number of patients available, and flaws in the randomization process. Hypothetically, patients without lung cancer could be randomized to smoke or not to smoke. However, given the ethical issues surrounding such a study and the time it would take to develop lung cancer, the study would clearly not be feasible.

Case reports, or case reports run together to form a series, lack any form of control. They are typically used to describe adverse drug reactions or an uncommon or new presentation of a condition. Although they may suggest a new association, they certainly do not have the power to prove causality (choice D is incorrect).

Greenhalgh T. How to read a paper: getting your bearings (deciding what the paper is about). Br Med J 1997; 315: 243–246

Laupacis A, Wells G, Richardson WS. User's guide to the medical literature, V: how to use an article about prognosis. JAMA 1994; 272:234–237

199. D. Coccidiomycosis.

This patient has traveled extensively in areas endemic for dimorphic fungi, including Tennessee and Alabama (blastomycosis), Iowa (histoplasmosis), and Arizona and California (coccidiomycosis). Travel to an endemic region and the lack of ability to respond to antibiotics is usually the first clue that an infection with one of the dimorphic fungi may be present. Her peripheral eosinophilia and the lung biopsy results showing the spherules associated with coccidiomycosis confirm the diagnosis (choice D is correct).

Pulmonary eosinophilia is a heterogeneous group of disorders that meet one or more of the following criteria: (1) peripheral blood eosinophilia with pulmonary abnormalities on radiographs; (2) eosinophilia in lung tissue from a transbronchial or open lung biopsy; and (3) increased eosinophils in BAL fluid. The causes of pulmonary eosinophilia are broad and include helminthic infections, medications, acute or chronic eosinophilic pneumonia, Churg-Strauss syndrome, allergic bronchopulmonary aspergillosis, and nonhelminthic infections. Coccidiomycosis is one of a few nonhelminthic infections that causes a pulmonary eosinophilia. The initiation of steroids would have led to improvement with medication-related eosinophilic lung disease, acute or chronic eosinophilic pneumonia, Churg-Strauss vasculitis, or allergic bronchopulmonary aspergillosis. The patient's symptoms worsened when starting corticosteroids, so an infectious etiology should be considered. Given her travel in the United States and her poor response to antibiotics, dimorphic fungal infections are very likely.

When symptomatic, coccidioidomycosis manifests itself as a community-acquired pneumonia (many patients are asymptomatic, as well). Most cases of coccidiomycosis are self-limited, but a minority of patients develop disseminated disease to skin, bone, meninges, and other organs. Individuals of Asian (Korean, Filipino, and Japanese) and African-American heritage are at increased risk of dissemination. Diagnosis is by tissue pathologic examination, which shows large spherules, or culture findings from the sputum, as in this case. All laboratory samples of suspected or confirmed cases of coccidiomycosis must be handled under special hoods because of the likelihood of transmission to laboratory workers. Treatment is with fluconazole for mild pulmonary or disseminated disease. For severe cases or cases with meningeal involvement, amphotericin (lipid preparation) is used.

More than 50% of patients with blastomycosis are asymptomatic. The remainder will first develop pulmonary disease with an associated dermatitis. Pulmonary disease is frequently cavitary, and there is no association with eosinophilia (choice A is incorrect). In 25% of cases, dissemination occurs and the disease becomes chronic. Diagnosis is by identification of the thickened budding yeast in the tissue. The treatment of choice is amphotericin in severe cases or itraconazole for more mild or limited disease. Histoplasmosis enters through the pulmonary system, and >95% of individuals remain asymptomatic. Disease syndromes include acute and chronic pneumonia, cavitary pneumonia, fibrosing mediastinitis, and acute and chronic disseminated disease. Histoplasmosis does not cause eosinophilia (choice B is incorrect). Diagnosis is with an antigen assay or identification of the very small organisms in tissue samples. The treatment of choice is amphotericin for severe disseminated cases or itraconazole for milder cases. Sporotrichosis causes cutaneous disease in immunocompetent hosts and can cause pulmonary or disseminated disease in immunocompromised individuals (choice C is incorrect). Alcoholism and diabetes are also associated with pulmonary disease, and patients usually demonstrate upper lobe cavity formation that mimicks TB. Treatment is with itraconazole or amphotericin B, depending on the severity of disease and the amount of immunosuppressive therapy.

Saubolle MA, McKellar PP, Sussland D. Epidemiologic, clinical, and diagnostic aspects of coccidiomycosis. J Clin Microbiol 2007; 45:26–30
Allen JN, Davis WB. Eosinophilic lung diseases. Am J Respir Crit Care Med 1994; 150:1423–1438
Lombard CM, Tazelaar HD, Krasne DL. Pulmonary eosinophilia in coccidioidal infections. Chest 1987; 91:734–736
Bradsher RW. Pulmonary blastomycosis. Semin Respir Crit Care Med 2008; 29:174–181
Hage CA, Wheat LJ, Loyd J, et al. Pulmonary histoplasmosis. Semin Respir Crit Care Med 2008; 29:151–156

200. B. Surgical resection should be attempted.

The management of most thymomas is relatively straightforward: surgical resection remains the primary mode of therapy (choice B is correct). However, the literature is controversial regarding histology and pathology, staging and its usefulness, the need for adjuvant therapy, and, recently, the role of video-assisted surgery in the treatment of this tumor.

It appears that invasiveness of the tumor, not the pathologic diagnosis, remains the single most consistent factor in predicting outcome (choice A is incorrect). Various staging systems have been defined based on the degree of invasiveness; these systems are totally independent of histologic and cytologic findings. Surgery is the treatment of choice for thymoma whenever a complete resection can be accomplished, and incomplete resection may have advantages over biopsy alone. There is reasonable evidence indicating that all thymomas except for completely encapsulated stage I tumors should be treated with postoperative adjuvant radiation therapy, with the goal of reducing the incidence of local relapse (choice C is incorrect). Myasthenia gravis associated with thymoma is no longer considered an adverse prognostic factor in thymoma and may actually confer a survival advantage (choice D is incorrect). This may be due to the preponderance of early-stage tumors discovered incidentally in patients with myasthenia gravis. However, other associated autoimmune diseases, such as polymyositis and autoimmune hemolytic anemia, are associated with poorer survival.

Blumberg D, Port JL, Weksler B, et al. Thymoma: a multivariate analysis of factors predicting survival. Ann Thorac Surg 1995; 60:908–914

Ciernik IF, Meier U, Lutolf UM. Prognostic factors and outcome of incompletely resected invasive thymoma following radiation therapy. J Clin Oncol 1994; 12:1484–1490

Kohman LJ. Controversies in the management of malignant thymoma. Chest 1997; 112:296S–300S

Laboratory Reference Values

	Conventional Unit Range	**SI Unit Range**
I. Whole Blood, plasma serum chemistries		
Acid phosphatase, serum	< 5.5 U/L	< 90 nkat/L
Adrenocorticotropic hormone (ACTH), plasma	< 120 pg/mL	< 26 pmol/L
Alanine aminotransferase (ALT), serum	10–40 U/L	0.17–0.68 μkat/L
Albumin, serum	3.5–5.0 g/dL	35–50 g/L
Alkaline phosphatase, serum	30–120 U/L	0.5–2.0 μkat/L
δ-Aminolevulinic acid, serum	15–23 μg/dL	1.1–8.0 μmol/L
Ammonia (as nitrogen), serum, plasma	15–45 μg/dL	11–32 μmol/L
Amylase, serum	27–131 U/L	0.46–2.23 μkat/L
Androstenedione, serum	75–205 ng/dL	2.6–7.2 nmol/L
Angiotensin-converting enzyme, serum	< 40 U/L	< 670 nkat/L
Anion gap, $Na^+ - (Cl^- + HCO_3^-)$, serum, plasma	8–16 mEq/L	8–16 mmol/L
Antibodies to double-stranded DNA	< 20% DNA bound	
Antideoxyribonuclease B	< 280 U	
Antihistone antibodies	< 1:16	
Antimicrosomal antibodies	< 1:100	
Antimitochrondrial antibodies	< 1:5	
Antinuclear antibody fluorescent test	< 1:80	
α_1-Antitrypsin, serum	78–200 mg/dL	14.5–36.5 μmol/L
Antistreptolysin O titer	< 200 Todd U	
Arterial studies, blood (breathing air at sea level) Oxygen, Po_2 Carbon dioxide, Pco_2 HCO_3^- pH Oxygen saturation Alveolar-arterial oxygen gradient, $(A\text{-}a)O_2$ Carboxyhemoglobin Mixed venous Po_2 Oxygen saturation	 80–100 mm Hg 35–45 mm Hg 21–28 mEq/L 7.35–7.45 95% or greater ≤ 20 mm Hg < 20% 35–40 mm Hg 70–75%	 11–13 kPa 4.7–5.9 kPa 21–28 mmol/L 7.35–7.45

Laboratory Reference Values, continued

	Conventional Unit Range	SI Unit Range
Ascorbic acid (vitamin C)	0.4–1.5 mg/dL	23–85 µmol/L
Aspartate aminotransferase (AST)	10–30 IU/L	0.17–0.51 µkat/L
Bicarbonate, serum	21–28 mEq/L	21–28 mmol/L
Bilirubin, serum Total Direct (conjugated)	 0.3–1.2 mg/dL 0.1–0.3 mg/dL	 5.0–21.0 µmol/L 1.7–5.1 µmol/L
Calcitonin, plasma	3–26 pg/mL	0.8–7.6 pmol/L
Calcium, total, serum	8.2–10.2 mg/dL	2.05–2.55 mmol/L
Calcium, ionized, serum	4.60–5.08 mg/dL	1.15–1.27 mmol/L
Carbon dioxide (total), serum, plasma	22–28 mEq/L	22–28 mmol/L
Carcinoembryonic antigen (CEA), serum	< 3.0 ng/mL	< 3 µg/L
β-Carotene, serum	10–85 µg/dL	0.2–1.6 µmol/L
Catecholamines, plasma	Dopamine: < 87 pg/mL Epinephrine: < 60 pg/mL Norepinephrine: 110–410 pg/mL	< 475 pmol/L < 330 pmol/L 650–2423 pmol/L
Chloride, serum, plasma	96–106 mEq/L	96–106 mmol/L
Cholinesterase, serum	5–12 mg/L	14–39 nmol/L
Chorionic gonadotropin (β-hCG), serum (nonpregnant)	5.0 mIU/mL	5.0 IU/L
Complement, serum C3 C4 CH_{50}	 1200–1500 µg/mL 14–48 mg/dL 110–190 U/mL	 1.2–1.5 g/L 0.35–0.60 g/L > 1/64
Cortisol, serum, plasma	5–25 µg/dL	140–690 nmol/L
C-peptide, serum	0.5–2.5 ng/mL	0.17–0.83 nmol/L
Creatine kinase (CK), serum	40–150 U/L	0.67–2.5 µkat/L
Creatine kinase-MB fraction, serum	0–7 ng/mL	0–7 µg/L
Creatinine, serum, plasma	0.6–1.2 mg/dL	53–106 µmol/L
Cyclosporine, serum	100–400 ng/mL	83–333 nmol/L
Cytomegalobody antibody titer- IgG IgM	 < 1:8 < 1:8	

Laboratory Reference Values, continued

	Conventional Unit Range	SI Unit Range
Dehydroepiandrosterone sulfate (DHEA-S), serum	50–450 μg/dL	1.6–12.2 μmol/L
11-Deoxycortisol, plasma	< 0–2 μg/dL	0–60 nmol/L
Digoxin, plasma	0.5–2.0 ng/mL	0.6–2.6 nmol/L
Epinephrine, plasma	< 60 pg/mL	< 330 pmol/L
Ethanol (ethyl alcohol), serum, whole blood	< 20 mg/dL	< 4.3 mmol/L
α-Fetoprotein, serum	< 10 ng/mL	< 10 μg/L
Fibrinogen, plasma	200–400 mg/dL	5.8–11.8 μmol/L
Gastrin, serum	25–90 pg/mL	12–45 pmol/L
Glucose, serum	70–110 mg/dL	3.9–6.1 mmol/L
γ-Glutamyltransferase (GGT), serum	2–30 U/L	0.03–0.51 μkat/L
Hemoglobin A_{1C} (glycated hemoglobin), whole blood	4–7% (% of total hemoglobin)	0.04–0.07 (proportion of total hemoglobin)
Immunoglobulins, serum IgA IgE IgG IgM	 40–350 mg/dL 0–1500 μg/L 650–1600 mg/dL 54–300 mg/dL	 400–3500 mg/L 0–1.5 mg/L 6.5–16.0 g/L 550–3000 mg/L
Insulin, serum	2.0–20 μIU/mL	14–140 pmol/L
Iron, serum	60–150 μg/dL	10.7–26.9 μmol/L
Iron-binding capacity, serum	250–450 μg/dL	44.8–80.6 μmol/L
Lactate, plasma	5.0–15 mg/dL	0.6–1.7 mmol/L
Lactate dehydrogenase (LDH), serum	100–200 U/L	1.7–3.4 μkat/L
Lead, serum	< 10–20 μg/dL	< 0.5–1.0 μmol/L
Lipase, serum	31–86 U/L	0.5–3.2 μkat/L
Magnesium, serum	1.3–2.1 mEq/L	0.65–1.05 mmol/L
β_2-Microglobulin, serum	1.2–2.8 mg/L	1.2–2.8 mg/L
Mixed venous oxygen - see Arterial		
Norepinephrine, plasma	110–410 pg/mL	650–2423 pmol/L
5'-Nucleotidase, serum	0–17 U/L	
Osmolality, serum	275–295 mOsm/kg	275–295 mmol/kg
Phosphorus (inorganic), serum	2.3–4.7 mg/dL	0.74–1.52 mmol/L

Laboratory Reference Values, continued

	Conventional Unit Range	SI Unit Range
Potassium, serum	3.5–5.0 mEq/L	3.5–5.0 mmol/L
Protein (electrophoresis)		
Proportion of total protein, serum		
Albumin	52–65%	0.52–0.65 (proportion of 1.0)
α_1-Globulin	2.5–5.0%	0.025–0.05 (proportion of 1.0)
α_2-Globulin	7.0–13.0%	0.07–0.13 (proportion of 1.0)
β-Globulin	8.0–14.0%	0.08–0.14 (proportion of 1.0)
γ-Globulin	12.0–22.0%	0.12–0.22 (proportion of 1.0)
Concentration, serum	3.2–5.6 g/dL	32–56 g/L
α_1-Globulin	0.1–0.4 g/dL	1–4 g/L
α_2-Globulin	0.4–1.2 g/dL	4–12 g/L
β-Globulin	0.5–1.1 g/dL	5–11 g/L
γ-Globulin	0.5–1.6 g/dL	5–16 g/L
Quinidine, serum	2.0–5.0 µg/mL	6.2–15.4 µmol/L
Rheumatoid factor, latex test	< 1:80	
Salicylates, serum, plasma	150–300 µg/mL	1086–2172 µmol/L
Sodium, serum	136–142 mEq/L	136–142 mmol/L
Theophylline, serum, plasma	10–20 µg/mL	56–111 µmol/L
Thyroglobulin, serum	3–42 ng/mL	3–42 µg/L
Thyroidal iodine (^{123}I) uptake	5–30% of administered dose at 24 h	
Thyroid-stimulating hormone (TSH), serum	0.4–4.2 mIU/L	0.4–4.2 mIU/L
Thyroxine, serum		
Total (T_4)	5.5–12.5 µg/dL	71–160 nmol/L
Free (FT_4)	0.9–2.3 ng/dL	12–30 pmol/L
Triiodothyronine resin uptake (T_3U)	25–35%	0.25–0.35
Triiodothyronine, reverse (rT_3)	13–50 ng/dL	
Triiodothyronine, serum		
Total (T_3)	60–180 ng/dL	0.92–2.76 nmol/L
Free (FT_3)	1.4–4.4 pg/mL	0.22–6.78 pmol/L
Transaminase, serum glutamic (SGOT)	0–35 U/mL	5–40 U/L
Transaminase, serum glutamic pyruvic (SGPT)	0–30 U/mL	<55 U/L
Urea nitrogen, serum	8–23 mg/dL	2.9–8.2 mmol/L
Uric acid, serum	4.0–8.0 mg/dL	240–480 µmol/L

Laboratory Reference Values, continued

	Conventional Unit Range	SI Unit Range
Vitamin B_{12}, serum	160–950 pg/mL	118–701 pmol/L
Zinc, serum	75–120 µg/dL	11.5–18.5 µmol/L
II. Cerebrospinal Fluid		
Cell count	0–5 mononuclear cells/mm^3	
Gamma-globulin	0–5 mg/dL	0–50 mg/L
Glucose	50–75 mg/dL	2.75–4.13 mmol/L
Pressure (initial)	70–180 mm CSF	
Total proteins	15–45 mg/dL	150–450 mg/L
III. Gastrointestinal		
D-xylose absorption (after ingestion of 25 g of D-xylose)	Serum: 25–40 mg/dL; urinary excretion: 4.5–7.5 g during a 5-h period	2.2–3.7 mmol/L 33–55 mmol/5 h
Fecal fat (as stearic acid)	2.0–6.0 g/d	2–6 g/24 h
Fecal nitrogen	<2 g/24 h	
Fecal weight	<250 g/24 h	
Gastric secretion	Basal acid output: 0–10 mEq of HCl/h Maximal acid output after pentagastrin stimulation: 3–30 mEq of HCl/h	
Gastrin, serum	25–90 pg/mL	12–45 pmol/L
IV. Hematologic		
Activated partial thromboplastin time (APTT), whole blood	25–40 s	25–40 s
Antithrombin III, plasma	21–30 mg/dL	210–300 mg/L
Bleeding time (template)	<10 min	
Clotting time (Lee-White)	5–15 min	
Carboxyhemoglobin, toxic, whole blood	>20%	>0.2 (proportion of 1.0)
Cluster Designation (CD) CD_4/T_4 (helper) CD_8/T_8 (suppressor/cytotoxic) CD_4/CD_8 ratio	 36–55% 517–1169/mL 19–29% 256–650/mL 1.2/2.6	

Laboratory Reference Values, continued

	Conventional Unit Range	SI Unit Range
Coagulation factors, plasma		
Factor I (fibrinogen)	150–350 mg/dL	1.5–3.5 g/L
Factor II (prothrombin)	70–130%	0.70–1.30 (proportion of 1.0)
Factor V	70–130%	0.70–1.30 (proportion of 1.0)
Factor VII	60–140%	0.60–1.40 (proportion of 1.0)
Factor VIII	50–200%	0.50–1.30 (proportion of 1.0)
Factor IX	70–130%	0.70–1.30 (proportion of 1.0)
Factor X	70–130%	0.70–1.30 (proportion of 1.0)
Factor XI	70–130%	0.70–1.30 (proportion of 1.0)
Factor XII	70–130%	0.70–1.30 (proportion of 1.0)
Erythrocyte (RBC) count, whole blood	$3.9–5.5 \times 10^6/\mu L$	$3.9–5.5 \times 10^{12}/L$
Erythrocyte survival rate (^{51}Cr)	$T_{1/2}$=28 days	
Ferritin, serum	15–200 ng/mL	33–450 pmol/L
Fibrin degradation products, plasma	<10 μg/mL	<10 mg/L
Folate (folic acid), serum	3–16 ng/mL	7–36 nmol/L
Glucose-6-phosphate dehydrogenase, whole blood	10–14 U/g hemoglobin	0.17–0.24 nkat/g hemoglobin
Hematocrit, whole blood	41–50%	0.41–0.50 (proportion of 1.0)
Hemoglobin, whole blood	14.0–17.5 g/dL	140–175 g/L
Electrophoresis:		
Hgb A	96–98%	
Hgb A_2	2.0–3.0%	0.02–0.03 (proportion of 1.0)
Hgb F	<1%	
Hemoglobin, plasma	0.5–5.0 mg/dL	5–50 g/L
Leukocyte (WBC) count, whole blood	4500–11000/μL	$4.5–11.0 \times 10^9/L$
Differential count (number fraction), whole blood		
Neutrophils-segmented	56%	0.56 (proportion of 1.0)
Neutrophils-bands	3%	0.03 (proportion of 1.0)
Lymphocytes	34%	0.34 (proportion of 1.0)
Monocytes	4%	0.04 (proportion of 1.0)
Eosinophils	2.7%	0.027 (proportion of 1.0)
Basophils	0.3%	0.003 (proportion of 1.0)
Differential count, whole blood		
Neutrophils-segmented	1800–7800/μL	$1.8–7.8 \times 10^9/L$
Neutrophils-bands	0–700/μL	$0–0.70 \times 10^9/L$
Lymphocytes	1000–4800/μL	$1.0–4.8 \times 10^9/L$
Monocytes	0–800/μL	$0–0.80 \times 10^9/L$
Eosinophils	0–450/μL	$0–0.45 \times 10^9/L$
Basophils	0–200/μL	$0–0.20 \times 10^9/L$

Laboratory Reference Values, continued

	Conventional Unit Range	SI Unit Range
Mean corpuscular hemoglobin (MCH), whole blood	26–34 pg/cell	26–34 pg/cell
Mean corpuscular hemoglobin concentration (MCHC), whole blood	33–37 g/dL	330–370 g/L
Mean corpuscular volume, whole blood	80–100 μm^3	80–100 fL
Partial thromboplastin time (activated)	30–40 s	
Platelet count, whole blood	130–350 × $10^3/\mu L$	150–350 × $10^9/L$
Prothrombin time (PT), plasma	10–13 s	10–13 s
Reticulocyte count, whole blood	0.5–1.5% of RBCs	0.005–0.015 (proportion of RBCs)
Ristocetin cofactor activity of plasma	50–150%	
Sedimentation rate, erythrocyte (Westergren)	Male: 0–15 mm/h Female: 0–20 mm/h	0–5 mm/h 0–7 mm/h
Thrombin clotting time (TCT)	Normal 8–10 s; therapeutic range 0.2–0.4 U heparin	
Volume, blood Plasma Red blood cell	Male: 44 mL/kg body weight Female: 43 mL/kg body weight Male: 25–35 mL/kg body weight Female: 20–30 mL/kg body weight	
V. Urine		
Aldosterone (RIA)	6–25 μg/24 h	50–235 nmol/d
Alpha-amino nitrogen	100–290 mg/24 h	
Amino acids	200–400 mg/24 h	
Amylase	1–18 U/h	
Calcium	100–300 mg/24 h	1.25–8.75 mmol/d
Catecholamines	Epinephrine: < 10 μg/24 h Norepinephrine: < 100 μg/24 h Total: < 100 μg/24 h	< 140 nmol/d < 825 nmol/d
Chloride	170–250 mEq/24 h	10–200 mmol/L
Chorionic gonadotropin (β-hCG)	< 2 mIU/24 h	
Copper	0–100 μg/24 h	< 1.0 μmol/d

Laboratory Reference Values, continued

	Conventional Unit Range	**SI Unit Range**
Coproporphyrin	< 200 μg/24 h	
Cortisol	20–100 μg/24 h	56–280 nmol/d
Creatine	Male: 0–40 mg/24 h Female: 0–100 mg/24 h	
Creatinine	15–25 mg/kg body weight/24 h	8.8–22 mmol/d
Creatinine clearance	90–140 mL/min	1.3–2.0 mL/s
17-Hydroxycorticosteroids	Male: 3–10 mg/24 h Female: 2–8 mg/24 h	8–28 μmol/d 5.5–17 μmol/d
5-Hydroxyindoleacetic acid (5-HIAA)	2–6 mg/24 h	10.4–31.2 μmol/d
77-Ketosteroids	3–12 mg/24 h	10–42 μmol/d
Lead	< 80 μg/24 h	< 0.6 μmol/d
Metanephrines	0–300 μg/24 h	0.0–4.9 μmol/d
Normetanephrines	50–800 μg/24 h	
Osmolality	38–1400 mOsm/kg H_2O	50–1400 mmol/kg
Oxalate	< 50 mg/24 h	190–480 μmol/kg
Protein	< 100 mg/24 h	< 0.15 g/d
Urea clearance, maximal	40–60 mL/min	
Urea nitrogen	12–20 g/24 h	
Uric acid	250–750 mg/24 h (varies with intake) 1.5–4.2 mmol/d	0–7 mm/h
Uroporphyrin	10–60 μg/24 h	< 31 nmol/d
Vanillylmandelic acid (VMA)	2.1–7.6 mg/24 h	11–38 μmol/d
VI. Hemodynamic Measurements		
Pressures Right atrium mean Right ventricle - Systolic/end diastolic Pulmonary artery - Systolic/diastolic/mean Pulmonary artery occlusion, mean Left atrium, mean Left ventricle, Systolic/end diastolic Mean systemic	 0–8 mm Hg 15–30/2–7 mm Hg 15–30/5–12/9–16 mm Hg 5–12 mm Hg 5–12 mm Hg 100–190/3–12 mm Hg 70–105 mm Hg	

Laboratory Reference Values, continued

	Conventional Unit Range	SI Unit Range
Volumes Systolic volume Systolic index	 60–130 mL 35–70 mL/m^2	
Flows Cardiac output Cardiac index Oxygen consumption	 2.5–6.0 L/min 2.4–3.0 $L/min/m^2$ 110–350 mL/min 110–150 $mL/min/m^2$	
Resistances Systemic vascular resistance Pulmonary vascular resistance Total pulmonary resistance	 800–1600 $dynes \cdot s \cdot cm^{-5}$ 20–130 $dynes \cdot s \cdot cm^{-5}$ 100–300 $dynes \cdot s \cdot cm^{-5}$	
VII. Miscellaneous		
Sweat test for chloride	$<$ 60 mEq/L	$<$ 60 mmol/L

Key Words Index

Congratulations *CHEST!*

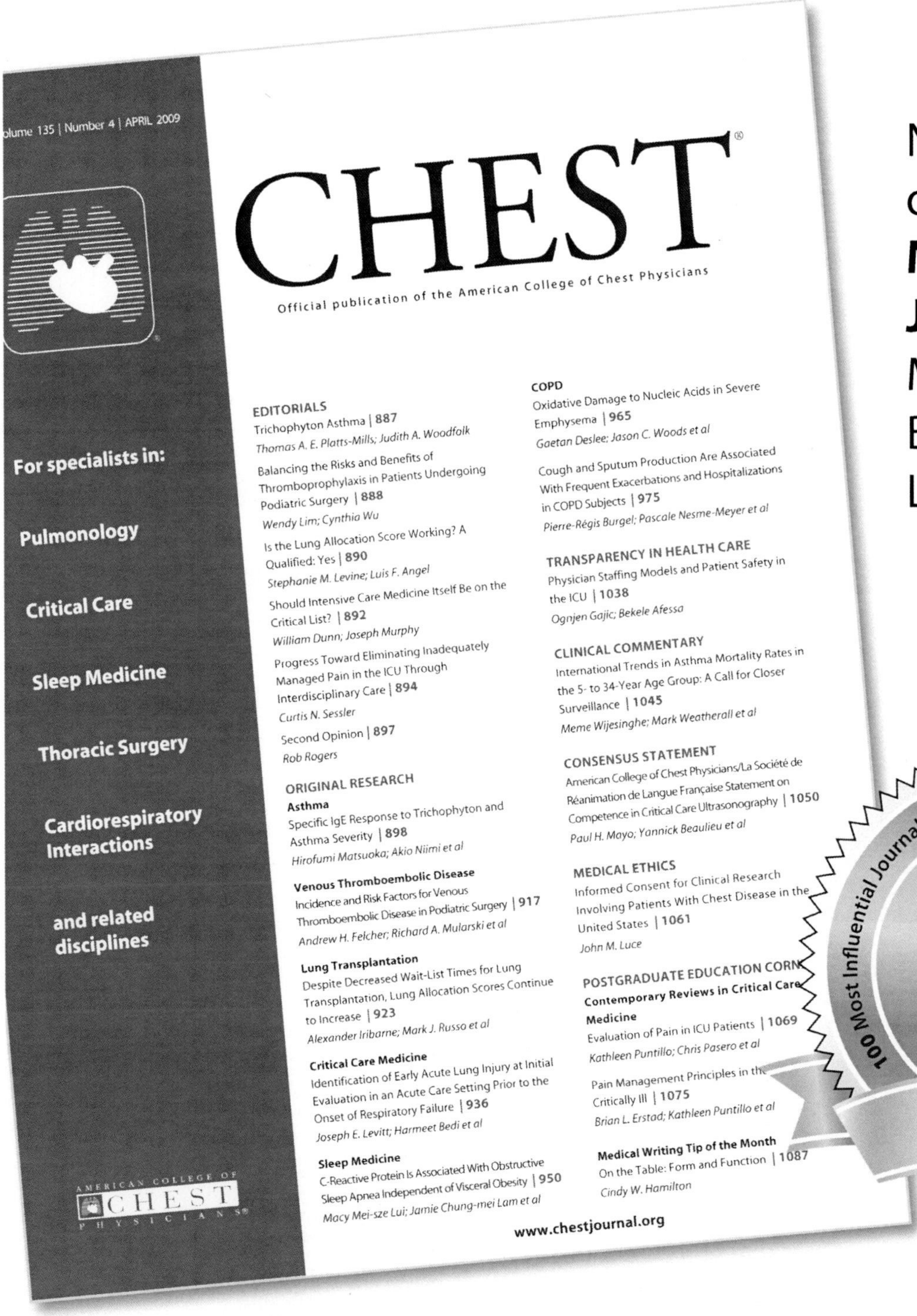

Volume 135 | Number 4 | APRIL 2009

CHEST®

Official publication of the American College of Chest Physicians

For specialists in:

Pulmonology

Critical Care

Sleep Medicine

Thoracic Surgery

Cardiorespiratory Interactions

and related disciplines

AMERICAN COLLEGE OF CHEST PHYSICIANS

www.chestjournal.org

Named One of the **100 Most Influential Journals** in Medicine and Biology Over the Last 100 Years

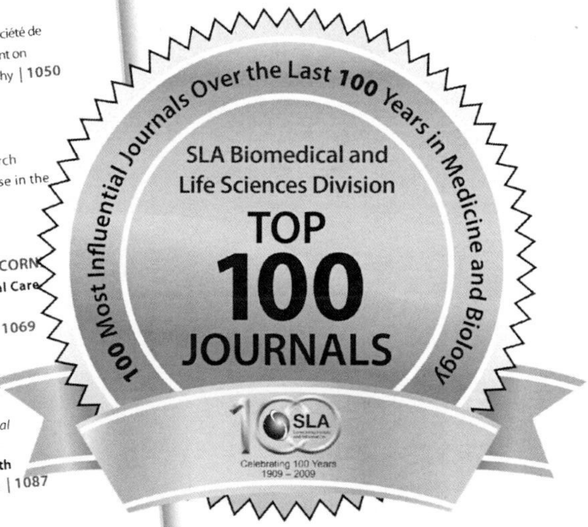

CHEST was voted one of the 100 most influential journals over the last 100 years in medicine and biology by the Biomedical and Life Sciences Division of the Special Libraries Association in conjunction with its centennial observance. *CHEST* won the respiratory medicine area in the clinical medicine category, scoring three times higher than its closest competitor.

Congratulations to *CHEST* and the ACCP.